INSTANT NEUROLOGICAL DIAGNOSIS

Digital Media Accompanying the Book

Individual purchasers of this book are entitled to free personal access to accompanying digital media in the on-line edition. Please refer to the access token card for instructions on token redemption and access.

The corresponding media can be found on *Oxford Medicine Online* at:

oxfordmedicine.com/instantneurologicaldiagnosis2e

If you are interested in access to the complete online edition, please consult with your librarian.

INSTANT NEUROLOGICAL DIAGNOSIS

DIAGNOSIS

Second Edition

CHRISTOPHER H. HAWKES
Honorary Professor of Neurology
Barts and the London School of Medicine & Dentistry
London, UK

KAPIL D. SETHI
Professor Emeritus of Neurology
Medical College of Georgia
Augusta University
Augusta, Georgia, USA

THOMAS R. SWIFT
Professor Emeritus of Neurology
Medical College of Georgia
Augusta University
Augusta, Georgia, USA

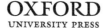

OXFORD
UNIVERSITY PRESS

OXFORD

UNIVERSITY PRESS

Oxford University Press is a department of the University of Oxford. It furthers
the University's objective of excellence in research, scholarship, and education
by publishing worldwide. Oxford is a registered trade mark of Oxford University
Press in the UK and certain other countries.

Published in the United States of America by Oxford University Press
198 Madison Avenue, New York, NY 10016, United States of America.

© Oxford University Press 2019

First Edition published in 2016

Library of Congress Cataloging-in-Publication Data
Names: Hawkes, Christopher H., author. | Sethi, Kapil D., author. |
Swift, Thomas R., author.
Title: Instant neurological diagnosis / by Christopher H. Hawkes,
Kapil D. Sethi, Thomas R. Swift.
Description: Second edition. | New York, NY : Oxford University Press, [2019] |
Includes bibliographical references and index.
Identifiers: LCCN 2018054869 | ISBN 9780190930868 (alk. paper)
Subjects: | MESH: Diagnostic Techniques, Neurological | Nervous System
Diseases—diagnosis | Handbook
Classification: LCC RC348 | NLM WL 39 | DDC 616.8/0475—dc23
LC record available at https://lccn.loc.gov/2018054869

1 3 5 7 9 8 6 4 2

Printed by Webcom, Inc., Canada

CONTENTS

PREFACE TO THE SECOND EDITION

We are extremely pleased with the reception of our first edition, testified by the fact it was the top seller in the Oxford University Press bookstall at the American Academy of Neurology (AAN) for 3 years in a row. It is hoped that our first edition has led to faster diagnosis and has improved the quality of teaching and patient care. Although feedback has been strongly positive, we are aware of the need to update some sections. All chapters have now been revised and the number of videos increased. The "Movement Disorders" chapter alone has 110 videos that demonstrate the majority of disorders you are likely to come across in a lifetime. One new chapter has been added: "The Fast Neurological Examination." This chapter synthesizes the bare essential techniques required for a patient whose problem, based on the history, is unlikely to be associated with abnormal physical signs—such as non-urgent headache or "funny turns."

In mid-2018, we were disappointed to learn that the AAN had decided to suspend NeuroBowl! This has been an annual event for the past 20 years and probably the most popular entertainment/learning occasion of the whole educational program. The reasons are not known, but we look forward to the reinstatement of NeuroBowl for the 2020 program.

Once more we emphasize the need to use these diagnostic short-cuts (Handles and Red Flags) with caution. They are powerful, save a lot of time, and, if you need an ego boost, they may demonstrate superior clinical acumen to your colleagues. You must never, ever bet your shirt on any Handle—just in case you turn out to be wrong and suffer the consequent humiliation: eating humble pie.

We wish to send our thanks to all those colleagues who have helped review relevant chapters and contributed photographs or videos.

We hope this second edition enhances your enjoyment of clinical neurology!

Please email any one of us with your feedback.

—Christopher H. Hawkes
Honorary Professor of Neurology
Barts and the London School of Medicine &
Dentistry
London, UK
c.hawkes@qmul.ac.uk

—Kapil D. Sethi
Professor Emeritus of Neurology Medical College of
Georgia
Augusta University
Augusta, Georgia, USA
ksethi@augusta.edu

—Thomas R. Swift
Professor Emeritus of Neurology
Medical College of Georgia
Augusta University
Augusta, Georgia, USA
tswift@augusta.edu

ACKNOWLEDGMENTS

Many colleagues have provided input for the first and second editions and were listed in the first edition. We wish to acknowledge further valuable support from the following:

Robert Hadden, King's College Hospital, London
Farooq Manyar, Barts Health, London
Richard Perry, National Hospital for Neurology and Neurosurgery, Queen Square, London.

Michael Rose, King's College Hospital, London
Jason Warren, National Hospital for Neurology and Neurosurgery, Queen Square, London
Brian Weinshenker, Mayo Clinic, Rochester, Minnesota
Paul Reading, James Cook University Hospital, Middlesbrough
Charles Marshall, Barts Health, London

Chapter 1: First Encounters

The neurological examination begins *before* your patient knows it. Your first task, as always, will be inspection. **Do not look at the referral letter or case notes at this stage!** Much information can be gleaned by simple observation. For further clues, consult the article "Bedside Sherlock Holmes" (Fitzgerald and Tierney, 1982). Here are some useful tips, but by no means exhaustive:

1. **Watch the patient enter your consulting room.** So many clinicians waste this vital moment by reading the case notes or the referral letter. Don't do this now. Focus!
2. **Watch how the patient turns to close the door.** Turning on the spot is a maneuver taken for granted by healthy people but it is actually quite complex. A tendency to overbalance on turning is a useful sign of cerebellar or extrapyramidal disorder—typically Parkinson's disease (PD), brainstem ischemia, or hydrocephalus.
3. **Watch the patient as he or she walks toward you and (maybe) shakes your hand.** Note whether the hand is released quickly or perhaps slowly, as in myotonia. Observation alone will allow you to make a basic assessment of the motor system. Tremor, chorea, or dystonia may be more obvious on walking than formal testing; you may detect poor arm swing and you could observe involuntary movement when the hand is extended to shake yours. Observe how the patient removes his or her glasses; this sometimes reveals incoordination. The earliest sign of parkinsonism and hemiparesis may be decreased arm swing or just reduced blink frequency.
4. **Look at the patient's face.** You can make a preliminary evaluation of a patient's emotional state by observing whether he or she is frowning or appears relaxed. If glasses are worn you should determine whether they are clean and symmetrically placed on the nose. Many headache sufferers have spotlessly clean, perfectly adjusted spectacles. Conversely, people who neglect their health will have their glasses at an angle and the lenses may be smudged. Someone who wears dark sunglasses indoors may have severe migraine or photosensitivity from local ocular conditions (e.g., optic neuritis, cataracts), but it is more often a sign of psychogenic disorder. Apart from establishing whether there is good eye contact you might detect facial asymmetry or impoverished facial expression (hypomimia), which is again a feature of parkinsonism. The anxious/stressed person will frown continually and display horizontal "worry lines" over the forehead. The face may show birthmarks, as in the Sturge Weber syndrome (Figure 1.11), or spider nevi, as in liver disease. Inspect the shape of the nose to determine if it is enlarged, as in rhinophyma—the traditional hallmark of a beer drinker, although this association is disputed (see Figure 1.6, right,); whether the anterior contour is depressed (saddle nose), as in granulomatous disorder, congenital syphilis, or leprosy (see Figure 1.6, left and middle); or if the nose is displaced from boxing and other facial trauma.
5. **Inspect the clothes.** The patient with early to mid-stage Alzheimer disease will be tidily dressed, whereas the person with frontal dementia is less concerned about his or her appearance and likely to have food marks or dirt on the clothing. Those with migraine tend to be smartly dressed. An expensive-looking suit frayed at the edges suggests recent decline in social circumstances. Lose-fitting clothes testify to recent weight loss; conversely, tight-fitting clothes are a feature of weight gain.
6. **Look at the fingernails.** Well-groomed nails suggest that the patient has good manual dexterity and pride in their

appearance. The shape and color are sometimes diagnostic, as explained later. Heavily bitten nails imply anxiety disorder, whereas a particularly long finger nail ("coke nail," usually fifth) makes a useful scoop for measuring cocaine and implies the patient is a drug dealer (Figure 1.1a). Clubbing of just one finger usually indicates trauma, but unidigital clubbing may be a sign of sarcoidosis (Figure 1.1b). Aortic aneurysm, brachial plexus, or median nerve lesions and gout are alternative possibilities. The subungual glomus tumor (Figure 1.1c) is a dull, red swelling beneath the nail causing repeated stabbing pains in the finger, aggravated by cold. They are often investigated needlessly for painful polyneuropathy. Horizontal white lines in the nails (Mees lines) indicate arsenic poisoning (Figure 1.1d). Sub- and periungual fibromas are seen in tuberous sclerosis (Figure 6.1). Pitted nails are found in psoriatic arthritis, which may be associated with unrelenting spinal pain. Koilonychia (Figure 1.1e) is an important sign for clinicians as it often suggests iron deficiency, which, especially in males, may be a sign of underlying malignant disease. Of particular relevance for the neurologist is the association of koilonychia with restless legs syndrome. Plummer's nail (Figure 1.1f) is a sign of hyperthyroidism that is caused by separation/elevation of the nail from its bed, thus allowing accumulation of dirt below the nail. Figure 1.1g shows the blue nails sign (courtesy Dr. Bruce Bouts). Here it is from a case of argyria (see Figure 1.10), but similar changes occur in Wilson disease and exposure to some antimalarials.

7. **Inspect jewelry.** This might give an approximate guide to a patient's wealth. In a depressed patient, absence of a wedding ring especially with an untanned area over the fourth finger hints at recent separation or divorce. A loose-fitting ring implies recent weight loss, whereas a tight ring points to weight gain, upper limb edema, or acromegaly. A MedicAlert or similar bracelet will have key information about your patient's illness and medication (e.g., epilepsy, diabetes, or allergy). Copper bracelets are worn by people with arthritis.

8. **Listen to the patient's voice.** Is it slurred, as in upper motor neuron lesions, or jerky, as in cerebellar disorder? If it is very quiet this suggests dysphonia and the possibility of parkinsonism or myasthenia. Nasal speech points to nasal/sinus disease or weakness of the soft palate, as found in myasthenia or cleft palate.

9. **Smell the breath.** The most common odors are cigarettes and alcohol. Patients with classic PD are rarely current smokers, and, if so, you should reappraise the diagnosis. If a patient is thought to be a heavy drinker and there is only a faint or no smell of alcohol, you should suspect consumption of vodka. Heavy drinkers progress to vodka because it lacks a distinctive odor. A minty smell in the breath might indicate deliberate masking of bad breath. Poor dental or mouth hygiene results in halitosis and a coated tongue. Marked halitosis is a feature of amphetamine abuse (Figure 1.35). The distinctive acetone odor in diabetic ketoacidosis and fecal smell of liver disease are well known but unlikely to cross the path of most clinical neurologists.

With all this you might be able to make an instant diagnosis, but, if not, you should have a general idea regarding the problem a patient is about to relate to you.

Study the following photographs (Figures 1.1–1.45). Each one conveys a particular disease that you might be able to diagnose simply by looking at patients as they answer your questions or as they walk into your consulting room. The answer is given in the figure legend, but you should first try to make a diagnosis based solely on the illustration.

The enophthalmos found in Horner's syndrome is probably an illusion (see Chapter 2). Sometimes there are dilated conjunctival vessels, but this is not apparent in Figure 1.32. If the patient has been in a car accident within the previous 2 weeks, then the Horner's syndrome is an important Handle for carotid or vertebral dissection. Many neurologists forget to look for this sign.

Now look at Figure 1.33—also a right-sided Horner's syndrome. The ptosis and miosis are quite mild and easily overlooked. If the patient is examined in a bright room, then both pupils will be small

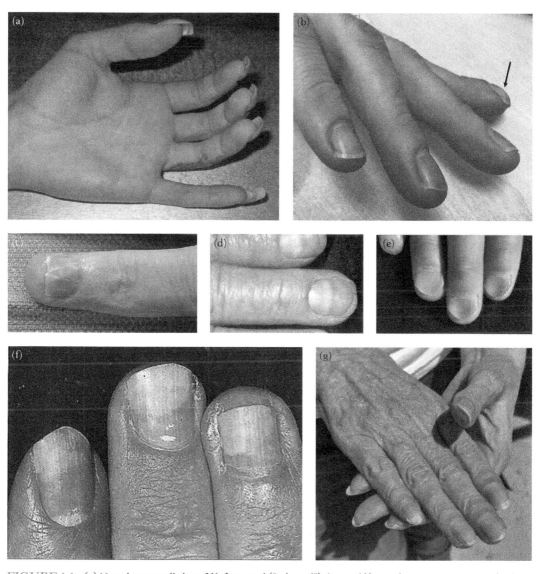

FIGURE 1.1: (**a**) Note the unusually long fifth finger nail ("coke nail") that could be used as a measuring scoop for drugs of abuse. (**b**) Unidigital clubbing of the right index finger (arrow). Here it is due to trauma, but this sign may be a feature of sarcoidosis, brachial plexus, and median nerve lesions. (**c**) Subungual glomus tumor. These tumors appear as a dull, red swelling beneath the nail. Patients present with repeated stabbing pains in the finger that are aggravated by cold. (**d**) Mees lines. A classic feature of arsenic exposure but also seen with thallium poisoning. (**e**) Koilonychia: spoon-shaped nails. An important sign of iron deficiency that is often associated with restless legs syndrome. (**f**) Plummer's nail, a sign of hyperthyroidism. This is caused by separation/elevation of the nail from its bed, thus allowing accumulation of dirt below the nail. Dirty elbows in an otherwise clean person are said to be typical of hyperthyroidism. Subungual glomus tumor reproduced with permission from Charles Eaton (www.eatonhand.com/img/img00090.htm). (**g**) This shows the blue nails sign (courtesy Dr. Bruce Bouts). Here it is from a case of argyria (see figure 1.10) but similar changes occur in Wilson disease and exposure to some antimalarials.

and you might miss the diagnosis—as all honest neurologists will tell you. Thus,

- ▶ Darkness exaggerates pupillary asymmetry due to a Horner's syndrome but conceals that due to a third cranial nerve (CN III) lesion.

Conversely,

- ▶ Strong light will conceal pupillary asymmetry due to a Horner's syndrome but it will accentuate that due to a CN III disorder.

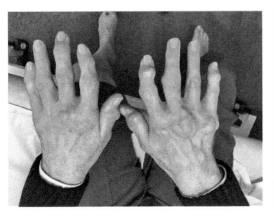
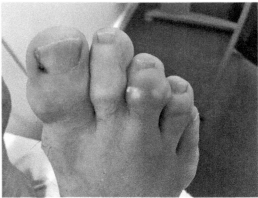

FIGURE 1.2: The hands and feet of a patient with gout arthropathy. Note the crystalline (yellow) swellings on the small joints (tophi). This is seen best on the interphalangeal joint of the right middle toe. Typically, gout causes severe pain in the hallux at night. The few neurological associations include carpal tunnel syndrome or spinal compression. Hyperuricemia and gout are features of the Lesch-Nyhan syndrome (Chapter 8)

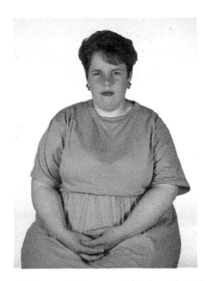

FIGURE 1.3: This 22-year-old overweight woman had recurrent facial acne but otherwise in good health apart from headache which disturbed sleep or troubled her on waking in the morning. She had bilateral tinnitus which was worse at night. She had taken repeated courses of the tetracycline antibiotic minocycline for acne. Funduscopy showed mild papilledema. Tinnitus and morning headache are both features of intracranial pressure (ICP). Diagnosis: idiopathic intracranial hypertension (IIH, pseudotumor cerebri). Patients with raised ICP due to tumor generally have many other symptoms. A sixth-nerve palsy is recognized in IIH, especially when the pressure is unduly high.

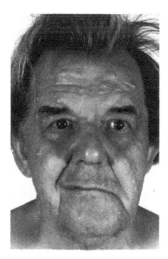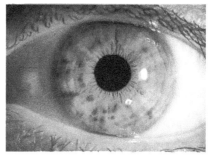

FIGURE 1.4: **Left**: A 65-year-old man referred because of possible facial palsy. He has an appearance typical of neurofibromatosis type 1. The left facial weakness was caused by a neuroma in the left cerebellopontine angle. Note the larger left palpebral fissure due to weakness of orbicularis oculi and the mouth droop. **Right**: Small dark brown spots in the iris (Lisch nodules) are characteristic of neurofibromatosis. Reproduced from Figure 46.8 in the chapter "The Phakomatoses," by MM Ariss, NK Ragge, M Moodley, and EI Traboulsi, in EI Traboulsi, ed., *Genetic Disease of the Eye* (2nd ed.), Oxford University Press. DOI:10.1093/med/9780195326147.003.0046.

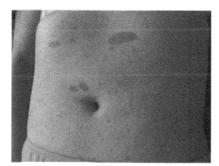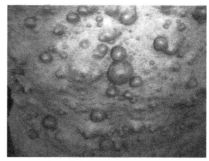

FIGURE 1.5: Neurofibromatosis (type 1). **Left**: Multiple café au lait spots and freckling over the anterior abdominal wall. You should next look for axillary freckling, check the fundi for papilledema or sign of optic nerve glioma, and take a family history. **Right**: Extensive neurofibromata, which are soft to touch. Photos courtesy Jose Biller, Chicago.

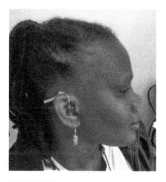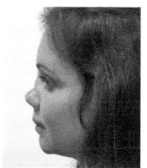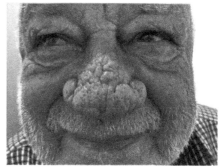

FIGURE 1.6: Occasionally, inspection of the nose gives a diagnosis. Here are some examples. **Left**: A typical saddle-nose deformity and a hearing aid that was required for bilateral perceptive deafness. Classically, this indicates congenital syphilis, but a variety of granulomata may cause this combination, particularly Wegener's granulomatosis, systemic lupus, leprosy, and sarcoid. Repeated snorting of cocaine damages the nasal septum and causes it to collapse. **Middle**: Wegener's granulomatosis in a 35-year-old female. Note the saddle-nose deformity due to erosion of the nasal septum. Most patients with this disorder are hyposmic. **Right**: Rhinophyma, the bulbous swelling of the nasal tip that is characteristic of heavy alcohol intake, usually beer. It is easily correctable by plastic surgery.

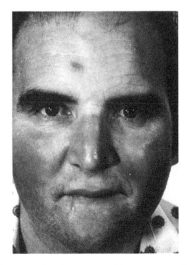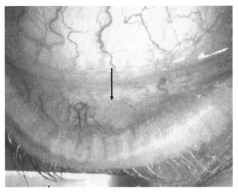

FIGURE 1.7: **Left**: This 55-year-old man was troubled by breathlessness with reddening of the face, including the nose, resembling frostbite. This is known as lupus pernio and it is characteristic of sarcoidosis. Skin biopsy will usually reveal the diagnosis, or if you are lucky you may see conjunctival nodules (**right**), which might give the answer on biopsy. Figure of lower lid reproduced with permission from *Training in Ophthalmology*, Figure 5.28, in the chapter Medical Ophthalmology, by E Hughes and M Stanford. Oxford University Press. DOI:10.1093/med/9780199237593.003.0005.

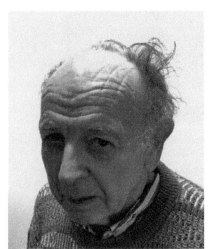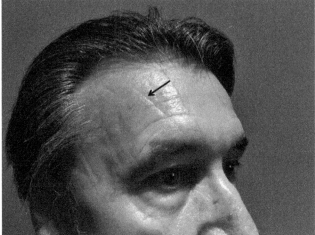

FIGURE 1.8: The forehead diagonal crease sign (arrows) in two patients, both of whom have Parkinson's disease. On the left there are three diagonal creases. This is caused by sleeping heavily on one side. It should alert you to sleep apnea syndrome or Parkinson's disease. In patients who complain of a tingling arm, it raises the possibility of brachial plexus compression from lying heavily on the side of the forehead creases.

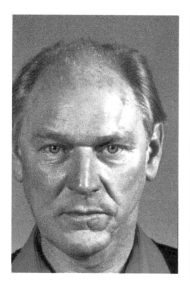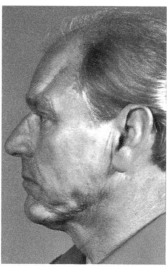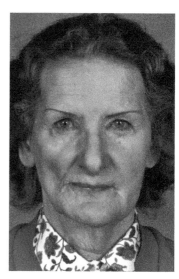

FIGURE 1.9: **Left and center**: You might not perceive this abnormality if you look at the full face view. On the side view, it is easy to see the apparent scar (not a crease) above the left eyebrow, shrinkage of the left mandible, and overlying skin. This is hemifacial atrophy or Parry-Romberg syndrome. The scar is likened to a saber cut as it is so sharply defined (*en coup de sabre*). This lesion may be concealed beneath the hair, so you need to palpate the scalp to find it. Atrophy of the jaw and facial skin on one side is characteristic. **Right**: A 74-year-old woman was referred because of possible right facial palsy, but it is clear there is atrophy of the right facial structures (muscle and bone). Milder cases of Parry-Romberg syndrome may go unnoticed until middle age or later, as here.

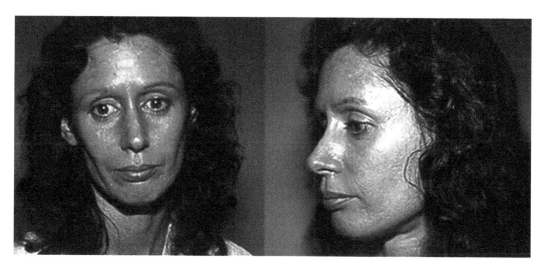

FIGURE 1.10: This woman has a dusky-gray silver complexion which developed from repeated use of colloidal silver-containing nose drops as a cold remedy over many years. Diagnosis: argyria. Argyria may occur also from recurrent application of silver nitrate nose drops for epistaxis and as naturopathic therapy for multiple sclerosis. Neurological complications are not well identified but include headache, peripheral neuropathy, and seizures. Figure reproduced with permission from Rosemary Jacobs.

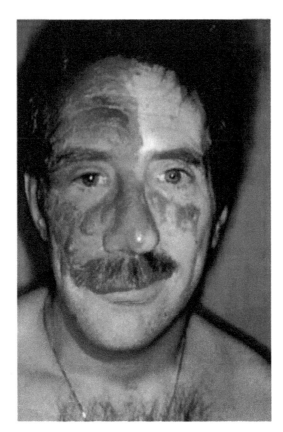

FIGURE 1.11: Note the port-wine stains over the face that correspond to the trigeminal dermatomes. This man had a lifelong history of seizures. This is the Sturge-Weber syndrome. Reproduced from Figure 13.17 in the chapter Capillary Malformations, Hyperkeratotic Stains, Telangiectasias, and Miscellaneous Vascular Blots, by JB Mulliken, in *Mulliken and Young's Vascular Anomalies: Hemangiomas and Malformations* Mulliken JB, ed., Oxford University Press. DOI:10.1093/med/9780195145052.003.0013.

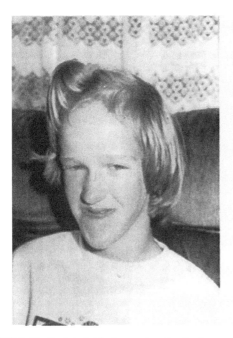 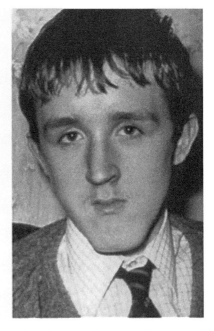

FIGURE 1.12: Both individuals are tall and suffer from epilepsy. Note the narrow face, pointed jaw, down-slanting palpebral fissures (right patient) and dolichocephaly (left subject). Diagnosis Sotos syndrome, caused by mutation in the NSD1 gene. Reproduced with permission from Agwu et al. (1999).

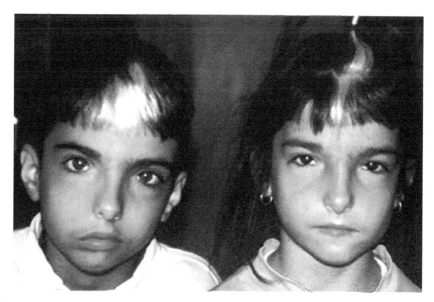

FIGURE 1.13: A brother and sister with an obvious white forelock. Both have deafness. Note the widely spaced eyes (hypertelorism). Diagnosis: Waardenburg syndrome. Reproduced courtesy Professor Dr. RA Schwartz, New Jersey Medical School.

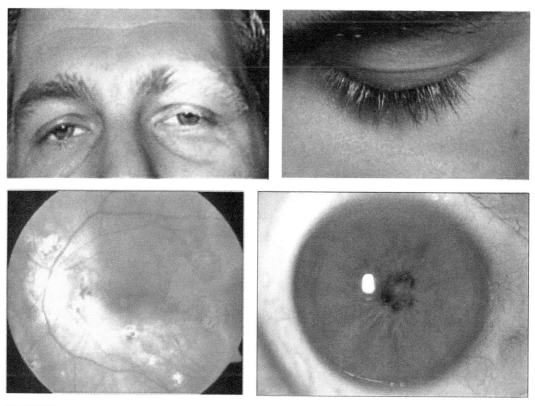

FIGURE 1.14: **Top left and top right**: Initially this patient was thought to have suffered an episode of optic neuritis. It was in fact uveitis. A major clue is the loss of pigment in the left eyebrow and eyelashes, known as poliosis. Diagnosis: Vogt-Koyanagi-Harada syndrome.**Bottom left**: The fundus shows a characteristic "sunset glow" sign due to loss of pigment from the retinal pigment epithelium. **Bottom right**: this shows depigmentation of the limbus (Sugiura's sign). Note: patients are often deaf. Vogt-Koyanagi-Harada syndrome image courtesy HA van Dijk, HL Fred, MD, OpenStax College. Sunset glow image reproduced with permission from Ho Su Ling, Figure 3 in Chan et al. (2010).

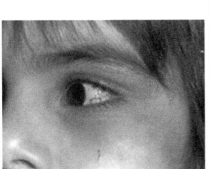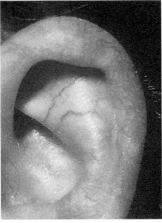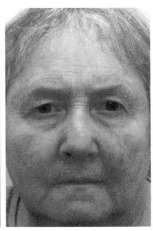

FIGURE 1.15: **Left and center**: A young child with cerebellar ataxia and recurrent chest infection. Note the telangiectasia on the sclera and pinna. Diagnosis: Ataxia telangiectasia (AT). **Right**: A 60-year-old woman, troubled with imbalance for the preceding 8 years. There were no conjunctival telangiectases but they were present over her cheeks. The diagnosis of AT variant was confirmed by genetic testing. Patients with AT are at high risk of lymphoma and leukemia. Left and center, reproduced from Figure 5.37 in the chapter Disorders of the Dermis, by V Sybert. Oxford University Press. DOI:10.1093/med/9780195397666.003.0005. Right photograph, courtesy Marios Hadjivassiliou, Sheffield, UK.

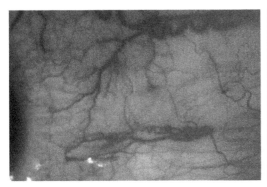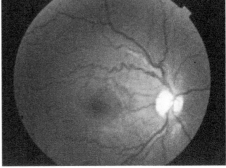

FIGURE 1.16: The photos reveal tortuous conjunctival and retinal blood vessels. With a slit lamp you may observe vortex keratopathy (cornea verticillata; see Chapter 11, Figure 11.15). This is typical of Fabry's disease. There may be retinal infarcts as well. Reproduced with permission from Sodi et al. (2007). Approved via Rights Link BMJ publishing group.

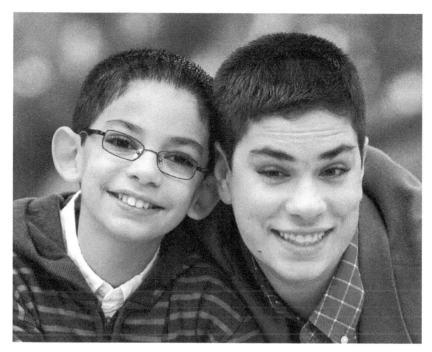

FIGURE 1.17: Two brothers aged 8 and 14. Note the large, protuberant ears in the younger brother (on left) and possibly elongated face in the older sib. Both have fragile X syndrome with the full mutation. Other features are learning difficulties, autism spectrum disorder, and macro-orchidism. Note that tremor and ataxia do not affect children with the full mutation; they are seen in older patients with the premutation. Reproduced with permission from Mrs. Paula Fasciano.

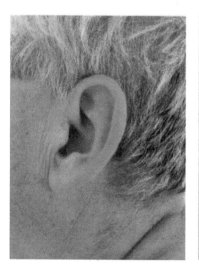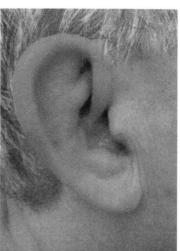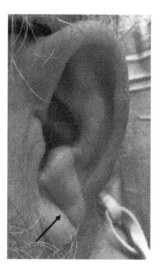

FIGURE 1.18: **Left and center:** The ears are inflamed, particularly in the upper pinna region. Typically, the earlobe is less inflamed. The ears eventually become floppy due to erosion of cartilage and the same process causes a saddle-nose deformity. Diagnosis: relapsing polychondritis. Note that the eyes may become red from episcleritis, thus a patient will have a red eye and red ear. Some present with recurrent episodes of nonbacterial meningitis, limbic encephalopathy, or stroke. You might confuse a nondeformed red ear with the "red ear syndrome," which is a variety of trigeminal autonomic cephalalgia. **Right:** Note the diagonal crease on the ear lobe (arrow)—Frank's sign. Although disputed, this sign is a proposed feature of cardiovascular disease. Relapsing polychondritis, courtesy Dr. Eris Jouvent, Paris. Frank's sign reproduced with permission from Xu and Pham (2014).

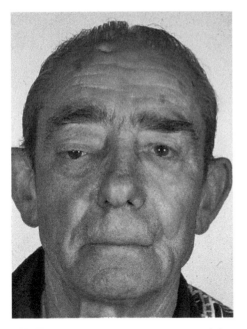

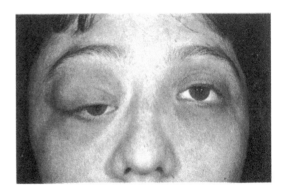

FIGURE 1.20: Note swelling in the upper outer aspect of the right eye displacing it down and inward (nonaxial proptosis) secondary to lacrimal gland swelling. This could be a tumor, but in neurological practice, sarcoidosis is high on the list. Reproduced with permission from *A Colour Atlas of Clinical Neurology*, 2nd ed., M Parsons. Mosby Year Book Europe, 1993.

FIGURE 1.19: Note swelling in the upper medial sector of the right orbit which is displacing the eye down and out. This is caused by mucocele of the right frontal sinus eroding the bone, entering the orbit and displacing the eye. It is a cause of nonaxial proptosis, as described in Chapter 2.

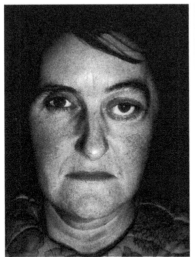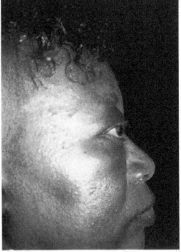

FIGURE 1.21: **Left**: The left eye is pushed forward and downward (nonaxial proptosis). Note the hyperostosis in the left temple. Diagnosis: meningioma of lateral third of sphenoid wing. The presence of hyperostosis helps distinguish this type of proptosis from intraorbital tumors and inflammatory lesions of the orbit. **Right**: The same condition causing marked temporal bony swelling and proptosis. Left image reproduced with permission from *A Colour Atlas of Clinical Neurology*, 2nd ed., M Parsons. Mosby Year Book Europe, 1993. Right image reproduced from *Clinical Ophthalmology*, J Kanski and B Bowling, Figure 19.56B, p. 828. With permission from Elsevier Saunders Ltd.

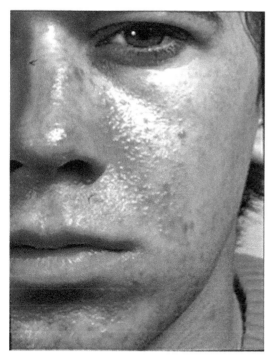

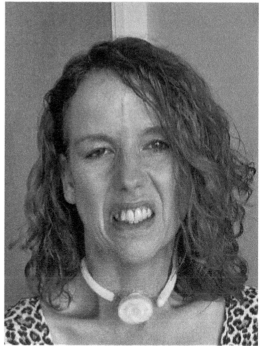

FIGURE 1.22: This patient was referred on account of seizures. If you look carefully at the nasolabial groove and chin you will see multiple soft cyst-like swellings. Diagnosis: tuberous sclerosis. If you are busy reading the notes and not concentrating on the patient's face, you might overlook this vital sign.

FIGURE 1.23: A patient with a "vertical" smile due to weakness of buccinator muscles bilaterally. It is highly characteristic of myasthenic syndromes but occurs in other myopathies that involve the face. The "myasthenic snarl" shown here is that of someone with DOK7 syndrome, one of the congenital myasthenic disorders (see Chapter 7). Reproduced with permission from Finlayson et al. (2013).

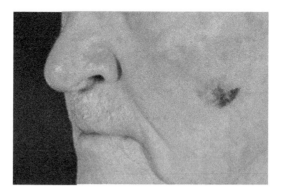

FIGURE 1.24: The figure shows a dark, sinister-looking cutaneous lesion on the face. This is a malignant melanoma. Your next questions should relate to the possibility of metastases, especially to the brain or liver. Extremely rare is a paraneoplastic retinopathy (cancer associated retinopathy) that results in phosphenes and peripheral constriction of the visual fields, which is often misdiagnosed as migraine (see Chapter 2).

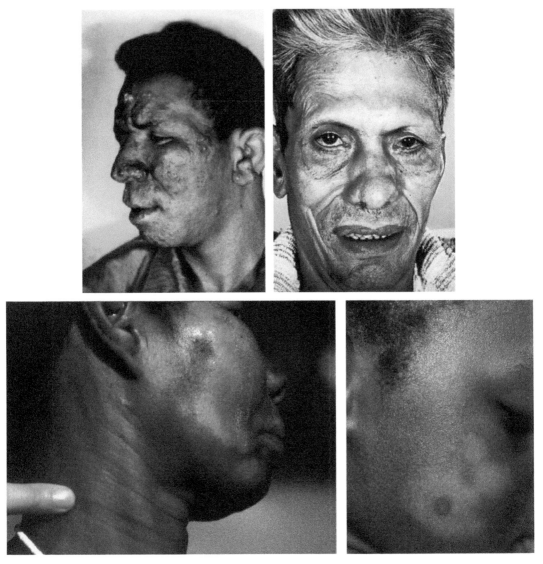

FIGURE 1.25: **Top pictures:** Facial appearance characteristic of advanced lepromatous leprosy, sometimes called leonine (lion-like) face. This results from multiple nodules, plaques, and thickened dermis. Sometimes there is collapse of the nasal bridge, as in top right picture. The absence of forehead wrinkles and constricted left palpebral fissure in the top right picture suggests upper facial weakness, a very characteristic feature of leprosy. **Lower left:** Marked thickening of the right great auricular nerve that runs just below the ear, over sternomastoid. **Lower right:** A depigmented macule typical of tuberculoid leprosy. The skin is anesthetic without hair follicles or sweat glands. Top photos courtesy USPHS Hospital Carville. Lower figures courtesy Jose Biller, Chicago.

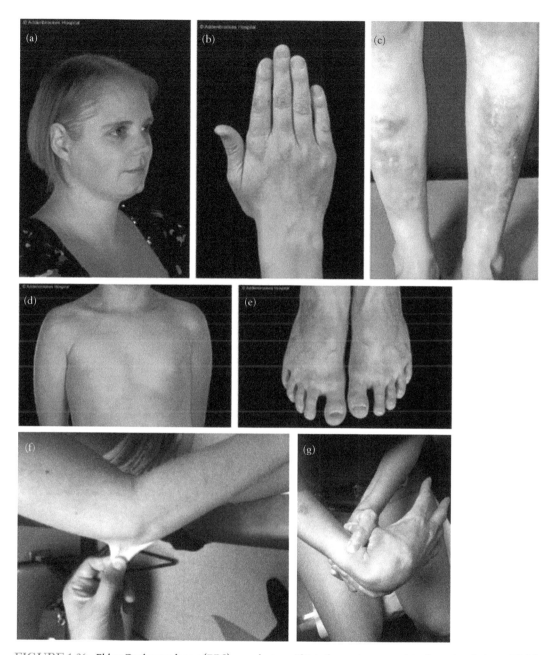

FIGURE 1.26: Ehlers Danlos syndrome (EDS), vascular type. This is the most severe variety, formerly called type IV. (**a**) Acrogeria, or premature aging, is a specific feature of vascular EDS; note the large eyes, thin, short nose (Madonna face), lobeless ears, and scar over the chin; (**b**) premature atrophy and wrinkling on the dorsum of the hands affecting the same child; (**c**) pretibial bruising and hemosiderosis. (**d**) Network of veins on upper chest due to cutaneous atrophy in 7-year-old boy; (**e**) similar features present on the dorsum of feet. (**f** and **g**) In another patient, note the marked skin elasticity and hypermobile joints. This patient could dislocate both shoulders at will. Such patients and those with Marfan's syndrome are at risk of a dural tear, low tension headache, and hemosiderosis. Reproduced from Figure 20.2.2 in the chapter Inherited Defects of Connective Tissue: Ehlers-Danlos Syndrome, Marfan's Syndrome, and Pseudoxanthoma Elasticum, by NP Burrows. Oxford University Press. DOI:10.1093/med/9780199204854.003.2002_update_002.

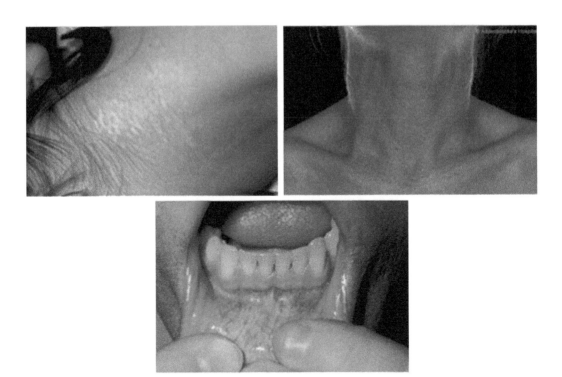

FIGURE 1.27: Skin lesions in pseudoxanthoma elasticum (PXE). See also Chapter 2, Figure 2.49. (**Upper left**) Typical flexural skin lesions in the lateral neck. (**Upper right**) More widespread changes on anterior neck with secondary cutis laxa. (**Lower**) Mucosal infiltration of the lower lip in PXE. Reproduced from Figure 20.2.11 in the chapter Inherited Defects of Connective Tissue: Ehlers–Danlos Syndrome, Marfan's Syndrome, and Pseudoxanthoma Elasticum, by NP Burrows. Oxford University Press. DOI:10.1093/med/9780199204854.003.2002_update_002.

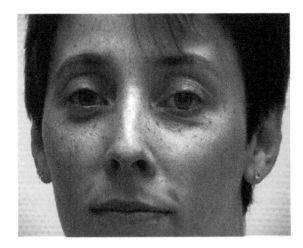

FIGURE 1.28: Spotty hyperpigmentation of the facial skin (lentiginosis) lips and eyelids suggests a diagnosis of the Carney complex. This is an autosomal dominant disorder due to mutation in the *PRKAR1A* gene on 17p23. Other features include multiple neoplasia, myxomas of the heart, oral mucosa, and endocrine overactivity (adrenocortical disease, hypercortisolism, excess growth hormone). The neurological complications result from embolic strokes. Photo courtesy Jose Biller, Chicago.

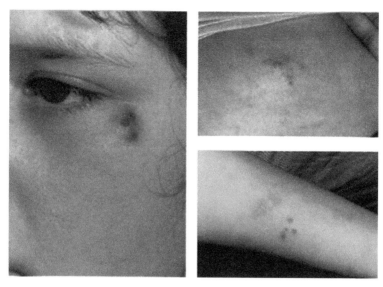

FIGURE 1.29: A child who displayed multiple dark blue, rubbery lesions on the skin and tongue characteristic of the blue rubber bleb nevus syndrome. Lesions also involve the gut and nervous system associated with liability to hemorrhage from venous malformations or dural AV fistulas. Reproduced with permission from Figure 5.39 in the chapter Disorders of the Dermis, by V Sybert. Oxford University Press. DOI:10.1093/med/9780195397666.003.0005.

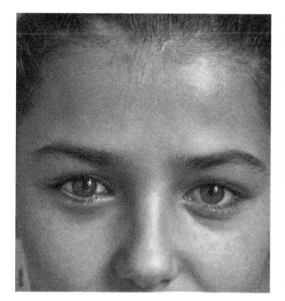

FIGURE 1.30: Hemolachria. This 11-year-old girl had a 2-year history of epistaxis accompanied by blood-stained tears from the right eye. There was hyperemia of the nasal mucosa. Hemolachria has several etiologies. In the related disorder hematohidrosis, the sweat is blood-stained. See Video 1.1, Hematohidrosis. Figure reproduced with permission from Ozcan et al. (2013).

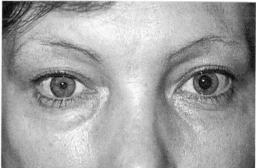

FIGURE 1.31: First try to work out which is the abnormal eye! With the small right pupil, you might think it is a right Horner's syndrome, but it is not because there is no ptosis. The face is well illuminated by the studio lights (see reflection on cornea) and the left pupil is large, so that is the abnormal side. Also note that the light reflection is at 11 o'clock on both sides, which suggests there is no weakness of the extraocular muscles (Hirschberg's sign, Figure 2.53). These are the eyes of a 35-year-old woman who complained of intermittent blurred vision and something odd about the left eye. She was healthy apart from occasional migraine (a frequent comorbidity). Diagnosis: tonic pupil where the pupil constricts to accommodation but slowly to light and redilates even more slowly. Also known as light-near dissociation. If the tendon reflexes are diminished, this is termed Holmes-Adie syndrome.

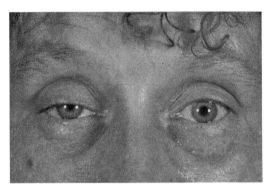

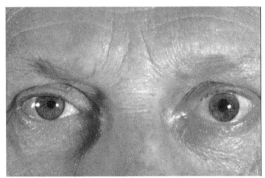

FIGURE 1.32: There is a partial right ptosis and a small pupil on that side. Perhaps the right cheek is dryer than the left, as there is less shine on the skin. Diagnosis: right Horner's syndrome, remembered by the mnemonic miosis, ptosis, and anhidrosis.

FIGURE 1.33: **Right**: Horner's syndrome. Note the right ptosis and small pupil. There is hyperemia of the conjunctival vessels (sympathectomy effect) and the *appearance* of enophthalmos.

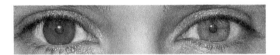

FIGURE 1.34: Unequal iris color from birth. Diagnosis: congenital anisochromia in this case. Congenital anisochromia occurs also in Sturge–Weber, Waardenburg, and Parry–Romberg syndromes. If anisochromia is acquired, darkening iris color in a blue-eyed person is an important sign of Wilson's disease, but the changes should affect both eyes. Other causes are Fuchs heterochromic iridocyclitis, a unilateral inflammatory disorder. Also, some prostaglandin analogs, such as latanoprost, bimatoprost, and travoprost, used for glaucoma treatment may darken a blue iris, but these drops are usually inserted into *both* eyes. Congenital anisochromia reproduced from Speakslowly, on en.wikipedia, cropped by Shannernanner under Creative Commons Attribution License.

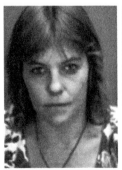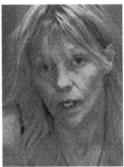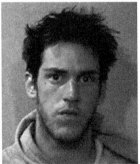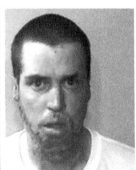

FIGURE 1.35: Drug effects before and after. **Left pair**: Beware the agitated, talkative patient with a runny nose, depressed nasal bridge, staring eyes, and sunken face of this woman. This may be cocaine addiction. Note the changed facial appearance over the space of 4 years. **Right pair**: Crystal meth addict. Note changed facial appearance with loss of subcutaneous tissue, acne, and aging effects in this man. Oral hygiene is usually poor—"meth mouth."

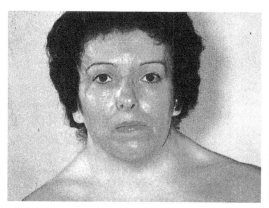
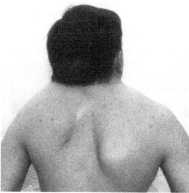

FIGURE 1.36: **Left**: This middle-aged woman presented because of cerebellar ataxia. The neck had been short since childhood due to congenital fusion of several cervical vertebrae—the Klippel-Feil anomaly. Diagnosis: late presenting Chiari malformation, a disorder regularly associated with a short neck and caused by a small posterior fossa. Cough headache and down-beating nystagmus on lateral gaze are characteristic. Reproduced with permission from *A Colour Atlas of Clinical Neurology*, 2nd ed., M Parsons. Mosby Year Book Europe. 1993. **Right**: A low hairline because of the short neck, again related to the Klippel-Feil anomaly.

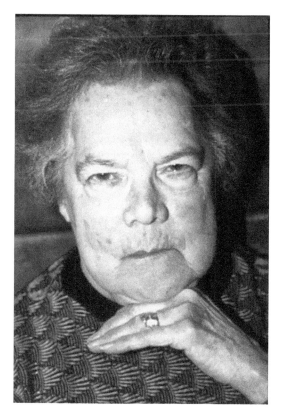

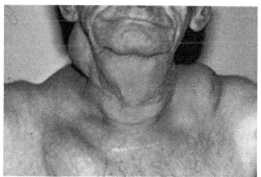

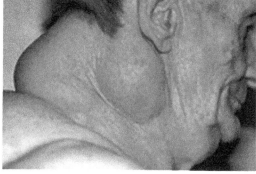

FIGURE 1.37: The jaw-supporting sign. An 83-year-old woman who repeatedly supported the jaw when talking. This maneuver also helped prevent her neck from flopping forward. There was ptosis as well (blepharoptosis and true ptosis). Diagnosis: myasthenia gravis. This sign may be seen rarely in myotonic dystrophy and oromandibular dystonia, but there is no fatigue in either.

FIGURE 1.38: Note the numerous deposits of fat around the neck. They form a collar-like expansion that may impair breathing. Patients present to neurologists because of obstructive sleep apnea or polyneuropathy. Many abuse alcohol. Diagnosis: Madelung's disease (a mitochondrial disorder), also known as multiple symmetric lipomatosis. The large neck should alert you to this diagnosis by inspection alone. Reproduced with permission from Figure 6.5 in the chapter Disorders of Subcutaneous Tissue, by V Sybert. Oxford University Press. DOI: 10.1093/med/9780195397666.003.0006.

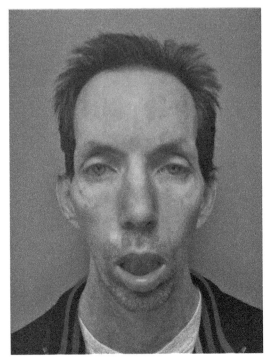

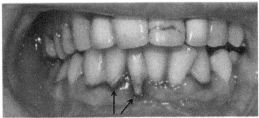

FIGURE 1.40: This 35-year-old woman spent 1 week on an acute surgical unit because of confusion and recurrent colicky abdominal pain. Nothing abnormal was found on multiple bowel investigations, but then basophilic stippling of red cells on the blood film was observed. This was ignored and attributed to anemia! Eventually, the physicians were consulted who noted the blue-gray discoloration at the dentogingival junction. Diagnosis: lead poisoning with lead line (arrows). Lead toxicity is a rare cause of basophilic stippling. Dental caries can mimic a lead line but usually oral hygiene is poor, and that was not the case here. This patient was exposed to lead through drinking cider from a poorly glazed Italian mug. Lead was used in the glazing process and, if undertaken incorrectly, it can be leeched out by solvents such as alcohol, as in this case. Reported in Zuckerman and Pham (1989).

FIGURE 1.39: Note the frontal balding, ptosis, temporalis wasting, and open mouth. This is dystrophia myotonica. Reproduced with permission from Figure 2.1 in Wicklund (2013).

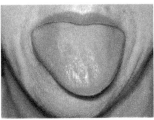

Note:

- Lines similar to lead lines occur with mercury or thallium poisoning.
- A red line at the base of the teeth suggests pulmonary TB.
- A purple line suggests gold poisoning.

A persistently large tongue may be found also in the following:

- Lymphoma
- Myxedema
- Riboflavin deficiency
- Mercury poisoning
- Acromegaly
- Myopathies, for example, limb-girdle and Duchenne dystrophies, acid maltase deficiency
- Mucopolysaccharidoses

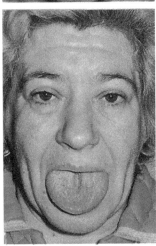

FIGURE 1.41: **Top**: Macroglossia in a patient with systemic AL amyloidosis. Ageusia is common. Reproduced with permission from Figure 47.11 in the chapter Dermatology, by CN Wieland and LA Drage. Oxford University Press. DOI:10.1093/med/9780199948949.003.0047. **Bottom**: Macroglossia in a woman with acromegaly. Note the coarse features. Reproduced with permission from *A Colour Atlas of Clinical Neurology*, 2nd ed., M Parsons. Mosby Year Book Europe. 1993.

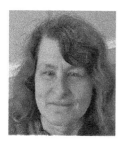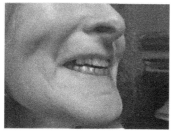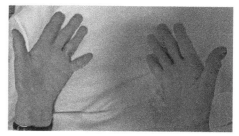

FIGURE 1.42: A 50-year-old lady with progressive paraparesis. **Left**: Strabismus, close-set eyes (hypotelorism), and microphthalmia. **Center**: Microdontia and enamel hypoplasia. **Right**: Small little fingers, scar from separation of fourth and fifth finger syndactyly, with absence of proximal phalanx of the right little finger. This is the oculo-dento-digital dysplasia (ODDD) syndrome. Presentation may be neurological, as in this case. Reproduced with permission from Adam Zeman, Exeter, UK.

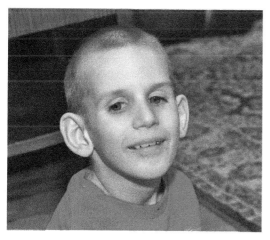

FIGURE 1.43: This is an 8-year-old boy. Note the deep-set eyes, thin dry hair, large ears, sallow complexion, ataxia and premature aging appearance (progeria). He has Cockayne syndrome. Other features comprise microcephaly, retinitis pigmentosa with visual and hearing impairment, photosensitivity. Photograph courtesy Amy and Friends, Cockayne Syndrome Support, UK.

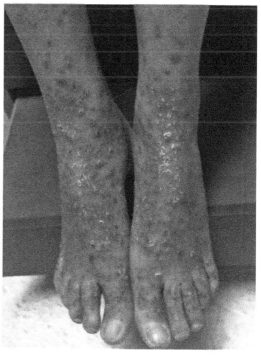

FIGURE 1.44: Multiple insect bites in a patient with hereditary sensory neuropathy. He was unaware that he was standing on a fire-ant mound and that the insects were biting until a passerby alerted him.

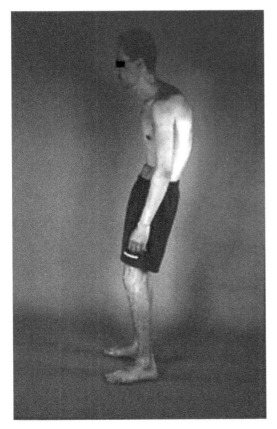

FIGURE 1.45: Note the pronounced thoracolumbar kyphosis and straightening of the lumbar spine. There is flexion contracture of the hips. This is the question mark spine of ankylosing spondylitis. It must not be confused with camptocormia (see Chapter 8). Patients with ankylosing spondylitis have recurrent episodes of uveitis and they are at major risk of cervical fracture in traffic accidents. They are liable to myelopathy, radiculopathy, and ossification of the posterior or anterior longitudinal ligaments. There is a probable link with multiple sclerosis. Reproduced with permission from Figure 10.4.1 in the chapter Spondyloarthropathies, by S Bawa, P Wordsworth, and I Atukorala. Oxford University Press. DOI:10.1093/med/9780199550647.003.010004.

Macroglossia occurs subacutely in angioneurotic edema and in superior vena caval obstruction. Some patients have symptoms of obstructive apnea.

Hypersalivation. See Video 1.1, Hypersalivation. This shows a patient troubled with severe hypersalivation due to PD. Apart from parkinsonism, this phenomenon is seen in relatively few other conditions, namely amyotrophic lateral sclerosis (ALS), rabies, and pseudobulbar palsy. The feature is characteristic of the later stages of PD but it may

be an early sign of multiple system atrophy (MSA). In all these disorders, swallowing is impaired, but saliva production is usually unchanged. Hypersalivation may be an acute phenomenon, as in mercury and organophosphorus poisoning.

In the related disorder **hematohidrosis**, the sweat is blood-stained (see Video 1.2, Hematohidrosis).

SUMMARY

- Inspection: watch the patient enter the room, how they turn to close the door, and as they walk toward you and shake your hand. Inspect the face, clothes, fingernails, and jewelry. Listen to the voice, smell the breath.
- Abnormal fingernails: coke nail, unidigital clubbing, subungual glomus tumor, Mees lines, koilonychia, Plummer's nails, blue or gray nails
- Hands and feet of patient with gout
- Woman with morning headache, tinnitus, acne, and mild papilledema: idiopathic intracranial hypertension.
- Facial palsy and Lisch nodules plus café au lait spots and freckling over the anterior abdominal wall; multiple soft lumps, freckling over abdomen: neurofibromatosis type 1
- Saddle nose deformity: congenital syphilis, Wegener's granulomatosis, systemic lupus, leprosy, sarcoid, and cocaine abuse; rhinophyma
- Red cheeks and nose that look like frostbite: lupus pernio (sarcoid); episcleral nodules from sarcoid deposits
- Forehead diagonal crease sign: caused by PD, heavy sleep on one side; possibly sleep apnea.
- Linear scar-like defect on forehead with shrinkage of facial soft tissues: hemifacial atrophy or Parry-Romberg syndrome
- Silvery-gray discoloration of facial skin: argyria
- Port-wine stain on face and epilepsy: Sturge-Weber syndrome
- Seizures and characteristic facial appearance of Sotos syndrome
- White forelock, deafness, and hypertelorism: Waardenburg syndrome
- Uveitis and poliosis, sunset glow in fundus, Sugiura's sign: Vogt Harada Koyanagi syndrome
- Cerebellar ataxia, recurrent chest infection, scleral and ear telangiectasia: ataxia

telangiectasia syndrome; telangiectasia may be confined to cheeks; high risk of lymphoma and leukemia

- Tortuous conjunctival and retinal vessels: Fabry disease
- Learning difficulty; large protuberant ears; long, thin face; large testes: fragile X syndrome (full mutation)
- Episodic inflammation of pinna, floppy ears, episcleritis, recurrent nonbacterial meningitis, red eye and red ear: relapsing polychondritis; Frank's sign
- Swelling of upper inner aspect of orbit with proptosis down and out: orbital mucocele, orbital tumor
- Swelling in upper outer aspect of orbit with proptosis down and in: lacrimal gland tumor or sarcoid; look for episcleral nodules
- Proptosis, eye pushed down with swelling of temple: meningioma of lateral third of sphenoid wing
- Seizures and multiple soft swellings in nasolabial fold: tuberous sclerosis
- Vertical smile: myasthenia gravis
- Melanoma on face with headache and blurred vision: metastases or cancer-associated retinopathy
- Leonine face, thickened accessory nerve, depigmented skin macules: leprosy
- Marked skin elasticity, hypotonic painful muscles, fatigue, hemorrhage from cerebral arteries or aneurysms: Ehlers Danlos syndrome type IV
- Thickened, lax neck skin, mucosal infiltration: pseudoxanthoma elasticum
- Lentiginosis, embolic strokes, myxoma of the heart and skin, multiple neoplasia: Carney complex
- Multiple dark blue lesions of skin and tongue: blue rubber bleb nevus syndrome
- Hematohidrosis and hemalachria
- Blurred vision with large pupil unreactive to light: tonic pupil. Association with migraine; if absent deep tendon reflexes, it is called Holmes-Adie syndrome
- Miosis, ptosis, and anhidrosis: Horner's syndrome; sometimes dilated conjunctival vessels
- Horner syndrome following recent car accident: carotid or vertebral artery dissection
- Darkness exaggerates pupillary asymmetry due to a Horner's syndrome but conceals that due to a CN III lesion; conversely, strong light conceals pupillary asymmetry due to a Horner's syndrome but accentuates that due to a CN III disorder
- One brown and one blue eye: congenital anisochromia, Sturge-Weber, Horner, Waardenburg, and Parry-Romberg syndromes; also Wilson's disease, Fuchs heterochromic iridocyclitis, use of prostaglandin analog drops for glaucoma
- Agitated patient with staring eyes and a runny nose: cocaine addict; patient with sunken, face, acne, aged look, and poor oral hygiene: crystal meth addict
- Imbalance and short neck: Chiari malformation with Klippel-Feil anomaly; cough headache and down-beating nystagmus are characteristic
- Jaw-supporting sign: myasthenia gravis, myotonic dystrophy, oromandibular dystonia
- Numerous fat deposits in neck, trunk, and limbs: Madelung's syndrome; associated with neuropathy and possibly alcoholism
- Frontal balding, ptosis, temporalis wasting, and open mouth: dystrophia myotonica
- Gray-black line at gingival margin, intestinal colic, basophilic stippling: lead line from lead poisoning. Similarly colored lines occur with mercury or thallium poisoning; red line suggests pulmonary TB; purple line occurs with gold poisoning
- Macroglossia: lymphoma, systemic amyloid, myxedema, riboflavin deficiency, mercurialism, acromegaly, myopathies, and mucopolysaccharidoses
- Progressive paraparesis, hypotelorism, microphthalmia, microdontia, and finger abnormalities: oculo-dento-digital dysplasia (ODDD) syndrome
- Child with sunken eyes, ataxia, and progeria: Cockayne syndrome
- Multiple painless insect bites in a patient with hereditary sensory neuropathy
- The question mark spine of ankylosing spondylitis
- Drooling saliva (Video 1.1, Hypersalivation): parkinsonism, ALS, rabies, and pseudobulbar palsies; occasionally an early feature of MSA or PD Acute phenomenon in mercury or organophosphorus poisoning
- Hematohidrosis in Von Willebrand disease

SUGGESTED READING

Agwu JC, Shaw NJ, Kirk J, Chapman S, Ravine D, Cole TR. Growth in Sotos syndrome. *Arch Dis Child.* 1999;80(4):339–342.

Chan EW, Sanjay S, Chang BCM. Headache, red eyes, blurred vision and hearing loss. *CMAJ.* 2010; 182:1205–1209.

Finlayson S, Beeson D, Palace J. Congenital myasthenic syndromes: an update. *Pract Neurol.* 2013;13: 80–91.

Fitzgerald FT, Tierney LM Jr. The bedside Sherlock Holmes. *West J Med.* 1982;137:169–175.

Ozcan KM, Ozdas T, Baran H, Ozdogan F, Dere H. Hemolacria: case report. *Int J Pediatr Otorhinolaryngol.* 2013;77:137–138.

Sodi A, Ioannidis AS, Mehta A, Davey C, Beck M, Pitz S. Ocular manifestations of Fabry's disease: data from the Fabry Outcome Survey. *Br J Ophthalmol.* 2007;91:210–214.

Wicklund MP. The muscular dystrophies. *Continuum (Minneap Minn).* 2013;19:1535–1570.

Xu R, Pham J. Frank's sign: a coronary artery disease predictor. *BMJ Case Rep.* 2014;2014.

Zuckerman MA, Savory D, Rayman G. Lead encephalopathy from an imported Toby mug. *Postgrad Med J.* 1989;65:307–309.

Chapter 2: Cranial Nerves

This chapter describes the main Handles and Flags in the cranial nerve territory that require various combinations of history and examination.

OLFACTORY NERVE (CN I)

Anosmia

▶ Intermittent anosmia suggests a *conductive* defect. Continual anosmia favors a *perceptive* (neurological) defect

Most clinicians do not ask about the sense of smell and even less frequently do they bother to test it. Simply asking a patient is better than nothing at all, but it should be emphasized that only ~40% of patients with anosmia will be aware of their defect, and virtually no-one is aware if the defect is unilateral. Apart from peripheral problems that cause anosmia, such as sinus disease, polyps, and head or facial trauma, it is recognized that degenerative conditions such as PD (Parkinson's disease) and Alzheimer's disease may be associated with early and significant smell impairment.

If air does not reach the olfactory receptor region in the nose because of variable obstruction to air entry by polyps, congestion, or the like, this is *conductive* anosmia. Measures that relieve congestion, such as ephedrine, steroid sprays, exercise, or heavy lifting, will improve the sense of smell temporarily. Conversely, continuous anosmia is usually *perceptive*—that is, a disorder of the olfactory nerve itself or its central connections.

▶ **Anosmia and Dementia**
This is a feature of the following:

- Alzheimer disease
- Lewy body dementia and late-stage PD
- Frontotemporal and semantic dementia
- Huntington disease
- Frontal pole tumor (may be unilateral initially and rarely reported)

- Prion disorder (e.g., CJD; Creutzfeld-Jacob disease)
- *Unilateral* anosmia accompanied by frontal type dementia should be an olfactory groove meningioma that compresses the frontal pole and, initially, just one olfactory bulb/tract (Figure 2.1).

▶ **Anosmia with Mirror Movements**
This occurs in young adults with:

- *Kallman's syndrome,* a mainly X-linked recessive disorder in which (male) patients are congenitally anosmic and hypogonadal.
- *Parkinson's disease.* Mirror movements are occasional features. Smell impairment is common and severe.

▶ **Anosmia and Retinitis Pigmentosa Suggest Refsum Syndrome**
Thus, if you are investigating the cause of retinitis pigmentosa (Figure 2.2), then test smell sense as it is usually very poor in Refsum's syndrome (Gibberd et al. 2004). There are always other corroborative features:

- Short stature
- Deafness
- Ichthyosis
- Peripheral neuropathy
- Unsteadiness

▶ **Anosmia, Myelopathy, Ataxia, and Deafness**
This combination (or at least three of the four) usually indicates

- Superficial siderosis or
- Mitochondrial disorder

A history of head injury, multiple or difficult brain or spinal surgical procedures, and intracranial/

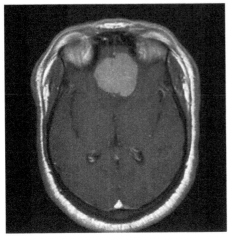 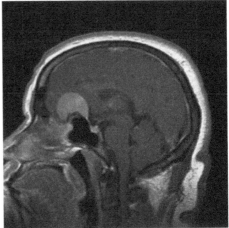

FIGURE 2.1: MRI scan that shows a large, high T2 signal mass in the inferior frontal region. The lateral view shows it arising from the floor of the anterior fossa. Diagnosis: olfactory groove meningioma.

spinal bleeding will clinch a diagnosis of superficial siderosis (Figure 2.3). Cognitive decline sometimes accompanies this

▶ Anosmia in Asian or South American Person Suggests Leprosy

Leprosy is a strong possibility, especially if nasal congestion is present and there is no other cause of obstruction such as polyps. This mycobacterium grows best in cooler areas like the dorsum of the hands or feet and inside the nose, which is 1°C lower than normal body temperature. Leprosy is also unusual in

that it causes patchy bilateral lower motor neuron facial weakness, which is often more severe in the cooler areas of the face such as the zygomatic area and brow (Figure 2.4). This may cause the eyebrows to assume a devilish appearance. Thus,

> ▶ Anosmia with bilateral, mainly upper facial palsy suggests leprosy.

▶ Intermittent Olfactory Hallucinations

In the absence of local nasal disease this suggests the following:

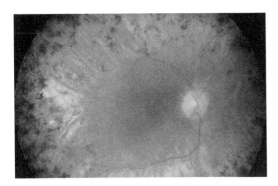

FIGURE 2.2: Retinitis pigmentosa. If there is anosmia then the number one diagnosis is Refsum's disease. Reproduced with permission from *Training in Ophthalmology*, Figure 4.44, in the chapter Medical Retina, by B Patil and P Puri. Oxford University Press. DOI:10.1093/med/9780199237593.003.0004.

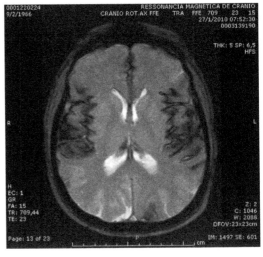

FIGURE 2.3: Axial MRI brain scan to show superficial siderosis. This appears as a dark signal on T2-weighted images. Courtesy Ildefonso Rodriguez.

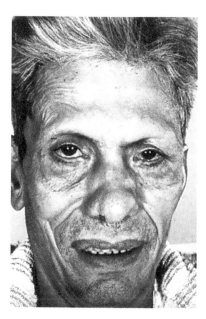

FIGURE 2.4: The face in lepromatous leprosy. There is bilateral facial weakness with contraction of the right frontalis muscle but not over the central forehead region, which is cool and therefore susceptible to bacterial invasion. There are buccinator wrinkles (indicating preserved innervation to this muscle) as the branches to buccinator are deep and therefore warm and less likely to be attacked by the mycobacterium. There is a saddle-nose deformity due to destruction of the nasal septum. The nasal cavity is about 1°C cooler than the face and thus more susceptible to bacterial growth. Courtesy USPHS Hospital Carville, LA.

- Anteromedial temporal lobe tumor or vascular lesion (Figure 2.5)
- PD
- Olfactory reference syndrome
- Transient epileptic amnesia (TEA)
- Complex partial seizures

The tumor is usually a glioma that irritates the amygdala (Figure 2.5), producing what are essentially focal seizures (uncinate fits). Most odors experienced are unpleasant, such as burning rubber, and usually difficult to describe. Disagreeable olfactory hallucinations are a rare feature of PD either in the prodromal or established disease phase. In the olfactory reference syndrome, psychotic or depressed patients imagine that an unpleasant odor emanates internally or that others are doing this with malicious intent. TEA is described in Chapter 13 (Dementia).

▶ Hyperosmia

This means increased sensitivity to odors. It occurs

- Around the time of a migraine attack.
- In the initial months of pregnancy. Some women can tell very early that they are pregnant because of a heightened sense of smell. Perhaps not the best way for a neurologist to diagnose pregnancy!
- Possibly in Addison's disease
- As a drug withdrawal effect. This is reported after cessation of benzodiazepine medication.

▶ Loss of Smell After Head Injury Suggests That the Injury Is Severe

The majority lose smell sense though shearing of olfactory fibers as they pass though the cribriform plate. This can happen in isolation, but there is often evidence of severe trauma such skull base fracture. Rarely, even minor head injury causes anosmia. Many complain of taste loss (ageusia), but usually this means that the patient has *misinterpreted loss of taste to mean loss of smell*. Rarely, extensive skull base fractures damage the olfactory and facial nerves, leading to anosmia and genuine ageusia.

▶ If there is no skull base fracture and on testing *you find that there really is loss of both smell and taste, then the lesion must be central.* This would be either in the anterior insula or frontal pole (orbitofrontal cortex). Both these areas are concerned with transmission and interpretation of smell and taste.

◀ *Normal smell sense in apparent PD.* At least 80% of patients with classic PD have reduced sense of smell, especially those with the nontremulous forms (Hawkes et al. 1997). Not all patients are aware of a smell problem, but if on *quantitative testing* someone with suspected PD has a normal smell sense, then this is a Red Flag. You should consider *parkinsonism* in, for example:
  - Progressive supranuclear palsy (PSP)
  - Corticobasal syndrome
  - Multiple system atrophy (MSA)
  - Essential tremor

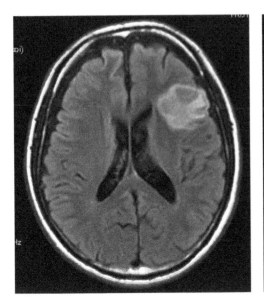 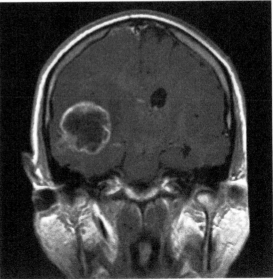

FIGURE 2.5: **Left**: Axial T1-weighted enhanced MRI scan that shows an oligodendroglioma in the left frontotemporal deep white matter. **Right**: MRI T1-enhanced coronal section that shows a large infiltrating glioblastoma multiforme occupying much of the right temporal lobe. Both of these lesions could cause olfactory hallucinations and complex partial seizures.

OPTIC NERVE AND VISIBLE PARTS OF EYE (CN II)

Eye examination is extremely valuable for localization and diagnosis. It is the only part of the nervous system ordinarily visible. Here are some Handles arranged according to the order in which you would test the eye: inspection, acuity, fields, pupils, and funduscopy. Always assess the pupils and fundi last as your patient may experience persisting blurred vision if you examine them first, and this will make acuity and field testing inaccurate.

Visual Acuity

▶ Looking through a pinhole improves virtually all refractive errors.
▶ Bilateral impaired visual acuity in a healthy teenage girl is usually a functional eye problem.
  A common presentation is that of a girl who complains of blurred vision in the absence of other objective eye signs. She may be unable to read anything better than the top letter of an eye chart, but this fails to improve when the chart is brought closer. The field may be tunnel- or spiral-shaped as described later in the chapter. This is a functional eye problem. Simple reassurance may not help, and some require psychiatric assistance.

▶ Distorted central vision in one eye is a macular problem.
  The patient complains that straight lines appear curved (metamorphopsia). Most are referred to the eye clinic, but occasionally you will be first in line. It is detected best by asking the patient to look with each eye separately at a grid of multiple vertical and horizontal lines—the Amsler chart (Figure 2.6).
▶ In a young adult, metamorphopsia is usually due to central serous retinopathy (CSR).
  Typically, the patient is an obsessional male aged 20–50 years who has distorted central vision, micropsia, or complaint of a central gray patch just in one eye. He may be receiving steroids or have taken them recently. Funduscopy reveals a collection of fluid, like a blister at the macula (Figure 2.7). Optic neuritis is a frequent misdiagnosis.
▶ In the middle-aged or elderly patient, the major causes of metamorphopsia are as follows:
  · Age-related macular degeneration
  · Diabetic macular edema
  · Epiretinal membrane (cellophane maculopathy)

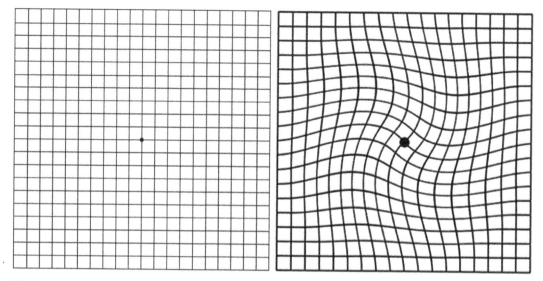

FIGURE 2.6: Amsler chart as seen by a healthy person, on the **left**. The distortion seen by a patient looking at the **right** chart is typical of a macular problem, in this case, age-related macular degeneration.

In general:

- Macular edema (e.g., CSR) makes objects appear abnormally small: micropsia.
- Macular scarring (e.g., epiretinal membrane) makes objects appear abnormally large: macropsia.

Field Defects

Before starting a formal assessment of visual fields in a partially sighted patient, you should observe how the patient negotiates the room furniture.

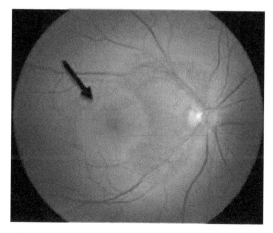

FIGURE 2.7: Central serous retinopathy demonstrating the "blister" of fluid underneath the macula.

▶ Patients with *Leber's optic atrophy* usually require no help because visual loss is mainly central (macular) and peripheral vision (for large objects) is retained.

▶ Patients with *Usher's or Refsum's syndrome* have difficulty navigating a room alone because there is involvement of the peripheral visual field (and later the central field).

Thus, if the patient carries a white stick but can still avoid items of furniture, then some peripheral vision must be present. If help is required to find the chair, then there is likely to be macular *and* peripheral field involvement.

Also, while you are watching the subject enter the room, be alert to the following phenomena:

▶ The patient who is blind in both eyes but appears unconcerned, denies it, or may not even be aware of it, has cortical blindness. This results typically from bilateral occipital infarcts (Anton's syndrome), border zone ischemia from prolonged cerebral hypoperfusion, and the "top of the basilar syndrome" (see Chapter 9, Stroke). Patients like this are sometimes accused of inventing their symptoms.

▶ In cortical blindness the pupillary light reflexes are normal. This happens because the tract for the light reflex runs through the

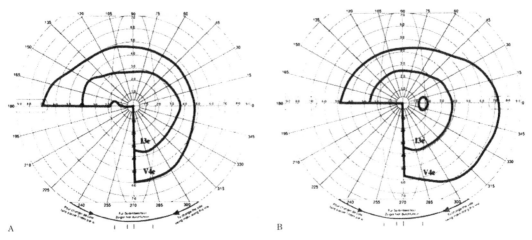

A   B

FIGURE 2.8: A perfectly congruous left homonymous inferior quadrantanopia that respects the vertical meridian as all postgeniculate lesions should. It is congruous because you could take one of the field defects and it would superimpose almost exactly on the other one. *Homonymous* means that the defect is in the same-named part of the visual field. Such defects are characteristic of optic radiation lesions, here an occipital infarct. Reproduced with permission from McFadzean and Hadley (1997).

midbrain; there is no cortical pathway for the light reflex arc.

Congruity

▶ A perfectly congruous homonymous field defect suggests a lesion in the occipital cortex (Figure 2.8). Note: Slight incongruity is found in parietal lesions.

▶ A markedly incongruous homonymous field defect is usually due to an optic tract lesion (Figure 2.9).

The word *congruous* means exactly the same shape and size—thus you could superimpose exactly the defects from the two eyes. The presence of congruity is a reflection of the anatomical arrangement of fibers in the optic radiation. In the optic tract they are not fully organized into their respective topographic positions. This is a general guideline with some exceptions.

Tunnel Vision

This refers to concentric constriction of the peripheral visual field.

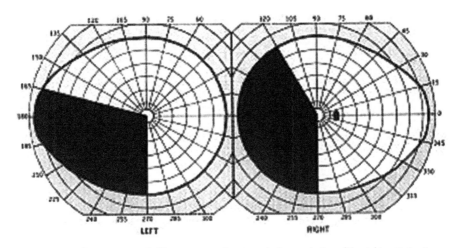

LEFT   RIGHT

FIGURE 2.9: A markedly incongruous left homonymous hemianopia due to a lesion of the right optic tract.

▶ The usual cause of persisting bilateral tunnel vision is a functional (psychogenic) disorder.

there are several organic conditions associated with this:

- Glaucoma
- Temporarily as part of a migraine aura
- Alcohol intoxication
- Retinitis pigmentosa
- Retinal ischemia due to severe anemia
- Markedly raised intracranial pressure (ICP)
- Vigabatrin
- Cancer-associated retinopathy (CAR; see later discussion)

The patient with functional tunnel vision is usually a young woman, and field measurement may reveal a spiral pattern; that is, an increasingly smaller field on sequential testing (Figure 2.10, *upper*), crossing of isopters, or constant diameter irrespective of screen distance—the "cylindrical" field. A genuine field defect is never spiral, and it enlarges like a cone with increasing distance of the eye from the screen. The Humphrey field analyzer plot may show the "clover leaf" pattern (Figure 2.10, *lower*).

Cancer-Associated Retinopathy

▶ Bilateral peripheral constricted fields, continuous phosphenes, night blindness, history of cutaneous melanoma or other cancers

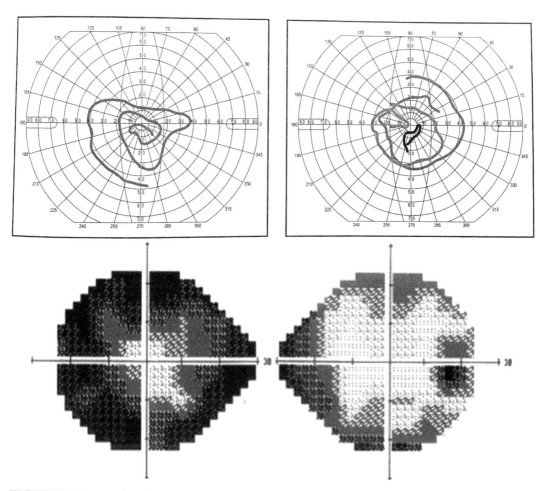

FIGURE 2.10: **Top:** Plots of visual fields in functional eye disorder. The "spiral visual field" becomes smaller toward fixation (left eye) with crossing isopters in the right eye.**Bottom:** Humphrey field analyzer plot that shows the "clover leaf" pattern, characteristic of functional disorder. Top image reproduced with permission from *The Neuro-ophthalmology Survival Guide*, Figure 2.26, by A Pane, M Burdon, and NR Miller. Mosby Elsevier, 2007. Bottom image reproduced with permission from Mollan et al. (2014).

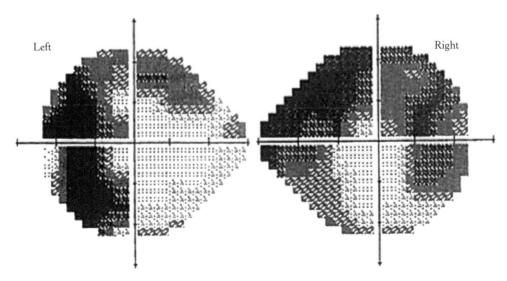

FIGURE 2.11: Humphrey field analyzer that shows large field defects in both eyes giving a partial tunnel vision field defect. This is from a patient with paraneoplastic retinopathy. There may be continuous phosphenes. Reproduced with permission from Dobson and Lawden (2011), figure 1.

suggests CAR. This is a paraneoplastic syndrome.

◀ *The continual phosphenes often lead to misdiagnosis of migraine.*

There is dysfunction of retinal bipolar cells, and the field defect is that of concentric constriction (Figure 2.11). These patients may have antibodies that bind to recoverin, a protein involved in photopsin recovery.

◀ *"Visual snow" may produce similar phosphenes* (Figure 2.12).

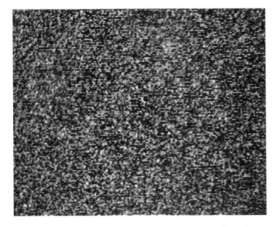

FIGURE 2.12: Visual snow phenomenon. The subject sees persisting horizontal lines like a badly adjusted old TV set.

This is a newly described benign disorder that may occur in isolation, but it is common in migraine. Features include:

- Continual, bilateral, dots or lines like TV static
- Normal visual fields
- Palinopsia (after images)

▶ Bitemporal hemianopia usually indicates a pituitary tumor that has spread upward to compress the undersurface of the chiasm (Figures 2.13 and 2.14).

    This is more a localizing rather than diagnostic sign, but it is extremely valuable and almost exclusive to disorders of the optic chiasm.

Other causes of bitemporal hemianopia include:

- Craniopharyngioma
- Meningioma
- Aneurysm
- Fusiform enlargement of both internal carotid arteries.
- Trauma

Also note:

▶ The upper temporal field is affected first with pressure from below, as in a pituitary tumor.

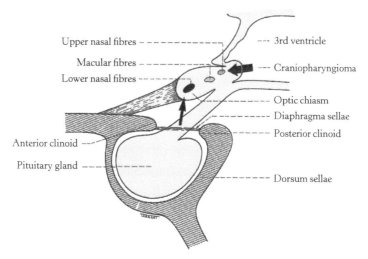

FIGURE 2.13: The relationship between the optic chiasm and pituitary gland. If a pituitary tumor expands upward and the chiasm is in its normal position, there will be pressure on the lower nasal fibers in the chiasm, resulting in a visual field defect in the upper temporal regions. Note the central position of macular fibers, which provides some protection in the early phase of compression. Reproduced from *Clinical Ophthalmology*, J Kanski and B Bowling, Figure 19.44. Elsevier Saunders, 2011.

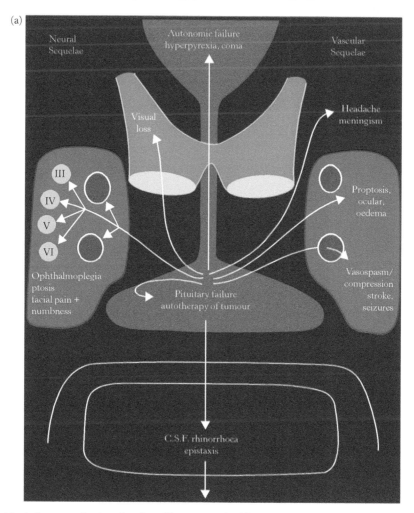

FIGURE 2.14: **A**: Summary of various disorders of the pituitary gland depending in its direction of expansion. **B**: The anatomical relations of the pituitary fossa. A, figure courtesy Adam Zeman, Exeter, UK. B, reproduced from *Training in Ophthalmology*, Figure 9.5, in the chapter Neuro-ophthalmology, by V Sundaram and J Elston. Oxford University Press. DOI:10.1093/med/9780199237593.003.0009.

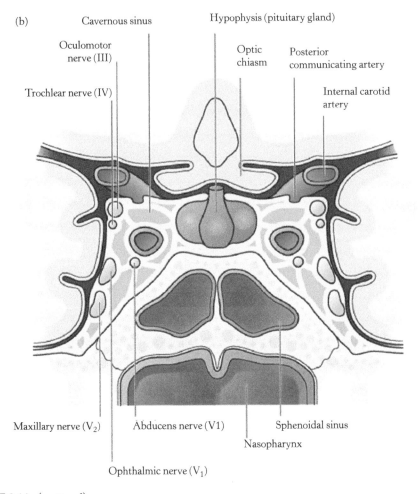

(b)   Cavernous sinus   Hypophysis (pituitary gland)

Oculomotor nerve (III)   Optic chiasm   Posterior communicating artery

Trochlear nerve (IV)   Internal carotid artery

Maxillary nerve (V$_2$)   Abducens nerve (V1)   Sphenoidal sinus

Nasopharynx

Ophthalmic nerve (V$_1$)

FIGURE 2.14: (continued)

▶ The lower temporal field is involved initially when there is pressure from above, as in a craniopharyngioma (Figure 2.15).

▶ In the early stages, the patient notices little impairment of visual acuity and presentation is late. This happens because the macular fibers are relatively protected in the central part of the chiasm (Figure 2.13).

▶ Initially, the upper temporal field loss is quite subtle but it can be detected by use of a red target.

Apart from a tendency to collide with a doorway entrance, etc., other Handles for a chiasmal lesion are as follows:

▶ *Hemi-field slide phenomenon* (Figure 2.16).
A patient may report difficulty reading because of a tendency for the right and left fields to move in opposite directions around the vertical meridian

▶ *Post-fixational blindness.*
This results in difficulty with depth appreciation, as explained in Figure 2.16.

◀ *Post-fixed chiasm* (Figure 2.17).
If the chiasm is more posterior than normal, a pituitary tumor will compress the optic nerve first, possibly simulating optic neuritis or producing a junctional scotoma (see later in this section).

◀ *Pre-fixed chiasm* (Figure 2.17).
Here the chiasm is further forward than normal, hence the optic tract is compressed. This causes an incongruous homonymous hemianopia (Figure 2.9). The field defects are different with each presentation.

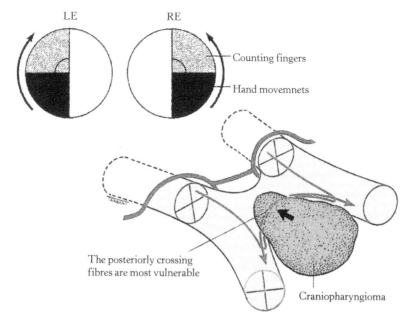

FIGURE 2.15: The applied anatomy of the optic chiasm and how a craniopharyngioma compresses the upper chiasm to cause a bitemporal field defect that is more severe in the lower sector. Reproduced with permission from *Clinical Ophthalmology*, J Kanski and B Bowling, Figure 19.53. Elsevier Saunders, 2011.

▷ Optic atrophy in one eye with a junctional field defect in the other is likely a compressive lesion (Figure 2.18).

The term "junctional" refers to the optic nerve where it joins the chiasm. The lesion may be a tumor or aneurysm.

Pressure on the optic nerve at its junction with the chiasm, causes (a) ipsilateral optic atrophy and a central scotoma, or (b) pressure on the posterior part of the optic nerve, compromising Wilbrand's knee. This contested piece of anatomy is now proved to exist on the basis of light imaging studies (Shin et al. 2014). It contains the lower nasal fibers from the opposite eye which are responsible for the contralateral upper temporal field.

◁ A *pituitary tumor* can cause a junctional field defect if the chiasm is post-fixed. See Figure 2.18.

The importance of this sign is that if the unilateral optic atrophy is ascribed incorrectly to optic neuritis, then a diagnosis of optic nerve or pituitary tumor will be delayed. Field testing should reveal an upper temporal defect in the opposite eye (Figure 2.18).

◁ *Homonymous hemianopia* cannot be caused by a frontal lobe lesion.

This very basic piece of applied anatomy can be useful in localizing a lesion. Thus, a patient with an uncomplicated frontal lobe tumor cannot have a field defect; if there is such a defect, there must be a second lesion. Conversely, a suspected, say, complete right middle cerebral artery thrombosis should cause a left hemiplegia and left homonymous hemianopia. If there is no field defect, then this is a Red Flag and you should look elsewhere, such as the brainstem, for an explanation. Rarely, exceptions occur if there are anomalies of vascular supply.

▷ Pie in the sky field defect suggests a Meyer's loop lesion (Figure 2.19).

Meyer's loop is part of the optic radiation that sweeps forward into the posterior temporal lobe and then back to join the main optic radiation fibers in the parietal lobe. In the case of a *right* Meyer's loop defect, the *fibers* have arisen from the right inferior temporal *retina* and the left inferior nasal *retina*, thus producing wedge-shaped defects in the contralateral upper nasal and

(a)   Standard perimetry   (b)   Near target perimetry

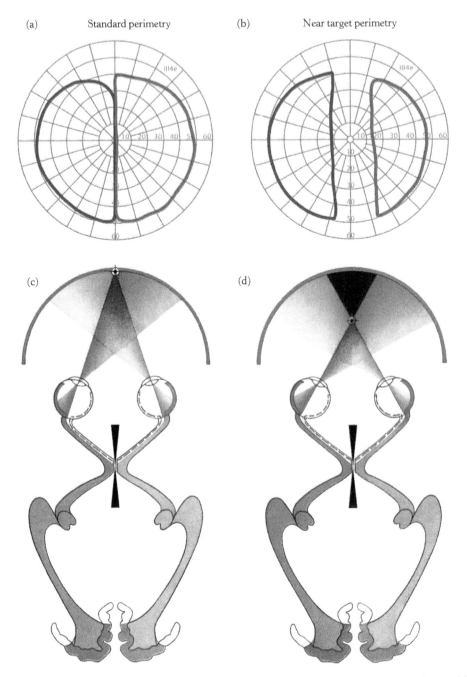

FIGURE 2.16: (**A and C**) Standard perimetry shows complete bitemporal hemianopia. The monocular visual fields of the right eye (blue) and the left eye (rust red) are superimposed. (**B and D**) Perimetry during convergence on a near target demonstrates post-fixational blindness with a gap between the two nasal hemifields (black wedge). There is sometimes difficulty fusing the two nasal fields such that they slide up and down in the vertical plane—the hemi-field slide phenomenon. Reproduced with permission from Weber and Landau (2013).

temporal visual *fields* of both eyes. This bears a fanciful similarity to a pie serving. Neurosurgeons are well aware of this important anatomy, which is highly relevant in temporal lobe resection. Such resection should not extend further back than 6 cm from the temporal pole to ensure there is no interference with vision. Thus, a pie

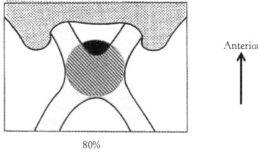

Anterior

80%

Prefixed

Postfixed

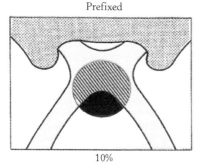
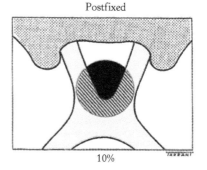

10%   10%

FIGURE 2.17: The anatomical variability of the chiasm in relation to the pituitary gland. Anterior is toward the top of the page. A pituitary tumor that expands upward where the chiasm is pre-fixed, as in 10% of healthy people, will allow pressure on the optic tract and classically an incongruous hemianopia. If the chiasm is post-fixed (10% healthy people), the pituitary tumor will press on the posterior region of the optic nerve and cause impaired vision due to a central scotoma in one eye and a junctional field defect in the other. See Figure 2.18. Reproduced with permission from *Clinical Ophthalmology*, J Kanski and B Bowling, Figure 19.45. Elsevier Saunders, 2011.

in the sky field defect tells you there is a lesion in the posterior temporal zone. Absence of this field defect suggests that a temporal lobe lesion is sited anteriorly. See Figure 2.19.

▶ Hypophysitis, meningeal infiltration; pancreatic, lacrimal, or parotid gland swelling suggests IgG-4 related disease.

Altitudinal Visual Field Loss

Patients often describe a curtain- or shutter-like effect that descends over their visual field lasting a few seconds, sometimes associated with a horizontal line in their visual field.

▶ Binocular altitudinal symptoms favor thromboembolism in the occipital cortex.
▶ Lower binocular altitudinal field loss suggests a lesion in the upper part of the optic radiation.
▶ Upper binocular altitudinal field loss points to a defect in the lower optic radiation or occipital cortex (Figure 2.20).

Rarely, such symptoms relate to inferior pressure on the chiasm or optic nerves from enlarged, tortuous internal carotid arteries or from bilateral symmetric infarction of the upper pole of each optic disk, as in anterior ischemic optic neuropathy. Monocular symptoms are characteristically thromboembolic and of carotid origin, and the defect is likely in the lower visual field.

Note:

▶ Advancing field defects move like the hands of a clock (Figure 2.21).
▶ *Equatorial field loss* characterizes a lesion of the lateral geniculate body (Figure 2.22). The fibers at this point are not completely arranged into their required positions in the optic radiation. A geniculate (especially anterior) defect is usually highly incongruous and typically lies around the equatorial zone.

Other Characteristic Field Defects

Other field defects are depicted in Figures 2.23 and 2.24.

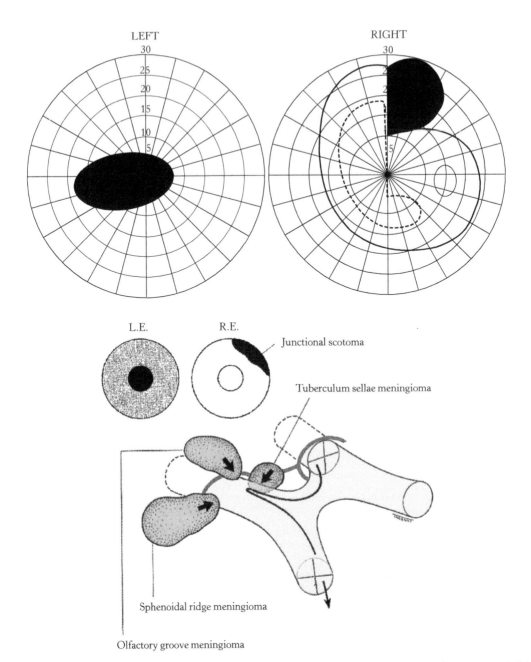

FIGURE 2.18: Top: Junctional scotoma field pattern due to a lesion in the posterior region of the left optic nerve. The left eye has a cecocentral field defect (i.e., involving the blind spot and central field) due to optic nerve pressure/ischemia, while the right eye displays an incomplete upper temporal defect from pressure/ischemia on Wilbrand's knee. **Bottom:** The various causes of junctional scotomas. The fibers of Wilbrand's knee are shown looping forward into the left optic nerve where it joins the chiasm. Top, reproduced with permission from RH Spector. The visual fields. Chapter 116. In *Clinical Methods: The History, Physical, and Laboratory Examinations,* 3rd ed. HK Walker, WD Hall, JW Hurst, eds. Boston: Butterworths; 1990. Bottom, reproduced with permission from *Clinical Ophthalmology,* J Kanski and B Bowling, Figure 19.55. Elsevier Saunders, 2011.

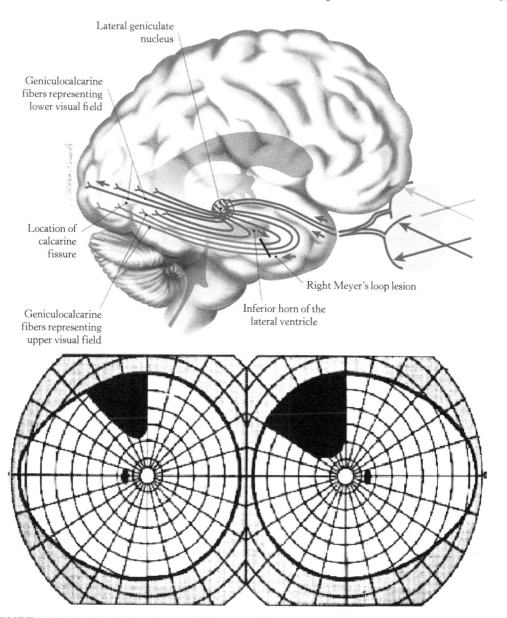

Lateral geniculate nucleus

Geniculocalcarine fibers representing lower visual field

Location of calcarine fissure

Geniculocalcarine fibers representing upper visual field

Right Meyer's loop lesion

Inferior horn of the lateral ventricle

FIGURE 2.19: **Top:** Meyer's loop shown in the lower-most fibers colored green. This is part of the optic radiation that sweeps forward initially into the posterior temporal lobe on its way to the main optic radiation in the parietal lobe. **Bottom:** The characteristic pie in the sky field defect. This is caused by a right posterior temporal lesion, which is the only part of this lobe that contains visual fibers. These fibers are responsible for vision in the contralateral upper field. Top image reproduced with permission from Linda Wilson-Pauwels, Cranial Nerves, PMPH-USA.

▶ A temporal field defect that crosses the vertical meridian must arise from the retina or optic nerve.

This Handle is useful if you consider that there might be an early bitemporal hemianopia, which always respects the vertical meridian. If the field loss crosses into the nasal field, then there must be a retinal or optic nerve defect because the fibers in the retina and optic nerve are not sorted out into their correct somatotopic position until they reach the chiasm. Figure 2.25 shows a tilted disk and its associated field defect.

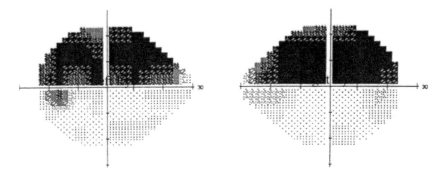

FIGURE 2.20: Automated perimetry using Humphrey field analyzer, showing bilateral superior altitudinal field defects likely due to a lesion in the lower optic radiation or occipital cortex.

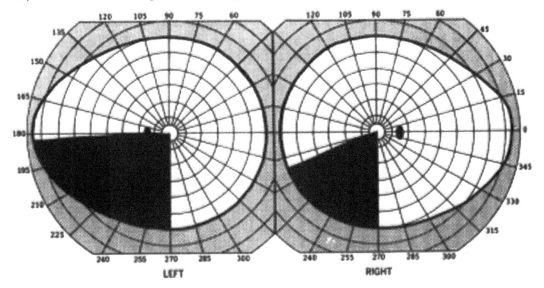

FIGURE 2.21: Left inferior quadrantanopia due to a defect in the right upper parietal optic radiation. The field loss is slightly incongruous, in keeping with parietal lesions. If the defect in the right eye progresses, it does so like the hands of a clock—moving from 8 o'clock to 9 o'clock in the right eye to complete the quadrant and obey the congruity rule.

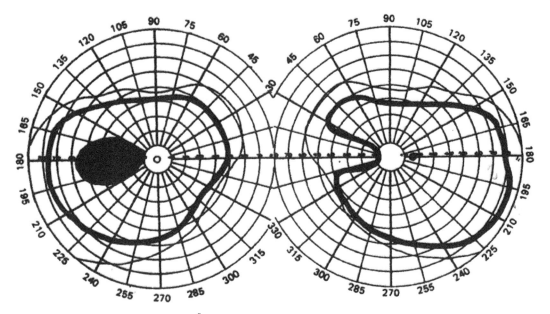

FIGURE 2.22: Wedge-shaped equatorial left hemianopia due to a geniculate field defect. Reproduced with permission from Luco et al. (1992).

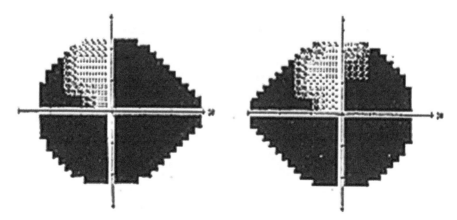

FIGURE 2.23: Bilateral homonymous hemianopia. There is a complete right homonymous hemianopia with an incomplete but congruous left homonymous hemianopia. This is typical of bilateral occipital infarction.

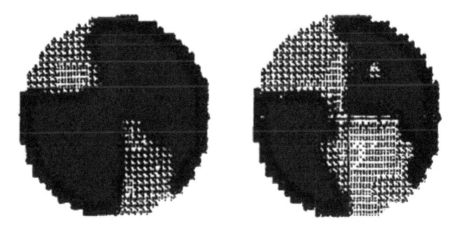

FIGURE 2.24: Checkerboard field defect produced by severe defects in the lower left and upper right fields with relative sparing of the upper left and lower right fields. The severe defects could be caused by two discrete lesions: one below the left calcarine fissure (affecting the upper right quadrant) and the other above the right calcarine fissure (affecting the lower left quadrant).

Transient Painless Monocular Visual Loss

This section will deal chiefly with the nonpainful varieties of transient monocular visual loss (TMVL) that are more likely to be of neurological origin. Please refer to Table 2.1. Remember these Handles are for *transient* loss of vision, not the permanent varieties.

▶ TMVL lasting under 1 minute is a feature of severe papilledema due to raised ICP.

The visual obscurations usually take place when standing up, especially from a stooped forward position, because perfusion of the optic disk, already compromised by venous congestion secondary to raised ICP, is aggravated further by stooping.

Comparable symptoms are found in retinal vein occlusion (Figure 2.26) or optic nerve meningioma.

If there is poor arterial perfusion of the eye due to giant cell arteritis (GCA) or postural hypotension, the obscurations are also provoked by standing up, particularly from a hot bath. The visual impairment typically affects both eyes in postural hypotension but just one eye in GCA. Thus, for TMVL lasting *less than* 1 minute:

▶ On standing after stooping suggests papilledema.
▶ On getting out of a hot bath is more likely cranial arteritis.

  Both conditions call for urgent action to prevent permanent visual loss.

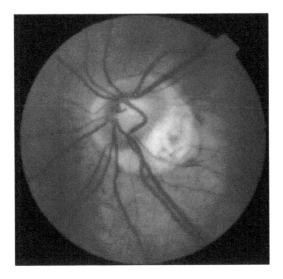

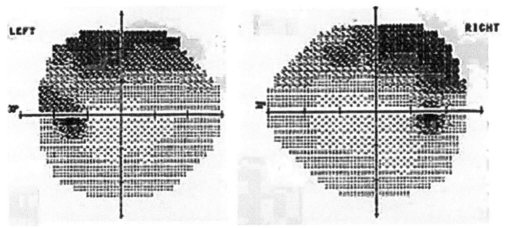

FIGURE 2.25: **Top:** Tilted left optic disk. The optic nerve should emerge from the globe at about 90 degrees tangential to its surface. Sometimes it leaves at a more oblique angle as shown here, where the optic nerve fibers are exiting more superiorly and to the left than normal. There is a semilunar yellow area at 4 o'clock next to the disk which is exposed sclera. **Bottom:** Visual fields in a patient with a tilted optic disk. Note the defect in the upper temporal regions that extends into the upper nasal zone. This is not typical of a chiasmal lesion, as they should respect the midline. Reproduced with permission from Williams et al. (2005).

Also:

▶ If the visual impairment is bilateral on rising from a hot bath and lasts under 1 minute, likely this is due to low systemic blood pressure.

▶ TMVL lasting more than 1 minute in a patient *over* 50 years of age favors a thrombo-embolic lesion (see Table 2.1). If your patient is under 50 years, then vasospasm is more likely.

Cholesterol Emboli (Hollenhorst Plaques)

Emboli, consisting of a loosely bound mixture of platelets and cholesterol, may dislodge from atheromatous plaques in the major neck arteries or branches of the thoracic aorta. If they lodge within a brain artery, they usually cause a transient ischemic attack (TIA). When they enter the ophthalmic artery, there is painless monocular blindness. The extent of field loss depends on which retinal vessel is occluded. If your patient reports monocular visual loss, you may be able to see the emboli with an ophthalmoscope

TABLE 2.1: CAUSES OF TRANSIENT VISUAL IMPAIRMENT

Lesion	Duration of visual impairment	Monocular or binocular	Triggers	Comment
Giant cell arteritis	<1 minute	Monocular	Change in posture, e.g., standing from a hot bath or use of vasodilators	Due to poor perfusion of optic disk
Venous congestion of optic disk	<1 minute	Either	Standing up, especially after stooping forward	Usually denotes papilledema from raised ICP. Possibly meningioma of optic nerve sheath or retinal vein occlusion
Low systemic blood pressure	<1 minute	Binocular	Change in posture, e.g., standing from a hot bath or use of vasodilators	Due to poor perfusion of the optic disk. If duration >1 minute then thromboembolism is more likely
Embolus in internal carotid artery territory	>1 minute	Monocular	Possibly vigorous exercise	Patient >50 years. Descending shutter illusion over a few seconds. Severe internal carotid artery stenosis may cause unilateral visual impairment on going outdoors
Embolus in vertebrobasilar artery territory	>1 minute	Binocular. can be hemianopic	Neck movement	Patient >50 years. Symptoms due to occipital lobe ischemia. Field defect may be altitudinal or complete bilateral loss (cortical blindness)
Retinal artery spasm	>1 minute	Monocular	Exercise	Patient <50 years. Usually no headache. May be multiple attacks per day

The first three rows refer to disorders lasting less than 1 minute. ICP, intracranial pressure.

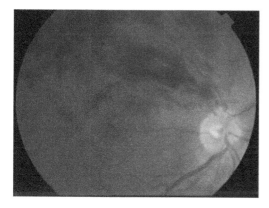 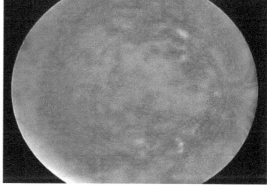

FIGURE 2.26: **Left:** Superior temporal branch retinal vein occlusion. **Right:** Central retinal vein thrombosis. This results in a "bloodstorm" appearance with profuse flame hemorrhages between the nerve fibers in all quadrants. Cotton-wool spots representing microinfarcts are often also present. Left image courtesy Dr. Irina Gout, Prince Charles Eye Unit, Windsor. Right image reproduced from *Oxford Textbook of Medicine* (5th ed.), DA Warrell, TM Cox, and JD Firth, eds., Figure 25.1.8 in the chapter The Eye in General Medicine, by P Frith. Oxford University Press.

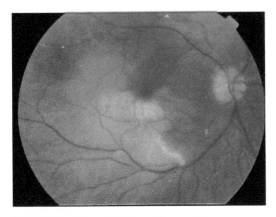

FIGURE 2.27: Hollenhorst plaques. These appear as bright yellow dots at the bifurcation of a retinal artery. There are at least six in this image. Figure courtesy Jose Biller, Chicago.

(Figure 2.27). The light-reflective cholesterol content causes the emboli to glint at arterial bifurcations. The time point at which the embolus dissolves coincides with return of vision.

In retinal artery vasospasm, the attack lasts typically 5–20 minutes, often associated with scintillations. Although there is usually no headache, some consider this to be a migraine variant ("retinal migraine"). Episodes are often multiple over the course of one day and may be triggered by exercise. Thus:

▶ TMVL lasting more than 1 minute in a patient *under* 50 years is likely due to retinal artery spasm.

Note that scalp tenderness is not confined to cranial arteritis; it is common in migraine and cervical spondylosis. The vascular sensitivity of arteritis and migraine may extend into the neck vessels—so-called *carotidynia*.

There is a related Handle associated with severe internal carotid stenosis, as follows:

▶ In the absence of cataract, temporary monocular glare or visual impairment when going from indoors out into bright sunlight favors severe carotid stenosis (see Chapter 9, Stroke, for other signs of severe carotid stenosis).
For this symptom, there has to be narrowing of the internal *and* external carotid arteries given the efficient anastomoses between these two divisions of the common carotid. This phenomenon is

thought to reflect the inability of a borderline retinal circulation to sustain increased retinal metabolic activity associated with exposure to bright light—sometimes known as "retinal bleaching." See Chapter 9 (Stroke) for further Handles that point to internal carotid artery insufficiency.

Apart from enquiry about headache, which is a fairly consistent symptom in GCA, a useful question is whether there are tender scalp nodules or jaw pain on chewing ("jaw claudication") and girdle pain (suggesting polymyalgia rheumatica). Hence:

▶ TMVL with tender scalp nodules, girdle pain, or jaw claudication indicates cranial arteritis.
▶ The superficial temporal artery and/or its branches may be tender, thickened, and pulseless, such that it can be rolled under the finger like a piece of cord.

Note that:

▶ Occlusion of the ophthalmic artery usually causes no field defect, provided the collateral supply from the external carotid territory is good (see Figure 2.28).
If there is vascular disease compromising the external carotid circulation from, for example, atheroma or arteritis, then occlusion of the ophthalmic artery will result in complete loss of vision.
▶ Occlusion of the central retinal artery (CRA) is usually embolic and causes complete monocular loss of vision (see Figure 2.29).

Funduscopy shows a cherry-red spot at the macula (Figure 2.29), which happens because you can see the normal vascular supply to the choroid that arises from the posterior ciliary arteries. There is usually no blood supply to the macula from the central retinal artery. An exception applies in 15–30% of individuals in whom the macula is fed by a cilioretinal artery. If this artery is present and the cause of CRA occlusion is nonarteritic, there will be severe peripheral field loss with a very small area of preserved central vision. In GCA, which often affects the ophthalmic artery and its branches—namely, the central retinal and posterior ciliary arteries (Figure 2.28)—the visual defect tends to be more severe and carries a worse prognosis than the nonarteritic variety (Hayreh and Zimmerman 2005).

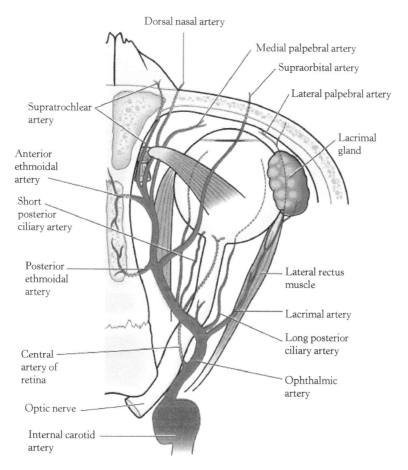

Dorsal nasal artery

Medial palpebral artery

Supraorbital artery

Lateral palpebral artery

Supratrochlear artery

Lacrimal gland

Anterior ethmoidal artery

Short posterior ciliary artery

Posterior ethmoidal artery

Lateral rectus muscle

Lacrimal artery

Long posterior ciliary artery

Central artery of retina

Ophthalmic artery

Optic nerve

Internal carotid artery

FIGURE 2.28: Vascular supply to the right optic nerve and retina. Reproduced with permission from *Training in Ophthalmology*, V Sundaram, A Barsam, A Alwitry, P Khaw, eds. Figure 10.4 in the chapter Orbit, by C Daniel, V Sundaram, and J Uddin. Oxford University Press. DOI:10.1093/med/9780199237593.003.0010.

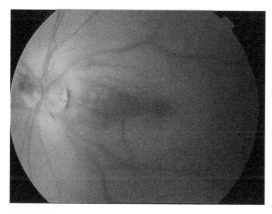

FIGURE 2.29: Cherry-red spot with pale retina secondary to central retinal artery occlusion. Courtesy Dr. Irina Gout, Prince Charles Eye Unit, Windsor.

▶ Cherry red spot is also found in lipid storage diseases, pantothenate kinase–associated neurodegeneration (PKAN) (Chapter 8), metachromatic leukodystrophy, and as the toxic effect of quinine, dapsone, carbon monoxide, or methanol.

▶ Anterior ischemic optic neuropathy (AION) is never embolic (Figure 2.30).

It is thought more likely that hypotension, especially during sleep in association with overtreated systemic hypertension, causes decreased perfusion in the anterior ciliary arteries and produces permanent, primarily central blindness. Many cases are associated with the use of amiodarone and sildenafil.

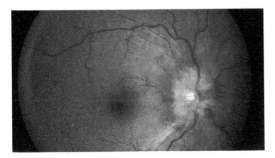

FIGURE 2.30: Anterior ischemic optic neuropathy. The ciliary vessels are not seen. The disk is swollen and will become pale.

Also note:

◀ If the optic disk is not swollen early on, then the diagnosis of AION is wrong

Retinitis Pigmentosa

Here are some useful combinations of retinitis pigmentosa (RP) (Figure 2.2) with other disorders.

▶ Anosmia suggests Refsum's disease.
▶ Cerebellar signs favor SCA7 (spinocerebellar atrophy type 7), AVED (ataxia with vitamin E deficiency), and Kearns-Sayre syndrome.
▶ Dystonia points to HARP (hypoprebetalipoproteinemia, acanthocytosis, retinitis pigmentosa, and pallidal degeneration), NARP (neuropathy, ataxia, and retinitis pigmentosa), and PKAN (pantothenate kinase–associated neurodegeneration).
▶ Deafness: Usher's syndrome.

Pupil and Iris

▶ A unilateral dilated pupil with normal accommodation that constricts after prolonged exposure to light and redilates slowly is a tonic pupil (Figure 2.31). If the tendon reflexes are depressed, this is the Holmes-Adie syndrome.

Also note:

▶ An acute-onset tonic pupil in someone over 50 years of age may be a sign of GCA.

The likely cause of tonic pupil is loss of neurons that control pupillary constriction in the ciliary ganglion resulting in denervation hypersensitivity. A tonic pupil is an acceptable diagnosis if pupillary constriction to light is fairly brisk, but the pupil must *redilate* very slowly. Also:

· The pupil often has irregular margins or may be oval.
· Many suffer from migraine as well.
· After several years the opposite eye may be affected similarly and cause confusion with the Argyll-Robertson pupil (Figure 2.32).
▶ Insertion of weak (2.5%) methacholine drops (cholinergic) will cause pupillary constriction on the abnormal side but have no effect on the healthy side.
▶ Tonic pupil with areflexia and segmental anhidrosis is the *Ross syndrome.*
   There is loss of facial flushing (after exertion for example) on the side of the tonic pupil. Chronic cough is an occasional symptom. (Figure 2.33, *left*).
▶ Loss of facial flushing after exertion usually accompanied by ipsilateral Horner syndrome is the *Harlequin syndrome* Figure 2.33, *right*)
▶ Check the driver license photo!

It is not unusual for the neurologist to evaluate a patient in the emergency department who swears the dilated pupil occurred a few days ago, when in fact it had always been dilated, as shown by earlier photographs.

Eventually, accommodation is abolished as well, and the pupil becomes small and fixed to light. When both pupils are small, as in the later stages, confusion might arise with an Argyll-Robertson pupil. The latter is rarely present in isolation, and serological tests will put aside any lingering doubt.

▶ A dilated pupil fixed to all stimuli in an otherwise healthy person usually means self-administration of mydriatic.

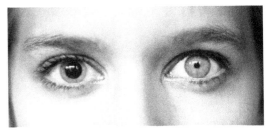

FIGURE 2.31: Tonic pupil. The right pupil is large, reacts sluggishly to light but constricts with accommodation, and dilates slowly in the dark.

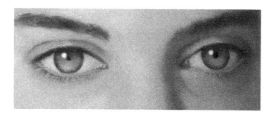

FIGURE 2.32: Argyll Robertson pupils. Note both pupils are small with irregular margins and the iris is pale, possibly atrophic particularly in the right iris. Reproduced from card-25976913-front.jpg under Creative Commons Attribution License.

Such patients are often medically qualified and use eye drops such as atropine, cyclopentolate, or tropicamide, to which they could have easy access. They may need psychiatric help, but before such referral, a brain scan would be wise, just in case you are dealing with a partial cranial nerve (CN) III lesion.

▶ A unilateral fixed dilated pupil may happen by accident if the patient has been in contact with common garden plants.

One example is *Brugmansia* sp. (Angel's trumpet) that contains antimuscarinics (cholinergic). This will differ from the tonic pupil because accommodation is impaired as well.

Relative Afferent Pupillary Defect and the Swinging Flashlight Test

An *afferent* defect is one that involves the ingoing light signals in CN II, as opposed to an *efferent* defect, which is a feature of a CN III lesion. When the light is swung from one eye to the other, the normal pupil should contract rapidly enough for both pupils to remain much the same size.

▶ The relative afferent pupillary defect (RAPD) sign is positive when you observe paradoxical dilatation to light shone in that pupil.

Usually, there is little or no constriction to direct stimulation of the affected eye, but there is constriction when the healthy opposite side is stimulated. Classically, an RAPD indicates a disorder of the optic nerve from any cause, including demyelination and optic nerve injury. In such trauma the pupil will contract consensually when the normal side is stimulated but then dilates passively when the light is switched back to the abnormal side.

▶ An afferent pupillary light defect is found on rare occasions in the eye contralateral to a lesion of the optic tract.

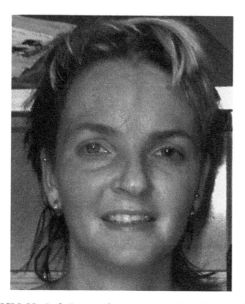
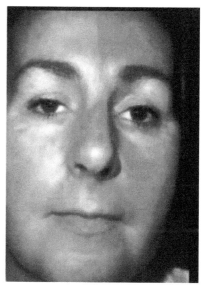

FIGURE 2.33: **Left**: Ross syndrome: tonic pupil on the patient's left side with ipsilateral absence of facial flushing following exercise. **Right**: Harlequin syndrome. There is a right Horner's syndrome with absent facial flushing on that side. Left image reproduced with permission from Dr. G Hagemann, Berlin. Right image reproduced with permission from PD Drummond and JW Lance (1987).

This happens because more than 50% of optic nerve fibers cross at the chiasm. In theory, this can help distinguish a hemianopic defect due to a tract lesion from a cortical hemianopia. As mentioned earlier, the field defect in a tract lesion is usually incongruous.

◀ There may be no RAPD if optic nerve involvement is bilateral.

Bilaterally Small Pupils

▶ Bilaterally small pupils reactive to accommodation but not to light.
This is light-near dissociation (LND) and usually indicates Argyll Robertson pupils (ARP; Figure 2.32). A useful mnemonic is
  o ARP, **A**ccommodation **R**eflex **P**resent. Reverse it:
  o PRA, **P**upillary **R**eflex **A**bsent.
In ARP, the pupil size is usually small. Rarely it may be normal or even large. Their margins are irregular and the iris is pale and atrophic.

▶ If the pupils are *large* and show LND, this favors:

· Tonic pupils
· Juvenile tabes dorsalis
· Dorsal midbrain problem, such as Parinaud's syndrome

In tabes dorsalis there is often primary optic atrophy. Ptosis is absent in a tonic pupil, but ptosis may be present in the other varieties. Bilaterally small pupils with retained accommodation reflexes occur in a long-standing tonic pupil and may be difficult to tell apart from ARP. Thus:

▶ LND with small pupils is likely Argyll Robertson pupils or long-standing tonic pupils.

Other causes of bilaterally small "pinpoint" pupils are as follows:
Acute:

▶ With tearing, salivation, runny nose, and sweating suggests mushroom poisoning or exposure to organophosphates. In both instances there are increased (muscarinic) cholinergic effects.
▶ Opiate exposure

▶ Brainstem stroke—classically pontine hemorrhage

Chronic:

▶ With bilateral ptosis and anhidrosis, suggests Horner's syndrome on both sides. This is rare and found in
  o Diabetic autonomic neuropathy
  o Amyloidosis
  o Pure autonomic failure
  o Multiple system atrophy
▶ With proximal myopathy, suggests Stormorken syndrome (see Chapter 7, Myopathy).
Miosis is congenital and severe; see discussion of myopathy in Chapter 7.
▶ Aging.
Many elderly people have small pupils, probably because of minor ocular inflammatory disorders.
▶ Poor visual acuity in one eye with normal pupillary light reflexes suggests Leber's optic neuropathy.
As long as you are happy that there is no functional (psychogenic) visual loss, this combination is characteristic of Leber's disease. It may occur because the melanopsin-expressing retinal ganglion cells are relatively preserved. This Handle is particularly useful if you are dealing with optic neuritis, where the light reflex is usually abnormal. This paradoxical preservation of pupillary light reflex should alert the clinician to Leber's disease.

Tadpole Pupil
This suggests migraine, tonic pupil, Horner's syndrome, or a midbrain lesion. This is a rare abnormality of pupil shape (see Figure 2.34, *left*) and usually asymptomatic. The pupil is tadpole-shaped but everything else is usually normal—reaction to light, accommodation, and imaging. It is probably due to focal spasm of the iris dilator muscle. In migraine it occurs either during or between attacks. The midbrain variety is sometimes called "midbrain corectopia" and usually caused by acute hemorrhage in the dorsal midbrain (Figure 2.34, *right*).

Horner's Syndrome
Please refer to Chapter 1 for photographs and basic details of this condition. Remember the mnemonic for

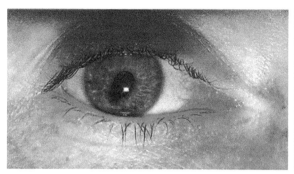 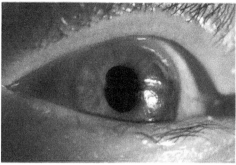

FIGURE 2.34: **Left**: Tadpole pupil affecting right eye. A benign, usually transient phenomenon. **Right**: Oval pupil after an acute left midbrain hemorrhage. Left image reproduced from Koay et al. (2004). Right image reproduced with permission from Mittal et al. (2013).

Horner's syndrome: **M**iosis, **P**tosis, and **A**nhidrosis. Occasionally, there appears to be enophthalmos, which is detected by looking at the intersection of the lower lid with the iris. Thus, on the affected side, the lower lid covers more of the iris than the normal side. The apparent enophthalmos is probably due to relaxation of Muller's muscle, which is sympathetically innervated and supplies the lower lid—so-called *upside-down ptosis*—and (as confirmed by exophthalmometer measurement) the eye does not really withdraw into the orbit. Please refer to Figure 2.35 for basic anatomy of the sympathetic supply to the eye.

Here are some guides to localization of an ipsilateral Horner's syndrome when associated with a disorder of the following:

▶ Pituitary, hypothalamus, or brainstem is a lesion of the first-order neuron.
▶ Cervical spinal cord or brachial plexus is a lesion of the second-order neuron.
▶ Carotid artery (common or internal) or CN VI is a lesion of the third-order neuron (postganglionic). Note that in this variety there may be distension of the conjunctival capillaries and lack of sweating.

An ipsilateral Horner's syndrome:

▶ With weak wasted hand, depressed triceps jerk (C7 and C8) with sensory loss in a C8 distribution is a second-order lesion in keeping with a compressive brachial plexus disorder.
This includes *Pancoast tumor* or *cervical rib*, both of which affect the lower trunk of the brachial plexus (C8 and T1).

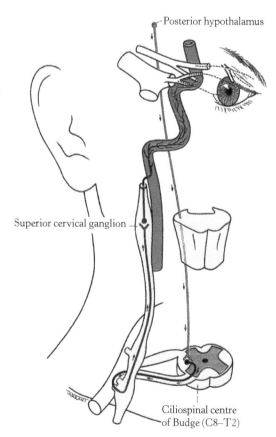

FIGURE 2.35: Pathway involved in Horner's syndrome. The first-order neuron is from the hypothalamus to spinal cord relay. Second-order neuron is from spinal cord relay to the superior cervical ganglion. Third-order neuron is from the superior cervical ganglion along the carotid sheath to the eye. Reproduced with permission from *Clinical Ophthalmology*, J Kanski and B Bowling, Figure 19.35. Elsevier Saunders, 2011.

The proximity of the sympathetic nerve fibers to the common or internal carotid artery (third-order) makes it vulnerable to carotid dissection, aneurysm, or arteritis. Thus:

▶ Horner's syndrome with neck pain is usually caused by internal carotid artery dissection or Eagle syndrome (see Chapter 9, Stroke). There is often a contralateral hemiparesis and ipsilateral hypoglossal palsy.
▶ Horner syndrome with eye pain and CN VI palsy is likely due to pressure from an intracavernous aneurysm. Other causes within the cavernous sinus include inflammatory disorders, such as *Tolosa Hunt syndrome* and pituitary tumors.

Also note:

▶ In brachial plexus avulsion injury with a flail arm, the presence of Horner's syndrome suggests that the avulsion is proximal to the plexus; that is, in the nerve roots or dorsal root ganglion.
    Lesions here recover poorly in comparison to those that are distal to the dorsal root ganglion, where continuity with the spinal cord is preserved.

Reversed Horner's Syndrome
An example of reversed Horner's syndrome (*Pourfour du petit syndrome*) is shown in Figure 2.36.

▶ Blue eyes that both become brown is likely Wilson's disease.

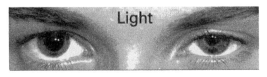

FIGURE 2.36: Reversed Horner syndrome affecting patient's right eye. It is sometimes known as "Pourfour du Petit" syndrome after the French neurologist who described it and characterized by upper lid retraction, pupillary dilation, and increased sweating. It might be confused with thyrotoxicosis, but the pupillary changes would be unusual. It is probably due to irritation of the cervical sympathetic, here because of parotid surgery. Figure reproduced with permission from Mattes et al. (2009).

Newborn babies have blue eyes that may become brown later (depending on the parental eye color), but apart from this physiological change (and use of colored contact lenses!), there are very few neurological causes of this other than Wilson's disease. In this disorder, there is progressive deposition of copper in Descemet's membrane where the peripheral cornea joins the sclera (Figure 2.37). This produces a golden-brown ring, the *Kayser-Fleischer ring*. This starts in the upper part of the iris at 12 o'clock (where it is concealed from cursory inspection), then at 6 o'clock, and finally forms a complete ring. The platelet count is often low in Wilson's disease, and there may be secondary amenorrhea, as detailed in the movement disorders section (Chapter 8).

Glaucoma patients with blue eyes who use *prostaglandin analog eye drops* such as latanoprost, travoprost, or bimatoprost may notice darkening of iris color, as this medication is usually applied to both eyes. The eyelashes become longer and thicker—a cosmetically appealing side effect.

One other condition is associated with long thick eyelashes: the *Oliver McFarlane syndrome* (see Table 12.2). Thus:

▶ Long, thick eyelashes suggest use of prostaglandin eye drops or the Oliver McFarlane syndrome
▶ One brown eye and one blue eye since birth (heterochromia or anisochromia) suggests:
    ○ Congenital Horner's syndrome with loss of iris pigment, making it pale
    ○ Sturge-Weber syndrome
    ○ Waardenburg syndrome
    ○ Parry-Romberg syndrome

Anisochromia may be an isolated phenomenon (Figure 1.34 and Figure 2.38). Note that it may be acquired from local eye trauma secondary to hyphema, melanocytic infiltration from iris nevus/melanoma, or Fuchs heterochromic iridocyclitis.

Funduscopy
Kestenbaum's Sign in Borderline Primary Optic Atrophy
Primary optic atrophy refers to a pale optic disk with clear margins. There are several *neurological* causes for this: demyelination; ischemia; optic nerve trauma;

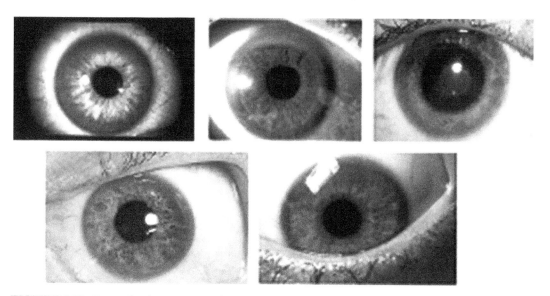

FIGURE 2.37: Kayser-Fleischer rings. **Top left**: A 17-year-old woman with secondary amenorrhea, psychiatric problems, cervical dystonia, and thrombocytopenia. She was lucky to be blue-eyed, as this made it easier to see the brown discoloration in the corneal limbus (in Descemet's membrane). **Top center**: The Kayser-Fleischer ring in a brown-eyed person. Note that the ring appears gray, but it is usually difficult to see without a slit lamp. **Top right**: The characteristic sunflower cataract. **Bottom left**: A 32-year-old man who complained of long-standing slurred speech and tremor. **Bottom right**: A 25- year-old blue-eyed woman with arm tremor, thought to have MS. The tremor was in fact a rest tremor, not intention type, and she had mild parkinsonism secondary to Wilson's disease. Top center and top right images reproduced with permission from Walshe (2011). Bottom left image reproduced from Wikipedia, courtesy HL Fred, MD, and HA van Dijk, under Creative Commons Attribution License.

congenital and inherited disorders; tabes dorsalis; and toxins such as alcohol, methylated spirit, and quinine.

It is sometimes difficult to decide whether a disk is "pale," but there is a useful sign for these borderline cases—*Kestenbaum's sign* (Figure 2.39).

If you ignore the larger arteries or veins and their branches that cross the disk margin, there should be at least 10 small blood vessels crossing its edge. If there are five or fewer, then it is likely the disk is ischemic or atrophic, and Kestenbaum's sign is positive. Not only might this help diagnostically, but

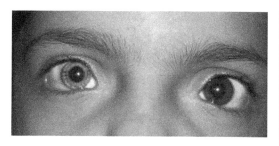

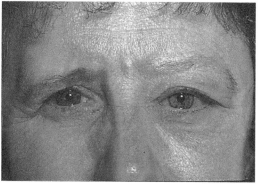

FIGURE 2.38: Congenital anisochromia. **Left**: In a young child. **Right**: An elderly woman with the same condition. Left image from Wikimedia under GNU Free Documentation License.

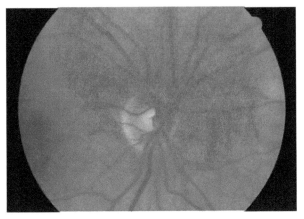
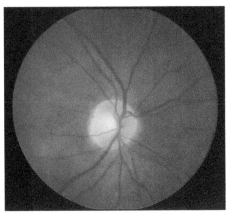

FIGURE 2.39: **Left**: Normal optic disk. **Right**: Kestenbaum's sign in borderline optic atrophy. You might pass this optic disk as normal. However, if you count the number of small blood vessels traversing the disk margin, there are only 2–3 which are not obviously arteries or veins (or branches thereof), which is well below the normal number of at least 10. In fact, the hook-shaped vessel at 10 o'clock is the cilioretinal artery, so there are just two small capillaries. If you look carefully, the pink hue is present only on the nasal disk sector (to the right in this picture), so you might diagnose optic atrophy on the basis of slight temporal pallor alone, but will you remember this say, 3 months later? Kestenbaum's sign gives you an objective measure that could be useful for monitoring purposes (Hawkes & Neffendorf 2014).

it can assist with serial monitoring (Hawkes and Neffendorf 2014).

▶ Optic atrophy in one eye and papilledema in the other is the *Foster Kennedy* syndrome (one person).

Classically, it indicates a frontal tumor pressing on one optic nerve (producing pallor) while raising ICP, causing papilledema in the other and occasionally anosmia in the side of optic atrophy. In reality, it happens more frequently because of anterior ischemic optic neuropathy which is long-standing in one eye (causing optic atrophy) and subacute in the other—where the optic disk is swollen because of ischemia—the *pseudo Foster Kennedy syndrome* (Figure 2.40).

Causes of Unilateral Central Visual Loss That May Simulate Demyelinating Optic Neuritis

▶ Neuroretinitis.

This is an inflammatory process involving the optic discs of typically one but occasionally both eyes, with exudative changes in Henle's

fiber layer producing a partial or complete macular star (Figure 2.41). It is usually painless. The main causes are as follows:

o Cat scratch disease (*Bartonella*)
o Syphilis, Lyme disease
o Sarcoid

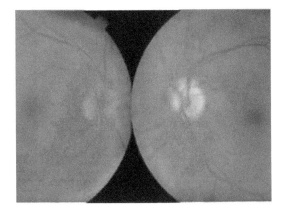

FIGURE 2.40: The pseudo Foster Kennedy syndrome. This shows optic atrophy in the right eye and papilledema on the left eye. This results from previous ischemia or demyelination in one eye (here the one on the right), followed by recent ischemia or demyelination in the other eye—here on the left. Reproduced with permission from www.neuroophthalmology.ca.

Neuroretinitis

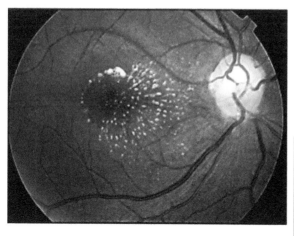
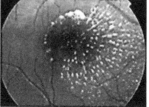

FIGURE 2.41: Neuroretinitis. This is an inflammatory process involving the optic discs and retina. The optic nerve is swollen, particularly on the temporal side. Exudates from leaking capillaries extend into the outer plexiform layer (Henle's layer) which spreads further to the macula in a star-like pattern. The same appearance occurs in hypertensive encephalopathy. Courtesy Dr. Irina Gout, Prince Charles Eye Unit, Windsor.

▶ Neuromyelitis optica (Devic's disease). Pupillary light reflexes are impaired and there is a RAPD.

▶ Leber's optic atrophy (Figure 2.42). The pupillary light reflexes may be preserved, as explained earlier.

▶ White dot syndromes. There are several varieties mostly affecting young females. Most are painless, cause varying degrees of impaired visual acuity and may be associated with flashing lights. The retinal appearances are distinctive (Figure 2.43).

▶ Ischemic optic neuropathy.

▶ Central serous retinopathy. Patients complain of a central gray patch and distortion of straight lines (*metamorphopsia*; see Figures 2.6 and 2.7). It is caused by accumulation of fluid beneath the macula.

▶ Vogt-Koyanagi-Harada syndrome.

This is really an autoimmune uveitis. A major diagnostic Handle is *poliosis* (i.e., patchy depigmentation in the hair, eyebrows, or eyelashes; see Figure 1.14).

▶ *Smartphone blindness.*
A patient complains of transient unilateral blurring of vision after using their smartphone at night. This happens if the subject lies in bed in darkness say, on their left side, viewing the phone only with their right eye, with their left eye occluded by the pillow.

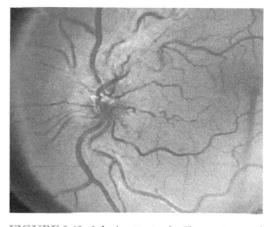

FIGURE 2.42: Leber's optic atrophy. There are increased numbers of tortuous blood vessels near the disk and peripapillary telangiectases. Later the optic disk becomes pale.

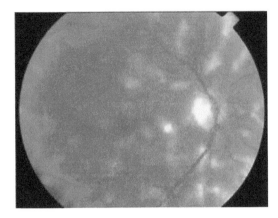

FIGURE 2.43: Birdshot chorioretinopathy. There are multiple pale-yellow ovoid spots affecting the macula and mid-peripheral retina. Courtesy Dr. Irina Gout, Prince Charles Eye Unit, Windsor.

The left eye will be dark adapted. When the phone is switched off, the subject finds that vision in the room is blurred in the right eye (which is not dark-adapted) but vision is normal in the dark with the left eye, which has been dark adapted. The blurring lasts for no more than a few minutes but remarkably has resulted in multiple concerns about visual health.

Consecutive (Sequential) Optic Neuropathy

This means loss of vision in one eye followed by similar loss in the other—after a variable time interval, but typically weeks. There are four main etiologies:

- Leber's optic neuropathy
- Neuromyelitis optica (Devic's disease)
- Ischemic optic neuropathy
- Neuroretinitis (Figure 2.41)

Papilledema

Papilledema means swelling of the optic disk caused by raised ICP and should not be used to describe optic disc swelling due to infectious, infiltrative, or inflammatory lesions of the optic nerve. The term *papillitis* is appropriate when there is evidence of inflammation, infiltration, or hemorrhage of the disk. The optic discs in far-sighted (long-sighted) patients may appear swollen (pseudo-papilledema) due to their small size and the crowded appearance of the blood vessels.

Here are some tips to help exclude papilledema from other conditions:

▶ Look at the nasal disk margin (Figure 2.44). In a normal disk, there should be a clear demarcation between the disk margin and the retina.
▶ Look at the veins over the optic disk. In papilledema, they are distended and there is no spontaneous pulsation. The optic disc cup will be filled with edema fluid.

Hence:

▶ Pulsating retinal veins virtually excludes raised ICP.
▶ Visual acuity is preserved unless the disk swelling is severe.

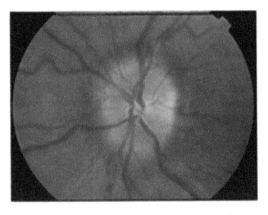
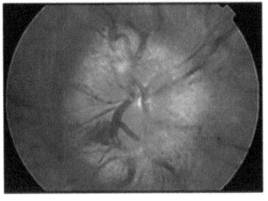

FIGURE 2.44: **Left**: Mild papilledema. Note the blurring of the disk margins, filling of the optic cup, and hyperemia on the nasal side of the disk (to the right of the picture). The veins are not distended but they did not pulsate in keeping with raised intracranial pressure. **Right**: Advanced (vintage/champagne cork) papilledema. The veins are distended and there is hemorrhage on the disk. Courtesy Dr. Irina Gout, Prince Charles Eye Unit, Windsor.

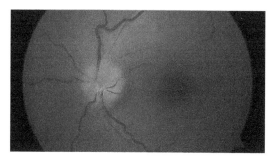

FIGURE 2.45: Acute optic neuritis. Note the blurred margins of the optic disk and filling of the optic disk cup. Photo courtesy Dr. Harinder Singh.

This leads to our next Handle:

▶ Disk swelling with normal visual acuity usually indicates papilledema (Figure 2.44) from raised ICP, whereas a swollen disk *with* impaired visual acuity suggests an inflammatory process such as *acute optic neuritis* (Figure 2.45) or *central retinal vein thrombosis* (Figure 2.26).
   When papilledema is long-standing or particularly severe, visual acuity will be impaired and the blind spot is enlarged.

The Swollen Optic Disk

The optic disk may be swollen from raised ICP, retinal vein thrombosis (partial or central), or inflammation such as optic neuritis. To distinguish these three causes of disk swelling, pay attention to the presence of hemorrhages as follows:

▶ Hemorrhages on the disc and in the retina are likely a result of retinal vein occlusion (Figure 2.26). Raised ICP is improbable and inflammation least likely.

▶ Hemorrhages on the disc alone suggest decompensated papilledema. Inflammation would be rare, and retinal vein occlusion rarer still.

▶ No hemorrhages anywhere favors inflammation (Figure 2.45) or compensated papilledema. Partial retinal vein occlusion would be a remote possibly.

Pseudopapilledema

This may result from

• Disk crowding, as in healthy far-sighted (long-sighted, hypermetropic) people (see earlier discussion)
• Drusen of the optic disk (Figure 2.46)

The patient with drusen is healthy and the disk changes are usually noticed at a routine eye checkup, particularly on autofluorescence and B-scan ultrasonography. Field defects may occur if the drusen are large.

▶ **Papilledema with Recent-Onset Low Back Pain Suggests Three Possibilities:**

• *Tumor of the cauda equina, such as ependymoma.*
   This tumor is often associated with a high cerebrospinal fluid (CSF) protein that causes papilledema through obstruction of CSF flow. Back pain and signs in the lower limbs are from the tumor itself.

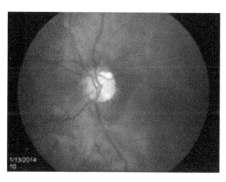 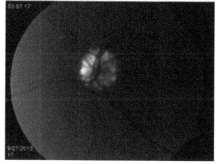

FIGURE 2.46: Pseudopapilledema due to optic disk drusen. **Left:** The disk margins are blurred, thus resembling true papilledema, but close inspection shows that the disk edges are lumpy due to drusen of the optic disk. **Right:** Fundus autofluorescence reveals hyperfluorescence of individual drusen around the disk margin. Photo courtesy Dr. Harinder Singh.

- *Idiopathic intracranial hypertension.*
  This may be due to lumbago if the patient is obese, or to increased pressure in the lumbar thecal sac.
- *Guillain-Barré syndrome.*
  Cervical or lumbar pain is common, and rarely there may be papilledema, again due to a high CSF protein level.

Other Related Conditions

▶ Back pain with recurrent uveitis suggests *Behçet disease.*
  The back pain results from sacroiliitis.

▶ Papilledema and headache in an overweight, otherwise healthy young adult woman (see Figure 1.2) is usually due to idiopathic intracranial hypertension (IIH, *pseudotumor cerebri*).
  The raised intracranial pressure often causes pulsatile tinnitus—a useful corroborative sign of raised pressure especially when the optic disks are equivocal. The MRI brain scan may reveal the following:
  - Empty sella
  - Enlarged, tortuous optic nerves due to distension of the subarachnoid space surrounding this nerve (see Figure 5.8)
  - Flattening of the globe where the optic nerve is attached

▶ Papilledema in an overweight man who snores suggests *obstructive sleep apnea.*

During hypoxic sleep, there is generalized venous congestion that results in raised ICP and papilledema. Patients with chronic bronchitis ("blue bloaters") may present in this way.

▶ Papilledema after radical neck dissection.
  This may occur after bilateral surgical ligation of the internal jugular veins or occasionally following ligation of just the dominant (typically right) internal jugular vein. The papilledema is usually bilateral (Shah et al. 2007) and results from raised ICP secondary to intracranial venous hypertension.

Miscellaneous Characteristic Fundal Appearances

Miscellaneous characteristic fundal appearances are shown in Figures 2.47 through 2.52.

OCULOMOTOR, TROCHLEAR, AND ABDUCENS NERVES (CN III, IV, AND VI)

▶ *Hirschberg's sign.* This will tell you if there is weakness of extraocular muscles. Look at the reflection on the cornea from a pen torch. It should be symmetrical. If there is weakness of an extrinsic eye muscle, the light reflection will be asymmetric (Figure 2.53).

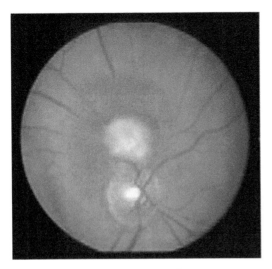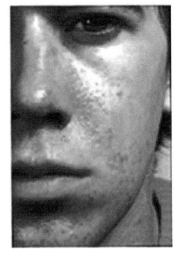

FIGURE 2.47: **Left:** Typical retinal phakoma (also known as retinal astrocytoma or mulberry lesion) from a patient with tuberous sclerosis. **Right:** Facial tubers along the nasolabial groove. This patient presented because of seizures, which are near universal in tuberous sclerosis.

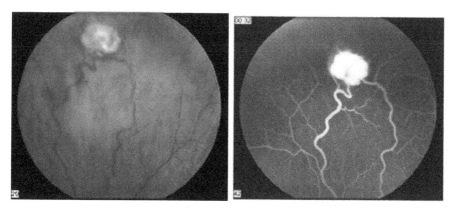

FIGURE 2.48: **Left**: Retinal angioma in Von Hippel-Lindau disease. This shows the feeding vessel to a very peripheral angioma at 12 o'clock. **Right**: The fluorescein angiogram demonstrates this more clearly. **Note**: Unless the pupil is dilated, neurologists will just see the tortuous vessels near the disk, because the angioma is peripheral, and to visualize it needs indirect ophthalmoscopy with a dilated pupil. Reproduced with permission from Figures 46.20 and 46.21 in the chapter The Phakomatoses, by MM Ariss et al. Oxford University Press.

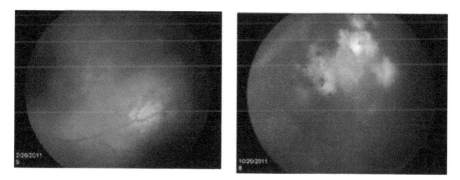

FIGURE 2.49: Toxoplasmosis. **Left**: Acute. There is a moderate exudate consisting of hypopigmented and hyperpigmented areas with ill-defined borders. **Right**: Chronic. There is an old pigmented scar, with clumps of pigment and pale areas typical of chronic toxoplasmosis. The organism encysts within the retina and may reactivate sporadically in this way. Photos courtesy Dr. Harinder Singh.

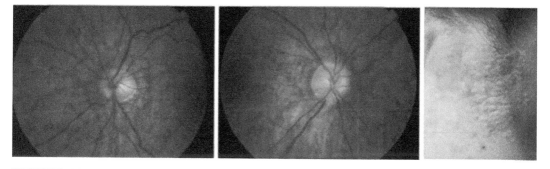

FIGURE 2.50: **Left and center**: Pseudoxanthoma elasticum (PXE). Fundus photograph from a patient with yellow-colored angioid streaks radiating from the optic disk. See also Insert Figure 1.27. Other causes of angioid streaks are sickle cell anemia, lead poisoning, Ehlers-Danlos syndrome, and thrombotic thrombocytopenic purpura. **Right**: The leather-wrinkled skin of the neck in PXE. Left and center images courtesy Dr. Irina Gout, Prince Charles Eye Unit, Windsor. Right image reproduced from Wikipedia under the Commons License Attribution Agreement.

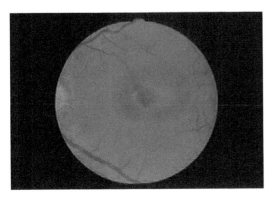

FIGURE 2.51: Bull's eye maculopathy. Macular damage is due to chloroquine or hydroxychloroquine and results in a concentric target-like pigmentary appearance. Reproduced with permission from *Oxford Textbook of Medicine* (5th ed.), DA Warrell, TM Cox, and JD Firth, eds., Chapter 25, The Eye in General Medicine, by P Frith.

Monocular Diplopia

▶ If local ocular causes are excluded, then monocular diplopia is usually psychogenic.

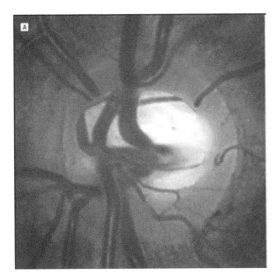

FIGURE 2.52: Bow-tie cupping (band atrophy) of the optic disk. This phenomenon results from retrograde degeneration of nasal retinal nerve fibers at the level of the chiasm or optic tract. At the optic disk, the temporal retinal fibers are predominantly located superiorly and inferiorly, whereas the nasal fibers occupy most of the nasal and temporal disk margins. Thus, retrograde degeneration of nasal fibers located either within the optic tract or where they cross in the center of the chiasm can be diagnosed by the selective pattern of optic disk atrophy producing a bow-tie or band-like effect of pallor or cupping, as seen here. Figure reproduced with permission from Hildebrand GD, et al. (2010).

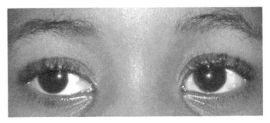

FIGURE 2.53: Hirschberg's sign. Note the reflected light is in the center of the left pupil but it is at 2 o'clock on the edge of the right pupil. This suggests outward deviation (esotropia) of the right eye which could be overlooked in a rushed examination. See also Figure 2.57 and 2.61).

▶ If you find variable and confusing responses to the cover tests, think of *myasthenia gravis* or *malingering*.
The main local ocular causes are retinal detachment, severe unilateral refractive error, cataract, corneal scar, and vitreous opacity. Remember that the correct way to analyze diplopia is to determine the direction of gaze that causes maximal separation of objects and then establish which is the more peripheral of the two by covering one eye at a time ("cover test"). Before this, it is important to occlude one eye at a time to determine whether the double vision is present in just one eye alone. If this is done first—and so many forget—then there is no need for the "cover" tests.

Variable and confusing responses to the cover tests suggest myasthenia gravis or malingering. The extraocular muscles fatigue and may confuse both you and your patient.

▶ *Oculomotor nerve palsy with contralateral hemiplegia* usually indicates a thrombotic lesion in the proximal portion of the posterior cerebral artery.

This is known as *Weber's syndrome* (see Chapter 9). Remember that the cerebral peduncle and dorsal midbrain are supplied by the posterior cerebral artery. Some have a homonymous hemianopia because the posterior cerebral artery supplies the optic radiation. So, here is a further Handle:

▶ Oculomotor palsy with contralateral hemiplegia and homonymous hemianopia suggests a proximal posterior cerebral artery lesion on the side of the CN III palsy.

Internuclear Ophthalmoplegia

See Video 2.1, Internuclear Ophthalmoplegia and Figure 9.17. Characteristically, in internuclear ophthalmoplegia (INO) there is slow inward movement of the medial rectus on conjugate lateral gaze, accompanied by jerky nystagmus mainly in the opposite lateral rectus muscle ("ataxic" nystagmus). Note:

▶ INO is detected more readily by saccadic eye movement rather than pursuit.

▶ Most have nystagmus on upgaze as well as horizontally.

This powerful sign localizes to the medial longitudinal fasciculus (MLF)—the dorsally situated pathway that traverses pons and midbrain. It is called "internuclear" because the lesion lies between the CN VI and CN III nuclei in the pons and midbrain, respectively.

The pontine center for bladder control (Barrington's nucleus) is fairly close to the MLF, thus:

▶ A pontine INO may be associated with bladder dysfunction.

Convergence is controlled by outgoing signals from the medial rectus nuclei within the oculomotor nerve complex. Hence, as a general rule:

▶ If convergence is normal, the lesion is in the pontine MLF.

▶ If convergence is impaired, the lesion is in the midbrain MLF.

If the INO is bilateral and there is a persistent divergent squint, it is called the *WEBINO syndrome* (wall-eyed bilateral INO).

Also note:

▶ In young adults, the vast majority of bilateral INO are due to multiple sclerosis (MS).

▶ In a patient over 60 years of age, particularly those with hypertension, the main cause is vascular disease, where the sign may be unilateral—that is, just in one direction of gaze.

Rarer associations include the following:

· Wernicke's encephalopathy
· Brainstem encephalitis
· Drug toxicity (e.g., phenytoin)
· Pontine or midbrain tumor; syringobulbia, Chiari malformation

· Traumatic brain injury
· Myasthenia gravis; this produces a pseudo-INO due to muscle fatigue.

Supranuclear Gaze Palsy

See Video 2.2, Supranuclear Paralysis of Upgaze (courtesy Shirley Wray). Conjugate eye movements are controlled by pathways from the cortical eye fields which descend to the midbrain vertical gaze center and pontine horizontal gaze center, mischievously known, respectively, as the "rostral interstitial nucleus of the medial longitudinal fasciculus" and "paramedian pontine reticular formation." A lesion of either pathway, which is the equivalent of the upper motor neuron, impairs voluntarily gaze in the desired vertical or horizontal direction. However, conjugate eye movement can be induced by employing the vestibulo-ocular reflex (VOR; doll's-head eye movement). To test vertical supranuclear gaze, ask the patient to look at your face, grasp the sides of his or her head, and move it fairly vigorously up and down for vertical VOR or side-to-side for horizontal VOR. Thus, a patient may be unable to move the eyes voluntarily either horizontally or vertically, but the eyes may turn reflexly in response to vigorous passive head movement due to input from the vestibular apparatus. If the patient cannot move the eyes voluntarily but has VOR, then this is a supranuclear gaze palsy.

Furthermore, if voluntary upgaze is absent, you can also test for supranuclear gaze weakness by asking the patient to close their eyes while you hold open the upper lids manually. If the eyes turn upward (Bell's phenomenon), this suggests supranuclear gaze palsy. This is shown in Video 2.2. Thus, if voluntary upgaze is absent, you can test for supranuclear gaze

· By moving the head up and down for the vestibulo-ocular reflex.
· By asking the patient to close the eyes while you hold the upper lids open.

Apart from vascular disease affecting the frontal lobes, the major causes of supranuclear gaze palsy are as follows:

· Progressive supranuclear palsy (PSP)
· Creutzfeld -Jacob disease (CJD)
· Ataxia telangiectasia (AT)
· Niemann-Pick disease type C (NPC; mainly for downgaze)
· Gaucher's disease (horizontal)

- Whipple's disease
▶ In a young person, vertical supranuclear *downgaze* palsy suggests NPC, while *horizontal* supranuclear gaze palsy favors Gaucher's disease (Video 2.3).
  Note that Video 2.3 only shows impaired horizontal pursuit; horizontal vestibular ocular reflexes were not recorded.

A history of vascular disease, such as hypertension, ischemic heart disease, or small strokes, will help with the common vascular type. Often this variety is associated with *marché a petits pas*—a slightly wide-based, short-stepped cautious gait; thus you should have been alerted to this possibility by watching the patient walk into your consulting room (see Video 8.22, Lower Body Parkinsonism).

PSP is a rare form of parkinsonism described later in Chapter 8 (Movement Disorders). Note these additional Handles for supranuclear gaze palsies:

▶ If it is difficult to test VOR because of neck muscle rigidity, then PSP is likely.
▶ Rapid progression, over months, favors CJD and there is relentless cognitive decline.
▶ Slow progression, over years, supports AT, NPC, and Whipple's disease.

In AT, the telangiectasia are often visible on the sclera (Figure 1.14), cheek, ears, or sublingually. In addition to supranuclear gaze palsy, some patients display ocular apraxia and use head thrusts to move the eyes in the desired direction (see Video 2. 18 for an example of head thrusts).

NPC usually commences in childhood, but some cases slip though the net and present late. Apart from vertical downgaze supranuclear palsy, other features include:

- Cerebellar ataxia, dysarthria
- Dysphagia, cognitive decline
- Cataplexy
- Deafness
- Neonatal jaundice and splenomegaly

NPC is sometimes diagnosed by astute adult neurologists and invariably turns up in grand rounds! Identification is extremely important given the possibility of treatment with, for example, cyclodextrin or miglustat.

Supranuclear horizontal gaze palsy may be seen in children with type 1 Gaucher's disease, which is due to a mutation in the glucocerebrosidase gene. There is a less severe adult form of Gaucher's disease that causes parkinsonism with a similar disorder of horizontal eye movement. Look for pingueculae in the conjunctiva, as these are allegedly characteristic and biopsy may be diagnostic (see Figure 8.10). Next time you are confronted with atypical PD, especially where there is Jewish ancestry and features suggesting multiple system atrophy, make sure you test *horizontal* VOR and inspect the conjunctiva for pingueculae—it might be Gaucher's disease.

Therefore:

▶ Supranuclear horizontal gaze palsy in a Jewish child or young adult may be type 1 Gaucher's disease.
▶ Pingueculae in the conjunctiva are sometimes found in Gaucher's disease, and biopsy may be diagnostic.
▶ Check for enlargement of the liver or spleen.

The clues for Whipple's disease are a history of alimentary problems (malabsorption, diarrhea, weight loss), involuntary ocular and facial movements (oculomasticatory myorhythmia), and joint pain, but most neurologists will be lucky to see a single personal case in their lifetime.

Downbeat Nystagmus

See Video 2.4, Downbeat Nystagmus (courtesy Shirley Wray). Downbeat nystagmus consists of a fast downward flick of the eyes followed by a slower upward movement, best detected on lateral gaze. The nystagmus in the video could be mistaken for ocular bobbing, a disorder of the ventral pons, but in this condition the movements are slower (see Video 2.6, Ocular Bobbing).

The main causes of downbeating nystagmus are the following:

- Drug toxicity
- Structural lesion at foramen magnum level, such as Chiari malformation, tumor, and syringomyelia
- Spinocerebellar ataxia type 6
- Brainstem ischemia if no obvious alternative cause is found

Upbeating Nystagmus

See Video 2.5, Upbeating Nystagmus (courtesy David Zee). Mild upbeating nystagmus is seen with excess alcohol, nicotine use, and selective serotonin reuptake inhibitor (SSRI) antidepressants. Marked upbeating nystagmus generally indicates a structural lesion in one of the following:

- Midbrain: midline
- Pons: trigeminal nerve root entry zone
- Medulla: perihypoglossal nucleus
- Cerebellum: anterior vermis

▶ Ocular Bobbing Suggests a Ventral Pontine Lesion

See Video 2.6, Ocular Bobbing (courtesy David Zee). Here, both eyes bounce rapidly downward from the neutral (or slightly down-facing) position and then slowly return back. It is a powerful Handle suggesting a ventral pontine disorder, such as:

- Vascular disorder: infarct/hemorrhage
- Tumor
- Demyelination, for example, central pontine myelinolysis or *CLIPPERS syndrome* (see Chapter 4)

This should be distinguished from ocular nodding (Video 2.10, Ping-Pong & Nodding). In this, the eyes turn downward and then very slowly return to their primary position, with a cycle lasting 12–17 seconds (Wang et al. 2017). This patient had bacterial meningitis, but the localizing value of ocular nodding is uncertain.

▶ Elliptical Nystagmus Favors MS, Cockayne Syndrome or Pelizaeus-Merzbacher Disease

See Video 2.7, Elliptical Pendular Nystagmus (courtesy Scott K. Sanders), and Video 2.8, Elliptical Nystagmus (courtesy Shirley Wray). This is usually a pendular nystagmus associated with movement of the eyes around the orbit in an elliptical path. The term is not strictly defined; some use it to describe nystagmus in an oblique path; others, to describe a circular path or a mixture. The Cockayne syndrome is sometimes associated with basal ganglia calcification (see Figure 1.43). *Pelizaeus-Merzbacher disease* is primarily a disorder of infancy associated with cognitive impairment, progressive spasticity, and ataxia. Milder forms may present to the adult neurologist.

Periodic Alternating Nystagmus

See Video 2.9, Periodic Alternating Nystagmus (courtesy David Zee). Periodic alternating nystagmus (PAN) is a congenital or acquired disorder. The main characteristic is nystagmus that changes the direction of the horizontal fast and slow phases. Thus, in the neutral position there is, for example, spontaneous conjugate horizontal left-beating jerk nystagmus for about 1 minute, which gradually ceases and the eyes return to the neutral position. After about 15 seconds, the nystagmus resumes, but this time it becomes right-beating. This pattern repeats continuously. PAN localizes to the *cerebellar nodulus*, but it is not disease specific and occurs in

- Neoplastic and paraneoplastic disorder
- Demyelinating conditions
- Phenytoin toxicity

Ping-Pong Gaze

This is probably a variant of PAN or roving eye movements in which the eyes are slowly moved conjugately in the horizontal plane from one side to the other; see Video 2.10, Ping-Pong (courtesy Wang et al. 2017). The second half of the video shows slow nodding movements. In this instance the cause of ping-pong gaze was bacterial meningitis, but in general, it is not specific for any particular disorder and may be found in several severe forms of brain dysfunction (cerebral or brainstem lesions or drug toxicity) associated with coma. It may arise from a disorder of the cerebellar vermis.

Brown Syndrome

See Figure 2.54 and Video 2.11, Brown Syndrome (courtesy David Zee). This is a congenital disorder caused by restricted movement of the superior oblique tendon in its pulley (trochlea), located in the upper medial part of the orbital wall. There may be diplopia on attempted upgaze when the abnormal eye is turned in. The eye cannot be elevated as usual by the *inferior* oblique because the *superior* oblique muscle cannot stretch as it should when the globe is elevated. In the adult, the trochlea may be compromised by tenosynovitis of the trochlea or by trauma, as occurs in traffic accidents and boxing. Thus:

- ▶ In a child, diplopia on upgaze when the abnormal eye is turned in suggests Brown syndrome caused by impaired relaxation of the superior oblique muscle in the trochlea.
- ▶ In an adult, diplopia on upgaze and downgaze with the eye turned out suggests orbital trauma or thyrotoxicosis caused by tethering of the inferior rectus.

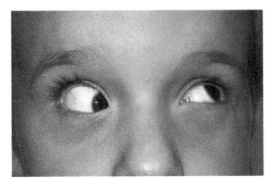

FIGURE 2.54: Child with right Brown syndrome. When the right eye is turned in, it cannot be elevated as usual by the right *inferior* oblique because movement of the right *superior* oblique is restricted in its pulley and cannot stretch as it should on upward movement of the globe in adduction. This results in diplopia on attempted upgaze. Reproduced from Figure 42.6 in the chapter The Genetics of Strabismus and Associated Disorders, by G Heidary, EI Traboulsi, and EC Engle. Oxford University Press. DOI:10.1093/med/9780195326147.003.0042.

The Brown syndrome should be distinguished from other disorders

- *Tethering of the inferior rectus muscle* (IR), which may result from trauma to the orbital floor (e.g., blow-out fracture)
- *Thyrotoxicosis* where the ocular muscles (particularly IR) become enlarged (Figure 2.55, *top*). If the IR is tethered, and the abnormal eye is turned out, there is diplopia on upgaze and downgaze because the IR cannot relax, and this impedes effective contraction of the superior rectus.

Recurrent Episodes of Diplopia Lasting Seconds

This condition is usually caused by one of the following:

- *Paroxysmal dystonic attacks.* This is typical of MS. There may be spells of dysarthria as well.
- *Myokymia* of the superior oblique. See Video 2.12, Myokymia of Superior Oblique (courtesy David Zee). There is rapid *shimmering* of objects rather than diplopia (see later discussion).
- *Vertebral artery dissection* with repeated embolization. This is relevant in the older patient.

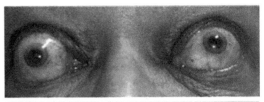

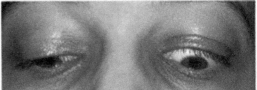

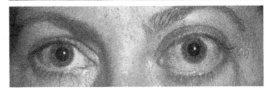

FIGURE 2.55: **Top**: Proptosis and lid retraction from acute thyrotoxicosis. Elevation of the right eye is restricted by tethering of the inferior rectus. **Middle**: Lid lag affecting the left eye. **Bottom**: Proptosis secondary to meningioma of left optic nerve sheath that was painful and developed in pregnancy. Middle image reproduced with permission from *Training in Ophthalmology*, edited by V Sundaram, A Barsam, A Alwitry, and P Khaw. Oxford University Press, 2009. Bottom image reproduced with permission from *A Colour Atlas of Clinical Neurology*, 2nd ed., MA Parsons. Mosby Year Book Europe, 1993.

Pendular Nystagmus

In this variety, the eyes swing from side to side, like a rapidly beating clock pendulum. Classically there is no jerk phase. See Video 2.13, Pendular Nystagmus. The likely causes are as follows:

- Congenital
- Blindness
- *Spasmus nutans.* A childhood-onset disorder with head tremor, myopia, and head tilt (see Video 2.21, Spasmus Nutans). There is severe impairment of visual acuity.
- Lesions of Guillain-Mollaret triangle resulting in palatal tremor (formerly called palatal myoclonus; see Video 2.22, Ataxia and Palatal Myoclonus)

Convergence-Retraction Nystagmus

See Video 2.2, Supranuclear Paralysis of Upgaze (courtesy Shirley Wray). This is a useful Handle that localizes to the dorsal midbrain. There is usually vertical supranuclear gaze palsy. On attempted vertical gaze, which is impaired, the eyes jerk medially and inward. This is caused by brisk contraction predominantly of the medial recti, which not only makes the eyes converge but also simultaneously pulls the eyes back into the orbit. In a complete *Parinaud's syndrome* there is:

- Vertical supranuclear gaze palsy
- Convergence-retraction nystagmus
- Light-near dissociation
- Lid retraction

The main causes are:

- Pineal tumor
- Dorsal midbrain vascular or demyelinating lesions
- Hydrocephalus

Superior Oblique Myokymia

See Video 2.12 (courtesy David Zee). Patients present with repeated, brief illusions of movement, *shimmering*, or diplopia affecting one eye. The primary action of superior oblique is downgaze, thus activities such as reading or walking downstairs will provoke myokymia. The main causes are as follows:

- In the young, midbrain demyelinating or neoplastic lesions.
- In the elderly, vascular compression of the trochlear nerve in its root exit zone.
- It may be an isolated finding in apparently normal individuals.
- ◀ Beware the patient with self-induced rapid eye movement that may simulate myokymia; see Video 2.14, Voluntary Flutter (courtesy David Zee). This happens usually on convergence and has to be distinguished from superior oblique myokymia, which relates only to downgaze.

See-Saw Nystagmus

See Video 2.15, See-Saw Nystagmus (courtesy Shirley Wray). This may be pendular or jerky and characterized by elevation and intorsion of one eye with synchronous depression and extorsion of the other eye. Following this, the opposite happens—there is a mirror-image change in direction during the next half-cycle. The bridge of the patient's nose may be considered the axis of the movement.

Following are the main causes of pendular see-saw nystagmus:

- Congenital
- Acquired causes are those that interfere with crossing axons at the optic chiasm and produce bitemporal hemianopia, such as a pituitary tumor.

Jerk see-saw nystagmus occurs with lesions in the region of the interstitial nucleus of Cajal, located at the most rostral termination of the medial longitudinal bundle within the dorsal midbrain.

Paroxysmal Tonic Downgaze of Infancy

This rare but highly characteristic eye movement disorder affects infants under 1 year of age; see Video 2.16, Paroxysmal Tonic Downgaze of Infancy. There are paroxysms of sustained conjugate downgaze sometimes associated with "eye popping," in which there is brief lid retraction synchronous with downgaze, as shown in the video. Some infants have paroxysms of upgaze. Otherwise, neurological examination and investigations are usually normal and the condition resolves spontaneously in about 6 months.

Chaotic Eye Movement

See Video 2.17 (courtesy David Zee). The eyes move rapidly and conjugately in all directions and there are myoclonic jerks of the limbs. It is often termed the *opsoclonus-myoclonus syndrome*. Causes include the following:

- In children: neuroblastoma
- In adults: neoplastic/paraneoplastic, autoimmune, or viral disorder

Oculomotor Apraxia

See Video 2.18, Congenital Oculomotor Apraxia (courtesy Shirley Wray). Some patients have difficulty with conjugate gaze (usually horizontal) even though there is no diplopia or weakness of any external eye muscle. This can be overcome by using head thrusts, which in essence employ the vestibulo-ocular reflex to initiate conjugate gaze. The major causes of oculomotor apraxia are as follows:

- Congenital
- Ataxia telangiectasia (see Chapter 1) in association with cerebellar ataxia and telangiectases of the conjunctiva or ear

• Ataxia with oculomotor apraxia syndromes (AOA, type I and II). See Chapter 12 on ataxia.

Third-Nerve Palsy with Normal Pupillary Responses

This is usually a medical disorder (Figure 2.56). In a total CN III nerve palsy there is complete ptosis, paralysis of all eye movement except functions of CN IV and VI, and a maximally dilated pupil that is paralyzed to all stimuli—the efferent pupillary defect. The primary action of the superior oblique muscle (CN IV), which is downgaze in the adducted position, cannot be tested properly because the eye is pulled out laterally by the intact abducens muscle (CN VI). The superior oblique has a secondary function which is inward rotation of the eyeball (intorsion). If the eye is in the neutral or abducted position, you can detect intorsion (and intactness of the superior oblique) by asking the patient to attempt downgaze. This is best seen by looking for intorsion of a conjunctival blood vessel.

Sometimes the third-nerve palsy is complete, except that the pupil reacts normally. In general, this indicates a medical cause (diabetes, vascular) rather than surgical (aneurysm, tumor). Thus preservation of fourth-nerve function can be a useful confirmatory sign of a medical third-nerve lesion. Pupil sparing is thought to occur because the pupillary fibers have a dorsal blood supply that is separate from the blood supply of the main nerve trunk (Figure 2.57), whereas a tumor would affect CN III and CN IV. A significant

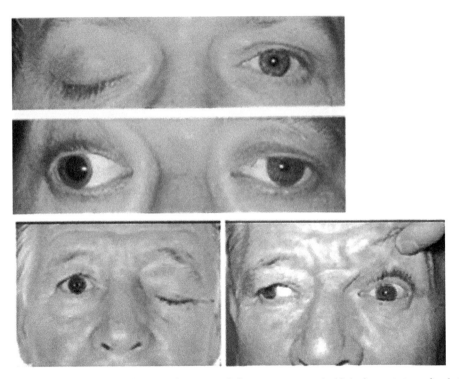

FIGURE 2.56: **Top photo** shows obvious right ptosis and allows you to guess the likely diagnosis immediately. **Middle photo**: When the upper lid is elevated manually, the right eye is passively abducted by an intact lateral rectus muscle, and the pupil is large, nonreactive to light, unlike the healthy left side. Diagnosis: complete right oculomotor paralysis, usually resulting from compressive lesions such as a posterior communicating artery aneurysm, pressure from the uncus or parasellar tumor. Note the positive Hirschberg's sign: the reflected light is near the center of the pupil in the normal left eye but at 3 o'clock and off-center in the abnormal right eye. Do not be put off by proptosis (up to 3 mm), as orbital muscle hypotonia from a complete third nerve lesion allows the eye to sag forward a little. **Bottom photo**: Another patient showing complete left ptosis, again suggesting a third nerve palsy. When the eyelid is elevated and the patient is asked to look right, the left eye does not adduct in keeping with medial rectus weakness and a third nerve lesion, but against expectation, the pupil is small and reacting to light from the studio lamps. This is a pupil sparing third nerve palsy and usually denotes diabetes and other vascular causes which can be in the nerve itself or in the brainstem. Middle photo reproduced from *Diagnosis in Color: Neurology*, M Parsons and M Johnson.

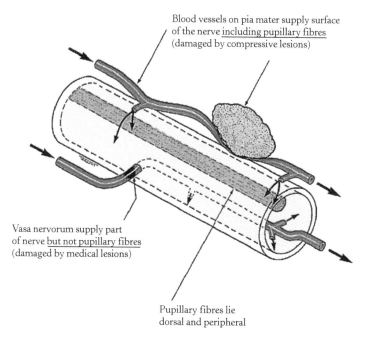

Blood vessels on pia mater supply surface
of the nerve <u>including pupillary fibres</u>
(damaged by compressive lesions)

Vasa nervorum supply part
of nerve <u>but not pupillary fibres</u>
(damaged by medical lesions)

Pupillary fibres lie
dorsal and peripheral

FIGURE 2.57: The dual blood supply of the oculomotor nerve. The pupillary fibers lie relatively protected in the dorsal sector of the nerve, thus it requires significant compression to involve this area as well as the main nerve trunk. The vasa nervorum to the main trunk are occluded in vascular pathology resulting from atheroma, vasculitis, and diabetes. Reproduced with permission from *Clinical Ophthalmology*, J Kanski and B Bowling, Figure 19.63. Elsevier Saunders, 2011.

proportion of patients with pupil-sparing CN III will have lacunar infarcts in the midbrain. Thus:

▶ A pupil-*sparing* CN III lesion is likely medical (diabetic, vascular) and the superior oblique is spared.

▶ A pupil-*involving* CN III lesion is likely surgical (tumor, aneurysm) and the superior oblique is affected.

◀ Beware the apparent partial CN III palsy with pupil sparing and variable diplopia. *It might be ocular myasthenia.* Also, note that myasthenia occasionally causes a pseudo-INO due to fatigue of the lateral rectus muscles. There may be misdiagnosis of MS.

Proptosis

Apart from thyroid disorder, which is often easily recognizable (Figure 2.55, *top* and *middle*), think of the following (main) causes:

- In people from the Far East: nasopharyngeal carcinoma
- In Westerners: cavernous hemangioma

- In children: dermoid cyst
- In neurofibromatosis: optic nerve glioma or meningioma of optic nerve sheath (Figure 2.55, *bottom*)
- Bony swelling of the temporal fossa: sphenoid ridge meningioma (Figure 2.58).
- Pulsatile proptosis: carotid-cavernous fistula (Figure 2.59)
- Granulomatous disorders affecting the orbital cavity: sarcoidosis, Wegener's granulomatosis, Erdheim Chester disease (see Figure 13.5)
- In patients with facial infection: cavernous sinus thrombosis (Figure 2.60); apart from proptosis and a swollen eye, there is headache, fever, and lesions of CN III, IV, or VI.

TROCHLEAR NERVE (CN IV)

See Video 2.19, Fourth-Nerve Palsy (courtesy Shirley Wray). Unilateral disorder of the trochlear nerve (CN IV) causes difficulty in downgaze resulting in diplopia on reading or walking downstairs. The diplopia is improved by tilting the head toward the shoulder of the unaffected side (*Bielschowsky's sign*;

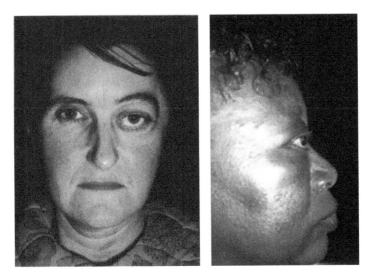

FIGURE 2.58: Two examples of sphenoid wing meningioma. **Left**: The left eye is pushed forward and downward (non-axial proptosis). Note the hyperostosis in the left temple. The presence of hyperostosis helps distinguish this type of proptosis from intraorbital tumors and inflammatory lesions of the orbit. **Right**: Reactive hyperostosis in a woman with a right sphenoid ridge meningioma. The eye is pushed forward by hyperostosis of the posterior orbit. Left image reproduced with permission from *A Colour Atlas of Clinical Neurology*, 2nd ed., MA Parsons. Mosby Year Book Europe, 1993. Right image reproduced with permission from *Clinical Ophthalmology*, J Kanski and B Bowling, Figure 19.56b. Elsevier Saunders, 2011.

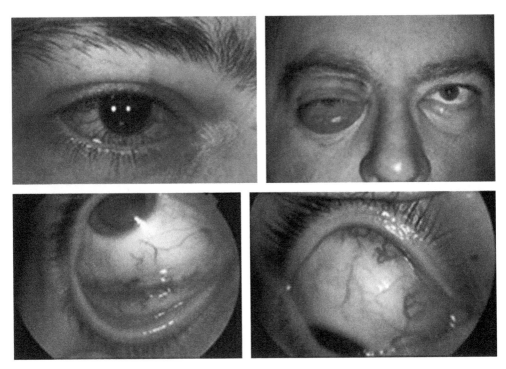

FIGURE 2.59: **Top**: Advanced case of carotico-cavernous fistula. The classic signs are chemosis, pulsatile exophthalmos and ocular bruit. The main causes are head trauma (even mild) or rupture of an intra-cavernous aneurysm. Note the extensive arterialized episcleral vessels, an important feature not seen in comparable disorders such as thyroid eye disease, orbital pseudotumor and cavernous hemangioma. **Bottom**: Another patient showing more subtle arterialization of episcleral vessels visible in upper and lower conjunctival sacs. Top image reproduced from *Clinical Eye Atlas*, DH Gold and RA Lewis, Figure 13.5. Oxford University Press. Bottom image courtesy Dr. Irina Gout, Prince Charles Eye Unit, Windsor.

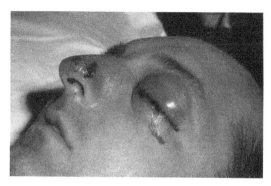

FIGURE 2.60: Cavernous sinus thrombosis. This patient developed a boil on his nose (see scarring on left nostril) followed 24 hours later by left proptosis. This strongly suggests cavernous sinus thrombosis. Typical features include periorbital edema, chemosis, headache, and proptosis. The sixth cranial nerve is most frequently affected, probably because it is within the sinus, but any of the nerves that traverse the sinus wall or are adjacent to it may be damaged, namely CN III, IV, V (ophthalmic and maxillary divisions). Funduscopy revealed papilledema and retinal hemorrhages. Reproduced with permission from *Diagnosis in Color: Neurology*, M Parsons and M Johnson. Mosby Publications (2001).

see Video 8.86, Bielschowsky). The main causes are as follows:

- Head injury
- Midbrain lesions such as hydrocephalus, vascular, neoplastic
- Raised ICP
- Mononeuritis, for example, diabetic
- Cavernous sinus and orbital disease

The trochlear nerve intorts the eye. This movement may be useful to determine whether CN IV is affected. In an oculomotor nerve palsy, ask the patient to look down and then inspect a conjunctival blood vessel for evidence of intorsion. In general:

▶ Preservation of CN IV with normal pupillary reflexes favors a medical CN III lesion.
▶ Involvement of CN IV with paralysis of pupillary reflexes suggests a surgical (compressive) disorder.

Note that the superior oblique is a weak abductor of the eye, so you cannot assume that CN VI is partially intact if there is weak abduction.

ABDUCENS NERVE (CN VI)

The only action of the lateral rectus muscle is abduction. Lesions of its nerve produce diplopia on horizontal gaze (Figure 2.61).

Apart from pontine vascular disease, the main alternative causes of *isolated* CN VI palsy are:

- Diabetes (mononeuritis)
- Multiple sclerosis
- Idiopathic intracranial hypertension, hydrocephalus
- Skull base fracture

Tumors cause a sixth-nerve lesion in two ways:

- As a false localizing sign due to raised ICP
- By direct pressure; for example, from a clivus tumor or aneurysm

If the only other sign is a Horner's syndrome on the same side as the CN VI lesion, then the disorder is likely in the cavernous sinus—that is, in the vascular sheath of the intracavernous part of the internal carotid artery where the sympathetic and sixth nerve are together (see Figure 2.14b). Thus:

▶ Horner's syndrome and ipsilateral CN VI palsy suggest a cavernous sinus lesion.

Duane Syndrome

This is a congenital disorder probably due to faulty innervation and contracture of the muscles responsible

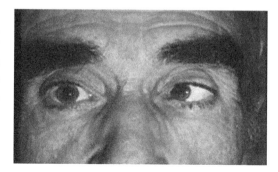

FIGURE 2.61: This 68-year-old patient is looking to his right. He has a clear right sixth nerve palsy due to a pontine hypertensive vascular lesion, which is the most common cause in elderly patients and resolves spontaneously in most instances. Reproduced with permission from *A Colour Atlas of Clinical Neurology*, MA Parsons. Mosby Year Book Europe, 1992.

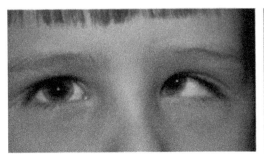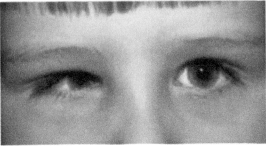

FIGURE 2.62: Child with bilateral Duane syndrome. In the left figure there is incomplete abduction of the right eye simulating a right CN VI lesion but note the narrowing of the *left* palpebral fissure due to retraction from a left Duane syndrome. In the right figure there is attempted gaze to the left with apparent left CN VI palsy, but there is now narrowing of the *right* palpebral fissure, reflecting the right Duane syndrome.

for horizontal gaze. Diagnosis may be delayed until adult life. It may be uni- or bilateral and is easily mistaken for CN VI palsy. If there is a unilateral Duane lesion on, say, the left, there is impaired abduction of the left eye, simulating CN VI palsy but without diplopia due to suppression. On conjugate horizontal gaze to the right, there is narrowing of the left palpebral fissure due to retraction of the affected eye on adduction (see Figure 2.62 and Video 2.20, Duane Syndrome).

TRIGEMINAL NERVE (CN V)

▶ *Jaw supporting sign* (see Figure 2.63).

This maneuver is performed to support a weak jaw and neck, but it may be obvious only after prolonged conversation. It is highly characteristic of:

- Myasthenia gravis, where both jaw and neck muscles are weak and fatigue and, rarely, in:
  - Myotonic dystrophy
  - Oromandibular dystonia (as a sensory trick), but there is no fatigue.

▶ Unremitting cheek pain with normal examination usually indicates depression.

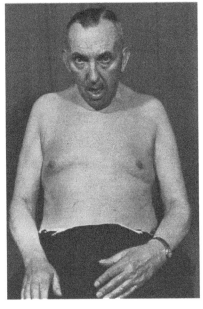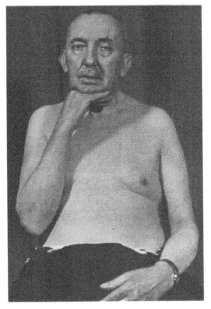

FIGURE 2.63: The jaw supporting sign, which is almost pathognomic of myasthenia gravis. It is performed to support weak neck *and* jaw muscles. A similar sign may be observed in myotonic dystrophy and oromandibular dystonia, but in the latter the neck muscles are not weak. Reproduced from *An Atlas of Clinical Neurology*, JD Spillane, Figure 269. Oxford University Press.

If sinonasal disease is excluded and there are no physical signs, then a patient with continuous cheek pain present day and night usually has depression. The typical person is a middle-aged woman. Even if depression cannot be substantiated, the pain usually responds to antidepressants.

▶ Intermittent central facial paresthesia in a young adult suggests hyperventilation/panic disorder.

Typically, the lips, tongue, or nose are involved, as well as the extremities. The tingling will last for minutes or hours.

Also note that in *panic attacks*, the hands may be tightly clenched before assuming the classic *main d'accoucheur* position of carpopedal spasm.

Do not be dissuaded by a history of asymmetric pins-and-needles sensations. The clue in the history lies in the *periodicity* of the complaint. In most cases of organically based disease, facial numbness is continuous, although its intensity may vary. Care should be taken in elderly hypertensive patients with basilar insufficiency because pontine ischemia may also produce this, and it may be a form of TIA. Metabolic causes have to be considered, such as:

· Hypoglycemia
· Hypocalcemia
· Lambert-Eaton myasthenic syndrome
◀ Beware the anxious patient with intermittent facial tingling due to hyperventilation superimposed on organically based numbness in the face or elsewhere; that is, two separate conditions. This can be a difficult diagnosis, particularly in young patients who are worried about the possibility of MS.

If doubt remains,

· Ask the patient to overbreathe for 2 minutes to determine whether this replicates his or her symptoms.

Trotter's Triad

On the side of the lesion, this comprises

· Facial or ear pain
· Conductive deafness
· Palatal palsy

The cause is usually a nasopharyngeal tumor. Unilateral or bilateral sixth-nerve palsy may follow.

Persistent Isolated Facial Numbness

Often this is partial and unexplained, but there is a brief checklist:

· *Trigeminal neuropathy*; for example, diabetes, Sjögren's syndrome, tabes dorsalis (central face), trichloroethylene exposure
· *Focal-onset sensory motor neuronopathy syndrome* (FOSM). This is a newly described disorder that starts with bilateral lower facial sensory impairment, gradually spreading over the face and upper body, followed by bulbar and limb lower motor neuron features (Vucic et al. 2006). See Chapter 7.
· Demyelination
· Sarcoidosis
· Tumor of the trigeminal nerve in its intracranial course; syringobulbia (peripheral face)

Numb Chin Sign (Roger's Sign)

This is sometimes ominous and may indicate the following:

· Local dental problems. Neoplasm in the jaw or skull base
· Metastases or paraneoplastic effect of breast and other cancers
· Sickle cell anemia
· Sarcoidosis, diabetes, MS

Trigeminal Trophic Syndrome (Idiopathic Trigeminal Neuropathy

See Figure 2.64. This rare disorder consists of facial anesthesia/dysesthesias and nonhealing skin ulcers, typically around the nose. There is often neuropathic pain in the face. Response to treatment is poor. A similar condition occurs in the following:

· Leprosy
· Sjögren's syndrome
· Lesch-Nyhan syndrome
· Tourette syndrome

FACIAL NERVE (CN VII)
· *Cupid bow sign.*
This fanciful but memorable sign (Figure 2.65) refers to droop of the upper lip in patients who have experienced facial palsy of either lower or upper motor neuron

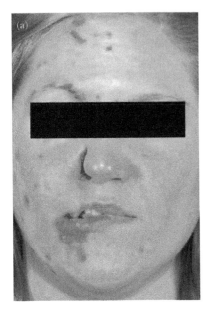
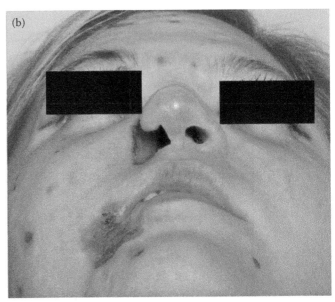

FIGURE 2.64: Trigeminal trophic syndrome. Note the multiple areas of self-inflicted wounds. Reproduced with permission from Golden et al. (2014), Figure 1.

variety. Sometimes it is the only evidence of previous facial weakness. Other clues are:
  o asymmetrical blinking
  o contracture of the orbicularis (Figure 2.65)
- Herpes zoster infection causes facial palsy but the vesicles may not be visible in the ear.

You need to check the palate. See Figure 2.66.

Bilateral Facial Weakness
Acute-onset bilateral facial palsy is usually due to trauma or Guillain-Barré syndrome. Long-standing bilateral facial weakness is caused by the following:

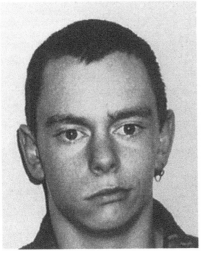
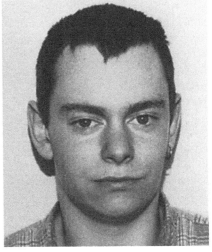

FIGURE 2.65: Cupid bow sign. **Left**: Five days after acute Bell's palsy. Note the drop of the right upper lip that produces asymmetry of Cupid's bow. The right palpebral fissure is slightly large because of orbicularis oculi weakness. **Right**: Three months later. The right palpebral fissure is now smaller than the left, suggesting mild contracture of the orbicularis oculi, but Cupid's bow is symmetrical. Reproduced from Figure 20.9. in the chapter The Lower Cranial Nerves and Dysphagia, by P Shaw and D Hilton-Jones. Oxford University Press. DOI:10.1093/med/9780198569381.003.0429.

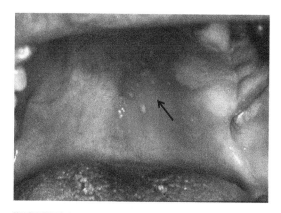

FIGURE 2.66: A 73-year-old male with a left Bell's palsy. There were no vesicles in the external meatus but there were vesicles on the left palate (arrow). Diagnosis: Ramsay Hunt syndrome (one person). The vesicles are due to herpes zoster infection, which is here involving the palate, supplied by CN IX. Note the black tongue most likely due to heavy smoking and poor oral hygiene.

- Sarcoidosis
- HIV
- Lyme disease
- Melkersson-Rosenthal syndrome (Figure 2.67)
- Leprosy
- Recurrent idiopathic Bell's palsy
- Amyloid neuropathy. This is associated with corneal lattice dystrophy (see Chapter 11).

Melkersson-Rosenthal syndrome is an autosomal dominant condition characterized by recurrent facial palsy, facial edema, and fissured "scrotal" tongue (Figure 2.67). If there is bilateral patchy *upper* facial weakness, then leprosy is most likely. The nerve to the buccinator is spared as this muscle is deep and warm, thus causing the characteristic buccinator wrinkles (Figure 2.4). Upper facial weakness happens because the forehead skin is cooler and provides a more favorable growth environment for the mycobacterium.

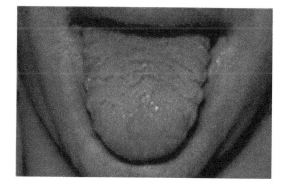

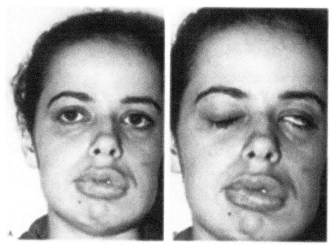

FIGURE 2.67: **Top**: Fissured ("scrotal") tongue characteristic of Melkersson-Rosenthal syndrome. Other features are recurrent facial palsies and swelling of the upper lip. It is sometimes familial and there is a gene locus on 9p11. Reproduced with permission from Figure 8.5 in the chapter Urticaria, by V Sybert. Oxford University Press. DOI:10.1093/med/9780195397666.003.0008. **Bottom**: This shows bilateral facial swelling and weakness of the left facial muscles. Reproduced from Kesler et al. (1998), Figure 1.

▶ Tears when eating ("crocodile tears") after Bell's palsy results from faulty reinnervation of CN VII.

Regenerating secretomotor fibers (in chorda tympani) destined for the salivary glands are misdirected into the lacrimal gland and cause ipsilateral tearing while eating.

Taste Disorder

The chorda tympani nerve carries taste sensation from the anterior two-thirds of the tongue and travels with the facial and lingual nerves. Taste is most often affected in Bell's palsy, although many are unaware when it is unilateral. During surgery the chorda tympani nerve is vulnerable in three places: medial to the lower third molar tooth, deep to the temporomandibular joint, and as it crosses the neck of the malleus (Figures 2.68 and 2.69).

Thus, unilateral loss of taste in the anterior two-thirds of the tongue may relate to the following:

• Extraction of the lower third molar tooth with trauma to the lingual nerve.
• Temporomandibular joint surgery with damage to the chorda tympani
• Middle ear surgery (e.g., stapedectomy) with damage to the chorda tympani.

• Tonsillectomy. Taste loss in the posterior tongue occurs after tonsillectomy as CN IX lies in the tonsillar bed. It usually recovers within 6 months.

Note:

▶ *Ciguatera poisoning.*
This poison damages the voltage-gated sodium channels, which are held wide open, leading to intense paresthesia and temperature reversal such that cold objects appear hot. Often there is metallic dysgeusia because of the damage to the sodium channels in the tongue.
▶ Metallic dysgeusia is a feature of exposure to many metals, including arsenic, mercury, manganese, and thallium.
▶ Preferential loss of taste for meat is said to be characteristic of gastric cancer.

VESTIBULO-COCHLEAR NERVE (CN VIII)

First, a point about taking the history from a patient who complains of "dizziness." This is a vague word, but thanks to a study of more than 100 dizzy patients (Drachman and Hart 1972), the meaning of this term

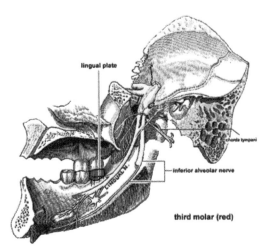

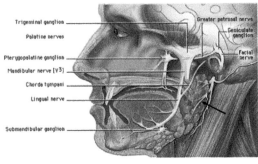

FIGURE 2.68: **Left**: The position of the lingual nerve in relation to the third molar tooth shown in red. The lingual nerve carries taste afferents from the anterior two-thirds of the tongue in the chorda tympani. **Right**: The course of the lingual nerve and chorda tympani. It passes deep to the temporo-mandibular joint and attaches to the lingual nerve at an oblique angle. The greater petrosal nerve, which supplies taste buds in the soft palate, is labeled. The glossopharyngeal nerve innervates the posterior foliate and circumvallate papillae in the posterior two-thirds of the tongue (black arrow). In the tonsillar bed it may be damaged during tonsillectomy. Reproduced with permission from the Yale Center for Advanced Instructional Media, Figure 6.16b.

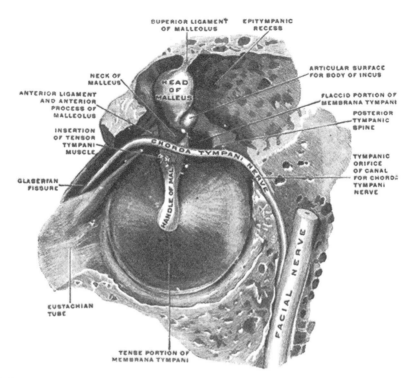

FIGURE 2.69: The middle ear viewed from inside the middle ear. It shows the course of the chorda tympani as it crosses the neck of the malleus and then joins the facial nerve at an acute angle. During middle ear surgery, such as stapedectomy, the chorda tympani may be injured. Reproduced from Wikimedia Commons.

has been clarified and may be divided into four different categories:

- *Presyncope*, where the patient thinks a faint is imminent. "Woozy" is a popular term.
- *Imbalance*, where the patient walks unsteadily, as in cerebellar or sensory ataxia
- *Spinning*, which is apparent rotation of the self or external environment. Some stressed patients complain that their "brain is spinning." This is more likely an anxiety disorder.
- *Anxiety*, which most often relates to overbreathing and panic in stressed subjects. It may lead to syncope.

The first letters of these four categories spells **PISA**, which will help you remember the list and allow a better analysis of the patient's complaints. The term *vertigo* is not well defined and is best avoided.

◀ A patient may have more than one variety of "dizziness," especially if he or she is anxious about physical symptoms.

▶ A noisy hearing aid usually means bilateral deafness.
  That is, if the patient had one good ear, he or she would turn down the volume of the hearing aid. This can be a useful Handle if you are considering an acoustic neuroma; such tumors are unilateral unless there is neurofibromatosis type 2.

Tinnitus

The *continuous* high-pitched whistling or buzzing tinnitus in the elderly is common.

▶ Pulsatile or continuous tinnitus may indicate elevation of intracranial pressure. It constitutes a guide to progress in patients with idiopathic intracranial hypertension (IIH, pseudotumor cerebri). It is more common on the right because the right jugular vein is usually dominant.
▶ Sometimes, the tinnitus of IIH may be abolished by pressure on the jugular vein.

Other causes of pulsatile tinnitus include the following:

- Turbulence from a nearby arteriosclerotic artery
- Overactive diploic circulation (e.g., Paget disease of bone, hemoglobinopathies)
- Carotid artery aneurysm/dissection or extensive collateral circulation
- Carotid-cavernous fistula
- Glomus jugulare tumor
- Persistent stapedial artery (associated with nose bleeds, deafness, and, rarely, seizures)
- Palatal tremor (clicking tinnitus)
- Myokymia of stapedius or tensor tympani muscles (fluttering tinnitus)

▶ A glomus tumor is associated with conductive deafness and occasionally vascular swelling, visible on the ear drum (Figure 2.70), which is, of course, diagnostic.

▶ Deafness with ataxia may be due to:
- Superficial siderosis. There often is a history of head injury or bleeding from aneurysm or vascular malformation in the brain or spinal cord. There is myelopathy, and most are anosmic
- Mitochondrial disease (e.g., Kearns-Sayre syndrome).

The deafness may be exercise-related.
- Refsum's syndrome

▶ Deafness with retinal infarcts suggests Susac's syndrome.

This is a presumed vasculitic autoimmune disorder usually affecting young women. See Figures 9.27 and Figure 9.28 for retinal and MRI imaging changes which are characteristic.

▶ Deafness with a short fourth metatarsal bone is probably Refsum's disease (Figure 2.71).

Occasionally there is shortening of metacarpal bones as well. There will be other features, of course, including ichthyosis, short stature, anosmia, peripheral neuropathy, and retinitis pigmentosa. Other rare causes of the combination of deafness and a short fourth metatarsal bone are:
  o Pseudohypoparathyroidism
  o Albright's hereditary osteodystrophy
  o Turner syndrome (fourth and fifth metatarsal bones may be short)

▶ Sudden unilateral sensorineural hearing loss is usually unexplained but may have a vascular or viral basis.

It is important to exclude lesions in the middle ear such as a blocked Eustachian tube, infection, and the like, but these problems will have been dealt with by the otolaryngologist. If it is sensorineural deafness, inspection of the audiogram will give some basic guidance (Figure 2.72). Thus, a down-sloping (high tone loss) suggests a vascular cause. An up-sloping

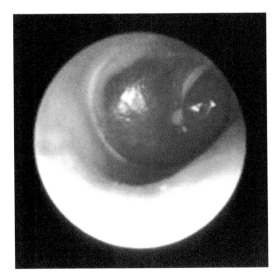

FIGURE 2.70: Glomus jugulare tumor. There is a dark red mass filling the middle ear and pushing the tympanic membrane outward. Reproduced from http://me.hawkelibrary.com/new/main.php?g2_itemId=1374.

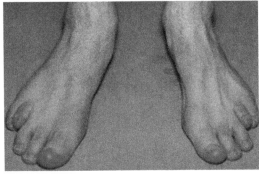

FIGURE 2.71: Refsum disease to show the short fourth metatarsal bone. Reproduced from *Atlas of Clinical Neurology*, 2nd ed., GD Perkin, FH Hochberg, and DC Miller, Figure 2.5. 1993, Wolfe Publishing.

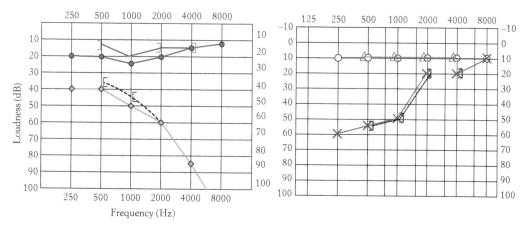

FIGURE 2.72: Acute sensorineural hearing loss. **Left**: High tone loss producing a down-sloping curve (green) that is typical of a vascular cause. **Right**: Up-sloping low tone curve (blue) typical of viral cause or Ménière's disease. Vertical axis: loudness in decibels. Horizontal axis: frequency in Hz.

curve (low tone loss) favors a viral cause or Ménière's disease.

Often the cause of acute deafness is unexplained. Possible etiologies include the following.

Vascular:

- Thrombosis of vertebral artery, anterior inferior cerebellar artery, internal auditory artery.
- *Fabry's disease.* Usually there is a painful peripheral neuropathy. Examine the skin (especially pelvic) for angiokeratomas (Figures 1.16, 9.26, and 11.19).
- Susac syndrome. There are retinal artery branch occlusions and a subacute encephalopathy (see Chapter 9). Paradoxically, the deafness is cochlear and affects low frequencies.

Inflammatory:

- Demyelination. Acute onset deafness is well recognized in MS.
- With interstitial keratitis and vertigo, this suggests *Cogan's syndrome* or *syphilis* (Figure 2.73). Both conditions have presumed autoimmune origin
- Sarcoidosis, systemic lupus erythematosus
- Viral infection: almost any, particularly herpes group. Also HIV
- Bacterial infection (e.g., Lyme disease)

Cerebellopontine angle tumors:
Typically acoustic neuroma, meningioma, or neurofibroma

▶ Deafness provoked by exercise suggests a mitochondrial disorder. It is important to exclude mundane causes such as transient blockage of the Eustachian tube.

Fabry's Disease

Patients with *Fabry's disease* present to neurologists on account of strokes or painful peripheral neuropathy. There are other features discussed in Chapter 11 (Peripheral Neuropathy).

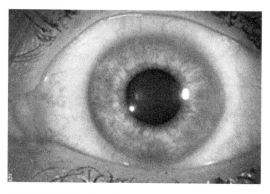

FIGURE 2.73: Cogan's syndrome. This is a combination of interstitial keratitis, sudden sensorineural deafness, and vertigo. Courtesy Dr. Irina Gout, Prince Charles Eye Unit, Windsor.

▶ Cochlear deafness is an important complication that may help clinch a diagnosis of Fabry's disease.

Vestibular Disorders

▶ Spinning sensation on turning (particularly when lying in bed) suggests *benign paroxysmal positional vertigo (BPPV)*.
  Usually the posterior semicircular canal is affected, and there is a history of head trauma.

Most instances of positional vertigo (i.e., spinning of environment) are peripheral, but, on rare occasions, they are central as a result of brainstem tumors or vascular and inflammatory processes. The vertigo may be provoked by positional tests, for example, the *Dix-Hallpike maneuver*:

With the body supine and the head hanging 30 degrees below horizontal and tilted to the affected side, in *peripheral* positional vertigo:

- Nystagmus is rotatory and upbeating lasting 20–60 seconds.
- Clockwise nystagmus indicates abnormality on the left side, counterclockwise on the right.
- Vertigo and nystagmus develop after a latent period of 5–10 seconds.
- Response fatigues if repeated.

In *central* positional vertigo:

- Nystagmus is up- or downbeating, occasionally torsional.
- There is no latency.
- Spinning can be elicited repeatedly (i.e., no fatigue).
▶ Spinning vertigo with prominent vomiting may happen in the first few hours of acute labyrinthitis but if persistent may indicate a posterior fossa tumor.
▶ Pure downbeating nystagmus is always of central origin.
▶ "Dizzy" sensation provoked by noise is the *Tullio phenomenon*.
  Patients experience rotation, nausea, or nystagmus on exposure to loud noise. The main causes are a fistula in the middle or inner ear or dehiscence of the superior canal.

▶ Abrupt-onset spinning lasting seconds or minutes is likely vestibular paroxysmia. There is nystagmus during an attack.
  A possible explanation is microvascular compression of the vestibular nerve analogous to trigeminal neuralgia. Patients respond to carbamazepine and related medication.

GLOSSOPHARYNGEAL AND VAGUS NERVES (CN IX AND X)

In the head, these nerves are concerned with movement of the palate and pharyngeal muscles plus sensation from the posterior tongue, epiglottis, soft plate, and tonsil (Figure 2.74).

Palatal Tremor/Myoclonus

See Video 2.22, Ataxia and Palatal Myoclonus, and Chapter 8, on movement disorders. This is a slow (1–3 Hz) tremor of the soft palate, sometimes associated with Holmes/rubral tremor, nystagmus, and diaphragmatic tremor.

- In the essential variety, patients report clicking sounds as the movement is at the edge of the palate near the opening of the Eustachian tube.

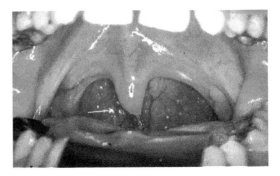

FIGURE 2.74: A left palatal palsy (CN IX and X) when the patient says "ah." The uvula is pulled over to the patient's right. If you obtain a good view of the pharynx you might observe an asymmetric "curtaining" effect of the muscles on the posterior pharyngeal wall (white arrow) as the right superior pharyngeal constrictor muscles sweep the "curtain" unopposed across the posterior pharynx. Reproduced with permission from *Clinical Examination*, O Epstein, GD Perkins, D de Bono, and J Cookson, Figure 12.120.

- Symptomatic tremor (from lesions of Mollaret's triangle) more often involves the uvula (levator veli palatini) and clicks are less common.
- Note the syndrome: progressive ataxia and palatal tremor (PAPT), probably related to *Alexander disease*. There is a mutation in the gene GFAP.

Thus:

▶ Palatal tremor with clicking is likely the essential variety.
▶ Palatal tremor without clicking favors symptomatic tremor, Alexander's disease/ PAPT.
▶ The tadpole sign on MRI may be diagnostic of Alexander's disease (Figure 2.75).
▶ Palatal tremor may occur after vertebral artery dissection.
▶ Facial or ear pain, conductive deafness, and palatal palsy is *Trotter's triad*. See CN VII section.

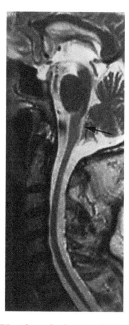

FIGURE 2.75: The tadpole sign of Alexander's disease. Sagittal T2 images show atrophy of cerebellum, brainstem (except pons), and spinal cord. The atrophic medulla is the upper part of the tail of the tadpole (arrow). The head of the tadpole is the pons. Reproduced with permission from Pareyson et al. (2008), Figure 1a.

▶ Unilateral palsy of the recurrent laryngeal and hypoglossal nerves is the *Tapia syndrome*. There is ipsilateral weakness of the vocal cord and tongue. It usually occurs after general anesthesia where there has been excess pressure from the cuff of a laryngeal mask. Most patients recover within 6 months.

ACCESSORY NERVE AND NECK MUSCLES (CN XI)

Painless Neck Flexion Weakness

Neck flexion is tested rapidly by asking the patient to flex the neck against the resistance of your hand on the forehead (Figure 2.76). There are six main causes, all beginning with the letter *M*:

- Myasthenia gravis
- Myotonic dystrophy
- Myositis (polymyositis or dermatomyositis)
- Motor neuron disease (amyotrophic lateral sclerosis; ALS)
- Mitochondrial myopathy
- Myxedematous myopathy

Here are two important Red Flags:

◀ If you are considering facioscapulohumeral or limb girdle dystrophy and the neck muscles are weak, then the diagnosis should be reviewed. The neck is rarely affected in either condition.

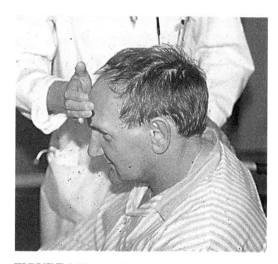

FIGURE 2.76: A rapid way of testing neck flexion muscles. The main causes of weakness begin with letter *M* as listed.

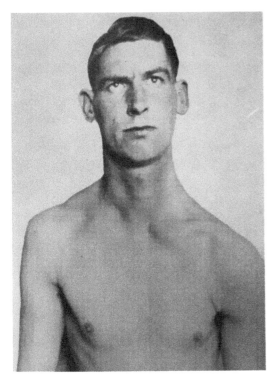

FIGURE 2.77: Idiopathic left accessory nerve palsy. Note the drop of the left shoulder and atrophy of the left sternomastoid muscle. Reproduced with permission from *An Atlas of Clinical Neurology*, JD Spillane, Figure 141. Oxford Medical Publications.

◀ If you think the diagnosis is myotonic dystrophy or polymyositis and the neck muscles are strong, your diagnosis will almost certainly be incorrect.

For causes of *head drop*, see Chapter 8 (Movement Disorders).

Isolated Accessory Nerve Palsy

This is a rare lesion (Figure 2.77) and sometimes no cause is found. These are the main etiologies:

- Local infection
- Trauma (e.g., accidents and neck surgery)
- Neck tumor
- Coronary artery bypass surgery
- Jugular foramen lesions (usually with CN IX and X)

Stiff Neck in a Sick Patient with Negative Kernig's Sign

Apart from neck trauma, which is usually given by the history, the causes of a stiff neck in a sick patient are few and there is a simple procedure to distinguish them. The most important cause of a stiff neck is meningitis, but it also occurs with raised ICP. Thus:

▶ If there is a stiff neck and Kernig's sign, you are probably dealing with meningeal irritation.
▶ If Kernig's sign is absent, then raised ICP is more likely.

This simple observation can be particularly useful when considering a lumbar puncture—something which clearly would be contraindicated with raised ICP secondary to a mass lesion but desirable in meningitis.

◀ When confronted with a sick patient who has neck stiffness but a negative Kernig's sign, request a brain scan first before undertaking a lumbar puncture.

Geste Antagoniste (Sensory Trick) in Cervical Dystonia

This is also called *spasmodic torticollis* (see Figure 2.78) and Chapter 8, on movement disorders). This form of dystonia causes involuntarily turning of the head. If the examiner tries to centralize the neck, it is usually difficult, and the sternomastoid muscle is hypertrophied unless treated previously with botulinum toxin. Some patients find that just touching with one finger on specific craniofacial locations (usually the chin) is sufficient to overcome their head turning. This remarkable sign is poorly understood and not seen in any other disorder. If the patient shows this phenomenon, the diagnosis can be made in seconds (see Chapter 8, Video 8.80, CD Sensory Trick).

Lhermitte's Sign, Reversed Lhermitte's Sign, and McArdle's Sign

These are considered in Chapter 4. The short neck from Klippel-Feil anomaly appears in Chapter 1.

HYPOGLOSSAL NERVE (CN XII)

Unilateral Tongue Weakness After Trauma

▶ A patient who sustains neck injury (typically from a traffic accident) and develops unilateral neck or temporal pain with tongue weakness a few hours or days later probably has internal carotid artery dissection.

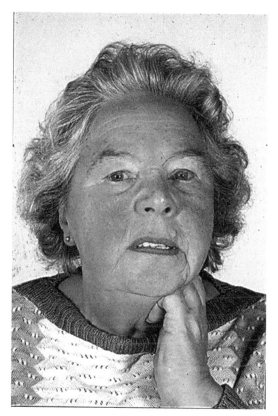

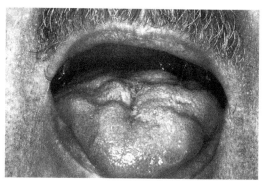

FIGURE 2.79: A 75-year-old man presented with a 6-month history of slurred speech and difficulty swallowing, especially liquids. The tongue is wasted and furrowed due to continual fasciculations. Diagnosis: bulbar amyotrophic lateral sclerosis. In a younger person with a more chronic course one would consider syringobulbia, low-grade medullary tumor, or bulbospinal neuronopathy (Kennedy syndrome).

FIGURE 2.78: Cervical dystonia showing the *geste antagoniste* or sensory trick used to overcome the head turn. There was marked hypertrophy of the right sternomastoid muscle.

The reason is that the hypoglossal nerve curves around the carotid sheath on its way to the tongue. For the same reason, an ipsilateral Horner's syndrome may accompany the dissection. MRI of the internal carotid artery shows the "crescent sign," as explained in Chapter 9 (Stroke).

▶ If there is a contralateral hemiparesis, this should involve the face because there is cortical ischemia.
▶ If the contralateral hemiparesis spares the face, the lesion must be in the medulla, where the exiting hypoglossal nerve is next to the pyramid.
▶ Even in the absence of trauma, think of internal carotid dissection in any case of recent-onset hypoglossal nerve weakness.

Note that any of the lower motor cranial nerves may be involved in a carotid dissection. Horner's syndrome or hypoglossal palsy are the most common features.

Florid Bilateral Tongue Fasciculation

If this feature (Figure 2.79) has been present for several months, it usually indicates one of the following:

- ALS (bulbar varieties)
- Syringobulbia
- Medullary tumor
- Kennedy syndrome (X-linked bulbospinal neuronopathy)

Repeated Tongue Protrusion

See Chapter 8 (Movement Disorders). In brief, these are the main causes:

- Chorea-acanthocytosis
- Tardive dyskinesia
- PKAN
- Neuroferritinopathy
- Angelman syndrome
- Lesch-Nyhan syndrome
- NBIA1
- Trombone tongue of syphilis
- Whispering dysphonia

SUMMARY

Cranial Nerves

CN 1

- Intermittent anosmia: conductive defect. Continuous anosmia: perceptive defect
- Anosmia and dementia: Alzheimer's disease, Lewy body dementia (including PD),

frontotemporal and semantic dementia, Huntington's disease, frontal pole tumor, prion disorder
- Unilateral anosmia (if no local obstruction): olfactory groove meningioma
- Anosmia with mirror movements: Kallman's syndrome, PD
- Anosmia and retinitis pigmentosa: Refsum's syndrome
- Anosmia, myelopathy, ataxia, and deafness: superficial siderosis, mitochondrial disorder
- Anosmia in an Asian or South American: leprosy, usually accompanied by bilateral, mainly upper facial palsy
- Intermittent olfactory hallucinations: temporal lobe glioma, complex partial seizures, PD, olfactory reference syndrome, transient epileptic amnesia
- Hyperosmia: migraine, pregnancy, Addison's disease, drug withdrawal effect
- Loss of smell and taste after head injury: patient misinterpretation of loss of taste to mean loss of smell; lesion of orbitofrontal cortex or insula
- Normal smell sense in apparent idiopathic PD suggests parkinsonism, essential tremor, PSP, corticobasal syndrome, multiple system atrophy

CN II
Looking through a pinhole improves virtually all refractive errors.

Acuity
- Bilateral blurred vision in healthy teenage girl is likely functional.
- Distorted central vision in one eye (metamorphopsia) is a macular problem.
  In young adult: central serous retinopathy. Elderly: age-related macular degeneration, diabetic macular edema, or cellophane maculopathy
- With macular edema there is micropsia. With macular scar, there is macropsia.

Field Defects
- Partially sighted patient without difficulty navigating a room alone: Leber's optic atrophy (peripheral field spared). If help is required: Usher's or Refsum's syndrome (peripheral field involved)

- Patient who is blind in both eyes but appears unconcerned, denies it, or may not even be aware of it has cortical blindness typically from bilateral occipital infarcts. Pupillary light reflexes are normal.
- A congruous homonymous field defect suggests a lesion in the occipital cortex. An incongruous homonymous field defect is usually due to an optic tract or anterior geniculate lesion.
- Tunnel vision with spiral pattern is functional. True tunnel vision occurs in glaucoma, migraine aura, alcohol intoxication, retinitis pigmentosa, retinal ischemia due to severe anemia, raised ICP, cancer associated retinopathy (CAR).
- Bilateral peripheral constricted fields, continuous phosphenes, and night blindness with history of cutaneous melanoma or other cancers: CAR
- Continual phosphenes in CAR often misdiagnosed as migraine; distinguish from visual snow.
- Bitemporal hemianopia points to a chiasmal lesion: pituitary tumor, craniopharyngioma, meningioma, trauma, aneurysm or fusiform enlargement of the internal carotid arteries
- Upper temporal field is affected first with pressure from below, as in a pituitary tumor. The lower temporal field is involved initially with pressure from above, as in a craniopharyngioma. Detected best with red target
- In the early stages of bitemporal hemianopia, patient notices little impairment of visual acuity because of macular sparing.
- Bitemporal hemianopia causes hemi-field slide phenomenon and post-fixational blindness.
- Pituitary tumor with post-fixed chiasm presses on optic nerve; with prefixed chiasm there is pressure on the optic tract.
- Optic atrophy in one eye with a junctional field defect in the other is likely a compressive lesion (tumour or aneurysm).
- Homonymous hemianopia cannot be due to a frontal lobe lesion.
- Pie in the sky field defect suggests a posterior temporal lobe field disorder (Meyer's loop lesion).
- Altitudinal visual field loss: if binocular, indicates thromboembolism in occipital

cortex; if monocular, the cause is thromboembolic carotid disease.

- Lower binocular altitudinal field loss suggests a lesion in the upper part of the optic radiation.
- Upper binocular altitudinal loss points to a defect in the lower optic radiation or occipital cortex.
- Advancing field defects move like the hands of a clock.
- Equatorial field loss suggests a lateral geniculate lesion.
- Bilateral occipital infarctions produce bilateral homonymous hemianopia.
- Checkerboard field defect: focal lesions of opposite optic radiations
- A temporal field defect that crosses the vertical meridian is likely retinal and not chiasmal in origin. A tilted optic disk will cause an upper temporal field defect, but it crosses the midline.

Transient Monocular Visual Loss (TMVL)
- Learn Table 2.1.
- Bright yellow dots at the bifurcation of retinal arteries; cholesterol-platelet emboli (Hollenhorst plaques)
- In the absence of cataract, temporary monocular glare/visual impairment when going from indoors out into bright sunlight suggests severe carotid stenosis.
- TMVL, tender scalp nodules, girdle pain, or jaw claudication indicates cranial arteritis with features of polymyalgia rheumatica.
- The superficial temporal artery and/or its branches may be tender, thickened, and pulseless.
- Occlusion of the ophthalmic artery usually causes no field defect provided the collateral supply from the external carotid territory is adequate.
- Occlusion of the central retinal artery is usually embolic and causes complete monocular loss of vision with cherry-red spot, unless there is a good cilioretinal artery supply to macula.
- Cherry-red spot is also found in lipid storage diseases, PKAN, metachromatic leukodystrophy, or toxic effect of quinine, dapsone, carbon monoxide, or methanol.
- Anterior ischemic optic neuropathy (AION) is never embolic.

- If the optic disk is not pale, then the diagnosis of AION is wrong
- Retinitis pigmentosa with anosmia: Refsum's disease. With cerebellar signs: SCA7, AVED, or Kearns Sayre syndrome. With dystonia: HARP, NARP, PKAN. With deafness: Usher's syndrome

Pupil and Iris
- A unilateral dilated pupil with normal accommodation that constricts after prolonged exposure to light and redilates slowly is a tonic pupil. If the tendon reflexes are depressed, this is the Holmes-Adie syndrome. Confirm diagnosis with weak (2.5%) methacholine drops.
- Tonic pupil with areflexia, segmental anhidrosis and lack of facial flushing is the *Ross syndrome*.
- Loss of facial flushing after exertion usually accompanied by ipsilateral Horner's syndrome is the *Harlequin syndrome*.
- An acute-onset tonic pupil in someone over age 50 years may be a sign of GCA.
- A dilated pupil fixed to all stimuli in an otherwise healthy person: self-administration of mydriatic
- A unilateral fixed dilated pupil may happen by accident if the patient has been in contact with common garden plants.
- The RAPD sign is positive when you observe paradoxical dilatation to light shone in that pupil.
- Argyll Robertson pupils. Mnemonic is ARP: **A**ccommodation **Ref**lex **P**resent; reverse it to PRA; **P**upillary **R**eflex **A**bsent.
- Light-near dissociation with a large pupil favors a tonic pupil, juvenile tabetic pupil, or dorsal midbrain lesion.
- Light-near dissociation with a small pupil is likely Argyll Robertson or long-standing tonic pupils.
- Acute-onset bilaterally small pupils: with tearing, salivation, runny nose, and sweating suggests mushroom or insecticide poisoning, also opiate exposure, brainstem stroke.
- Chronically small pupils, bilateral ptosis, and anhidrosis suggests bilateral Horner's syndrome as found in diabetic autonomic neuropathy, amyloidosis, pure autonomic failure, and multiple system atrophy.
- Small pupils with proximal myopathy: Stormorken syndrome (Chapter 7)

- Poor visual acuity in one eye with normal pupillary light reflexes: Leber's disease
- Tadpole pupil causes: migraine, tonic pupil, Horner's syndrome, or midbrain lesion

Horner's Syndrome

- This causes miosis, ptosis, and anhidrosis. Enophthalmos is probably an illusion. Ipsilateral Horner's syndrome and disorder of
  - Pituitary, hypothalamus, or brainstem is a lesion of the first-order neuron.
  - Cervical spinal cord or brachial plexus is a lesion of the second-order neuron.
  - Carotid artery (common or internal) or CN VI is a lesion of the third-order neuron lesion (postganglionic). There may be distension of the conjunctival capillaries and lack of sweating.
- Ipsilateral Horner's syndrome with weak, wasted hand and depressed triceps jerk (C7 and C8) with sensory loss in a C8 distribution is a second-order lesion in keeping with a compressive brachial plexus disorder (i.e., Pancoast tumor or cervical rib).
- Horner's syndrome with neck pain is usually caused by internal carotid artery dissection. There is often a contralateral hemiparesis and ipsilateral hypoglossal palsy.
- Horner syndrome with eye pain and CN VI palsy is usually caused by pressure from an intracavernous aneurysm.
- In brachial plexus avulsion injury with a flail arm, the presence of Horner's syndrome indicates a lesion proximal to brachial plexus and a poor prognosis.
- Upper lid retraction, pupillary dilation, and increased sweating: reversed Horner's syndrome (*Pourfour du Petit* syndrome)
- Blue eyes that both become brown: Wilson's disease or use of prostaglandin analog eye drops for glaucoma
- Long thick eyelashes: use of prostaglandin analog eye drops for glaucoma or the Oliver McFarlane syndrome
- One brown eye and one blue eye since birth suggests a congenital Horner's syndrome, Sturge-Weber, Waardenburg, and Parry-Romberg syndromes.
- Acquired anisochromia: local eye trauma secondary to hyphema, melanocytic infiltration from iris nevus/melanoma; Fuchs heterochromic iridocyclitis

Fundus

- Kestenbaum's sign in borderline primary optic atrophy
- Optic atrophy in one eye and papilledema in the other: Foster Kennedy syndrome, bilateral anterior ischemic optic neuropathy; rarely, frontal pole tumor
- Unilateral central visual loss that may simulate demyelinating optic neuritis: neuroretinitis, neuromyelitis optica, Leber's optic atrophy, white dot syndromes, ischemic optic neuropathy, central serous retinopathy
- Consecutive (sequential) optic neuropathy: Leber's optic atrophy, neuromyelitis optica, ischemic optic neuropathy, neuroretinitis

Papilledema

- Pulsating retinal veins virtually excludes raised ICP.
- Visual acuity is preserved unless the disk swelling is severe.
- A swollen disk with reduced acuity favors acute optic neuritis or central retinal vein thrombosis.
- Hemorrhages on the disc and in the retina is likely retinal vein occlusion; raised ICP unlikely and inflammation least likely. Hemorrhages on the disc only suggests decompensated papilledema; inflammation rare and retinal vein occlusion least likely. No hemorrhages anywhere favors inflammation or compensated papilledema. Partial retinal vein occlusion would be a remote possibly.
- Pseudopapilledema. This may result from disk crowding, as in healthy far-sighted people, or drusen of the optic disk.
- Papilledema with recent-onset low back pain: ependymoma of the cauda equina, idiopathic intracranial hypertension, or Guillain-Barré syndrome
- Back pain with recurrent uveitis suggests Behçet's disease.
- Papilledema and headache in overweight, otherwise healthy young adult female: idiopathic intracranial hypertension. MRI may show empty sella, flattened globe at optic nerve entry point, and enlarged tortuous optic nerves.
- Papilledema in overweight male who snores: obstructive sleep apnea

- Papilledema after radical neck dissection: ligation of the dominant (usually right) internal jugular vein

Miscellaneous Characteristic Fundal Appearances

- Epileptic with retinal phakoma and skin lesions: tuberous sclerosis
- Retinal hemangioma due to Von Hippel–Lindau disease
- Exudate of hypopigmented and hyperpigmented areas with ill-defined borders: toxoplasmosis
- Leathery facial skin with angioid streaks: pseudoxanthoma elasticum
- Concentric target-like pigmentary appearance at macula: bull's eye maculopathy
- Bow-tie (band) atrophy of the optic disk: retrograde degeneration of nasal retinal nerve fibers suggests lesion of chiasm or opposite optic tract.

CN III, IV, and VI

- Monocular diplopia: if local eye disorder is, excluded this is usually psychogenic.
- Variable and confusing responses to the cover tests: myasthenia gravis or functional disorder
- Oculomotor nerve palsy with contralateral hemiplegia usually indicates a thrombotic lesion in the proximal portion of the posterior cerebral artery (Weber's syndrome).
- INO: Detected more readily by tests of saccadic eye movement rather than pursuit. If convergence is normal, the lesion is in the pontine MLF. If convergence is impaired, the lesion is in the midbrain MLF. Bladder disorder favors a pontine INO.
  - WEBINO syndrome: bilateral INO and persistent divergent squint
  - There is usually upbeating nystagmus as well as horizontal.
  - In young adults, the vast majority of bilateral INO are due to MS.
  - In the patient over 60 years, particularly those with hypertension, the main cause is vascular disease.
- Rare causes of INO: Wernicke's encephalopathy, brainstem encephalitis, drug toxicity, pontine or midbrain tumor, traumatic brain injury, syringobulbia, and Chiari malformation. Myasthenia gravis may cause a pseudo-INO due to muscle fatigue.

Supranuclear Gaze Palsy

- If voluntary upgaze is absent, test supranuclear gaze by moving the head up and down for the vestibulo-ocular reflex or ask patient to close the eyes while you clamp the upper lids open.
- Main causes: frontal lobe vascular disease, PSP, CJD, ataxia telangiectasia; NPC, Gaucher's disease, and Whipple's disease
- In a young person, vertical supranuclear downgaze palsy indicates NPC, while horizontal supranuclear gaze palsy favors Gaucher's disease.
- Difficulty in testing vertical VOR because of neck muscle rigidity is likely PSP.
- Rapid progression of supranuclear gaze palsy, over months, favors CJD and there is relentless cognitive decline. Slow progression, over years, supports AT, NPC, and Whipple's disease.
- AT features: supranuclear gaze palsy; telangiectasia on sclera, ears, or under tongue; oculomotor apraxia with head thrusts
- NPC features: supranuclear downgaze palsy, cerebellar ataxia, dysarthria, dysphagia, cognitive decline, cataplexy, deafness, and neonatal jaundice
- Supranuclear horizontal gaze palsy in Jewish child or adult may be type 1 Gaucher's disease. Pingueculae in the conjunctiva are typical and biopsy may be diagnostic. Check for enlarged liver or spleen.
- Whipple's disease: history of alimentary problems (malabsorption, diarrhea, weight loss), involuntary ocular and facial movements (oculomasticatory myorhythmia), and joint pain.
- Downbeat nystagmus causes: drug toxicity, structural lesion at foramen magnum level (Chiari malformation, tumor, and syringomyelia), spinocerebellar ataxia type 6, or brainstem ischemia
- Upbeating nystagmus: lesion of midline midbrain, trigeminal nerve root entry zone, perihypoglossal nucleus, or anterior vermis
- Ocular bobbing: central pontine disorders: infarct/hemorrhage, tumor, central pontine myelinolysis, or CLIPPERS syndrome
- Elliptical nystagmus: Pelizaeus-Merzbacher disease, Cockayne syndrome, and MS
- Periodic alternating nystagmus: lesion in cerebellar nodulus due to neoplastic or

demyelinating lesions and phenytoin toxicity; ping-pong gaze
- Brown syndrome: tethering of the superior oblique tendon in its pulley; congenital or due to local trauma in adults; causes diplopia on attempted upgaze with the abnormal eye turned in
- Tethering of inferior rectus causes diplopia on up *and* downgaze with eye turned out; caused by blow-out fracture or thyrotoxicosis.
- Recurrent brief (seconds) episodes of diplopia: usually paroxysmal (dystonic) attacks of MS or myokymia of the superior oblique. In older patient: vertebral artery dissection with repeated embolization
- Pendular nystagmus: congenital, blindness, spasmus nutans, lesions of Guillain-Mollaret triangle
- Convergence-retraction nystagmus: lesion of dorsal midbrain (tectum); causes are pineal tumor, dorsal midbrain vascular or demyelinating lesions, and hydrocephalus.
- Parinaud's syndrome: vertical supranuclear gaze palsy, convergence-retraction nystagmus, light-near dissociation, lid retraction. Main causes are pineal tumor, dorsal midbrain vascular or demyelinating lesions, thalamic hemorrhage, hydrocephalus.
- See-saw nystagmus: causes are congenital, chiasmal lesions, lesion of interstitial nucleus of Cajal
- Superior oblique myokymia: causes are demyelinating or neoplastic lesions in midbrain. In elderly patients, vascular compression of the trochlear nerve at its root exit zone, an isolated finding in healthy people.
- Beware the patient with self-induced rapid eye movement that may simulate myokymia.
- Chaotic eye movement (opsoclonus-myoclonus syndrome): in children it is due to neuroblastoma. In adults, neoplastic/paraneoplastic, autoimmune, or viral cause
- Oculomotor apraxia causes: congenital, ataxia telangiectasia, ataxia with oculomotor apraxia syndrome
- Third-nerve palsy with normal pupillary responses is usually medical (diabetes, vascular). A pupil involving CN III lesion is likely surgical (tumor, aneurysm) and the superior oblique is affected. An apparent partial CN III palsy with pupil sparing and variable diplopia might be ocular myasthenia.

- Proptosis causes: most are due to thyroid disorder. In those from the Far East, the most common cause is nasopharyngeal carcinoma; in Westerners, cavernous hemangioma. In children: dermoid cyst. Neurofibromatosis and proptosis suggest optic nerve glioma. Bony temporal fossa fullness: sphenoid ridge meningioma. Pulsatile proptosis: carotid-cavernous fistula. Granulomatous disorders affecting the orbital cavity: sarcoidosis, Wegener's granulomatosis, Erdheim Chester disease. Facial infection: cavernous sinus thrombosis

CN IV

- Difficulty in downgaze.
- Diplopia is improved by tilting the head toward the shoulder on the unaffected side (Bielschowsky sign).
- Superior oblique is a weak abductor of the eye, so you cannot assume that CN VI is partially intact if there is weak abduction.
- Main causes: head injury, midbrain lesions (hydrocephalus, vascular, neoplastic), raised ICP; mononeuritis (e.g., diabetic), cavernous sinus, and orbital disease.
- Preservation of CN IV with normal pupillary reflexes favors a medical CN III lesion.
- Involvement of CN IV with paralysis of pupillary reflexes suggests a surgical (compressive) disorder.

CN VI

- If isolated lesion: MS in young; hypertensive vascular lesion in elderly. Also: diabetic mononeuritis, IIH, hydrocephalus, skull base fracture. With ipsilateral Horner's syndrome: cavernous sinus lesion
- Tumors cause CN VI lesions as false localizing sign due to raised ICP or from direct pressure (e.g., clivus tumor or aneurysm)
- Horner's syndrome and ipsilateral CN VI palsy suggest a cavernous sinus lesion.

Duane Syndrome

- May be mistaken for CN VI palsy.
- The main clue is narrowing of the palpebral fissure and ptosis on lateral gaze.

CN V

- Jaw supporting sign: myasthenia gravis, myotonic dystrophy, oromandibular dystonia

- Unremitting dull cheek pain with normal examination: sinonasal disease, depression
- Intermittent central facial paresthesia in a young adult: hyperventilation, hypoglycemia, and hypocalcemia. In elderly: brainstem TIA. In panic attack, hands may be tightly clenched. Patients may have hyperventilation *and* organic disorder such as MS.
  - Consider metabolic causes, such as hypoglycemia, hypocalcemia
  - Lambert-Eaton myasthenic syndrome
- Trotter's triad: facial or ear pain, conductive deafness and palatal palsy. Usual cause is nasopharyngeal tumor
- Persistent isolated facial numbness: trigeminal neuropathy (diabetes, Sjögren's), tabes dorsalis, trichloroethylene exposure, FOSMN, demyelination, sarcoidosis, tumor of CN V
- Numb chin sign: local dental conditions; neoplasm of jaw or skull base, metastases or paraneoplastic effect of breast cancer, sickle cell anemia, MS, diabetes, and sarcoidosis
- Trigeminal trophic syndrome may be caused by idiopathic trigeminal neuropathy, leprosy, Sjögren's syndrome, Lesch-Nyhan syndrome, Tourette disorder

CN VII

- Cupid's bow sign helps identify previous facial palsy.
- Herpes zoster infection causes facial palsy, but the vesicles may not be visible in the ear. Check palate.
- Bilateral facial weakness causes: if acute: trauma or Guillain-Barré syndrome. Long-standing bilateral facial weakness: sarcoidosis, HIV, Lyme disease, Melkersson-Rosenthal syndrome (scrotal tongue), leprosy, recurrent idiopathic Bell's palsy, amyloid neuropathy
- Bilateral upper facial weakness suggests leprosy.
- Crocodile tears. Tears when eating due to faulty reinnervation following Bell's palsy.
- Unilateral loss of taste: following lower third molar tooth extraction suggests trauma to the lingual nerve. After temporomandibular joint surgery implies chorda tympani damage. Following middle ear surgery indicates damage to chorda tympani. After tonsillectomy indicates damage to CN IX.

- Metallic dysgeusia may follow ciguatera poisoning, exposure to metals, including arsenic, mercury, manganese, and thallium.
- Preferential loss of taste for meat: gastric cancer (possibly)

CN VIII

- Mnemonic PISA: **P**resyncope, **I**mbalance, **S**pinning, **A**nxiety
- A patient may have more than one variety of "dizziness," especially if anxious about physical symptoms.
- Noisy hearing aid usually means bilateral deafness.
- Pulsatile tinnitus causes: raised ICP; turbulence from a nearby arteriosclerotic artery, overactive diploic circulation (e.g., Paget's disease of bone, hemoglobinopathies); carotid artery aneurysm/dissection, carotid-cavernous fistula, glomus jugulare tumor, persistent stapedial artery, palatal myoclonus (clicking tinnitus), myokymia of stapedius or tensor tympani muscles (fluttering rather than pulsatile tinnitus)
- Deafness with ataxia: superficial siderosis, mitochondrial disease, Refsum's syndrome
- Sudden unilateral sensorineural hearing loss is usually unexplained but may have a vascular or viral basis.
- Exercise-induced deafness suggests a mitochondrial disorder.
- Deafness with retinal infarcts: Susac's syndrome
- Deafness with short fourth metatarsal bone: Refsum's disease, pseudohypoparathyroidism, Albright hereditary osteodystrophy, Turner syndrome (fourth and fifth metatarsals short)
- In acute-onset deafness, audiogram that shows down-sloping (high tone) loss has a vascular or age-related basis. If up-sloping (low tone), it is more likely viral.
- Strokes or painful peripheral neuropathy with cochlear deafness: Fabry's disease
- Sudden deafness and interstitial keratitis: Cogan's syndrome or syphilis
- Spinning sensation on turning in bed suggests benign paroxysmal positional vertigo.
- Positional tests:
  - Peripheral positional vertigo: nystagmus rotatory and upbeating, clockwise nystagmus indicates left-side abnormality;

counterclockwise the right. Vertigo and nystagmus develop after 5–10 seconds, response fatigues if repeated.

- o Central positional vertigo: nystagmus is up- or downbeating; no latency, spinning can be elicited repeatedly.
- Positional vertigo with prominent vomiting suggests a posterior fossa tumor.
- Pure downbeating nystagmus is always of central origin.
- "Dizzy" sensation provoked by noise is the Tullio phenomenon.
- Abrupt-onset spinning lasting seconds or minutes is likely vestibular paroxysmia.

CN IX and X

- Uvula deviates to the strong side: curtaining of posterior pharyngeal muscles
- Palatal tremor: palatal tremor with clicking is likely the essential variety. Palatal tremor without clicking favors symptomatic palatal tremor (brainstem lesions), Alexander's disease, or PAPT. MRI shows tadpole sign.
- Palatal tremor may occur after vertebral artery dissection.
- Palatal palsy with conductive deafness and facial pain (Trotter's triad) suggests nasopharyngeal tumor.
- Unilateral recurrent laryngeal and hypoglossal nerve palsy is the Tapia syndrome.

CN XI

- Painless neck flexion weakness: all beginning with letter M: myasthenia gravis, myotonic dystrophy, myositis, motor neuron disease (ALS), mitochondrial myopathy, myxedematous myopathy
- If you are considering facioscapulohumeral or limb girdle dystrophy and the neck muscles are weak, then the diagnosis should be reviewed. The neck is rarely affected in either condition.
- If you think the diagnosis is myotonic dystrophy or polymyositis and the neck muscles are strong, your diagnosis will almost certainly be wrong.
- Isolated accessory nerve palsy: local infection, neck trauma, neck tumor, coronary artery bypass surgery, jugular foramen lesions (with CN IX and X)

- Stiff neck in a sick patient with negative Kernig's sign: neck trauma, raised ICP
- Stiff neck in a sick patient with positive Kernig's sign: meningitis
- Geste antagoniste (sensory trick): cervical dystonia

CN XII

- Unilateral tongue weakness after trauma: internal carotid artery dissection
- Unilateral tongue weakness with contralateral hemiparesis due to internal carotid dissection should involve the face because there is cortical ischemia. If the hemiparesis spares the face, the lesion must be in the medulla.
- Florid bilateral tongue fasciculation: ALS, syringobulbia, medullary tumor, and bulbospinal neuronopathy (Kennedy syndrome)
- Repeated tongue protrusion: chorea-acanthocytosis, tardive dyskinesia, PKAN, neuroferritinopathy, Angelman syndrome, Lesch-Nyhan syndrome, NBIA1, trombone tongue of syphilis, whispering dysphonia

SUGGESTED READING

Dobson R, Lawden M. Melanoma associated retinopathy and how to understand the electroretinogram. *Pract Neurol.* 2011;11:234–239.

Drachman DA, Hart CW. An approach to the dizzy patient. *Neurology.* 1972;22:323–334.

Drummond PD, Lance JW. Facial flushing and sweating mediated by the sympathetic nervous system. *Brain* 1987;110:793–803.

Gibberd FB, Feher MD, Sidey MC, Wierzbicki AS. Smell testing: an additional tool for identification of adult Refsum's disease. *J Neurol Neurosurg Psychiatry.* 2004;75:1334–1336.

Golden E, Robertson CE, Moossy JJ, Sandroni P, Garza I. Trigeminal trophic syndrome: a rare cause of chronic facial pain and skin ulcers. *Cephalalgia.* 2014;35(7):636.

Hawkes CH, Shephard BC, Daniel SE. Olfactory dysfunction in Parkinson's disease. *J Neurol Neurosurg Psychiatry.* 1997;62:436–446.

Hawkes ED, Neffendorf JE. Kestenbaum's capillary number test—a forgotten sign? *Mult Scler Relat Disord.* 2014;3:735–737.

Hayreh SS, Zimmerman MB. Central retinal artery occlusion: visual outcome. *Am J Ophthalmol.* 2005;140:376–391.

Hildebrand GD, Russell-Eggitt I, Saunders D, Hoyt WF, Taylor DS. Bow-tie cupping: a new sign of chiasmal compression. *Arch Ophthalmol.* 2010;128(12):1625–1626.

Kesler A, Vainstein G, Gadoth N. Melkersson-Rosenthal syndrome treated by methylprednisolone. *Neurology.* 1998;51:1440–1441.

Koay KL, Plant G, Wearne MJ. Tadpole pupil. *Eye (Lond).* 2004;18:93–94.

Luco C, Hoppe A, Schweitzer M, Vicuna X, Fantin A. Visual field defects in vascular lesions of the lateral geniculate body. *J Neurol Neurosurg Psychiatry.* 1992;55:12–15.

Mattes D, Mayer M, Feichtinger M, Lindner S. Neurological picture: a case of Pourfour du Petit syndrome following tumour surgery of the mandible. *J Neurol Neurosurg Psychiatry.* 2009;80(1):69.

McFadzean RM, Hadley DM. Homonymous quadrantanopia respecting the horizontal meridian. A feature of striate and extrastriate cortical disease. *Neurology.* 1997;49:1741–1746.

Mittal MK, Rabinstein AA, Wijdicks EF. Pearls & oysters: oval pupil: two observations. *Neurology.* 2013;81:e124–e125.

Mollan SP, Markey KA, Benzimra JD, et al. A practical approach to, diagnosis, assessment and management of idiopathic intracranial hypertension. *Pract Neurol.* 2014;14(6):380–390.

Pareyson D, Fancellu R, Mariotti C, et al. Adult-onset Alexander disease: a series of eleven unrelated cases with review of the literature. *Brain.* 2008;131:2321–2331.

Shah VA, Yang GS, Smith R, Lee AG. Neurological picture. Intracranial hypertension after unilateral neck dissection. *J Neurol Neurosurg Psychiatry.* 2007;78:403–404.

Shin RK, Qureshi RA, Harris NR, et al. Wilbrand knee. *Neurology.* 2014;82:459–460.

Vucic S, Tian D, Chong PS, Cudkowicz ME, Hedley-Whyte ET, Cros D. Facial onset sensory and motor neuronopathy (FOSMN syndrome): a novel syndrome in neurology. *Brain.* 2006;129:3384–3390.

Walshe JM. The eye in Wilson's disease. *QJM.* 2011;104:451–453.

Wang Y, Huang YH, Yang SL. Ping-pong gaze and ocular nodding in bacterial meningitis. *Neurology* 2017;89(19):2021.

Weber KP, Landau K. Teaching NeuroImages: mind the gap! Postfixational blindness due to traumatic rupture of the optic chiasm. *Neurology.* 2013;80:e197–e198.

Williams A, Williams A, Austen D. The tilted disc syndrome. *Practical Neurol.* 2005;5:54–55.

Winston GP, Daga P, White MJ, et al. Preventing visual field deficits from neurosurgery. *Neurology.* 2014;83:604–611.

Chapter 3: Limbs and Trunk

Despite a creeping habit among neurologists not to have their patients undress, there are in fact many useful signs concealed by hats, scarves, stockings, trousers, and long sleeves that might allow an instant diagnosis.

As detailed in Chapter 1, the smart neurologist may have already made a basic assessment through the following observations:

- Watch the patient enter the consulting room for posture, turns, gait pattern, sitting, speech, and shaking your hand.
- Listen to their speech for volume (e.g., quiet in parkinsonism), nasality (sino-nasal disease, palatal weakness), clarity (indistinct in cerebellar and pyramidal lesions), fluency and language (impaired in various forms of dysphasia and dementia)

If the patient has not gone behind screens:

- *Watch your patient remove their socks.* This causes gentle plantar stimulation and may produce a patient-elicited extensor plantar response.
- *Discretely watch your patient undress and dress.* This might highlight a movement disorder or dressing apraxia, as there may be difficulty with fine movements such as undoing buttons or shoelaces, unbuckling a belt, removing/replacing a watch.
- *Observe the way a patient climbs onto the examination couch.* This can be instructive, especially where there is a question of malingering or fabrication of symptoms. For example:
   ▶ A patient with genuine weakness of a leg will use an arm to lift the weak limb onto (or off) the couch.
- *Undressing may reveal a problem with joints*—especially the shoulder or neck—and this may be relevant to the patient's complaints in the upper limb, such as cervical spondylosis or frozen shoulder.
- A frozen shoulder or low back pain is very common in Parkinson's disease, the

significance of which is so often appreciated only in retrospect. Note that it is frequently impossible to make an accurate assessment of muscle power if a nearby joint is painful.

What follows are a series of tips based on the history, simple inspection, and formal examination of the limbs. Inevitably, there will be some duplication of material here because of overlap with other chapters on specific diseases.

HANDLES AND FLAGS FROM THE HISTORY RELEVANT TO THE LIMBS

▶ Discomfort on standing, eased by walking is caused usually by orthostatic tremor, weak plantar flexion, parkinsonism, or restless legs syndrome.

In orthostatic tremor there is a rapid (~16 Hz) tremor that may be felt by placing the hands on the thighs or listening with a stethoscope for a "helicopter" sound over the patella. Patients may fall forward when trying to wash their face in a sink (wash basin sign). They dislike standing in a line or queue. The diagnosis is clinched by surface electromyography (EMG).

▶ Plantar flexion weakness (sometimes with "knee-bopping" sign).

When the patient stands, weak calf muscles are unable to provide sufficient anti-gravity resistance, and the knees are flexed to compensate. The knees tend to give way intermittently—see Chapter 11 on peripheral neuropathy. Selective plantar-flexion weakness is unusual in peripheral neuropathy, but it is a recognized feature of distal hereditary motor neuropathy and dysferlin myopathy. The "knee bopping," which is due to fatiguing muscles, has to be distinguished from the asterixis (negative myoclonus) seen in postanoxic myoclonus. Parkinsonism and restless legs syndrome are described in Chapter 8, Movement Disorders.

▶ Intermittent, often asymmetric, tingling in the hands, feet, or face is usually caused by hyperventilation, primarily in women.

The clue is that the tingling is *intermittent*, lasting a few minutes to hours, whereas the paresthesias from demyelination or peripheral neuropathy are continuous.

▶ In panic disorder, the hands may be clenched; but they are not clenched in organic causes of hyperventilation, such as metabolic alkalosis.

Having the patient take deep, rapid breaths for 2 minutes often reproduces their symptoms.

▶ If the *fingers* of both hands tingle, first suspect carpal tunnel syndrome (CTS). Note that if the *palms* tingle, CTS is excluded because the median nerve branch to the palm does not traverse the carpal tunnel. Suspect cervical spinal stenosis at C4 and C5.

◀ Be aware that circumoral tingling is seen in metabolic or ischemic disorders, such as:
  ○ Hypoglycemia
  ○ Hypocalcemia
  ○ Ciguatera poisoning
  ○ Brainstem transient ischemic attack (TIA) (older patients)
  ○ Lambert-Eaton myasthenic syndrome
  ○ Medication-induced alkalosis

Recurrent or continual distal tingling is recognized in patients receiving carbonic anhydrase inhibitors, such as acetazolamide or topiramate, in the treatment of idiopathic intracranial hypertension (acetazolamide), epilepsy, or migraine (topiramate).

▶ A patient who does not report tingling when prescribed acetazolamide is probably not taking it.

The most complex patients are those with true peripheral sensory loss with superimposed hyperventilation, say, from fear of multiple sclerosis (MS). It is wise to ask whether the tingling disappears completely or whether the intensity varies but never goes completely.

▶ Hyperemesis gravidarum with distal tingling is usually caused by thiamine deficiency.
It is very important to identify this disorder as it is easily treatable, but it becomes irreversible if therapy is delayed. The usual misdiagnosis is MS.

Shooting Leg Pains

If the pain shoots down the lower limb from the back, do not diagnose a prolapsed disk immediately.

▶ Usually, pain from an L5 or S1 radiculopathy spreads down to the foot. L5 lesions radiate from the hip into the great toe; S1 lesions spread from the buttock to the heel.

▶ If the pain stops short at the knee, then this is more characteristic of facet joint pathology or occasionally "wallet neuropathy." The latter results from compression on the posterior cutaneous nerve or sciatic nerve when sitting.

▶ Pain at right angles to the limb axis is a classic sign of tabes dorsalis.

▶ Longitudinal shooting pain in the absence of spondylotic lumbar radiculopathy suggests painful peripheral neuropathy due to any of the following:
  ○ Diabetes
  ○ Alcohol
  ○ Amyloid
  ○ Porphyria
  ○ Fabry's disease

▶ Allodynia so severe that any form of contact for physical examination is impossible points to Fabry's disease or severe alcoholic polyneuropathy. See Chapter 11.

▶ Neck pain and altered sensation on the ipsilateral half of the tongue provoked by head turning is the *neck-tongue syndrome*.
It is thought to result from stretching of lingual afferent nerve fibers traveling in the hypoglossal nerve to the C2 spinal roots. There are sometimes writhing tongue movements as well.

▶ Match-striking difficulty in a teenager because both hands move in the same direction suggests mirror movements and usually indicates
  ○ Klippel-Feil syndrome
  ○ Kallmann's syndrome
  ○ Cervical spondylosis (older patients)

Shower Signs

Marty Samuels, Professor of Neurology at the Brigham and Women's Hospital, Boston, describes the slippery surface of the shower cubicle as a

Romberg machine! The environment is potentially challenging, and history-taking may elicit some of the following:

- *Panic attack.* The shower is a confined space and may evoke tingling around the mouth, fingers, or toes.
- *Self-induced Romberg sign.* Shutting the eyes will remove visual compensation if there is impaired joint position sense.
- *Uhthoff's sign.* Increased body temperature may induce or aggravate symptoms such as numbness, fatigue, weakness, visual impairment, or limb incoordination, and it is characteristic of MS. The weakness of myasthenia gravis may also be aggravated by warmth.
- *Lhermitte phenomenon.* This is provoked by neck flexion and likewise very characteristic of MS and other cervical disorders. The reversed Lhermitte sign is provoked by neck extension (see Chapter 4, Demyelination).
- *Extracranial arterial dissection* induced by neck extension.
- *Imbalance or falling* due to peripheral or central vestibular dysfunction.
- *Impairment of consciousness* from presyncope induced by heat, pain, emotion, or micturition. There may be a rare variety of reflex seizure:- *Water-induced epilepsy*

FUNCTIONAL DISORDERS

In this section, we present a list of warning signs to alert you of the possibility of psychogenic disease. Some say that psychogenic disorder affects mostly those younger than 40 but should only be diagnosed by doctors older than 40!

There are several Red Flags and Handles related to movement disorders; they are discussed in more detail Chapter 8 (Movement Disorders). Never forget that your patient may be suffering from more than one condition (Hickam's dictum). Thus, someone with a physical problem may have superimposed psychogenic symptoms or signs, probably because they are extremely concerned about what is wrong.

- ▶ Use of dark glasses when indoors.
  This is usually unnecessary unless the patient is suffering a migraine attack or has chronic photophobia from, for example, optic neuritis.
- ▶ Adult who clutches a cuddly toy

- ▶ The over-friendly patient
  This refers to someone who usually has no important physical disease but is very familiar with the "system" and has been to multiple clinics. Typically, after shaking your hand, the patient asks how *you* are, talks about the weather, and settles into the chair for a long conversation. Such patients appear to derive satisfaction from the attention received at multiple clinics and perhaps take pride in or even boast of having symptoms that mystify their doctors. They rarely have anything seriously wrong.
- ▶ Effortful or sighing response during neurological examination
  This is the "huffing and puffing" sign. It implies that the patient is stressed or depressed or both.
- ▶ Use of inappropriate or revealing underwear
- ▶ Overly solicitous family members.
  Typically, there are several family members or friends accompanying the patient, who has multiple symptoms. Everyone is talking, sometimes at once, questioning your diagnosis or asking for more opinions and investigations. We suggest you heed their requests for investigation but try to refer to another doctor for a second opinion. The situation usually requires firm handling from a senior colleague.
- ▶ Adult still living with parents. This is not diagnostic of functional disease but should alert you to its presence
- ▶ The patient with back pain who prefers to stand during consultation usually has no important physical disease.
  The patient may be malingering if there is litigation. One of the authors treated such a patient who fooled everyone right up to the time of the court hearing, where he stood in the witness box in apparent agony, supporting himself on two elbow crutches. His case collapsed when normal mobility was shown by video surveillance. Despite this, you should be aware that sacroiliac pain is classically lessened by standing and worsened by sitting and lying. Also, some patients with free lumbar disk fragments prefer to stand.
- ▶ Mattress on the floor usually indicates pseudo-seizures (Figure 3.1)
- ▶ Slippers sign (Figure 3.2)

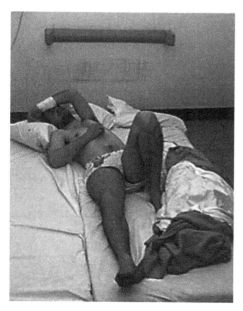

FIGURE 3.1: Mattress on the floor sign. In this instance the nurses reported that the "fits" were so severe it took several people to restrain the patient from injury and that he had to be placed on the floor for his own safety. Some severely affected, usually institutionalized, epileptic patients may require such care.

► Dragging gait pattern

In a genuine spastic hemiparesis, the patient walks with the foot plantar-flexed and inverted to varying degrees. To overcome the plantar-flexion, most patients rock the pelvis toward the good side and circumduct the affected limb at the hip to reduce floor contact by the plantar-flexed foot. If the weakness is functional, the foot is dragged along passively and there is no attempt to lift the foot clear of the floor by tilting the pelvis. Some patients adopt a skating pattern of walking in which they push one foot in front (Video 3.1, Psychogenic Gait). Other patients display violent lurching, rarely with falls, unless it is into the arms of an attendant

► Weakness in a nonpyramidal pattern

In a genuine upper motor neuron disorder, the "anti-gravity" muscles are strongest, probably because they are more powerful in healthy people. Thus, in the arms, the weak muscles are deltoid, triceps, supinators, wrist and finger extension, and dorsal interossei (abducting). In the lower limbs, the weaker muscles are flexors and abductors of the hip, knee flexors, and dorsiflexors and evertors of the ankle. If you have time and patience plus a

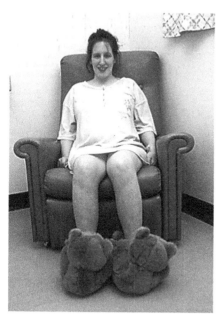

FIGURE 3.2: The slippers sign. Patients with "functional" disease sometimes prefer enormous slippers, often with an animal motif. This young woman had nonepileptic attacks connected to major social problems. There were no abnormal neurological signs.

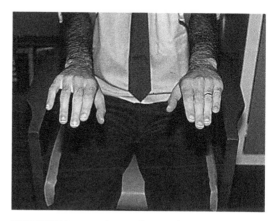

FIGURE 3.3: Myelopathy (Souques) hand sign. Note passive abduction of the fourth and fifth fingers in the right hand. This is a sign of corticospinal tract involvement, typically in the neck, but it occurs anywhere along the corticospinal tract and is seen in hemiplegia. It was described first by Souques in 1907. Ulnar nerve palsy can look like this but brief examination should distinguish the two.

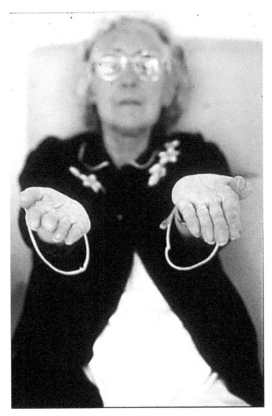

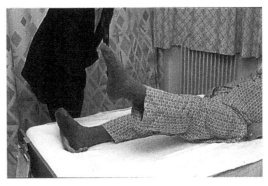

FIGURE 3.5: Hoover's sign. This is a useful way of detecting simulated lower limb weakness. The patient here is being asked to elevate the left leg. If there is genuine weakness there is involuntary downward pressure on the opposite (right) heel. If there is no such pressure, then the weakness is probably simulated.

FIGURE 3.4: Pronator sign in right arm. This is a classic sign of a corticospinal lesion. Note slight flexion at the elbow and possible adduction at the shoulder. Passive pronation is the most sensitive change and of great value in detecting simulated weakness where the arm usually drifts down without pronation.

cooperative patient, deviations of this pattern may be detected. As indicated later in this section, it is much easier to check for:

- o Passive finger abduction and pronator drift (Figures 3.3 and 3.4), as in genuine weakness
- o Passive vertical downward drift of the supinated outstretched arm without pronation, as in simulated weakness
- o Sudden "giving way" of muscles, as in psychogenic weakness

▶ Patients with a weak lower limb will usually need to lift it up when climbing onto the couch. In psychogenic weakness, this is not done (unless the patient is very sophisticated), but there is apparent weakness on formal testing. This is where the test described next—Hoover's sign—becomes so valuable.

▶ Hoover's sign
If you are suspicious about the validity of a patient's leg weakness, perform Hoover's

test, as shown in Figure 3.5. If the weakness is real, there will be involuntary hip extension on the opposite side that can be felt by placing your palm underneath the heel.

▶ All passive limb movements appear painful and associated with histrionic behavior.

HANDLES BASED ON SIMPLE INSPECTION OF LIMBS AND TRUNK

Upper Limbs

A really fast way to examine the arms is to ask patients to perform the following tests in sequence while you observe:

1. Myelopathy hand sign ("Souques sign"). Hold arms, fully extended straight out in front, palms down (Figure 3.3). The fourth and fifth fingers tend to abduct passively. This is really a feature of pyramidal tract dysfunction rather than specific for the spinal cord.
2. With the arms still extended and palms down, ask patients to spread out the fingers (Figure 3.6). Look for hyperextension at the metacarpophalangeal joints, a sign which usually indicates hypotonia, as in cerebellar disorder and chorea. It is most useful when asymmetric, because some healthy individuals (e.g., Asians) have hypermobile joints.
3. Ask patients to turn the arms, still fully extended, palm up and look for the pronator sign (Figure 3.4). Here the forearm pronates

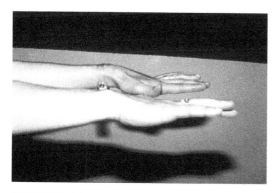

FIGURE 3.6: Asymmetric hyperextension. The patient is abducting all fingers. Note hyperextension at the left metacarpophalangeal joint. If this is asymmetric, it usually means hypotonia on the hyperextended side. Thus, it is found in cerebellar disorders and chorea. Symmetric hyperextension is common in Asians so the sign is not specific, but symmetric hyperextension may indicate generalized ligamentous laxity, and you should think of Ehlers-Danlos or Marfan's syndromes.

and there may be mild elbow flexion as well. This is a hallmark of a corticospinal lesion.

Camptodactyly (Figure 3.7) has superficial resemblance to an ulnar nerve lesion, but there is no weakness, sensory loss, or abnormality of neurophysiological tests.

In clinodactyly (Figure 3.8), the little finger is curved and short and there is no flexion deformity. Ectrodactyly is a more severe hand deformity shown in Figure 3.9.

Unidigital Clubbing

This means clubbing of just one fingernail (see Chapter 1, Figure 1.1b). It is characteristic of sarcoidosis, aortic aneurysm, brachial plexus, or median nerve lesions and gout.

Starfish Hand

Here the fingers are fully abducted and hyperextended at the metacarpophalangeal joints as a result of severe dystonia (see Figure 3.10).

Short Fourth Metatarsal Bone

The main cause of this is Refsum's disease (Figure 3.11). There are a few alternative associations:

- Pseudohypoparathyroidism
- Albright's hereditary osteodystrophy
- Turner syndrome: the fourth and fifth metatarsal bones and some of the metacarpal bones may be short.

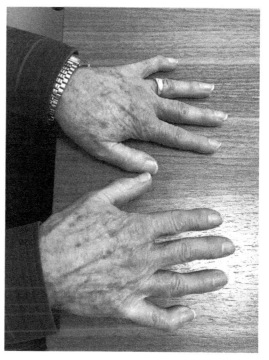

FIGURE 3.7: Camptodactyly. Literally this means "bent finger." Remember the similar term *camptocormia*, which means "bent spine." In camptodactyly there is, from birth, a fixed flexion deformity affecting the interphalangeal joints of (usually) the fifth finger. Shown here is clawing of the little fingers. It is benign and unilateral, mainly affecting women. There may be superficial resemblance to an ulnar palsy. It can be a useful Handle for the maternal myasthenic syndrome (Chapter 7), Schwartz-Jampel syndrome (Chapter 7), and Smith-Lemli-Opitz syndrome in which the index finger overlaps and patients have low cholesterol, cerebellar hypoplasia, and dystonia. Reproduced from Figure 9.6A in the chapter The Hands, by W Reardon. Oxford University Press. DOI:10.1093/med/9780195300451.003.0009.

Charcot Joint

This is a painless, grossly deformed joint (typically the ankle, shoulder, or elbow) consequent upon severe loss of joint sensation (Figure 3.12). The usual causes are:

- Diabetes
- Syringomyelia
- Leprosy
- Tabes dorsalis
- Rare causes are congenital insensitivity to pain and alcoholic polyneuropathy.

Patients with Marfan's syndrome (Figure 3.13) are liable to have the following traits:

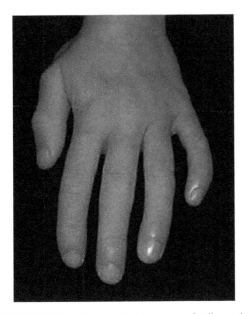

FIGURE 3.8: Clinodactyly. This is superficially similar to and easily confused with camptodactyly. In clinodactyly the little finger is curved in the horizontal plane like a letter C and is slightly shortened. In contrast to camptodactyly there is minimal flexion at the interphalangeal joints. It is found as an isolated phenomenon but also in various congenital disorders such as Down syndrome and Russell-Silver syndrome. Reproduced from Figure 9.4 in the chapter The Hands, by W Reardon. Oxford University Press. DOI:10.1093/med/ 9780195300451.003.0009.

- Upward lens dislocation
- Cardiac arrhythmias
- Prolapsing mitral valve and dilated aorta
- Spontaneous pneumothorax
- Orthostatic headache from dural tear or exertion.

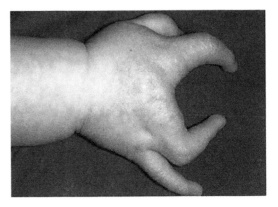

FIGURE 3.9: Ectrodactyly. Shown here is a typical "lobster-claw" malformation of the rare autosomal-dominant ectrodactyly, ectodermal dysplasia, and clefting (EEC) syndrome. There is camptodactyly of the digits on either side of the cleft. It is associated with progressive visual problems mostly due to corneal lesions. Reproduced from Figure 9.11 in the chapter The Hands, by W Reardon. Oxford University Press. DOI:10.1093/med/9780195300451.003.0009.

In the similar disorder of homocystinuria (Figure 3.14 (discussed later in the chapter), the lens is displaced downward. Many individuals with Marfan's syndrome are diagnosed late in life despite the apparently obvious phenotype.

Skin Abnormalities of Relevance to Neurological Diagnosis

Some skin abnormalities relevant to neurological diagnosis are shown in Figures 3.15–3.25.

Livedo Reticularis

The main diseases associated with livedo reticularis (Figure 3.20) are

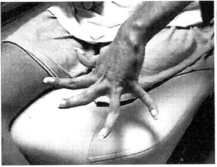
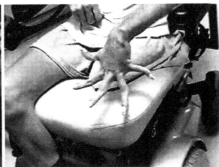

FIGURE 3.10: Starfish hand. This is basically a dystonic hand which, in this instance, followed a right middle cerebral artery stroke that involved the caudate nucleus. Reproduced with permission from Ho et al. (2007), Figure 1.

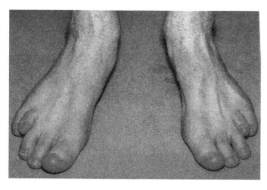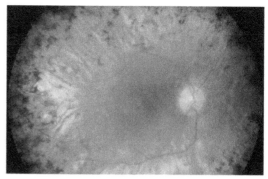

FIGURE 3.11: Refsum's syndrome. **Left**: Shortening of the fourth metatarsal bone. The fourth metacarpal bone in the hand is sometimes abnormally short as well. **Right**: Retinitis pigmentosa. If there is anosmia then the number one diagnosis is Refsum's disease. Left photo reproduced with permission from *Atlas of Clinical Neurology*, 2nd ed., GD Perkin, FH Hochberg, and DC Miller, Figure 2.12. Mosby Year Book Europe Ltd. Right image reproduced with permission from *Training in Ophthalmology*, Figure 4.44, in the chapter Medical Retina, by B Patil and P Puri. Oxford University Press. DOI:10.1093/med/9780199237593.003.0004.

- Autoimmune vasculitis (e.g., polyarteritis, lupus, phospholipid antibody syndrome)
- Dermatomyositis (Figure 3.16)
- Lymphoma
- Dopaminergic medication (e.g., amantadine and levodopa)
- Sneddon's syndrome
- Cryoglobulinemia
- Polycythemia rubra vera

Erythema Nodosum

Disorders of neurological relevance associated with erythema nodosum are as follows:

- Behçet's disease
- Rheumatoid arthritis

- Infection: TB, cat scratch disease, lepromatous leprosy (Figure 3.21), fungal or streptococcal throat infection
- Sarcoidosis (Figure 3.22)
- Crohn's disease
- Reaction to sulfonamide medication

HANDLES AND FLAGS ON FORMAL EXAMINATION

At this point, you will have inspected as much as possible and performed some very basic assessments of tone and involuntary movement. While it is not within the scope of this book to repeat the formal examination techniques, here are some useful tips and short-cuts.

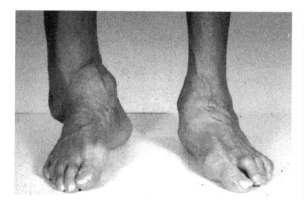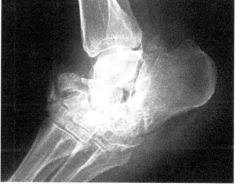

FIGURE 3.12: Charcot joint. **Left**: This was associated with gross deformity of the right ankle joint without pain. The usual causes are diabetes, syringomyelia, leprosy, and tabes dorsalis. Rare causes are congenital insensitivity to pain and alcoholic polyneuropathy. **Right**: Ankle X-ray of Charcot joint from another patient shows marked deformity of the joint. The shoulder and elbow joints may be affected as well. Left image reproduced with permission from *Atlas of Clinical Neurology*, 2nd ed., GD Perkin, FH Hochberg, and DC Miller, Figure 11.51. Mosby Year Book Europe Ltd.

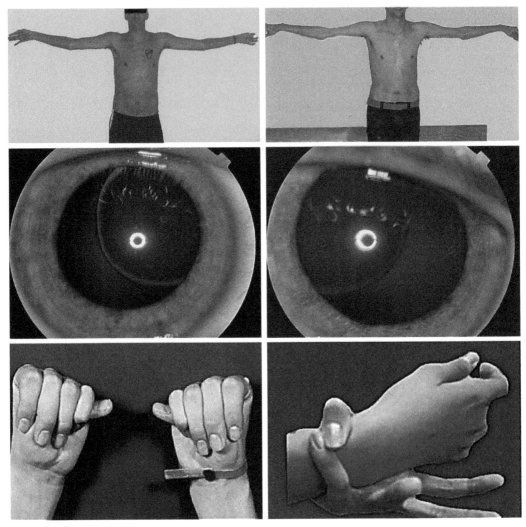

FIGURE 3.13: Marfan syndrome. **Top:** Note unusually long arms and pectus excavatum. **Center:** Dislocation of both lenses in an upward direction. Lower pictures show two tests of arachnodactyly. **Lower left:** Steinberg thumb sign where the entire thumbnail projects around the ulnar border of the hand. **Lower right:** Walker-Murdock wrist sign where the thumb and fifth finger overlap around the wrist. Top image reproduced with permission from Redruello et al. (2007), Figure 1a and 1b. Center image courtesy Dr. Irina Gout, Prince Charles Eye Unit, Windsor. Lower right image reproduced from Figure 52.6 in the chapter Marfan Syndrome, by NM Ammash and HM Connolly. Oxford University Press. DOI:10.1093/med/9780199915712.003.1056.

Motor Examination
Tone

We have mentioned already an indirect assessment of tone with the arms outstretched (Figures 3.3–3.4 and Figure 3.6)).

Another useful method for testing tone in the upper limb is for the examiner to undertake the following:

- Alternately pronate and supinate the patient's forearm. The forearm should be relaxed as much as possible. Try to flip the forearm from full pronation to full supination in one quick movement. A "catch" and release will be felt halfway through. Make sure the patient is not trying to "help" you with the test.

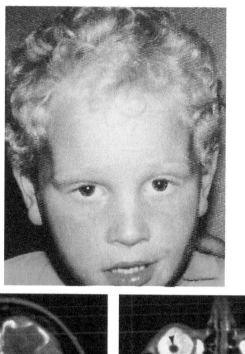

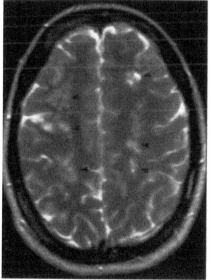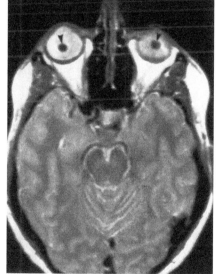

FIGURE 3.14: Homocystinuria. **Top**: Note the fine, silvery hair, blue eyes, pale complexion, and possible malar flush. **Bottom left**: Axial T2-weighted image shows multiple small focal areas of hyperintensity (arrowheads) in the centrum semiovale bilaterally. The risk of strokes (from arterial or venous occlusion) is increased. **Bottom right**: Axial proton density image shows both lenses (arrowheads) dislocated into the vitreous. Top image reproduced from *Clinical Ophthalmology*, J Kanski and B Bowling, Figure 9.31A. Elsevier Saunders, 2011. Lower figures reproduced with permission from Ruano et al. (1998), Figure 1a and 1b.

- Patients who appear to be helping you more than average, but often in the wrong direction, may have a frontal lobe problem. This can produce a false impression of increased tone, known as paratonic rigidity or *gegenhalten*.

In the lower limbs, a good way to evaluate tone is to grasp the limb at the knee and rock the relaxed limb from side to side (Figure 3.26). Others prefer to flip up the bent leg at the knee and observe the how quickly the leg descends.

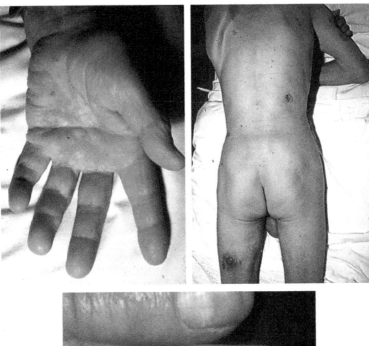

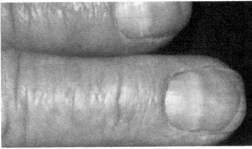

FIGURE 3.15: Arsenic poisoning. **Top:** Note the thickened scaly, yellow patches on the hands. Similar patches were present on the soles of his feet as well. This was an elderly epileptic patient who received arsenicals in the 1930s when they were used to treat refractory seizures. He developed a painful peripheral neuropathy some 20 years after discontinuing arsenicals. The lesions on the trunk and thigh are those of multiple squamous cell carcinomata—Bowen's disease—another recognized complication of chronic arsenic exposure. **Bottom:** A further clue to arsenic poisoning is the presence of horizontal white lines (Mees lines) in the nails. They are also seen with thallium poisoning. Note that arsenic is contained in some Ayurvedic medicines and skin cream for psoriasis.

Power

The formal methods are well known. For a short-cut in the upper limbs, ask patients to

- Pretend to play the piano while the arms are held outstretched and extended. This should be done with the forearm pronated after looking for the myelopathy hand sign. Rapid finger movements are a good test of the corticospinal tracts, as they are concerned with skilled movement.

In the lower limbs, request patient to

- Tap your hand with the ball of their foot (Figure 3.27)

Coordination

The best screening procedures in the upper limbs are:

- The finger–nose test
- Rapid alternating movement test: The patient is asked to pat their hand or thigh alternately with the dorsal and palmar surfaces of the hand as rapidly as possible.

An alternative, somewhat theatrical method, is to ask patients to tap rapidly on a desktop or similar hard surface so that you can hear the taps, which will be irregular in time and force if there is a cerebellar lesion. This is known as

- Listening to the cerebellum

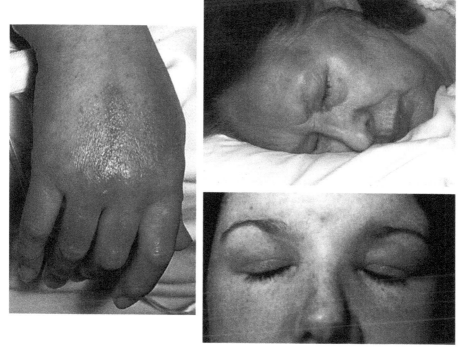

FIGURE 3.16: Dermatomyositis. **Left and top right**: A 63-year-old woman who presented acutely with a patchy rash over the hands. There was swelling of the whole hand, especially over the first metacarpophalangeal joints (Gottron's nodules), and painful proximal weakness of the shoulder and pelvic girdle. There is often a butterfly rash and purplish (heliotrope) discoloration of the eyelids. **Bottom right**: Dermatomyositis with heliotrope discoloration of eyelids. Left and top right images Courtesy John Pilling, Norwich. Bottom right image reproduced from Figure 19.7 in the chapter Rheumatology, by S Burge and D Wallis. Oxford University Press. DOI:10.1093/med/9780199558322.003.0019.

For lower limb coordination, the most useful procedure is the heel–shin test.

Muscle Stretch Reflexes

For those who have difficulty remembering the deep tendon reflex levels, here is the well-known

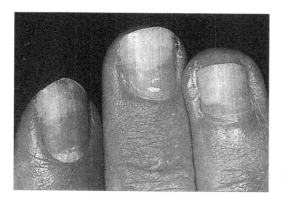

FIGURE 3.17: Plummer's nail in hyperthyroidism. This is caused by separation of the nail from the nail bed, thus allowing accumulation of dirt below the nail. Dirty elbows in an otherwise clean person are said to be typical of hyperthyroidism.

mnemonic. Note that there is considerable variability of root values in healthy people.

It requires you to count in pairs from 1 to 8.

- Sacral: 1 & 2. Ankle jerk
- Lumbar: 3 & 4. Knee jerk
- Cervical: 5 & 6. Biceps jerk
- Cervical: 7 & 8. Triceps jerk

There is no standard reflex for L5. Percussion of the medial hamstring muscle, which is supplied by L5, is favored by some clinicians although it requires practice (see later in this section).

Remembering myotome levels is more tedious. If you have learned the deep tendon reflex levels, then for the legs you need more information as follows (note: there is considerable normal variation in these levels and in specialists' opinions!):

- L2, L3: hip flexion; L4, L5: hip extension
- L3, L4: knee extension; L5, S1: Knee flexion
- L4, L5: ankle dorsiflexion; S1, S2: ankle plantar flexion

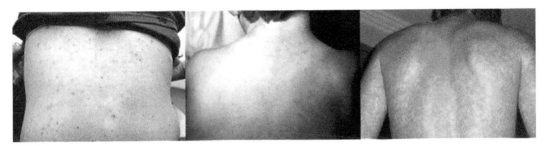

FIGURE 3.18: Erythematous macular or maculopapular rashes on the trunk and extremities are seen in infections with West Nile virus (A), enteroviruses (B), and Epstein-Barr virus (C). Reproduced with permission from Tsai et al. (2013), Figure 4.

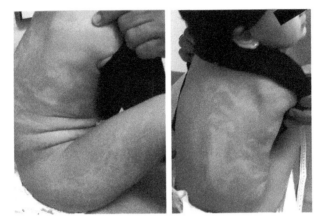

FIGURE 3.19: Unilateral hypopigmented whorled lesions following the lines of Blaschko, pathognomonic for hypomelanosis of Ito (incontinentia pigmenti achromians). This is a disorder of children who suffer from learning disability and seizures. Reproduced from Khaku et al. (2013).

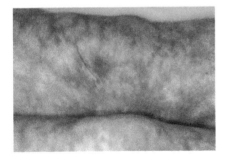

FIGURE 3.20: Livedo reticularis in systemic lupus erythematosus. Note the characteristic purple lace-like pattern due to distended medium-sized superficial veins in the skin. It may occur in healthy people. Reproduced from *OSH Paediatric Dermatology*, edited by S Lewis-Jones. Patterns, Shapes, and Distribution in Skin Disease, Figure 4.11. Oxford University Press DOI:10.1093/med/9780199208388.003.04.

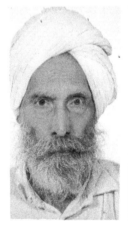
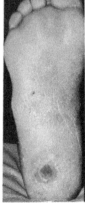

FIGURE 3.21: Leprosy. This Sikh man has a painless nonhealing foot ulcer most likely due to lepromatous peripheral neuropathy. Note that initially the sensory loss in the foot involves mainly the cooler skin of the dorsum of the foot and spares the skin of the sole until later stages. When pain and temperature sensations are lost on the sole, penetrating ulcers develop ("mal perforans") in areas sustaining the highest pressures, usually under the heel and metatarsal heads. Figure reproduced with permission from *A Colour Atlas of Clinical Neurology*, M Parsons. Mosby Year Book Europe, 1993.

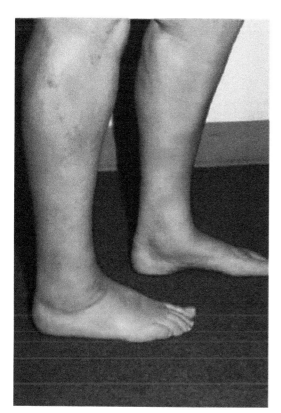

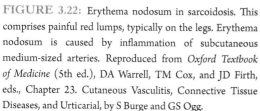

FIGURE 3.22: Erythema nodosum in sarcoidosis. This comprises painful red lumps, typically on the legs. Erythema nodosum is caused by inflammation of subcutaneous medium-sized arteries. Reproduced from *Oxford Textbook of Medicine* (5th ed.), DA Warrell, TM Cox, and JD Firth, eds., Chapter 23. Cutaneous Vasculitis, Connective Tissue Diseases, and Urticarial, by S Burge and GS Ogg.

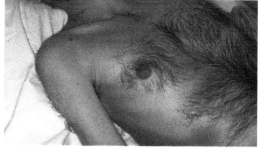

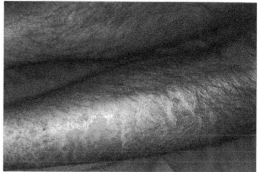

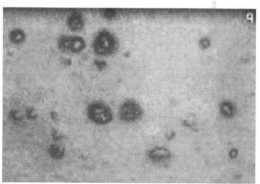

FIGURE 3.23: POEMS syndrome. Think of this syndrome if the patient has a polyneuropathy and hirsutism. (**top and center**). It stands for polyneuropathy, organomegaly, edema/endocrinopathy, M protein, and skin changes. Almost pathognomonic is the dark red cutaneous glomerular hemangioma. A pale red halo is characteristic (**bottom**). See also Figure 11.27. Figures reproduced courtesy of the Department of Internal Medicine, Lille Nord-de-France University, France.

▶ The medial hamstring jerk tests for L5. The examiner's fingers are percussed while they rest on the medial hamstring tendon. The patient must be sitting on the edge of the examination couch.

  Mnemonic: medial hamstring L5, lateral hamstring S1, lateral gastrocnemius S1, medial gastrocnemius S2. Alternatively: L5, S1, S1, S2. (Medial, Lateral, Lateral, Medial)

Also note:

▶ Inability to walk on heels: lesion of L5 or peroneal nerve
▶ Inability to walk on toes: lesion of S1 and S2

For the arms there is no easy mnemonic, but you will have already learned C5 and C6 for the biceps reflex and C7 and C8 for the triceps. So you have to remember the following:

▶ Most shoulder movements are C5 and C6, and the intrinsic hand muscles are C8 and T1.

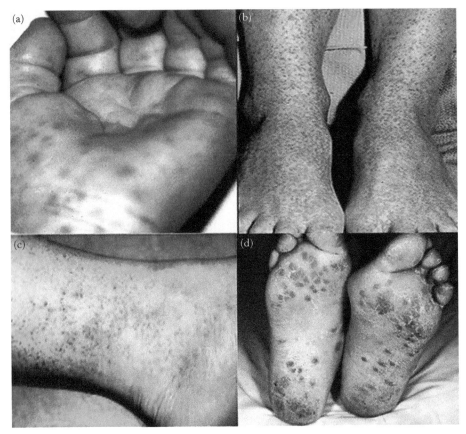

FIGURE 3.24: A macular or petechial rash with or without erythema is seen predominantly on the extremities and can become widespread in Rocky Mountain spotted fever (**A and B**), meningococcal meningitis (**C**), or secondary syphilis (**D**). In secondary syphilis the rash is typically bronze colored. Reproduced with permission from Tsai et al. (2013).

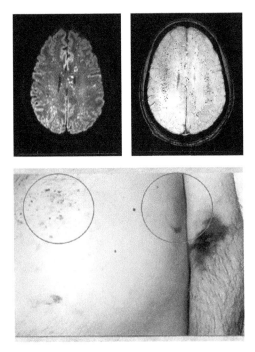

FIGURE 3.25: Fat embolism. **Top, Left**: diffusion weighted axial MRI. **Right**: SWI axial MRI to show "starfield pattern" due to bone marrow derived fat emboli in patient with sickle-cell disease. A similar pattern is seen in patients with fractured long bone. **Bottom**: Petechial skin changes due to emboli. Top image courtesy Karl Knights, Augusta. Bottom image reproduced with permission from Alex Rabinovich.

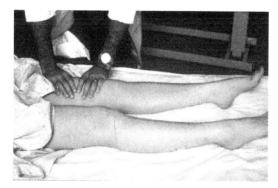

FIGURE 3.26: Testing lower limb tone by rocking the relaxed leg at the knee.

▶ There are no radial nerve–innervated intrinsic hand muscles.

▶ Finger extensors are primarily C7 and C8.

▶ Extensor carpi radialis is C5 and C6, but extensor carpi ulnaris is C7 and C8.

Some Handles have been mentioned already in the inspection section earlier in this chapter. Following are some additional tips.

The Easily Elicited Babinski Response

In some patients, it may be difficult to obtain a clear reaction to plantar stimulation because of withdrawal. In others, the toe elevates so easily that almost anyone can make the toe turn up, as shown in Figure 3. 28. This feature is characteristic of the following:

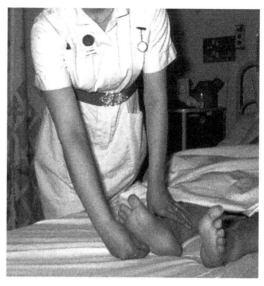

FIGURE 3.28: The easily elicited Babinski response. In some patients it may be difficult to obtain a clear reaction to plantar stimulation because of withdrawal. In others, the hallux dorsiflexes easily, as shown in the picture. This feature is characteristic of demyelinating disease, familial spastic paraplegia, HTLV-1 myelopathy, traumatic spinal cord section, and possibly radiation myelitis.

- Demyelinating disease
- Familial spastic paraplegia
- Traumatic spinal cord section
- Human T-lymphotrophic virus type 1 (HTLV-1) myelopathy
- Radiation myelitis?

Sensory Examination

This is the most tiresome part of the examination, for both you and your patient. A lot of information can still be obtained by omitting the various sensory modalities (pain, touch, joint position, etc.) and rubbing your fingers gently over affected areas of skin and asking: "Does this feel normal? Does it feel like the other side?"

You must have a rough idea of dermatome distribution; the classic map is shown in Figure 3.29. If you wish to screen the main dermatomes quickly, use "hot spots." These are areas where sensation should be normal if that dermatome is intact. It is easy to miss a sensory deficit because of overlap between adjacent dermatomes, but there is usually a small zone that belongs to just one dermatome; this we call a "hot spot," as shown in Figure 3.29. They can be useful if you wish to check for lumbar radiculopathy, say, from

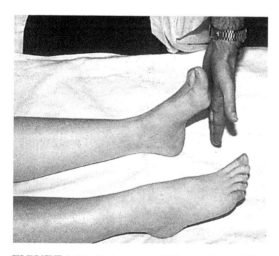

FIGURE 3.27: Testing pyramidal function by rapid foot tapping on the examiner's hand.

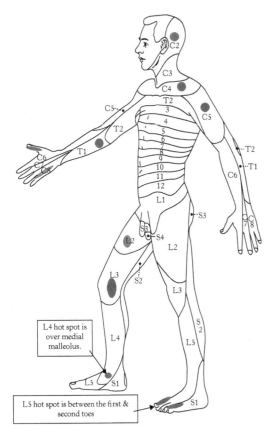

FIGURE 3.29: Dermatomes and "hot spots" shown in red. Note hot spots for the following: L4 is over the medial malleolus; L5 is between the first and second toes; S1 is over the little toe; L2 is over the medial thigh. Adapted from JK Wolk *Segmental Neurology*. Baltimore: University Park Press, 1981.

a prolapsed disk. In the lumbosacral area, the roots usually affected are L4, L5, and S1. To screen rapidly for this, check sensation over the medial malleolus (L4), interspace between hallux and second toe (L5), and dorsum of little toe (S1). The L5 hot spot is a real life-saver because, in the motor examination, the only muscle stretch reflex for L5 is the medial hamstring reflex (which is sometimes difficult), and you must rely on dorsiflexion of the great toe (L5).

Note that the hot spots do not distinguish a root lesion from a peripheral nerve disorder. Thus, the L4 hot spot over the medial malleolus could relate to a saphenous nerve problem.

Joint Position Sense

Most doctors test joint position sense (JPS) poorly. The term "proprioception" is not well-defined clinically and should be avoided. In a healthy young person, a movement of as little as 1 degree may be detected at the index finger and 3 degrees at the hallux. Make sure you grasp the digit at the sides and not by the dorsal and ventral surface, because in theory a patient may use other pathways (e.g., pressure sense) to detect the position of the digit, although they need to be pretty smart to do this. A major value of testing joint sense is to determine whether the large afferent fibers are affected. Thus:

▶ If a patient has glove-and-stocking sensory loss and JPS is spared, it is more likely to be a small fiber polyneuropathy.

▶ If JPS *is* affected, then the large fibers will be involved.

▶ Watch for the patient with extensive loss of joint position sense. Think of:
  ○ Vitamin B_{12} deficiency
  ○ Tabes dorsalis
  ○ Dorsal root ganglionitis, as in Sjögren's syndrome
  ○ Paraneoplastic disorders

Vibration Sense

In our view, this is not a particularly valuable part of the sensory examination, but if you wish to examine it, place the tuning fork on the distal phalanx of the index finger or the distal phalanx of the hallux. If vibration is felt at these levels, it will be normal elsewhere. It is impaired in most disorders of peripheral nerves but also, and paradoxically, in cortico-spinal tract lesions.

▶ If the sense of vibration continues for an unusually long time, that suggests demyelination.

▶ In pure corticospinal lesions, vibration sense is sometimes impaired when there is no evidence of peripheral nerve disorder.

Sensory Loss That "Splits" the Ring Finger

Classically, this is a sign of ulnar palsy if the medial side of the ring finger (and whole of the little finger) is numb. If digits 1–3 are numb and this extends to the *lateral aspect* of the ring finger, this characterizes a median nerve lesion.

Hemisensory Loss

Complete hemisensory loss is seen frequently in functional disorders (mainly on the nondominant side according to some), and a good discriminatory test is to place a tuning fork on either side of the forehead or sternum. There should, of course, be no difference between the two sides. Thus:

▶ A patient with simulated sensory impairment may claim that vibration feels different on the "numb" side of the sternum or forehead.

Hemisensory loss can be genuine; here are some Handles:

▶ Hemisensory loss that *spares* the trunk is frequent in stroke patients and implies a cortical or "parathalamic" lesion, probably because of the smaller area of cortical representation for trunk fibers.
▶ Hemisensory loss that *involves* the trunk is likely to be a lesion of the thalamus or its major afferents in the brainstem.
▶ Loss of axillary sensation probably indicates a lesion of the thalamus even if trunk sensation is normal.

Thickened Peripheral Nerves

The best places to palpate are over the ulnar groove at the elbow, the side of the neck for the great auricular nerve, at the wrist for the median nerve, dorsum of wrist and hand for radial nerve, and over the outer aspect of the fibular head for the common peroneal nerve. The main causes are listed in Chapter 11, but really, there are too many to qualify as a powerful Handle.

COMA

The unconscious patient is particularly challenging for a neurologist because there may be a sketchy history or none at all. Your initial assessment will depend greatly on the examination. If you have not done so already, you are strongly recommended to read *Plum and Posner's Diagnosis of Stupor and Coma* (Posner et al. 2007). What follows are the more useful bedside tests, assuming the patient is not intubated and has not been paralyzed with a neuromuscular blocker.

Smell the breath.
This may indicate:

- Alcohol excess
- Diabetic ketoacidotic coma with acetone smell
- Uremia with smell of urine
- Hepatic coma with odor of feces
- "Meth mouth" smell in a drug addict

Although the smell of alcohol may be relevant, in addition:

◀ There may be hepatic encephalopathy or a subdural hematoma that is deepening the level of unconsciousness. Remember that alcoholics when drunk fall over, injuring the head and limbs and thus creating multiple pathologies: subdural, extradural, and intracerebral hemorrhage; fat embolism from fractured femur (Figure 3.25).

Look at the skin.
- Cyanosis suggests a cardiac or respiratory problem.
- Bright red skin (cherry-red lips and cheeks) is typical of carbon monoxide (CO) poisoning (Figure 3.30, *left*). Watch out for the patient who lives in a mobile home or similar abode who is admitted with confusion. This may be CO poisoning from a faulty gas heater.
- Apart from the smell of breath, an alcoholic may be identified by the presence of spider nevi over the face and trunk (Figure 3.30, *right*).

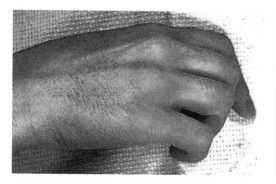 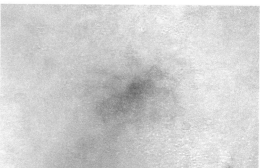

FIGURE 3.30: **Left**: Cherry-red skin discoloration in CO poisoning. **Right**: A spider nevus typical of hepatic cirrhosis.

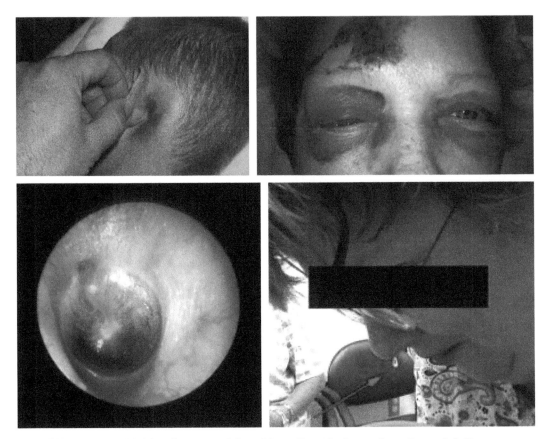

FIGURE 3.31: Signs of skull base fracture. **Top left**: Battle's sign. **Top right**: "raccoon" eyes. **Bottom left**: Hemotympanum. **Bottom right**: CSF rhinorrhea (red arrow). Top images reproduced with permission from Tarolli et al. (2014), Figure 1.

- Look for evidence of skull base fracture, manifest as bruising behind the ear (Battle's sign) or around the eyes (raccoon eyes), or blood behind the ear drum (hemotympanum) or cerebrospinal fluid leak from the nose or ear (Figure 3.31).
- Hemorrhage in the sclera or conjunctiva suggests thrombotic thrombocytopenic purpura. Patients are comatose because of widespread deep hemorrhages or infarcts in the cerebral hemispheres.
- Burn marks on the lip mucosa but not the skin of the lip itself suggest attempted suicide by drinking corrosive poison such as Lysol.
- Petechial rash associated with bone trauma points to fat embolism (Figure 3.25).
- Massive petechiae and ecchymoses suggest meningococcal septicemia.
- Excess sweating points to hypoglycemia or hypovolemic shock.

Observe the position of limbs and note the type of breathing.

- A hemiparetic lower limb is externally rotated, mimicking hip fracture.
- Hemiparesis can be detected by lifting the limb and allowing it to fall. More rapid decline on one side suggests weakness.
- Observe the breathing pattern: Slow breathing favors opiate or barbiturate poisoning. Deep rapid breathing (Kussmaul respiration) implies acidosis or pneumonia. Cheyne-Stokes breathing is typical of cortical lesions; it is less frequent in brainstem disorders.

Observe response to pain.

- Tickling the inside of the nose with cotton wool is very alerting; this involves the same pathway as pain.

- If there is no response, use pressure on the nail bed or finger pressure over the supraorbital ridge.
- Those in apparent coma may be *locked-in*; that is, they are quadriplegic from bilateral pyramidal tract lesions (usually ventral pontine vascular) but the midbrain is spared so that consciousness and pupillary reflexes (which are both midbrain functions) are preserved. Ask such patients to blink, close, or move their eyes to signal if pain is felt.
- Purposeful withdrawal to pain suggests light coma.

- Upper limb flexion and leg extension to pain is the "decorticate" response, localizing to the opposite cerebral hemisphere.
- Arm *and* leg extension following pain is the decerebrate posture and suggests brainstem involvement.
- Flex the head. If there is no neck trauma and Kernig's sign is positive, then neck stiffness points to meningitis or subarachnoid hemorrhage. Absence of Kernig's sign suggests raised intracranial pressure. Head flexion may elicit pain and a ciliospinal reflex, whereby both pupils dilate. Impaired pupillary dilation on one side localizes the lesion to the same side of the brainstem (Figure 3.32).

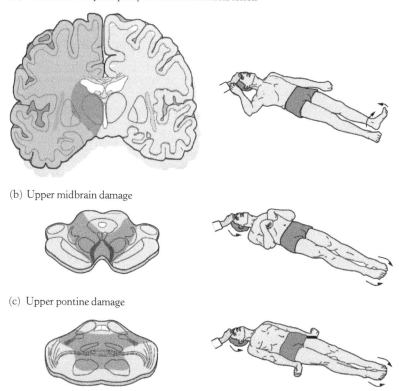

(a) Metabolic encephalopathy or unilateral cortical lesion

(b) Upper midbrain damage

(c) Upper pontine damage

FIGURE 3.32: Motor responses to noxious stimulation in patients with acute cerebral dysfunction. Approximate levels of associated brain dysfunction are indicated on left. Patients with unilateral forebrain or diencephalic lesions (**A**) often have a hemiparesis but can generally make purposeful movements with the opposite side. Lesions involving the junction of the diencephalon and the midbrain (**B**) may show decorticate posturing, including flexion of the upper extremities and extension of the lower extremities. As the process descends into the pons, there is generally a shift to decerebrate positioning (**C**), in which there is extension of both upper and lower extremities. Reproduced from Figure 2.10 in *Plum and Posner's Diagnosis of Coma and Stupor*, 4th ed., J Posner, CB Saper, N Schiff, and F Plum. Oxford University Press, 2007.

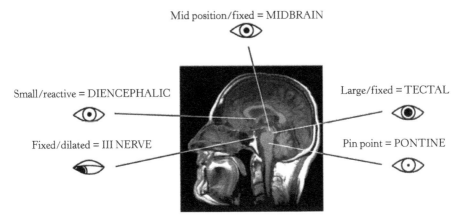

FIGURE 3.33: Summary of pupillary abnormalities in coma. Note: in metabolic coma, the pupils are small and reactive. Reproduced with permission from Bateman (2001).

Check pupils (Figure 3.33).

Inspect shape, size, and reactions to light.

- Unilateral, large unreactive pupil suggests pressure on the oculomotor nerve from tentorial herniation.
- Large pupils unreactive to light is likely a near terminal event from hypoxia, as long as anticholinergic medication such as atropine

has not been given (therapeutically or as an overdose).
- Both pupils pinpoint suggests a dorsal pontine/midbrain lesion or exposure to opiates.
- Coma with normal pupillary light reflexes has a metabolic cause, whereas coma with unresponsive pupils is either structural in origin (e.g., space-occupying lesion) or related to acute hydrocephalus.

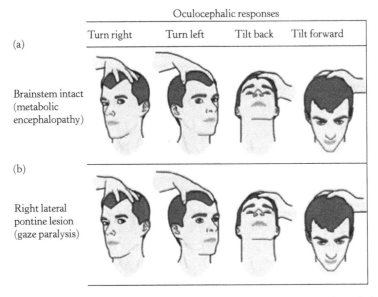

FIGURE 3.34: Ocular reflexes in unconscious patients. These movements should only be performed after the possibility of cervical spine injury has been eliminated. Normal VOR in a patient with metabolic encephalopathy (e.g., hepatic) are illustrated in row (**A**). The patient shown in row (**B**) has a lesion of the right side of the pons, causing a paralysis of conjugate gaze to the patient's right side. Reproduced and modified from *Plum and Posner's Diagnosis of Coma and Stupor*, 4th ed., J Posner, CB Saper, N Schiff, and F Plum. Oxford University Press, 2007.

- Pupil eccentric or oval nearly always means a structural lesion, typically in the midbrain.

Doll's head eye movements (vestibular-oculocephalic reflexes [VOR]). Figure 3.34.

- These movements are absent in the awake person and in metabolic coma, except for hepatic coma, where they are overactive and associated with hyperventilation.
- They appear in light coma resulting from cortical lesions because the normal cortically derived suppression is lost.
- Vertical dolling in a comatose patient suggests that the dorsal midbrain is intact because the vertical gaze center is preserved.
- Horizontal dolling in a comatose patient infers that the dorsal pons is functioning due to preservation of the horizontal gaze center.

If these passive eye movements are observed, further localization can be made (Figure 3.33).

Note:

▶ Horizontal roving eye movements are a feature of early coma and indicate that the brainstem is intact.

They cannot be mimicked in psychogenic coma, so they are a good sign of organic disease.

This information, in conjunction with pupillary reflexes, can be used to work out the level of a suspected brainstem lesion as follows:

▶ **With deepening coma, the brain fails in a top-down fashion:**
  - VOR that are initially brisk become increasingly difficult to elicit.
  - First, vertical dolling is lost due to midbrain failure.
  - Then the horizontal VOR are abolished due to pontine damage.

Ice-water caloric testing is of little clinical value other than in confirmation of suspected brain death.

SUMMARY

When the Patient Enters the Consulting Room

- Many useful signs are concealed by hats, scarves, stockings, trousers, and long sleeves.
- Watch the patient enter the consulting room for posture, turns, gait pattern, sitting, speech, and shaking your hand.
- Listen to their speech for volume, clarity, nasality, fluency, and language.
- Watch the patient remove their socks for possible self-induced Babinski sign.
- Discretely watch the patient undress. This may reveal movement disorder, dressing apraxia, or difficulty with fine movements.
- Observe how the patient climbs onto the examination table.
- A patient with genuine weakness of a leg will use an arm to lift up the weak limb.
- Undressing may reveal a problem with joints (relevant to spondylosis or Parkinson's disease).
- A frozen shoulder or low back pain is very common in Parkinson's disease.

History

- Discomfort on standing, eased by walking: orthostatic tremor, plantar flexion weakness, parkinsonism, restless legs syndrome
- Intermittent, often asymmetric tingling in hands and feet; hyperventilation, medication (acetazolamide, topiramate). Tightly clenched hands confirm panic disorder.
- If *fingers* of both hands tingle, suspect CTS. If the *palms* are included, suspect cervical spinal stenosis at C4 and 5.
- Intermittent circumoral paresthesia is usually caused by panic disorder. May relate to a metabolic problem (hypoglycemia, hypocalcemia), ciguatera poisoning, Lambert-Eaton myasthenic syndrome, brainstem TIA, medication-induced alkalosis
- Recurrent distal tingling is a side effect of carbonic anhydrase inhibitors such as acetazolamide or topiramate.
- A patient who does not report tingling when prescribed acetazolamide is probably not taking it.
- Hyperemesis gravidarum and distal tingling: thiamine deficiency
- Shooting leg pains: usually, L5 lesions radiate from the hip into the great toe; S1 lesions spread from the buttock to the heel.
- If the pain stops short at the knee, this is more characteristic of facet joint pathology or occasionally "wallet neuropathy." Here, the

posterior cutaneous nerve or sciatic nerve is compressed.

- Pain at right angles to the limb axis is a classic sign of tabes dorsalis.
- Longitudinal shooting pain suggests a small fiber polyneuropathy secondary to diabetes, alcohol, amyloid, porphyria, or Fabry's disease.
- Allodynia so severe that physical examination is not possible suggests advanced alcoholic polyneuropathy or Fabry's disease.
- Neck pain and altered sensation in the ipsilateral half of the tongue provoked by head turning: neck-tongue syndrome
- Match-striking difficult in a teenager: mirror movement from Klippel-Feil syndrome, Kallman's syndrome, or cervical spondylosis (older patients)
- Shower signs: panic attack, self-induced Romberg sign, Uhthoff's sign, classic or reversed Lhermitte signs, extracranial arterial dissection, vestibular dysfunction, faint, or water-induced epilepsy

Functional Disorders

See also Chapter 8 on movement disorders.

- Dark glasses when indoors
- Adult who clutches a cuddly toy or uses enormous animal slippers
- The over-friendly patient
- Effortful or sighing response during neurological examination
- Inappropriate or revealing underwear
- Overly solicitous family members
- Adult still living with parents
- The patient with back pain who prefers to stand during consultation (except for sacroiliac pain and those with free lumbar disk fragments)
- Mattress on the floor sign usually indicates pseudo-seizures
- Slippers sign
- Dragging gait pattern
- Weakness in a nonpyramidal pattern with sudden "give-way" on formal power testing or gradual downward drift without pronation. Check for pronator drift, passive finger abduction.

- A patient with a weak lower limb will usually need to lift it up when climbing onto the examination table.
- Hoover's sign
- All passive limb movements are reported to be painful and are associated with histrionic behavior.

Inspection of Limbs and Trunk

- Myelopathy hand sign (Souques sign, pyramidal), hyperextended fingers (hypotonia), pronator sign (pyramidal)
- Camptodactyly: flexion deformity of fifth finger that simulates ulnar nerve lesion. Seen in maternal myasthenic syndrome, Schwartz-Jampel syndrome, and Smith-Lemli-Opitz syndrome
- Clinodactyly: incurved fifth finger seen mainly in Down and Russell Silver syndromes
- Ectrodactyly as in the ectrodactyly, ectodermal dysplasia, and clefting (EEC) syndrome
- Unidigital clubbing suggests sarcoidosis, aortic aneurysm, brachial plexus, or median nerve lesions and gout.
- Starfish hand: dystonic hand, typically following a stroke affecting the caudate nucleus
- Short fourth metatarsal bone: Refsum's syndrome, pseudo-hypoparathyroidism, Albright's hereditary osteodystrophy, Turner syndrome
- Charcot joint: causes are diabetes, leprosy, syringomyelia, tabes dorsalis, congenital insensitivity to pain alcoholic neuropathy
- Marfan's syndrome: upward lens dislocation, hypermobile joints, arachnodactyly, cardiac arrhythmias, prolapsing mitral valve and dilated aorta, spontaneous pneumothorax, orthostatic headache
- Homocystinuria: fine, silvery hair and pale complexion, long fingers, lens displaces downward, increased risk of stroke

Skin Abnormalities

- Livedo reticularis: autoimmune vasculitis (e.g., polyarteritis, lupus, antiphospholipid syndrome), dermatomyositis, lymphoma, dopaminergic medication, Sneddon's syndrome, cryoglobulinemia, polycythemia rubra vera

- Erythema nodosum: Behçet's disease, rheumatoid arthritis, sarcoidosis, infections (TB, cat scratch disease, leprosy, fungal or streptococcal), Crohn's disease, and reaction to sulfonamide medication
- Arsenic poisoning: thickened scaly, yellow patches on the hands, Mees lines, painful peripheral neuropathy, multiple squamous cell carcinomata
- Dermatomyositis: patchy facial, knuckle, and elbow rash (Gottron's nodules), painful proximal weakness
- Plummer's nail in hyperthyroidism
- Erythematous macular or maculopapular rashes: West Nile virus, enterovirus, or Epstein-Barr virus
- Hypomelanosis of Ito: unilateral hypopigmented whorled lesions
- Non-healing, painless foot ulcer: leprosy, diabetes, or severe small fiber polyneuropathy
- POEMS syndrome: polyneuropathy, organomegaly, edema/endocrinopathy, M protein, and skin changes (hairy legs and cutaneous glomerular hemangioma)
- Macular or petechial rash on extremities: Rocky Mountain spotted fever, meningococcal meningitis, secondary syphilis (bronze rash on soles and palms)
- Fat embolism: widespread petechial skin lesions, multiple hyperintense punctate lesions on MRI (star-field pattern)

Handles and Flags on Formal Examination
Examination of the Motor System
- Tone: alternate pronation and supination for upper limb; rocking at knee or upward flip for lower limb
- Patients who appear to be helping you with tone testing by alternate pronation and supination, often in the wrong direction, may have a frontal lobe problem (paratonic rigidity or *gegenhalten*).
- Piano playing and foot tapping for indirect measurement of pyramidal function
- Limb coordination: finger–nose test, listening to the cerebellum, and heel–shin test.
- Deep tendon reflex levels: S1, S2 ankle; L3, L4 knee; C5, C6 biceps; C7, C8 triceps. For L5, percuss medial hamstring muscle.

- Myotome levels: Hip flexion/extension: L2 and L3 ; L4 and L5Knee extension/flexion: L3, L4; L5, S1. Ankle dorsiflexion/plantar-flexion: L4, L5; S1, S2.
- Most shoulder movements are C5 and C6, and the intrinsic hand muscles are C8 and T1. There are no radial nerve–innervated intrinsic hand muscles.
- Wrist extensors are C5 and C6. Finger extensors are primarily C7 and C8.
- Unable to walk on heels: lesion of L5 or peroneal nerve. Unable to walk on toes: lesion of S1 and S2
- The easily elicited Babinski response: demyelinating disease, familial spastic paraplegia, traumatic spinal cord section, HTLV-1 myelopathy, radiation myelitis?

Examination of the Sensory System
- Use hot spots.
- If a patient has glove-and-stocking sensory loss and JPS is spared, then it is more likely to be a small fiber polyneuropathy.
- If JPS *is* affected, then the large fibers will be involved.
- Watch for the patient with disproportionate loss of JPS. Think of vitamin B_{12} deficiency, tabes dorsalis, dorsal root ganglionitis (e.g., Sjögren's syndrome, paraneoplastic disorders).
- Place tuning fork on either side of the forehead or sternum to detect functional sensory loss.
- If the sense of vibration continues for an unusually long time, that suggests demyelination.
- In pure corticospinal lesions, vibration sense is sometimes impaired when there is no evidence of peripheral nerve disorder.
- Sensory loss that "splits" the ring finger: ulnar or median nerve lesion
- Hemisensory loss that *spares* the trunk is frequent in stroke patients and implies a cortical or "parathalamic" lesion.
- Hemisensory loss that *involves* the trunk is likely a lesion of the thalamus or its major connections.
- Loss of axillary sensation probably indicates a lesion of the thalamus even if trunk sensation is normal.

Coma

Smell the breath.

- Alcohol, acetone (diabetes), urine-like (uremia), feces (hepatic coma), meth mouth (drug addict). In alcoholics: may be hepatic encephalopathy or a subdural hematoma that is deepening the level of unconsciousness. Alcoholics when drunk fall over, injuring the head and limbs, thus creating multiple pathologies: subdural, extradural, and intracerebral hemorrhage; fat embolism

Look at the skin.

- Cyanosis: cardiac or respiratory problem
- Bright red skin: CO poisoning
- Alcoholics may have spider nevi over the face and trunk.
- Evidence of skull base fracture: Battle's sign, raccoon eyes, hemotympanum, or CSF leak from nose
- Hemorrhage in the sclera or conjunctiva: thrombotic thrombocytopenic purpura.
- Burn marks on the lip mucosa but not the skin of the lip: suicidal attempt by, for example, Lysol
- Petechial rash associated with bone trauma: fat embolism
- Massive petechiae and ecchymoses: meningococcal septicemia
- Excess sweating: hypoglycemia or hypovolemic shock

Observe the position of limbs and note the type of breathing.

- Hemiparetic lower limb is externally rotated, mimicking hip fracture Detect hemiparesis by lifting the limb and allowing it to fall.
- Slow breathing: opiate or barbiturate poisoning
- Deep rapid breathing: acidosis or pneumonia
- Cheyne-Stokes breathing: cortical lesions rather than brainstem disorders

Observe response to pain.

- Tickle the inside of the nose. Place pressure on the nail bed or finger, pressure over the supraorbital ridge.
- Locked-in state: apparent coma with quadriplegia. Pupillary reflexes are preserved and patient is conscious. Ask patient to blink or close the eyes to signal if pain is felt.
- Purposeful withdrawal to pain: light coma
- Limb flexion to pain: decorticate response localizing to the opposite cerebral hemisphere
- Arm and leg extension following pain: decerebrate posture; suggests brainstem involvement
- Flex the head. If no neck trauma, neck stiffness points to meningitis, subarachnoid hemorrhage, or raised intracranial pressure.
- Head flexion may elicit a ciliospinal reflex whereby the pupils dilate. Impaired pupillary dilation on one side localizes the lesion to the same side of the brainstem.

Check pupils.

- Inspect shape, size, and reactions to light.
- A unilateral large, unreactive pupil suggests pressure on CN III from tentorial herniation.
- Both pupils large and unreactive to light: near terminal event from hypoxia (as long as anticholinergic medication such as atropine has not been given)
- Both pupils pinpoint: probably dorsal pontine or midbrain lesion or exposure to opiates
- Coma with normal pupils has a metabolic cause; coma with unresponsive pupils is structural in origin or related to acute hydrocephalus.
- If pupil is eccentric or oval: structural lesion in midbrain

Doll's head eye movement (vestibular-oculocephalic reflexes [VOR])

- Absent in the awake person and in metabolic coma. Appears in light coma resulting from cortical lesions. In comatose patient with:

- Vertical dolling: intact dorsal midbrain
- Horizontal dolling: intact dorsal pons
- Horizontal roving eye movements suggest early coma with an intact brainstem and cannot be mimicked in psychogenic coma.

With deepening coma, brain dies in a top-down fashion:

VOR that are initially brisk become increasingly difficult to elicit. First, vertical dolling is lost, then the horizontal VOR.

SUGGESTED READING

Bateman DE. Neurological assessment of coma. *J Neurol Neurosurg Psychiatry.* 2001;71(Suppl 1):i13–i17.

Ho BK, Morgan JC, Sethi KD. "Starfish" hand. *Neurology.* 2007;69:115.

Khaku AS, Hedna VS, Nayak A. Teaching neuroimages: hypomelanosis of Ito. *Neurology.* 2013;80:e130.

Medeiros MO, Behrend C, King W, Sanders J, Kissel J, Ciafaloni E. Fat embolism syndrome in patients with Duchenne muscular dystrophy. *Neurology.* 2013;80:1350–1352.

Posner JB, Saper CB, Schiff N, Plum F. *Plum and Posner's diagnosis of stupor and coma,* 4th ed. New York: Oxford University Press, 2007.

Redruello HJ, Cianciulli TF, Rostello EF, et al. Monozygotic twins with Marfan's syndrome and ascending aortic aneurysm. *Eur J Echocardiogr.* 2007;8:302–306.

Ruano MM, Castillo M, Thompson JE. MR imaging in a patient with homocystinuria. *AJR Am J Roentgenol.* 1998;171:1147–1149.

Tarolli C, Scully MA, Smith AD. Teaching neuroimages: unmasking raccoon eyes—a classic clinical sign. *Neurology.* 2014;83:e58–e59.

Tsai J, Nagel MA, Gilden D. Skin rash in meningitis and meningoencephalitis. *Neurology.* 2013;80:1808–1811.

Chapter 4: Demyelination

The diagnosis of multiple sclerosis (MS) is reasonably straightforward, although we tend to remember instances where we made a diagnosis not suspected by others or where a provisional diagnosis of MS has turned out to be something else, such as phospholipid antibody syndrome, sarcoidosis, or neuromyelitis optica (NMO).

Neurologists used to rule out MS if the patient was of Afro-Caribbean or Asian origin. Indeed, this should still be regarded as a Red Flag, but if such a patient is born in the Western world, and particularly if they are second generation, then MS is an acceptable diagnosis provided the clinical profile and special tests are confirmatory. For further reading on difficult diagnoses, see Katz Sand and Lublin (2013).

HISTORY

Here are some early features of MS that are worth exploring when you take a history.

- ▶ Variation of symptoms according to body temperature or exercise is *Uhthoff's phenomenon.*

   Thus, a patient reports temporary weakness, fatigue, or worsening visual acuity after a hot bath, shower, exercise, or when the weather is hot. Importantly, the symptoms recover once body temperature reverts to normal. Temperature sensitivity is recognized also in:
   - ○ Peripheral nerve disorder, such as the peripheral neuropathy of diabetes that worsens with warmth in bed
   - ○ Myasthenia gravis

Thus, Uhthoff's sign is characteristic of central demyelination but not specific.

- ▶ Shock-like tingling induced by neck flexion spreading down the spine is *Lhermitte's phenomenon* and usually indicates cervical demyelination from MS.

The sensation may spread into the feet or down the arms. This may be a symptom noted by the patient on neck flexion. It may also be a *sign*; thus it is well worth testing by gently pushing the neck fully forward and asking whether there are appropriate symptoms. When positive, most often it indicates demyelination in the upper cervical spinal cord. There are a few rarer causes that you must be aware of, namely:
   - ○ Cervical spondylosis
   - ○ Vitamin B_{12} and copper deficiency
   - ○ Radiation myelitis
   - ○ Nitrous oxide poisoning
   - ○ Cervical cord tumor or trauma
   - ○ Syringomyelia
- ▶ Shock-like feeling on neck *extension* is the *reversed Lhermitte sign.*
   It is compatible with MS but probably more common in cervical spondylosis.
- ▶ Transient deterioration of arm (e.g., grip) or leg strength on neck flexion is *McArdle's sign.* Some patients prefer to walk with the neck extended to avoid this phenomenon. The cause may be conduction block in the pyramidal tracts or pressure on the cervical corticospinal tracts in those with spondylosis where there is narrowing of the cervical canal —both provoked by neck flexion.
- ▶ Symptom onset or relapse in puerperium
   It is unusual to have MS relapses during pregnancy (indeed, pregnancy appears to be relatively protective), but it is highly characteristic to experience a first attack or relapse in the puerperium. While systemic lupus erythematosus (SLE) and NMO tend to worsen toward the end of pregnancy, they also tend flare up more in the puerperium.
- ▶ Band-like numbness

Numbness that appears to compress the waist or trunk is characteristic; patients call this the "MS hug." Rarer causes include the following:
  o Vitamin B$_{12}$ deficiency
  o Arachnoiditis
  o Spinal tumor

▶ Useless hand syndrome
  See Video 4.1 (reproduced with permission from Kamogawa and Okuda, 2015). Here the patient complains that one hand is clumsy and that fine tasks cannot be performed. Usually it means a demyelinating plaque in the posterior columns at C2–C4 that causes deafferentation of the hand (or whole limb). Examination reveals severe loss of joint position sense (JPS) and pseudo-athetosis of the fingers, for example, when the arms are outstretched.

▶ Numbness in the vaginal or perineal area is usually due to MS.
  Rarely, it arises from a nonorganic disorder. Hemi-vaginal numbness is strongly suggestive of MS, and it is usually reported during intercourse.

▶ Paroxysmal sensory symptoms.
  The best recognized of these symptoms is *trigeminal neuralgia*. It is probably due to short-circuiting (i.e., ephaptic transmission) by a plaque at the trigeminal nerve root entry zone or its brainstem connections. It can be identical to the common variety seen in elderly patients. If your patient is a young adult who gives a good history of trigeminal neuralgia, then MS is a strong possibility. Lhermitte's phenomenon, as detailed earlier, could be viewed as a paroxysmal sensory symptom related to neck movement that provokes ephaptic transmission in the posterior columns.

▶ *Paroxysmal motor phenomena* affecting a limb, causing it to assume a dystonic position for a few minutes, is characteristic of MS. This includes:
  • Paroxysmal dystonia
  • Tonic spasms
  They may be unilateral and painful, often induced by hyperventilation, exercise, or sudden movement (Video 8.94, Demyelinating). Note that tonic spasms are more frequent in NMO than MS.

Other paroxysms consist of the following:

  • Speech arrest
  • Ataxia
  • Exercise-related dyskinesia
  • Itching

These episodic phenomena respond well to acetazolamide or carbamazepine.

▶ Early and persistent sphincter disturbances.
  In the early stages, such disturbances affect the bladder far more than the bowel and result in frequency, urgency, and nocturia, often refractory to treatment. Note that in amyotrophic lateral sclerosis (ALS), which occasionally simulates MS, the sphincters are hardly ever affected. The main exception is the primary lateral sclerosis variant.

▶ Painful optic neuritis (ON) suggests an intraorbital lesion.
  In typical ON, eye movement is unpleasant because it stretches a swollen optic nerve, evoking pain usually in the temple, sometimes causing flashes of light (phosphenes). If the lesion affects the *intracranial* part of the optic nerve or chiasm, there is usually no pain on turning the eye because there is no movement of the optic nerve.

▶ Eye pain is unusual in Leber disease but frequent in ON, NMO and chronic relapsing inflammatory optic neuropathy (CRION) (see Figure 4.1).
  A positive aquaporin-4 antibody will clinch a diagnosis of NMO and analysis of mitochondrial DNA will help with Leber's optic atrophy, but there are two further clues for Leber's disease that might assist while waiting for the genetic information:

▶ Peripapillary telangiectases
  These are corkscrew-shaped vessels around the disk margin (see Figure 4.2).

▶ Pupillary light reflexes *may be normal* even though visual acuity is reduced!
  This phenomenon may be due to relative sparing of the melanopsin-expressing retinal ganglion cells, which mediate the pupillary light response.

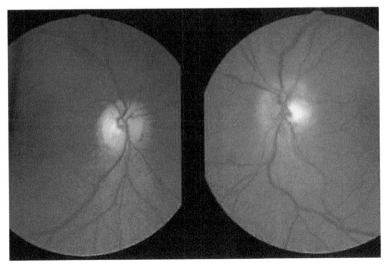

FIGURE 4.1: Fundus photograph from patient with CRION. **Left figure:** shows disk pallor. **Right figure:** shows disk swelling. Reproduced with permission from Kidd et al. (2003).

◄ When testing pupillary light reflexes, make sure you do not illuminate the contralateral eye and evoke a consensual response.

► Isolated dysgeusia.
  This is a rare presenting symptom of MS that relates to a lesion in the solitary tract (medulla), its ascending connections in the brainstem, or the thalamus (Combarros et al. 2000).

Red Flags in the Early Phase of Illness
◄ Consecutive ON (see also Chapter 2)
  This refers to ON in one eye followed by ON in the other eye after a period of days to months. In the elderly, *ischemic optic neuropathy* (arteritic or ischemic) is high on the checklist. In young and middle-aged adults, MS very rarely may be responsible. Apart from this, there are several alternative causes to be considered:

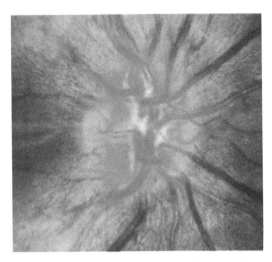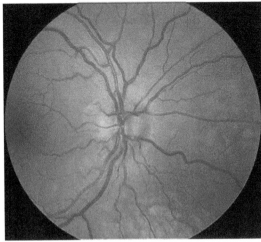

FIGURE 4.2: Leber's optic atrophy. **Left:** Acute changes. Note the dilated capillaries on the optic disk, swelling of the peripapillary nerve fiber layer, and distended tortuous vessels. **Right:** Subacute phase. Note the increased number of tortuous blood vessels near the disk, and peripapillary telangiectasias, an occasional phenomenon. Later the optic disk becomes pale.

- NMO (Devic's disease)
- Leber's optic neuropathy
- Neuroretinitis
- Myelin oligodendrocyte glycoprotein (MOG) antibody disease
- Chronic relapsing inflammatory optic neuropathy (CRION) Figure 4.1
- Sarcoidosis
- Systemic lupus erythematosus (SLE)/autoimmune optic neuritis (ON)

See Table 4.1 for clues on how to distinguish MS from MOG antibody–positive conditions

and aquaporin-4–positive disorders Devic's disease; NMO).

◀ *Prominent limb or trunk pain.* In the early stage of apparent MS this is unusual. Late in the disease course, a deep, burning leg pain is frequent, but if such pain appears early on, especially over the spine, then the diagnosis should be reviewed. Think instead of:
  - Spinal dural fistula
  - Vertebral disease/degenerative disk disease
  - NMO
  - Axonal polyneuropathy

TABLE 4.1: COMPARISON OF FEATURES THAT MAY DISTINGUISH MULTIPLE SCLEROSIS, MYELIN OLIGODENDROCYTE GLYCOPROTEIN (MOG)-POSITIVE DISORDERS AND AQUAPORIN-4 (AQP4)-POSITIVE CONDITIONS

Disease patterns	Multiple sclerosis	MOG antibodies present	AQP-4 antibodies present (Devic disease/neuromyelitis optica)
Age of onset	20–40 y	Bimodal: children & 30–40 y	35–50 y
Gender and race	F:M 3:1. White	F>M. White	F>>M. Asian
Paediatric presentation	Rare	More common in <12 y	Rare in children
Other autoimmune conditions	Rare	Occasional	Frequent
ADEM-like presentation	Rare	Common in children	Rare in children
Typical onset	Unilateral optic neuritis or short length myelitis	Bilateral or rapidly sequential optic neuritis	Optic neuritis or transverse myelitis (more than 3 vertebral segments)
Bilateral optic neuritis	Rare.	Frequent.	Occasional; usually consecutive
Early bladder involvement	Occasional	Frequent	Rare
Conus affected	Rare	Typical	Rare
Oligoclonal bands confined to CSF	Essential for diagnosis	Occasionally during acute attack then disappear	Occasional oligo- or mon-clonal bands that usually disappear
Seizures	Rare	Frequent	Rare
Area postrema involved	Rare	Occasional	Frequent
Response to steroids	Good	Good	Modest
MRI visual pathway involvement	Intra-orbital optic nerve	Peri-optic nerve sheath	Chiasmal lesions; frequent
MRI brain lesion pattern	Periventricular and juxta-cortical lesions; Dawson's fingers	If ADEM-type presentation: multiple enhancing white matter lesions, at the same stage of development; no chronic lesions	Around lateral, third, and fourth ventricles. Rarely, tumefactive cortical lesions
Probability of relapse	High	Moderate	High

Modified with permission from Narayan et al. (2018).

◀ *Any feature suggestive of parkinsonism; namely rigidity, akinesia, or rest tremor.* Tremor is common in MS, but it should be present only on voluntary movement—the famous *intention tremor* (now called *terminal kinetic tremor*), which is due to demyelination in the cerebellum or its connections. If the tremor occurs mainly *at rest*, this would not be characteristic, and the diagnosis should be reviewed. In some patients with advanced MS there is a slow rest tremor markedly aggravated by movement or maintaining a posture, known variously as *Holmes, rubral,* or *midbrain tremor.*

◀ You should think of the following possibilities where there is a combination of demyelinating disorder and parkinsonism:

- Young-onset leukodystrophy, such as hereditary diffuse leukoencephalopathy with axonal spheroids (HDLS)
- Familial pigmentary orthochromatic leukodystrophy (POLD). Possibly the same condition as HDLS.

The clinical features are not particularly suggestive of MS, but you might be misled by the MRI (Figure 4.3).

◀ *Possible MS in an Afro-Caribbean patient.* Although MS is now well recognized in Afro-Caribbean people, the diagnosis needs to be made with caution. Human T-lymphotrophic virus type 1 (HTLV-1) and NMO are overrepresented among non-Caucasians. HTLV-1 features are as follows:

- Early progressive and disabling spasticity
- History of blood transfusion, sexual contact, or infected breast milk many years before symptoms
- Visual impairment
- Sensorimotor neuropathy which might mask the characteristic hyperactive tendon jerks

HTLV-1 myelopathy can be confused with progressive MS (PMS) and primary lateral sclerosis. It is rare in Caucasians; if suspected, that would constitute a Red Flag. Thus:

◀ An Afro-Caribbean with progressive paraplegia and prior exposure to infection from blood transfusion, sexual contact, or breast milk should be tested for HTLV in the spinal fluid

◀ Unilateral, gradual-onset ON that is painless and progressive over several months is not MS. More likely this results from pressure on the optic nerve from

- Meningioma
- Pituitary tumor
- Optic nerve tumor

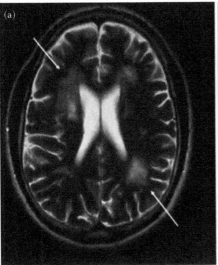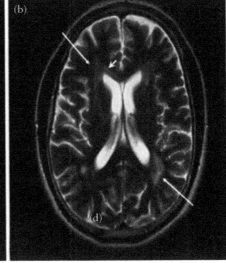

FIGURE 4.3: Hereditary diffuse leukoencephalopathy with axonal spheroids. Axial T2-weighted images (**a, b**) show localized, hyperintense foci in frontal and parietal lobes (long arrows), involving the periventricular, deep, and subcortical white matter, sparing the subcortical U-fibers. There is a hyperintense focus in the right forceps minor (short arrow, b). Reproduced from Rademakers et al. (2012).

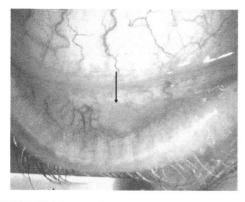

FIGURE 4.4: Sarcoid nodules in the conjunctiva. Biopsy of a nodule may be diagnostic. Reproduced from Figure 5.28 in the chapter Medical Ophthalmology, by E Hughes and M Stanford. Oxford University Press. DOI:10.1093/med/9780199237593.003.0005.

- Sarcoidosis. Look for conjunctival nodules (Figure 4.4), unidigital clubbing (Figure 1.1), inflamed tattoos or scars

(Figure 11.20 right), lupus pernio (Figure 11.20 left), and the "trident sign" on spinal MRI (Figure 4.5).

Progressive painless "optic neuritis" may be seen in mitochondrial disorders and is usually bilateral.

▶ MS usually improves during pregnancy but relapses or begins during the puerperium.

Conversely:

◀ Vascular lesions tend to enlarge, for example:
- Meningioma
- Pituitary tumor
- Glioma
- NMO
- Arteriovenous malformation or aneurysm

Therefore:

◀ Be cautious in diagnosing MS onset during pregnancy although SLE usually does *not*

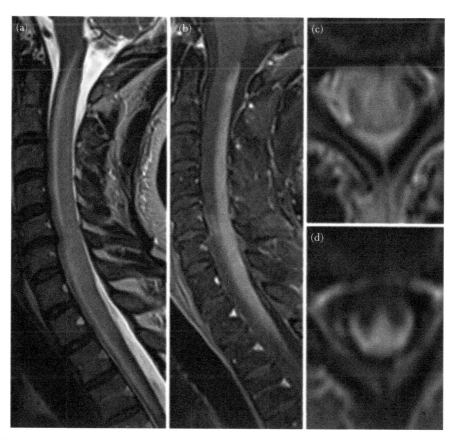

FIGURE 4.5: Spinal cord sarcoidosis and the trident sign. T2-weighted cervical spine MRI images show intramedullary T2 hyperintensity associated with cord edema on sagittal (A) and axial sequences (C). T1-weighted images show linear dorsal subpial gadolinium enhancement (B) which on axial sequences also involved the central cord/canal forming a "trident" appearance (D). Reproduced with permission from Figure 1 in Jolliffe et al. (2018).

cause MS-like symptoms. Many episodes of "lupus myelitis" or "lupus optic neuritis" are in fact comorbid NMO.

▶ NMO sometimes commences in the third trimester. Note that pregnancy does not suppress relapses, and there is significant risk of relapse of NMO (as well as MS) in the puerperium.

▶ *Bilateral painless optic neuropathy of rapid onset*. If you do not think this is Leber's optic atrophy or NMO, then consider a toxic or nutritional cause, such as:
  · Vitamin B$_{12}$ deficiency
  · Tobacco/alcohol amblyopia
  · Exposure to methanol (Figure 4.6), thallium, ethambutol, or quinine

Methanol (methyl-alcohol) exposure occurs in alcoholics who use this as a substitute for ethanol (ethyl-alcohol). There are major changes in the basal ganglia on MRI (Figure 4.6). Thallium poisoning is a rare but formerly popular homicide agent. Apart from effects on the eye, it causes a painful polyneuropathy. Ethambutol is used for treatment of TB, and optic neuropathy is one of its many toxic effects. Quinine derivatives taken for night cramp and formerly for arrhythmias or malaria may cause severe rapid loss of vision if consumed in excess. This may result from patient or physician error, occasionally, a self-inflicted overdose. Thus:

▶ Tinnitus and rapid bilateral loss of vision suggests quinine toxicity (cinchonism).

Further Red Flags:

◀ *Isolated third cranial nerve (CN III) palsy is an unusual presentation for MS (around 2%), whereas involvement of CN VI is frequent.*

◀ *Bilateral or sequential (over less than 2 weeks) and relapsing steroid-responsive ON is a Red Flag for ON of MS.* You should instead consider:
  · NMO
  · Sarcoidosis
  · SLE/autoimmune optic neuritis
  · CRION
  · MOG antibody disease

Note: Afro-Caribbean people are particularly susceptible to sarcoid optic neuropathy and NMO.

◀ *Complete and permanent blindness in both eyes.* In MS, it is very unusual to have complete blindness of such severity that the patient requires a white stick or dark sunglasses or has to be registered as blind (Figure 4.7). Hence:
A patient with alleged MS who requires a white stick probably has another condition, such as:
  · Neuromyelitis optica
  · Leber's disease

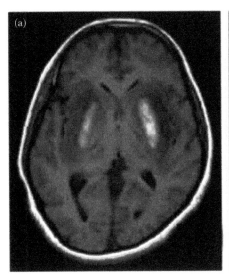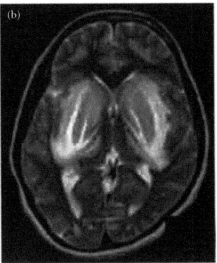

FIGURE 4.6: MRI axial sequences in methanol intoxication. (**a**) T1-weighted sequence shows hyperintense signal in the putamen bilaterally. (**b**) T2-weighted sequence shows isointense signal and the "lentiform fork sign," which is seen in severe metabolic disorders.   Reproduced with permission from Azeemuddin and Naqi (2012).

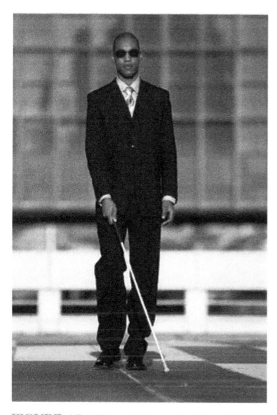

FIGURE 4.7: White stick sign—a Red Flag. This man is unlikely to have multiple sclerosis (MS). Blindness that is so severe that the patient requires a white stick is most unusual. You should also be cautious in diagnosing MS in an Afro-Caribbean male.

- Nonorganic disorder
- Toxic optic neuropathy

◀ *Strong family history.* Although there are well-documented pedigrees with multigenerational MS, it is quite unusual to find more than one relative similarly affected. You need to consider autosomal dominant conditions such as the following:

a. *Hereditary spastic paraplegia* (HSP). In the classic variety of HSP there are minimal or no sensory features, the upper limbs and cranial nerves are mostly spared, and progression is slow, thus simulating PMS. Also:
   - Spasticity is more prominent than weakness.
   - The plantar response is readily upgoing, as in MS.
   - MRI changes are late.

b. *Adult-onset autosomal dominant leukodystrophy* (ADLD; a B1 laminopathy). This mimics PMS with the addition of prominent autonomic features (bladder and bowel) and sometimes basilar migraine (Figure 4.8).

c. *Retinal vasculopathy with cerebral leukodystrophy* (RVCL). This is autosomal dominant and presents in middle age with visual disturbance, migrainous headache, Raynaud's phenomenon, or rash mimicking SLE and responsive to steroids. The retinal changes comprise microangiopathy, microaneurysms, and telangiectatic capillaries preferentially around the macula. It is associated with renal or hepatic impairment and due to mutations in *TREX1* (Richards et al. 2007). MRI shows cerebral pseudo-tumors and white matter lesions (Figure 4.9).

d. Spinocerebellar ataxia, Alexander disease, CADASIL (cerebral autosomal dominant arteriopathy with subcortical infarcts and leukoencephalopathy), and pigmented orthochromatic leukodystrophy (POLD)/HDLS

◀ *Seizures in the early disease phase.* Seizures are well-recognized in MS (prevalence around 5%), but they occur mostly in the later stages. Although an epileptic attack may be the presentation of MS, it is quite unusual and you should consider a vasculitic disorder or neoplasm.

◀ *Slowly progressive disorder from onset.* This pattern is consistent with PMS, but you need to consider:
   - HTLV-1
   - HSP
   - Leukodystrophies, such as adrenoleukodystrophy (ALD) and metachromatic leukodystrophy
   - Vitamin B_{12} deficiency
   - Copper deficiency myelopathy
   - Autosomal recessive spastic ataxia of Charlevoix-Saguenay (ARSACS) (see Chapter 12, Ataxia).

Copper myelopathy is easily overlooked but increasingly recognized with:

- Bariatric surgery
- Excess zinc salt intake. Zinc competes with copper for ceruloplasmin binding; free

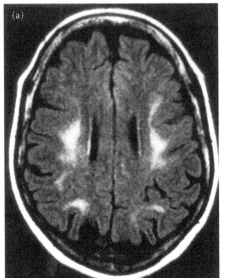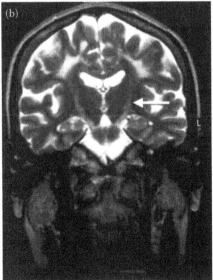

FIGURE 4.8: Adult-onset autosomal dominant leukodystrophy (ADLD). MRI (**A, B**) is from a 48-year-old woman with a 2-year history of urinary bladder dysfunction. Note that the frontoparietal white matter changes do not involve the periventricular area, as expected in typical MS. There is increased signal intensity in the corticospinal tracts in the internal capsules (B, arrow). From Melberg et al. (2006).

copper is excreted by the kidneys. Some types of dental adhesive used to contain zinc but these have since been withdrawn.

◄ Be aware that vitamin B$_{12}$ and copper deficiency may coexist.

◄ Recurrent migraines. Although the prevalence of headache in MS is slightly increased, it is worth considering other options:

• CADASIL. Transient ischemic attack (TIA)-like episodes in suspected MS

should make you alert to this disorder (Figure 4.10).

• Venous sinus thrombosis
• Mitochondrial encephalomyopathy, lactic acidosis, and stroke-like episodes (MELAS)
• SLE
• Lymphoma
• Retinal vasculopathy with cerebral leukodystrophy (RVCL; (Figure 4.9)

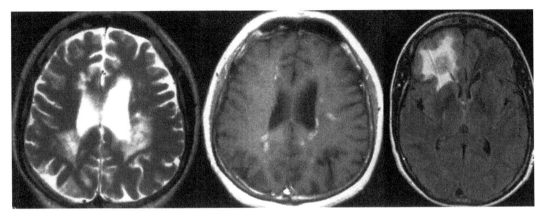

FIGURE 4.9: Retinal vasculopathy with cerebral leukodystrophy. MRI axial scans show leukoencephalopathy (**a**) with some enhancement (**b**) and a tumefactive appearance in the right frontal area (**c**). Reproduced with permission from Mateen et al. (2010).

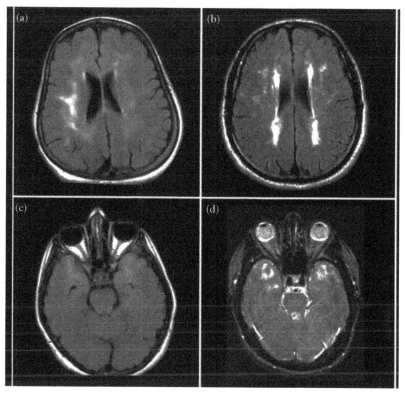

FIGURE 4.10: CADASIL. Axial FLAIR (**A, B, C**) and T2-weighted (**D**) brain MRI from four patients with CADASIL. There are periventricular diffuse white matter ischemic abnormalities and multiple lacunar lesions in the thalamus, pons, and basal ganglia. Note the characteristic inferior frontal and anterior temporal lesions. Reproduced with permission from Bohlega et al. (2007).

- Adult-onset autosomal dominant leukodystrophy (ADLD; Figure 4.8)

EXAMINATION

Optic Neuritis

▶ Eye movements are usually painful if the lesion involves the intraorbital part of the optic nerve.

Discomfort is felt especially in the temple or eye and occurs on looking away from the affected eye. The pupil should be tested carefully, in particular checking for the characteristic relative afferent pupillary defect (RAPD). If there is no pain, think of a retro-orbital lesion (e.g., chiasm).

◀ If the pupillary light reflexes are normal despite poor acuity, this favors Leber's disease.

If a patient has recovered from isolated ON, achieving 20/20, vision but there is color desaturation

in comparison to the unaffected eye or impairment of low contrast visual acuity, then demyelination is the likely explanation. Test for this with the Ishihara plates (Figure 4.11). Thus:

▶ Color desaturation or impaired low-contrast visual acuity may indicate previous ON although acuity is normal in that eye.
  Please refer to Chapter 2 for the differential diagnosis of unilateral ON; in brief, this is:

  - Neuroretinitis
  - NMO (Devic's disease)
  - MOG antibody disease
  - Leber's optic atrophy
  - White dot syndromes
  - Chronic relapsing inflammatory optic neuropathy (CRION)
  - Acute ischemic optic neuropathy
  - Central serous retinopathy

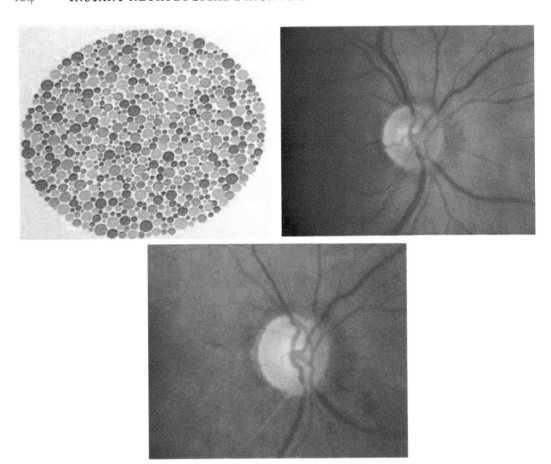

FIGURE 4.11: Top left: One of the Ishihara color plates. Remember to test for color vision in someone with a past history of possible optic neuritis. **Top right:** A normal optic disk. Note the healthy pale red rim to the optic disk. **Bottom:** Typical appearance of the optic disk after recent optic neuritis. Note temporal pallor, residual hemorrhages particularly at 4 o'clock and reduced number of small vessels crossing optic disk margin (Kestenbaum's sign).

- • Vogt-Koyanagi-Harada syndrome (Figure 1.14)
- • Smartphone blindness
- ▶ Poliosis

Look at the eyelashes, eyebrows, and scalp hair for reduced pigmentation (Figure 1.14). Depigmentation in any of these regions raises the possibility of the Vogt-Koyanagi-Harada syndrome. Some patients have deafness. It simulates ON, but it is really an autoimmune uveitis.

- ▶ Progressive spastic paraparesis with alopecia, loss of eyelashes, and premature baldness suggests adrenomyeloneuropathy (AMN).

Most patients are male, and the presentation mimics PMS, except that the ankle jerks are absent due to coexistent peripheral neuropathy. Some have pigmentation in the hand creases or tongue and other features typical of Addison's disease. The hardest cases to diagnose are middle-aged females with a heterozygous mutation in the *ABCD1* gene. They present with progressive paraplegia and normal brain/spinal cord MRI and cerebrospinal fluid (CSF). Diagnosis in either case is made by measurement of very-long-chain fatty acids, the short Synacthen test, and double-checking the family history (Bargiela et al. 2014). The MRI changes of the closely related disorder ADLD are shown in Figure 4.12.

- ◀ Be wary of the male patient with apparent PMS and absent ankle jerks. This suggests a peripheral neuropathy and raises the possibility of AMN or ADLD.

Nystagmus

Several varieties of nystagmus are observed in MS. The most characteristic is bilateral internuclear

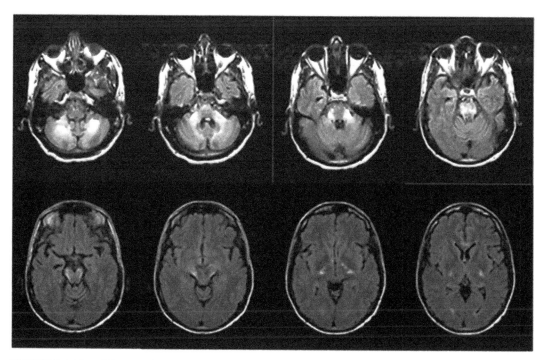

FIGURE 4.12: Adult-onset adrenoleukodystrophy. MRI FLAIR sequences show hyperintensity in the cerebellum, middle cerebellar peduncles, pons, cerebral peduncles, internal capsule, and genu of the corpus callosum. Reproduced from Elenein et al. (2013), Figure 1.

ophthalmoplegia (INO), best elicited by testing saccadic rather than pursuit movement (see Video 2.1). If the patient's eyes are divergent, this is the WEBINO syndrome (wall-eyed bilateral internuclear ophthalmoplegia; see Chapter 2). Note that most patients with INO have upbeat nystagmus on vertical gaze as well.

▶ Nearly all cases of *bilateral* INO are due to MS. Other instances are uni- or bilateral in association with the following:
  • Brainstem vascular or vasculitic disease (usually older patient and unilateral)
  • Anticonvulsant toxicity
  • Wernicke's encephalopathy
  • Infection: for example, brainstem encephalitis, AIDS
  • Tumor (pontine or midbrain)
  • Traumatic brain injury
  • Syringobulbia, Chiari malformation
  • Myasthenia gravis. This is really a pseudo-INO due to fatiguing extraocular muscles.

Rarer types of nystagmus in MS include periodic alternating nystagmus and elliptical nystagmus (see Chapter 2 and Video 2.7, Video 2.8, and Video 2.9).

Miscellaneous Signs That Might Raise the Question of MS

▶ Unduly prolonged sensation of vibration when tuning fork is placed on limb. It is presumed this is due to demyelination-induced short-circuiting of afferent signals in the posterior columns.
▶ Oral and genital ulceration (typically large) is characteristic of Behçet syndrome. This disorder that may cause confusion with MS especially if the history of ulcers is not elicited.

The pathergy test may be useful. In this, a sharp needle is inserted into the forearm skin; when positive, there is marked inflammatory reaction, often with pustule formation (Figure 4.13, *right*). This may be discovered coincidentally after routine phlebotomy. It is not specific for Behçet's disease and is likely to be negative in white people.

Other features of Behçet's syndrome include:

  • Recurrent uveitis
  • Arthritis
  • Skin lesions

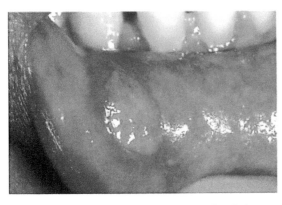
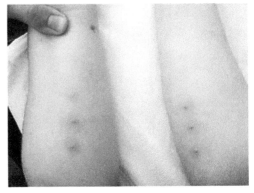

FIGURE 4.13: Behçet's disease. **Left**: An infected ulcer on the lower lip. Similar ulcers may be found on the genitalia. **Right**: A positive pathergy test for Behçet's syndrome. Reproduced from Figure 19.11.5.2 in the chapter Behçet's Syndrome, by H Yazici, S Yurdakul, and I Fresko. Oxford University Press. DOI:10.1093/med/9780199204854.003.191105_update_002.

- Testicular pain
- Venous thrombosis affecting the lower limb or cerebral veins
- Absent oligoclonal bands (OCBs) in spinal fluid
- Vascular lesions in the dorsal midbrain or posterior thalamus (pulvinar) are very typical.
▶ Muscle weakness accompanied by severe fatigue is highly characteristic of MS.

Fatigue is recognized increasingly as a prevalent and early symptom that likely relates to occult lesions in the hemispheric gray matter and may be accompanied by early cognitive deficits. On rare occasions, it is an initial symptom.

▶ Easily obtained Babinski sign
See Figure 4.14. The deep tendon reflexes in the lower limbs are typically very brisk and the plantar reflexes upgoing. In fact, MS is one of few conditions in which Babinski responses are most easily elicited. This is a useful diagnostic clue, and, apart from demyelinating conditions, it is found in:
 o Familial spastic paraplegia
 o HTLV-1 infection
 o Acute spinal cord transection
▶ Continuous extension of the hallux
In MS patients with severe spasticity, the great toes may be extended continuously, most likely because of minor sensory stimulation from contact with sheets or clothing.

This sign is seen in three other disorders apart from MS:

- Basal ganglia disorder: the "striatal toe" sign.
- Foot dystonia
- Inclusion body myositis, due to selective weakness of flexor hallucis longus (Figure 7. 22)
▶ Bilateral Babinski signs with unilateral symptoms
A Babinski sign may be present in the *asymptomatic* leg. This points to a subclinical lesion of the spinal cord or cortex. It is

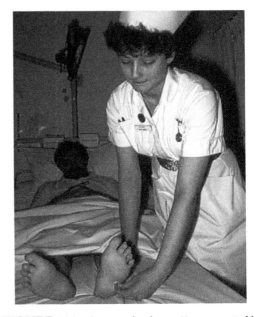

FIGURE 4.14: The easy Babinski sign. Here a nurse is able to obtain a Babinski response without difficulty and there is no withdrawal.

evidence of dissemination in space and may help confirm a diagnosis of MS.

◀ Babinski sign, brisk knee jerks, and impaired ankle jerks

If you find this in the absence of lumbar spondylosis, then you are dealing with a mixture of upper and lower motor neuron signs. MS is usually excluded when there are lower motor neuron signs, thus an absent ankle jerk would constitute a Red Flag. There is a long list of possibilities, but your immediate thought should be *vitamin B$_{12}$ deficiency* (subacute combined degeneration of the cord). The main causes are as follows:

○ Subacute combined degeneration of the cord
○ Friedreich's ataxia
○ Amyotrophic lateral sclerosis
○ Syringomyelia
○ Adrenomyeloneuropathy
○ HTLV-1 myelopathy
○ Taboparesis
○ Neurofibromatosis

Most are easily diagnosed by MRI and their specific tests.

Further rare instances of central demyelination and peripheral neuropathy waiting to trap the unwary clinician include:

· Chronic inflammatory demyelinating polyneuropathy (CIDP)
· Lyme disease
· Sarcoidosis
· Adrenomyeloneuropathy (AMN)
· Metachromatic leukodystrophy
· Krabbe's disease

▶ Temporal disk pallor in the asymptomatic eye

This suggests a previous subclinical episode of ON and could be viewed as a further lesion unless there is a single lesion in the chiasm, which is unusual for MS (but not for NMO). As mentioned earlier, there is often color desaturation in the affected eye even when visual acuity has returned to normal. Color desaturation in the unaffected eye would give further support to a previous episode of unrecognized optic nerve demyelination. The same principles apply to the visual evoked potentials; look critically at the latency, amplitude, and shape of the *asymptomatic* eye (Figure 4.15).

▶ Kestenbaum's sign

See Figure 2.39. It is sometimes challenging to decide whether an optic disk is abnormally pale. In this situation, look for Kestenbaum's sign. If you ignore the obvious arteries or veins and their branches that traverse the disk margin, there should be around 10 or more small

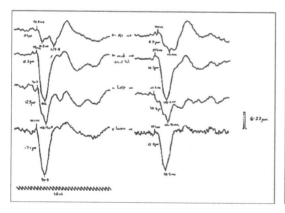
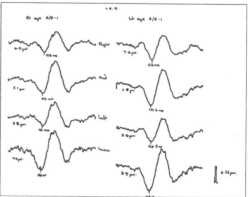

FIGURE 4.15: Visual evoked potentials: 32 degree whole-field, pattern-evoked visual potentials. Tracings from top to bottom rows are derived from: right occipital; mid-occipital; left occipital; Inion. Right eye recordings are on the left side of each figure. Time is the 10 mS sawtooth marker on lower left. Amplitude scale on the right side of each figure is 6.25 μV. **Left:** Healthy person. Note latency to P100 (the first major downward peak) is 99–100 mS in all four tracings, with amplitude of 10–15 μV. **Right:** Delayed P100 latency (~123 mS) from both eyes, with moderately well-preserved amplitude (5–7 μV) but broadened wave shape, in a 30-year-old patient with a history of unilateral optic neuritis. In most departments P100 latencies up to 108 mS are considered normal.

blood vessels crossing its edge. If there are five or less, then it is likely the disk is ischemic or atrophic, and Kestenbaum's sign is positive. Not only might this help diagnostically, but it can assist with serial monitoring.

Red Flags on Examination

◀ Prominent lower motor neuron signs, such as wasting early in the disease course, are unusual.

These findings should prompt diagnostic review. Most forms of weakness should be explicable in terms of a corticospinal tract lesion, and wasting beyond disuse atrophy would not be expected.

◀ Fasciculations

These are recognized in MS but they are stunningly rare. You should consider:

  o Benign fasciculation
  o Amyotrophic lateral sclerosis (ALS). There are isolated reports of confirmed MS and ALS.
  o Isaac syndrome. This may be associated with white matter lesions on brain MRI (Sedarous & Lange, 2013)

◀ Recurrent anterior uveitis with recent-onset back pain worse in the mornings suggests ankylosing spondylitis (Figure 4.16).

As long as mundane spondylotic causes of low back pain are excluded, this combination suggests ankylosing spondylitis. There may be heel pain, question mark spine (Figure 1.44), and inflammatory bowel disease. Rarely, ankylosing spondylosis and MS co-exist.

◀ Acute paraplegia with a sensory level that spares JPS is unlike MS and favors anterior spinal artery thrombosis.

Such patients are usually elderly arteriopaths and hypertensive. Typically, they have recovered from recent surgery to the abdominal aorta (e.g., an aortic graft procedure). The anterior spinal artery supplies the spinothalamic tracts but not the posterior columns; thus, JPS in the toes is preserved (see Chapter 9, Stroke). In demyelinating spinal cord conditions, the posterior columns are nearly always affected.

◀ Suspected MS with:

  · *Renal involvement*: Fabry's disease, SLE, RVCL
  · *Livedo reticularis*: phospholipid antibody syndrome (Hughes syndrome); SLE or Sneddon syndrome
  · *Deafness*: Susac syndrome, Fabry syndrome, brainstem vasculitic/neoplastic disorder, syphilis, Vogt Harada Koyanagi syndrome
  · *Recurrent, spontaneous abortion*: phospholipid antibody syndrome, Behçet's syndrome, SLE, or idiopathic thrombocytopenic purpura
  · *Cataract*. MS patients who have received multiple courses of steroids are susceptible to cataracts, and, of course, they are common with aging. There are rare instances of an MS-like clinical profile and cataract that include
    i. Cerebrotendinous xanthomatosis, a cerebellar syndrome that you can diagnose by examining the Achilles and other tendons for lumps (see Figure 8.6).

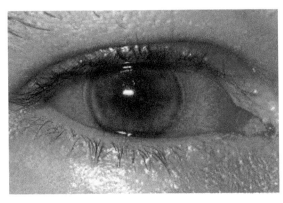 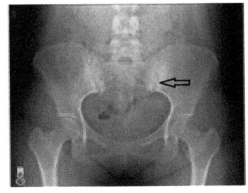

FIGURE 4.16: **Left:** Anterior uveitis. If this is associated with low back pain from sacroiliitis (arrow, **right** photo) the diagnosis is ankylosing spondylitis.

ii. Wilson's disease. This causes sunflower cataract (see Figure 2.37).

◀ *Retinitis pigmentosa*: Refsum's disease or mitochondrial disorder

◀ *Retinal infarcts*: Susac's syndrome and Fabry's syndrome

◀ *Parotid enlargement or galactorrhea*: sarcoidosis

◀ *Diabetes insipidus*: sarcoidosis, Devic's disease, Erdheim-Chester disease (polyostotic sclerosing histiocytosis). Erdheim-Chester disease is a diffuse histiocytosis associated with bone pain (due to cysts), exophthalmos, dementia, and retroperitoneal fibrosis. (For more details, see Chapter 13, Dementia.)

Red Flags on Investigation

◀ Absent oligoclonal bands (OCB)

If you suspect active MS and there are no OCB confined to the spinal fluid, the diagnosis should be reviewed. Band-negative MS is very unusual in the established phase of disease and probably excludes it. See Figure 4.17 for the various patterns of bands.

◀ Spinal tap lymphocyte count greater than 50/mm^3 or total protein level greater than 1 g/L (100 mg/dL)

Both of these features are atypical and likely exclude definite MS.

◀ Negative serum EBV IgG

All patients with MS have been exposed to Epstein-Barr virus (EBV) infection. There may not necessarily be a history of infectious mononucleosis, but there will be a positive serum IgG to this virus. If you suspect MS and the EBV IgG is negative, then the diagnosis is wrong.

Rare Syndromes That Might Be Confused with MS

CLIPPERS syndrome is chronic lymphocytic inflammation with pontine perivascular enhancement responsive to steroids. This affects the brainstem, particularly the pons and cerebellum, and may resemble MS. It presents as:

• Remittent ataxia
• Diplopia

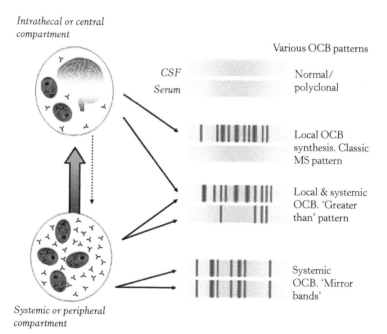

FIGURE 4.17: The four main types of abnormality found on cerebrospinal fluid (CSF) protein electrophoresis. Type 1 (**first row**) is normal. Type 2 (**second row**) shows bands in the CSF but not serum and it is characteristic of MS. Type 3 (**third row**) shows the "greater than" pattern where there is local and systemic synthesis but mainly in the CSF. Type 4 (**fourth row**) shows the mirror band pattern where there are identical bands in the blood and CSF due to a systemic immune reaction with spillover from the blood into the CSF. Courtesy G Giovannoni, London.

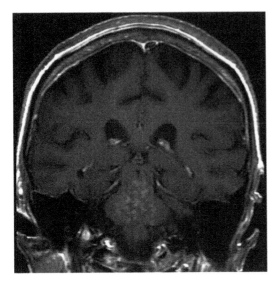

FIGURE 4.18: Coronal T1-weighted image with gadolinium demonstrating the "peppered pons" characteristic of chronic lymphocytic inflammation with pontine perivascular enhancement responsive to steroids (CLIPPERS). Reprinted with permission from Pittock et al. (2010).

- Peppered pons sign on MRI due to multiple punctate hyperintensities on gadolinium enhancement (Figure 4.18)

CLIPPERS should be distinguished from central pontine myelinolysis. The lesions in CLIPPERS are peppered rather than confluent.

▶ *Acute demyelinating encephalomyelitis (ADEM)-like disorder with very high blood ferritin is hemophagocytic lymphohistiocytosis (Griscelli syndrome)* (Figure 4.19). This presents like ADEM and is often triggered by EBV exposure. The MRI changes are similar to MS, with multiple white matter lesions in the cerebral and cerebellar hemispheres. Apart from high ferritin levels:

▶ Some have silvery hair (Figure 4.19, *left*).

▶ A *"disappearing" space-occupying lesion after steroids is likely primary central nervous system (CNS) lymphoma.* Occasionally, a patient presents with a deteriorating neurological disorder such as progressive hemiparesis, foot drop, ataxia, or focal seizures, and the scan shows what appears to be a large tumor and little else. A brain biopsy is sometimes required but even this may not clarify the diagnosis. Thus:

▶ If the MRI scan suggests a tumor that disappears after steroid treatment, then primary CNS lymphoma is likely (Figure 4.20). Although MS lesions often resolve after steroid treatment, cerebral lymphoma is particularly responsive.

- Lymphoma is a strong possibility, particularly if the patient is immunosuppressed from, for example, HIV/AIDS.

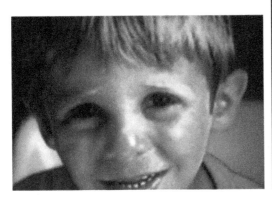

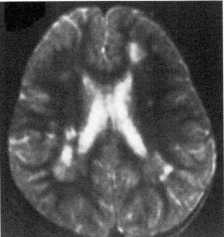

FIGURE 4.19: Hemophagocytic lymphohistiocytosis (Griscelli syndrome). **Left**: Note the silver-gray hair of scalp, eyebrows, eyelashes, and facial hair. **Right**: MRI T2-weighted image shows several white matter lesions that might be mistaken for multiple sclerosis. Reproduced from Figure 14.10 in the chapter Immune Deficiency Diseases, by V Sybert. Oxford University Press. DOI:10.1093/med/9780195397666.003.0014.

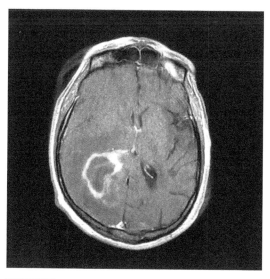
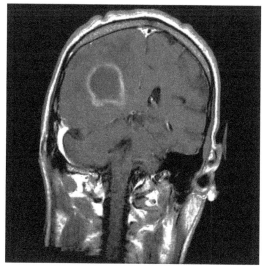

FIGURE 4.20: Primary central nervous system B-cell lymphoma. Axial and coronal enhanced T1 MRI scans show a ring-enhancing lesion in the right parietal region in a patient with HIV. Reproduced with permission from Dr. Frank Gaillard ID: 5474. Radiopedia.

Tumefactive MS refers to tumor-like lesions seen on MRI (Figure 4.21) that are due to MS. This finding may be mimicked by the following:

- ADEM
- RVCL
- Glioma

- Sarcoidosis
- Lymphoma
- Abscess

Fabry's disease (see Figure 4.22). The clinical features of Fabry's disease are delineated in Chapter 11 (Peripheral Neuropathy). Despite the

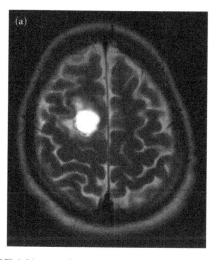
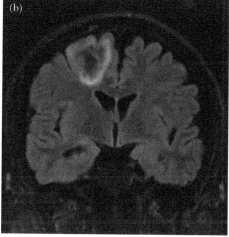

FIGURE 4.21: scan showing a single tumefactive demyelinating lesion due to multiple sclerosis or acute demyelinating encephalomyelitis (ADEM). (**a**) Axial T2 sequence and (**b**) coronal FLAIR sequence showing a well-circumscribed hyperintense tumefactive lesion in the right parietal lobe with mild surrounding edema. It can be difficult to tell this lesion apart from primary central nervous system lymphoma, as shown in Figure 4.20. Reproduced with permission from Hardy and Chataway (2013), Figure 1A and 1B.

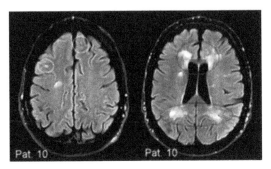

FIGURE 4.22: MRI axial FLAIR sequences in a 64-year-old female with mild Fabry's disease that was diagnosed 32 years after initial symptoms. There are multiple non-enhancing white matter lesions (circled) which do not affect the corpus callosum. Sparing of the corpus callosum is unusual for multiple sclerosis and constitutes a Red Flag. Reproduced with permission from Bottcher et al. (2013).

classic involvement of peripheral nerve, blood vessels, and skin, it may present as a milder form in middle-aged females, with a relapsing-remitting profile that can be mistaken for MS (Bottcher et al. 2013).

The main features are those of brainstem involvement (deafness, ataxia, gait disturbances, double vision, and vertigo) or intermittent paresthesia in keeping with neuropathy, but a history of stroke or skin lesions may be lacking in this late-onset variety.

Progressive multifocal leukoencephalopathy (PML). This disorder, caused by JC virus infection, needs consideration in any individual with impaired immunity such as patients with HIV/AIDS or those receiving long-term immunosuppression with steroids,

natalizumab, fingolimod, and dimethyl fumarate. Any part of the brain can be affected. The features are therefore varied but typically as follows:

- Cognitive and behavioral problems
- Weakness and ataxia
- Visual defects (particularly homonymous hemianopia)
- Speech and language disorder
- The MRI lesions are characteristically greater than 5 cm (Figure 4.23).
- Positive CSF polymerase chain reaction (PCR) for JC virus clinches the diagnosis.

Delayed posthypoxic leukoencephalopathy. Typically, a patient becomes comatose following a hypoxic event, such as:

- Cardiac arrest or strangulation
- Carbon monoxide poisoning
- Narcotic overdose

There is initial recovery followed *weeks later* by neuro-psychiatric changes such as disorientation, amnesia, hyperreflexia, parkinsonism, and akinetic mutism. The MRI shows diffuse white matter changes that spare the posterior fossa. If the full history is not available, confusion with another leukoencephalopathy may result.

Common variable immune deficiency (CVID). Such patients have recurrent lymphadenopathy; increased susceptibility to infection because of deficiency of IgG, IgA, and IgM; and idiopathic thrombocytopenic

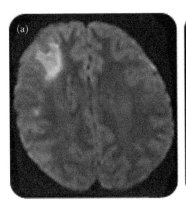
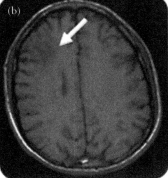
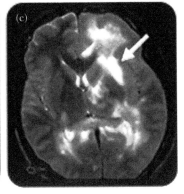

FIGURE 4.23: MRI of progressive multifocal leukoencephalopathy (PML). (**A**) FLAIR image shows a large subcortical lesion of right frontal lobe. A smaller lesion is observed posterior to this. (**B**) T1-weighted image shows hypointense lesion (arrow) in the right frontal lobe. (**C**) T2 image from another patient with extensive high signal intensity lesions in the white matter sparing the cortex. Reproduced with permission from Berger et al. (2013).

purpura (ITP). They may develop transverse myelitis with longitudinally extensive white matter changes on MRI reminiscent of NMO (Jabbari et al. 2015). Thus:

▶ Myelopathy with history of recurrent infection and ITP suggests CVID.

NMO (Devic's disease) is characterized by the following:

- Consecutive and painful ON. The chiasm is often affected.
- Cervical and/or thoracic cord demyelinating lesions, extending for 3 or more vertebral segments (Figure 4.24)
- Positive aquaporin-4 antibodies (preferably based on the more sensitive, cell-based assay). Note: the alternative ELISA assay may become negative after immunosuppression.
- Negative myelin oligodendrocyte glycoprotein (MOG) antibodies
- Oligoclonal bands confined to spinal fluid are rare, and, if present, they disappear. See Table 4.1.

Lesions involve the periventricular areas of the medulla and hypothalamus. These locations give rise to some of the presenting features that are diagnostically useful, namely:

- Area postrema syndrome. Nausea and vomiting; intractable, paroxysmal, frequently recurring hiccups or yawning, Note: hiccups from peripheral causes due to, for example, diaphragmatic irritation are usually of low recurrence frequency).
- Inappropriate ADH secretion and diabetes insipidus
- Pruritus and girdle pain. The cause is presumably related to demyelination in the spinothalamic tracts in the spinal cord.
- Onset in the third trimester or in puerperium
- Dysgeusia, deafness, narcolepsy, tonic spasms
▶ *An acute demyelinating condition of children or teenagers who lapse into coma is likely ADEM.* Typically, there is a history of exposure to vaccine or viral or bacterial infection within the preceding 2 weeks. Some clues for ADEM are as follows:
  - MRI shows multiple enhancing white matter lesions, usually at the same stage of development, and there is a deficit of chronic lesions (Figure 4.25).
  - MOG antibody is positive; aquaporin-4 antibody is negative.
  - If there are oligoclonal bands (~10%) in the CSF, they disappear.
  - Apparent ADEM in an adult is a Red Flag; most patients turn out to have MS.
  - ADEM-like presentation after EBV infection could be hemophagocytic lymphohistiocytosis (Griscelli syndrome; Figure 4.19). Remember, there is a raised blood ferritin and silvery hair.

SUMMARY

Handles for MS in History

- Uhthoff's phenomenon
- Lhermitte's sign, reversed Lhermitte sign
- McArdle's sign
- Symptom onset or relapse in puerperium
- Numbness around waist or perineum ("MS hug")
- Useless hand syndrome
- Numbness in the vaginal or perineal area
- Paroxysmal sensory or motor symptoms: trigeminal neuralgia, paroxysmal dystonia, tonic

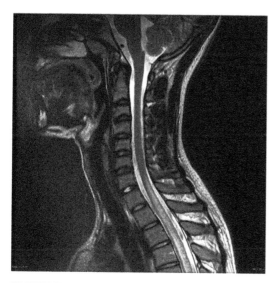

FIGURE 4.24: Devic's disease (NMO). Sagittal T2 MRI of cervical cord from a case of Devic's disease. This MRI shows a demyelinating lesion extending well over the minimum three vertebral segments, from the C7 vertebral level to upper thoracic cord. Reproduced with permission from Radiopedia, courtesy Dr. Frank Gaillard ID: 19649.

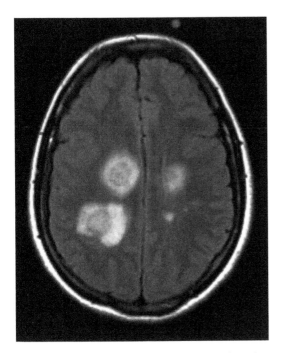

FIGURE 4.25: Acute demyelinating encephalomyelitis (ADEM). Axial FLAIR MRI demonstrates bilateral asymmetric lesions with open ring enhancement characteristic of demyelination. All lesions are at the same stage of development. Reproduced with permission from Radiopedia, courtesy Dr. Frank Gaillard. ID: 2576.

spasms, speech arrest, ataxia, exercise-related dyskinesia, or itching
- Early and persistent sphincter disturbances
- Painful ON indicates intraorbital, not intracranial, lesion
- Consecutive ON: Devic's disease, Leber's optic neuropathy, neuroretinitis, CRION, sarcoidosis, SLE, rarely MS
- Eye pain is unusual in Leber's disease but frequent in NMO and CRION.
- In Leber's disease there may be peripapillary telangiectases and normal pupillary light reflexes.
- Isolated dysgeusia

Red Flags in the Early Phase of Illness
- Consecutive ON
- Prominent limb or trunk pain in early stages: think of spinal dural fistula, vertebral disease, NMO, axonal polyneuropathy.
- Parkinsonism: rigidity, akinesia, or rest tremor; think of HDLS/POLD.

- Possible MS in Afro-Caribbean patient: HTLV-1 and NMO are more likely.
- Unilateral gradual-onset ON that is painless and progressive over several months: meningioma, pituitary or optic nerve tumor, sarcoidosis (trident sign on MRI), mitochondrial disorders (usually bilateral)
- MS onset or relapse is rare during pregnancy but common in the puerperium. Think of meningioma, pituitary tumor, glioma, NMO, arteriovenous malformation, or aneurysm.
- Be cautious in diagnosing MS onset during pregnancy. SLE usually does *not* cause MS-like symptoms. Many episodes of "lupus myelitis" or "lupus optic neuritis" are in fact comorbid NMO. NMO tends to relapse in the puerperium.
- Bilateral painless optic neuropathy of rapid onset: Leber's optic atrophy; toxic or nutritional amblyopia; vitamin B_{12} deficiency; tobacco/alcohol amblyopia; exposure to methanol, thallium, ethambutol, or quinine
- Tinnitus and rapid bilateral loss of vision suggests quinine toxicity (cinchonism).
- Isolated CN III palsy is rare.
- Painful, bilateral, or sequential ON that is steroid-dependent is unlikely to be MS. Consider NMO, sarcoidosis, SLE, autoimmune ON, and CRION.
- White stick sign: Complete permanent blindness in both eyes. A patient who requires a white stick probably does not have MS. More likely: NMO, Leber's disease, nonorganic disorder, toxic optic neuropathy
- Strong family history: think of HSP, ADLD, RVCL, spinocerebellar ataxia, Alexander's disease, CADASIL, and POLD/HDLS.
- Seizures in the early disease phase: vasculitic disorder or neoplasm
- Slowly progressive disorder from onset: may be PMS, but think of HTLV-1, HSP, leukodystrophies, vitamin B_{12} deficiency, and copper-related myelopathy.
- Recurrent migraines: CADASIL, venous sinus thrombosis, MELAS, SLE, lymphoma, RVCL, and ADLD

Examination
Optic Neuritis
- Painful eye movement on looking away from the lesion is suggestive of ON and likely

involves the intraorbital part of the optic nerve. If no pain, the lesion is likely retro-orbital (e.g., chiasm).

- Normal pupillary light reflexes in ON suggest Leber's optic neuropathy as long as contralateral eye is not illuminated.
- Color desaturation in the eye that has regained normal acuity after suspected ON helps confirm previous ON.
- Differential diagnosis for unilateral ON: neuroretinitis, NMO, MOG antibody disease, Leber's optic atrophy, white dot syndromes, CRION, acute ischemic optic neuropathy, central serous retinopathy, Vogt-Koyanagi-Harada syndrome, smartphone blindness
- Poliosis and apparent ON suggest Vogt Harada Koyanagi syndrome.
- Progressive spastic paraparesis with alopecia, loss of eyelashes, and premature baldness suggest AMN.
- Be wary of the male patient with apparent PMS and absent ankle jerks. This suggests a peripheral neuropathy and raises the possibility of AMN or ALD.

Nystagmus
- Bilateral INO : typical of MS brainstem lesion
- Other causes of INO: brainstem vascular or vasculitic disease, anticonvulsant toxicity, Wernicke's encephalopathy, infection (brainstem encephalitis, AIDS), tumor (pontine or midbrain), traumatic brain injury, syringobulbia, Chiari malformation, myasthenia gravis
- Rare types of nystagmus are periodic alternating nystagmus and elliptical nystagmus.

Miscellaneous Signs That Might Raise the Question of MS
- Unduly prolonged sensation of vibration when a tuning fork is placed on a limb: possible posterior column demyelination.
- Oral and genital ulcers with positive pathery reaction suggest Behçet's disease. Look for characteristic vascular lesions in the posterior thalamus.
- Muscle weakness accompanied by severe fatigue correlates with MS gray matter lesions and cognitive defects.

- Easily obtained Babinski sign: MS, familial spastic paraplegia, acute spinal cord transection. HTLV-1 infection
- Continuous extension of the hallux: MS, inclusion body myositis, parkinsonism (striatal toe sign), and foot dystonia
- Bilateral Babinski signs with unilateral symptoms suggest MS.
- Bilateral Babinski sign, brisk knee jerks, and impaired ankle jerks: causes include vitamin B_{12} deficiency, Friedreich's ataxia, ALS, syringomyelia, HTLV-1 myelopathy, taboparesis, neurofibromatosis, CIDP, AMN, metachromatic leukodystrophy, sarcoidosis, tropical spastic paraplegia, Lyme disease, Krabbe's disease
- Temporal pallor in the asymptomatic eye
- Kestenbaum's sign

Red Flags on Physical Examination or Investigation
- Prominent lower motor neuron signs (e.g., wasting or fasciculation) early in disease course
- Fasciculations: benign fasciculations, ALS, or Isaac syndrome
- Recurrent anterior uveitis and recent back pain: ankylosing spondylitis
- Acute paraplegia with sensory level that spares JPS suggests anterior spinal artery thrombosis.

Suspected MS with:
- Renal involvement: Fabry's disease, SLE, RVCL
- Livedo reticularis: phospholipid antibody syndrome (cardiolipin antibody or Hughes syndrome), SLE, or Sneddon syndrome
- Deafness: Susac syndrome, Fabry syndrome, brainstem vascular/neoplastic disorder, syphilis, Behçet's disease
- Recurrent spontaneous abortion: phospholipid antibody syndrome or thrombotic thrombocytopenic purpura
- Cataract: MS and multiple courses of steroids, cerebrotendinous xanthomatosis, Wilson's disease
- Retinitis pigmentosa: Refsum's disease or mitochondrial disorder
- Retinal infarcts: Susac's syndrome and Fabry's syndrome

- Parotid enlargement or galactorrhea: Sarcoidosis
- Diabetes insipidus: sarcoidosis, Devic's disease, Erdheim-Chester disease

Red Flags on Investigations

- Absent OCB confined to spinal fluid
- CSF lymphocyte count greater than 50/mm³ or total protein level greater than 1 g/L (100 mg/dL)
- Negative serum EBV IgG

Rare Syndromes That Might Be Confused with MS

- *CLIPPERS syndrome*: episodic ataxia, diplopia, peppered pons sign on MRI; distinguish from central pontine myelinolysis
- *ADEM-like disorder with very high blood ferritin is hemophagocytic lymphohistiocytosis (Griscelli syndrome).* Some have silvery hair.
- *Primary CNS lymphoma*: brain tumor that disappears after steroids
- *Tumefactive MS mimicked by* ADEM, RVCL, glioma, sarcoidosis, lymphoma, abscess
- *Fabry's disease*: be alert to the mild form in middle-aged females with a history of relapsing brainstem symptoms and paresthesia but no skin lesions or strokes.
- *Progressive multifocal leukoencephalopathy*: main features are cognitive and behavioral problems, weakness and ataxia, visual defects (particularly homonymous hemianopia), speech and language disorder. MRI lesions are typically greater than 5 cm. Positive CSF PCR for JC virus
- *Delayed posthypoxic leukoencephalopathy*: initially cardiac arrest/strangulation; carbon monoxide poisoning or narcotic overdose followed weeks later by neuropsychiatric syndrome. Diffuse white matter changes on MRI
- *Common variable immune deficiency (CVID)*: myelopathy with history of recurrent infection and ITP
- *Devic's disease (NMO)*: consecutive painful ON, cervical and/or thoracic cord demyelinating lesions extending over three or more vertebral segments, aquaporin-4 antibodies. Preferential involvement of chiasm and occasionally the conus. Absent Dawson's fingers. Presentation: area postrema syndrome (intractable paroxysmal hiccups or yawning, nausea, and vomiting), inappropriate ADH secretion and diabetes insipidus, pruritus and girdle pain, dysgeusia, deafness, narcolepsy, tonic spasms. OCB confined to spinal fluid are rare and, if present, usually disappear.
- NMO may start in the third trimester, unlike MS.
- *Acute demyelinating encephalomyelitis (ADEM)*: an acute demyelinating condition of children who lapse into coma is likely ADEM. MRI: multiple enhancing white matter lesions at the same stage of development. Few chronic lesions. Positive MOG antibody; negative Aq-4 antibody. If there are OCB confined to spinal fluid, they subsequently disappear. Apparent ADEM in an adult is a Red Flag; most have MS. ADEM-like presentation after EBV infection could be hemophagocytic lymphohistiocytosis (Griscelli syndrome).

SUGGESTED READING

Azeemuddin M, Naqi R. MRI findings in methanol intoxication: a report of three cases. *J Pak Med Assoc.* 2012;62:1099–1101.

Bargiela D, Eglon G, Horvath R, Chinnery PF. An under-recognised cause of spastic paraparesis in middle-aged women. *Pract Neurol.* 2014;14:182–184.

Berger JR, Aksamit AJ, Clifford DB, et al. PML diagnostic criteria: consensus statement from the AAN Neuroinfectious Disease Section. *Neurology.* 2013;80:1430–1438.

Bohlega S, Al Shubili A, Edris A, et al. CADASIL in Arabs: clinical and genetic findings. *BMC Med Genet.* 2007;8:67.

Bottcher T, Rolfs A, Tanislav C, et al. Fabry disease—underestimated in the differential diagnosis of multiple sclerosis? *PLoS One.* 2013;8:e71894.

Combarros O, Sanchez-Juan P, Berciano J, De PC. Hemiageusia from an ipsilateral multiple sclerosis plaque at the midpontine tegmentum. *J Neurol Neurosurg Psychiatry.* 2000;68:796.

Elenein RA, Naik S, Kim S, Punia V, Jin K. Teaching neuroimages: cerebral adrenoleukodystrophy: a rare adult form. *Neurology.* 2013;80:e69–e70.

Hardy TA, Chataway J. Tumefactive demyelination: an approach to diagnosis and management. *J Neurol Neurosurg Psychiatry.* 2013;84:1047–1053.

Jabbari E, Marshall CR, Longhurst H, Sylvester R. Longitudinally extensive transverse myelitis: a rare association with common variable immunodeficiency. *Pract Neurol.* 2015;15(1):49–52.

Jolliffe EA, Keegan BM, Flanagan EP. Trident sign trumps Aquaporin-4-IgG ELISA in diagnostic value in a case of longitudinally extensive transverse myelitis. *Mult Scler Relat Disord.* 2018;23:7–8.

Kamogawa K, Okuda B. Useless hand syndrome with astereognosis in multiple sclerosis. *Mult Scler Relat Disord* 2015;4(1):85–87.

Katz Sand IB, Lublin FD. Diagnosis and differential diagnosis of multiple sclerosis. *Continuum (Minneap Minn).* 2013;19:922–943.

Kidd D, Burton B, Plant GT, Graham EM. Chronic relapsing inflammatory optic neuropathy (CRION). *Brain.* 2003;126:276–284.

Mateen FJ, Krecke K, Younge BR, et al. Evolution of a tumor-like lesion in cerebroretinal vasculopathy and *TREX1* mutation. *Neurology.* 2010;75:1211–1213.

Melberg A, Hallberg L, Kalimo H, Raininko R. MR characteristics and neuropathology in adult-onset autosomal dominant leukodystrophy with autonomic symptoms. *AJNR Am J Neuroradiol.* 2006;27:904–911.

Narayan R, Simpson A, Fritsche K, Salama S, Pardo S, Mealy M, Paul F, Levy M. MOG antibody disease: a review of MOG antibody seropositive neuromyelitis optica spectrum disorder. *Mult Scler Relat Disord.* 2018;25:66–72.

Pittock SJ, Debruyne J, Krecke KN, et al. Chronic lymphocytic inflammation with pontine perivascular enhancement responsive to steroids (CLIPPERS). *Brain.* 2010;133:2626–2634.

Rademakers R, Baker M, Nicholson AM, et al. Mutations in the colony stimulating factor 1 receptor (CSF1R) gene cause hereditary diffuse leukoencephalopathy with spheroids. *Nat Genet.* 2012;44:200–205.

Richards A, van den Maagdenberg AM, Jen JC, et al. C-terminal truncations in human 3′-5′ DNA exonuclease TREX1 cause autosomal dominant retinal vasculopathy with cerebral leukodystrophy. *Nat Genet.* 2007;39:1068–1070.

Sedarous M, Lange DJ. Can white matter changes occur in disorders of peripheral nerve hyperexcitability? *Mult Scler Relat Disord.* 2013;2:388–390.

Chapter 5: Headache

If you ever feel slightly confused about making a diagnosis in a patient with headache, do not despair: you are in good company! Headache neurologists disagree strongly, but most other neurologists find its classification unwieldy, ever-changing, and expanding. History-taking can be a nightmare. The worst question you can ask a patient is, "How often do you get a headache?" You will be lucky to get a meaningful answer; in fact, for many clinicians, the best way to take a headache history is to say to the patient, "Tell me about your headache" and hope that something useful emerges. In essence, obtaining accurate information about severity, frequency, location, and characteristics (throbbing, stabbing, etc.) may be difficult in all but the most articulate patients. Furthermore, physical examination is usually normal.

Note:

▶ If the patient is troubled with headache when attending the clinic, ask them to shake the head. Migraine patients are reluctant to do this because the headache is worsened, although the sign is probably not specific. In general, migraineurs dislike sudden movement and may experience headache even on bending over.

▶ Pressure on both superficial temporal arteries for a few minutes often abolishes a migraine headache.

▶ Unless really acute, sinus disease does not often cause head pain but rather pain and tenderness over the affected sinus.

HANDLES AND FLAGS IN THE HISTORY

Reassuring Features

There are a few aspects of migraine that point away from serious pathology as follows:

▶ Pain is preferentially but not exclusively on one side of the head. Thus, the pain may be right-sided in most attacks, but there are a few on the left.

▶ Scalp tenderness on combing hair or sleeping on the side of pain. There may be carotid artery tenderness (carotidynia) as well. The main exception is giant cell arteritis, where there is scalp tenderness and jaw claudication, but the patient is older than 50 years. Occasionally, carotidynia and headache indicates arterial dissection.

▶ Sensory or motor symptoms that are *usually* on the same side as the headache

▶ There is a slow evolution of symptoms (typically over minutes), as found in hemisensory or hemiparetic migraine. See Chapter 9 (Stroke, Table 9.1).

▶ In general, the patient with migraine has symptom onset before 50 years of age (often going back to teenage or childhood years). The person with transient ischemic attack (TIA), which may simulate migraine, has symptom onset *after* age 50 years. Be aware that patients suffering migraine with aura may develop TIAs, and they are indeed at slightly higher risk of cerebrovascular events than are non-migraineurs.

▶ Typically, the patient is smartly dressed with a neatly typed diary of their headaches and severity. Many migraineurs pay great attention to detail concerning their clothing, home, and work environment.

Red Flags

Other features should sound alarm bells and warrant full investigation:

◀ *First or worst headache*—that is, someone who rarely suffers headache who experiences severe head pain for the first time

◀ *Cough headache*. Most headaches are *aggravated* by coughing or exertion, but if they are *provoked* by such action this is termed cough headache. In the primary variety, there is no obvious underlying pathology and it is benign. In the secondary or symptomatic form, there are a few possible causes:

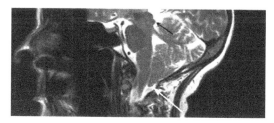

FIGURE 5.1: T2-weighted sagittal brain MRI of Chiari type I malformation. White arrow points to the tip of the cerebellar tonsils. Black arrow shows the beaked appearance of the inferior colliculus that results from partial fusion of the colliculi. Reproduced from Figure 18–2 in the chapter Developmental and Genetic Disorders, by RW Baloh, V Honrubia, and KA Kerber. Oxford University Press. DOI:10.1093/med/9780195387834.003.0018.

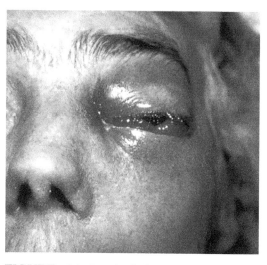

FIGURE 5.2: Periorbital fungal infection due to mucormycosis in diabetic. Reproduced courtesy PHIL, Thomas F. Sellers, Emory University.

- Chiari type 1 malformation (Figure 5.1)
- Colloid cyst of the third ventricle (see Figure 12.9)
- Posterior fossa tumor
- Sinus thrombosis

◀ *Continuous headache in an elderly person suggests cranial arteritis or chronic subdural hematoma.* Check for scalp tenderness and nodules and jaw muscle tenderness. Ask about jaw claudication as these are all features of giant cell arteritis. Shoulder and pelvic muscle tenderness often coexist and suggests polymyalgia rheumatica.

◀ A chronic subdural can be subtle: there are usually no focal signs, just headache and a story that the patient is not so alert as usual. History of a fall and use of anticoagulants are major clues for this diagnosis and warrant an urgent brain scan.

◀ *Periorbital headache and fever in a diabetic or immunosuppressed patient.* Number one on your list would be mucormycosis sinus infection (Figure 5.2).

◀ *Morning headache.* It is well known that occipital headache on wakening or during sleep may signal raised intracranial pressure (ICP) from, for example, space-occupying lesions and idiopathic intracranial hypertension (IIH). Less serious causes are as follows:
- Obstructive sleep apnea. The main Handles for this are:
  - Overweight person (usually male) who snores
  - Not refreshed on morning wakening and sleepy during the day
  - Apneic spells greater than 10 seconds
  - Collar size greater than 17 inches (43 cm) in males or more than 16 inches (40.6 cm) in females
  - Sometimes papilledema due to carbon dioxide retention
  - Occasionally, "weekend headache" if the patient likes to sleep longer at weekends. This may be mistaken for the weekend headache of migraine.
- Occipital headache from cervical spondylosis
- Typical migraine, often triggered by cervical spondylosis
- Bitemporal pain from bruxism.

◀ Headache with ipsilateral carotidynia suggests migraine or internal carotid dissection.

◀ *Coital headache.* Characteristically, this is a disorder of men, consisting of occipital thunderclap headache just *before or during* orgasm, lasting a few minutes. It should be investigated fully, although serious lesions such as aneurysm, vascular malformation, or tumor are rare.

Headache *after* orgasm is unusual and potentially more serious. Think of a dural tear leading to low-tension headache. Patients with connective tissue problems, for example, Marfan's syndrome and Ehlers

Danlos syndrome, are susceptible to low-pressure headache.

◀ *Thunderclap headache.* This is defined as abrupt-onset headache that reaches its peak in less than 1 minute.

Thunderclap headache associated with impairment of consciousness is a major Red Flag and suggests

- ○ Subarachnoid or intracranial hemorrhage
- ○ Colloid cyst of the third ventricle
- ○ Reversible cerebral vasoconstriction syndrome (RCVS)

Most instances of thunderclap headache *without alteration of consciousness* are benign, and it used to be a powerful Handle, but the number of recognized causes has increased over the years, now demoting it to a Red Flag.

Prior events or signs that may help elucidate a cause are as follows:

- ○ Head trauma: arterial dissection or intracranial hypotension
- ○ Horner's syndrome: with cranial nerve (CN) XII palsy suggests internal carotid artery dissection. It is sometimes associated with contralateral hemiparesis or pulsatile tinnitus. Note that the hypoglossal nerve crosses the origin of the internal carotid artery, where it is vulnerable to swelling or inflammation. Pulsatile tinnitus probably results from narrowing of the internal carotid lumen.
- ○ Exposure to vasoactive medication, such as recreational drugs, nasal decongestants, triptans. Such medication may result in RCVS.
- ○ Lumbar puncture: this causes intracranial hypotension and rarely cerebral venous thrombosis.
- ○ Childbirth: this may be associated with maternal cerebral venous thrombosis (postpartum), RCVS, eclampsia, or PRES (posterior reversible encephalopathy syndrome). Note these related Handles:

▶ Headache aggravated by lateral head movement but not flexion suggests venous sinus or jugular vein thrombosis. It is likely that lateral head movement causes compression of the ipsilateral internal jugular vein. Remember that the right internal jugular vein is usually dominant, thus head tilting to the right would be expected to cause more pain.

▶ Headache increased by neck flexion suggests meningeal irritation, cervical spine disorder, or raised ICP. If Kernig's sign is absent, then raised ICP is more likely.

▶ In RCVS, the headache is characteristically recurrent over the space of a few days and may be associated with seizures and focal signs.

Other associations with thunderclap headache:

- · Migraine, coital headache (see earlier discussion), pituitary apoplexy (Figure 5.3)
- · If an initial CT brain scan and LP are normal, think of
  - ○ Cervical artery dissection, RCVS, cerebral venous thrombosis, and pituitary apoplexy (Figure 5.3)

▶ A patient with suspected multiple sclerosis (MS) who develops migraine-like headache and TIAs may have the cerebral autosomal dominant arteriopathy with subcortical infarcts and leukoencephalopathy (CADASIL) syndrome.

▶ The patient with headache who dislikes lying down probably has raised ICP. Apart from space-occupying lesions, this symptom may indicate

- ○ Subarachnoid hemorrhage

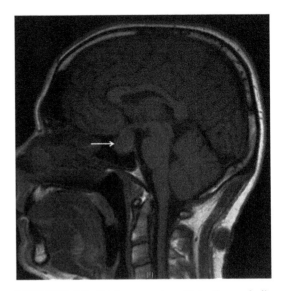

FIGURE 5.3: Pituitary apoplexy. Note the markedly enlarged pituitary gland (white arrow). Figure courtesy Jose Biller, Chicago.

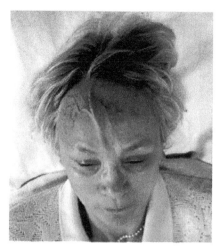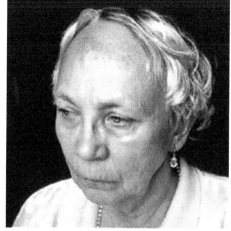

FIGURE 5.4: Caput medusa sign after cerebral venous sinus thrombosis. This woman was known to have thrombosis of the sagittal and transverse sinuses. When supine (**left**) there was facial flushing and headache due to impaired venous drainage. The symptoms were abolished by sitting or standing (**right**). Reproduced with permission from Meyer and Hoffman (2001), Figure 1.

- o Cerebral venous thrombosis (see Figure 5.4)
- o Idiopathic intracranial hypertension (IIH)
- ▶ *The patient with daily headache who keeps painkillers everywhere has medication overuse headache.* The disorder often starts with migraine, but the patient lapses into the habit of taking painkillers (particularly codeine-containing medications that are weakly addictive) on a regular basis, often at the suggestion of a primary care physician. To avoid being caught with headache, reserve tablets are kept at work, in a handbag, in the car, and in pockets. Before social occasions, the patient takes a painkiller to avoid having a headache later.
  - o The diagnosis is confirmed if the patient admits to taking painkillers more than 15 days per month.
  - o Be aware that a patient can still have an additional, underlying cause for their headache.
- ▶ Headache with bilateral papilledema after a long-distance run suggests cerebral venous sinus thrombosis. It results from dehydration and possibly low systolic blood pressure.
- ▶ *Headache with bilateral papilledema following radical neck dissection suggests thrombosis in a major venous sinus.* The surgery is undertaken typically for removal of malignancy or a glomus tumor and arises because the dominant (usually right) internal jugular vein is removed. This produces raised intracranial venous pressure, papilledema, and, occasionally, thrombosis in a major venous sinus (transverse or sigmoid).

- ▶ *Headache after brain radiotherapy may be the SMART syndrome* (stroke-like migraine attacks after radiation therapy). A few years after radiotherapy for brain tumor some patients develop headaches and hemiparesis for several weeks, raising the question of tumor recurrence. The weakness usually resolves spontaneously. See also Chapter 9 (Stroke).

CLUSTER HEADACHE

This is usually an easy diagnosis, with the following characteristics:

- · Middle-aged male
- · Awoken on successive nights during the early hours
- · Intense, strictly unilateral eye pain lasting up to 2 hours

Here are some useful Handles:

- ▶ Autonomic features: Horner's syndrome, tearing, red eye, nasal stuffiness on the side of the pain
- ▶ Triggered by alcohol, warmth, or exercise

▶ *Unilateral* photophobia
▶ Agitation: the patient has to get up and pace about, unlike migraineurs, who prefer to keep still
▶ Relief by 100% oxygen inhalation

Note that clusters may occur at the same month in the year, with headache-free intervals lasting months or years. Symptoms often overlap with paroxysmal hemicranias, but cluster headache does not respond to indomethacin.

▶ Hypnic headache has some similarities to cluster headache but affects the elderly (see later discussion in this chapter).

ORTHOSTATIC HEADACHE

This variety is characterized by pain on standing, relieved by lying flat. ICP falls when upright, causing headache, but rises when recumbent, resulting in pain relief within a few minutes. Most instances are due to spontaneous intracranial hypotension (SIH). Here are some Handles for diagnosis:

▶ The patient with headache who refuses to get out of bed
  Most occurrences follow lumbar puncture (LP) or trauma, but the condition may occur spontaneously and abruptly.
▶ Afternoon headache: in milder cases the headache is delayed until the afternoon
▶ Orthostatic tinnitus: the patient complains of tinnitus (sometimes pulsatile) on standing. Note that tinnitus may be a feature of *raised* ICP as well. See idiopathic intracranial hypertension later in this chapter.
▶ The patient with IIH whose headache initially improves after LP and then relapses
  This suggests low-pressure headache induced by LP, but note:
  ○ Post–LP headache may be due to cerebral venous sinus thrombosis.
  ○ If acetazolamide is given after the LP, persistent headache may ensue.
▶ Orthostatic headache following exertion may mimic subarachnoid hemorrhage.
  The suspected cause is a ruptured meningeal diverticulum or perineural tear that results in leakage of cerebrospinal fluid (CSF), but often no seepage is found. Typical appearances on MRI are shown

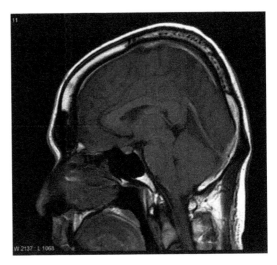

FIGURE 5.5: A 40-year-old male with orthostatic headache. Sagittal T1 MRI shows prominent dural thickening and enhancement throughout all compartments. There is sagging of the splenium of the corpus callosum and posterior fossa contents ("brain sag"). Reproduced with permission from Radiopedia, courtesy Frank Gaillard, case ID 4085.

in Figure 5.5; i.e., brain sag and meningeal enhancement.

Note:

▶ Patients with connective tissue disorders are particularly susceptible.
  Think of orthostatic headache in someone with joint hypermobility, for example, Marfan's syndrome or Ehlers-Danlos syndrome. These patients have increased risk of orthostatic headache, spontaneous pneumothorax, cerebral aneurysm, and arterial dissection.
▶ Orthostatic headache may follow bariatric surgery. The reason for this is not clear.
▶ Occasionally SIH is associated with raised prolactin level, galactorrhea, deafness, and CN VI palsy.

HANDLES FOR OTHER CHARACTERISTIC HEADACHES

▶ Multiple attacks of daytime orbital pain lasting up to 2 minutes with red eye and tearing is the SUNCT syndrome (short-lasting unilateral neuralgiform headache with conjunctival injection and tearing).

During attacks, there may be eyelid swelling.

▶ Multiple brief stabbing pains as if hit by a small hammer suggests ice-pick headache (idiopathic stabbing headache; jabs-and-jolts syndrome).

The stabs last for just seconds and are not confined to one side of the head, and there are no autonomic features. Most patients have migraine as well and respond to indomethacin if it can be tolerated.

▶ Attacks of moderate severity pain over a coin-shaped area, typically parietal, lasting for hours is nummular headache (Figure 5.6).

There may be exacerbations; this is a benign, usually self-limiting disorder probably due to extracranial pathology.

▶ Familial migraine with advanced sleep phase disorder

This is a newly discovered variety of familial migraine associated with an advanced shift in circadian rhythm. Characteristically, patients go to bed around 7 P.M. and wake at 4 A.M. It is due to a mutation in casein kinase 1 delta (CK1δ) (Brennan et al. 2013). The few patients described so far have chronic migraine, namely, headache on more than 15 days per month.

▶ Intense headache provoked by consuming very cold food or drink is cold stimulus headache.

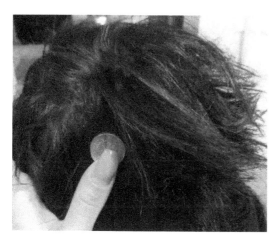

FIGURE 5.6: A patient with nummular headache demonstrates the site of pain with a coin. It is characteristically over the parietal region in a coin-shaped territory, as shown here.

"Ice cream headache" is a common variety. This is a benign disorder triggered by cold. It is short-lasting but may recur with subsequent exposure.

▶ Multiple attacks of sharp, shooting pain in the ear lasting for hours suggests geniculate (nervus intermedius) neuralgia.

This nerve supplies the external auditory meatus and upper concha. There may be triggering by cold, noise, swallowing, or touch, as in trigeminal neuralgia.

▶ More than five attacks per day of severe unilateral periorbital pain lasting up to 30 minutes with autonomic features suggests *chronic paroxysmal hemicrania.*

It is more common in women. Hemicrania continua is similar but the pain is constant, lasting more than 3 months.

▶ An elderly patient with recurrent uni- or bilateral headache without autonomic features who wakes up during rapid eye movement (REM) sleep likely has hypnic headache (alarm-clock headache).

It is helped by indomethacin or caffeine (coffee before sleep or even during the attack).

▶ Recurrent, severe, acute-onset posterior neck pain, fever, and raised inflammatory markers is likely the crowned dens (odontoid process) syndrome.

It is caused by deposits of hydroxyapatite or calcium pyrophosphate dihydrate in ligaments around the odontoid process, which create the appearance of a crown or halo surrounding the odontoid process on CT or MRI (Figure 5.7). Indomethacin or steroid treatment is beneficial.

▶ *Visual snow.* Around 30% patients with migraine experience this phenomenon. See Chapter 2.

▶ Headache that starts during flight take-off or particularly descent is likely *airplane headache.* Patients experience severe unilateral frontal headache. It lasts about 30 minutes and may be relieved by triptans or nonsteroidal anti-inflmmatory drugs (NSAIDs).

▶ Transient migraine-like headache with neurological defects (e.g., hemiparesis) lasting about 2 hours associated with CSF lymphocytosis is the HaNDL syndrome (transient headache and neurologic defects with CSF lymphocytosis). Some are confused

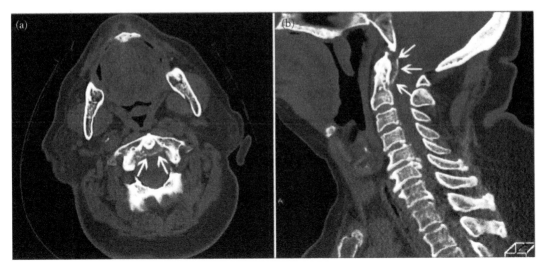

FIGURE 5.7: The crowned dens syndrome. (**A**) Thin curvilinear calcification (arrow) of the transverse ligament of the atlas. (**B**) Linear calcification (arrows) in the sagittal view. Reproduced with permission from Kuriyama (2014).

during the attack. Although there may be one or more episodes, it appears benign.

▶ Headache on bending suggests:
  ○ Migraine
  ○ Sinus disease
  ○ Aneurysms on circle of Willis
  ○ Raised ICP; see causes of cough headache and section on IIH.

Headache Syndromes That Respond Well to Indomethacin

· Chronic paroxysmal hemicrania
· Hypnic headache
· Ice pick headache
· Coital headache
· Crowned dens syndrome

IDIOPATHIC INTRACRANIAL HYPERTENSION

See Figure 1.2. The main features are as follows:

· Headache before breakfast or disturbing sleep. Worse on lying down, less when up and about
· Obese and female
· Continual or pulsatile tinnitus
· Papilledema
· Raised pressure on LP

Here are some further clues that might allow you to clinch a diagnosis:

▶ Headache may wake the patient from sleep because of raised ICP during recumbency.
▶ Headache may improve after LP.
  Sometimes the head pain returns on the following day, suggesting low-pressure headache induced by LP. Rarely, it signals cortical venous sinus thrombosis probably induced by low ICP and dehydration.
▶ Papilledema
  This may be mild or, very rarely, absent. Pulsations in the retinal veins over the optic disk disappear when the ICP exceeds 22 cm H_2O, hence absence of such pulsation helps confirm the presence of raised ICP. Be aware that some healthy people do not show retinal vein pulsation.
▶ Low back pain from increased pressure in the subarachnoid space surrounding the nerve roots or lumbago from obesity
▶ CSF rhinorrhea
  This is rare but it may relieve the headache. The CSF may be distinguished from nasal mucus as it tests positive for glucose or tau protein.
▶ MRI brain scan (Figure 5.8) may show the following:
  ○ Empty sella
  ○ Distended/tortuous optic nerve due to enlarged perineural subarachnoid space
  ○ Flattening of the posterior globe

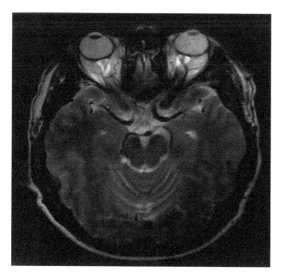 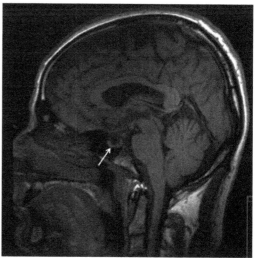

FIGURE 5.8: Left: Axial T2 MRI brain scan in a case of IIH. It shows distended and tortuous optic nerves due to enlarged perineural subarachnoid spaces. Where the optic nerve joins the eye there is flattening of the globe. **Right:** Sagittal T1 MRI shows an empty sella (white arrow). Courtesy Bart's Health Neuroimaging Department, London.

▶ Astronaut with headache relieved on return to Earth.

In microgravity, ICP rises and causes headache (Figure 5.9). One problem with proposed flights to Mars is that astronauts would risk blindness from papilledema by the time they arrived.

SUMMARY

- Head shaking by patients aggravates a migraine attack.
- Pressure on both superficial temporal arteries for a few minutes often abolishes a migraine headache.
- Sinus disease rarely causes severe head pain.

Reassuring Features

- Pain is preferentially *but not exclusively* on one side of the head.
- Scalp or carotid artery tenderness (if under age 50 years)
- Sensory or motor symptoms located usually on the same side as the headache
- Slow evolution of symptoms (minutes) if hemisensory or hemiparetic migraine
- Migraine symptom onset before 50 years of age; TIAs: symptom onset after age 50 years
- Smartly dressed patient with neatly typed diary of headaches and severity

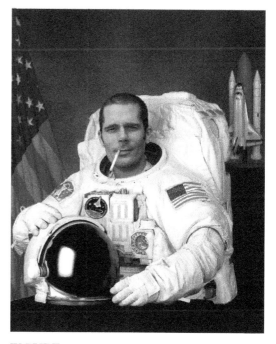

FIGURE 5.9: The astronaut Adam Carlsson, who would have experienced headache while in orbit. Back on Earth, he is relaxing as gravity improves the pain. Headaches in space are most likely due to idiopathic intracranial hypertension, from elevated intracranial pressure in microgravity. Reproduced from NASA photo division (NASA) [FAL], via Wikimedia Commons.

Red Flags

- First or worst headache
- Primary cough headache is usually benign. Secondary form is due to Chiari type 1 malformation, colloid cyst of the third ventricle, posterior fossa tumor, or sinus thrombosis.
- Continuous headache in an elderly person suggests cranial arteritis or chronic subdural hematoma.
- A chronic subdural can be subtle: there are usually no focal signs, just headache and a story that the patient is not so alert as usual. History of fall or use of anticoagulants is suspicious.
- Periorbital headache with fever in a diabetic or immunosuppressed patient points to mucormycosis sinus infection.
- Morning headache infers raised ICP, IIH, obstructive sleep apnea (overweight, not refreshed on wakening, apneic spells >10 seconds, male collar size >17 inches, papilledema), cervical spondylosis, bruxism, migraine
- Coital headache
- Thunderclap headache. If consciousness impaired: subarachnoid or intracranial hemorrhage; colloid cyst of the third ventricle. Without significant impairment of consciousness: RCVS; head trauma with internal carotid dissection, especially Horner' syndrome with CN XII lesion; vasoactive medication; LP; childbirth; migraine; coital headache; pituitary apoplexy; cerebral venous thrombosis
- Headache aggravated by lateral head movement but not flexion suggests venous sinus thrombosis. Headache increased by neck flexion suggests meningeal irritation, cervical spine disorder, or raised ICP.
- A patient with suspected MS who develops migraine-like headache and TIAs may have the CADASIL syndrome.
- The patient with headache who dislikes lying down usually has raised ICP. Think of space-occupying lesions, subarachnoid hemorrhage, cerebral venous thrombosis, or IIH.
- The patient with daily headache who keeps painkillers everywhere has medication overuse headache. Note that there may be additional, underlying physical problems.
- Headache with bilateral papilledema after a long-distance run suggests cerebral venous sinus thrombosis.
- Headache with bilateral papilledema following radical neck dissection suggests thrombosis in a major venous sinus.
- Headache after brain radiotherapy may be the SMART syndrome.

Handles for Cluster Headache

Main features:

- Middle-aged man awoken on successive nights with intense, strictly unilateral eye pain lasting about 2 hours
- Autonomic features
- Triggering by alcohol, warmth, or exercise
- *Unilateral* photophobia and agitation
- Rapid relief by 100% oxygen
- Clusters may occur at the same month in the year.
- Distinguish from hypnic headache

Orthostatic Headache

- Headache patient who refuses to get out of bed likely has orthostatic headache.
- Afternoon headache
- Orthostatic tinnitus
- Watch for the patient with IIH whose headache improves after LP, then relapses. This suggests low-pressure headache induced by LP but could be cerebral venous sinus thrombosis.
- Orthostatic headache following exertion may mimic subarachnoid hemorrhage.
- Patients with connective tissue disorders are susceptible; think of Marfan's or Ehlers-Danlos syndrome.
- May follow bariatric surgery
- Occasionally associated with raised prolactin level, galactorrhea, deafness, and CN VI palsy.
- Brain MRI may show "brain sag" and contrast MRI shows meningeal enhancement.

Handles for Other Characteristic Headache Patterns

- Multiple attacks of daytime orbital pain lasting up to 2 minutes with red eye and tearing suggest the SUNCT syndrome.
- Multiple brief stabbing pains as if hit by a small hammer is likely ice-pick headache, which has a good response to indomethacin.
- Coin-shaped area of pain in parietal area: nummular headache

- Familial migraine with advanced sleep phase disorder
- Intense headache provoked by consuming cold food or drink is cold stimulus headache.
- Multiple attacks of sharp shooting pain in the ear lasting for hours suggest geniculate (nervus intermedius) neuralgia.
- Recurrent periorbital pain lasting up to 30 minutes with autonomic features: chronic paroxysmal hemicrania
- Elderly patient with recurrent uni- or bilateral headache without autonomic features causing waking from REM sleep: hypnic headache
- Recurrent, severe, acute-onset posterior neck pain, fever, and raised inflammatory markers: crowned dens syndrome.
- Visual snow phenomenon is common in migraine.
- Severe unilateral frontal headache on take-off or landing is airplane headache.
- HaNDL syndrome
- Headache on bending: migraine, sinus disease, aneurysms on Circle of Willis, raised ICP. See causes of cough headache and section on IIH
- Headache syndromes that respond well to indomethacin: chronic paroxysmal hemicrania, hypnic headache, ice-pick headache, coital headache, crowned dens syndrome

Idiopathic Intracranial Hypertension

- Main features: morning headache, overweight, female, tinnitus; low back pain; papilledema may be mild; raised pressure on LP; headache improves after LP
- CSF rhinorrhea may relieve the headache.
- Brain MRI: empty sella, distended optic nerves, flattening of posterior part of globe
- Astronaut with headache while in orbit has IIH; disappears on returning to Earth

SUGGESTED READING

Brennan KC, Bates EA, Shapiro RE, et al. Casein kinase 1 delta mutations in familial migraine and advanced sleep phase. *Sci Transl Med.* 2013;5:183ra56.

Ducros A, Bousser MG. Thunderclap headache. *BMJ.* 2012;346:e8557.

Kuriyama A. Crowned dens syndrome. *CMAJ.* 2014;186:293.

Meyer BU, Hoffman KT. Caput medusae after sinus venous thrombosis. *Neurology.* 2001;57:137.

Chapter 6: Epilepsy and Sleep Disorders

Diagnosis of epilepsy may be straightforward, *provided* there is a competent eye witness report that would allow you to distinguish a seizure from ordinary syncope (e.g., where there may be a few jerky movements). Smartphone video recordings afford a very useful supplement to an eye witness account and should be encouraged. When there is no witness, you have to rely on traditional guides like postictal confusion, urinary incontinence, or tongue biting, which most patients will remember, but:

◀ *Urinary incontinence is not uncommon in everyday faints.*
◀ *Urinary incontinence and tongue biting occur in nonepileptic attack disorders.*

If the patient is hot and has been standing for a long time and then blacks out, particularly if there is hypoglycemia, strong emotion, or pain, then syncope is the first diagnosis. The presyncopal symptoms of nausea and clamminess are important to elicit.

Despite these popular guidelines, experts get it wrong, and rarely:

◀ Syncope and epilepsy may be present in the same patient.

We describe in this chapter some Handles that may assist in the diagnosis and, in particular, how to spot the person who is simulating an attack.

INSPECTION

Some patients who present with seizures can be diagnosed immediately if you know what to look for:

Tuberous Sclerosis (Bourneville's Disease, Epiloia)

This autosomal dominant condition is identified easily provided there are the usual hallmarks (Figure 6.1):

- Adenoma sebaceum
- Periungual fibromas (i.e., under or around the fingernails or toenails)
- Hypomelanotic macules (ash-leaf spots that show up best under ultraviolet light)

- Shagreen (leathery) patches over the back (Figure 6.1)

Sturge Weber Syndrome

In most cases this disorder is sporadic, but in some instances it is caused by a mutation in the gene that codes for guanine nucleotide-binding protein subunit alpha (GNAQ). The cardinal features are as follows:

- Port-wine skin lesion, generally in the distribution of the trigeminal nerve (Figure 6.2)
- Mental retardation
- Seizures
- Vascular lesions in the meninges overlying areas of cerebral cortex which show characteristic tramline calcification on CT scan (Figure 6.2)

Lipoid Proteinosis (Urbach–Wiethe Disease)

A young adult with epilepsy, beaded eyelid papules, and hyperkeratosis with verrucous lesions on the elbows has lipoid proteinosis (see Figure 6.3). This is a rare autosomal recessive disorder due to mutations in the extracellular matrix protein 1 gene. Life expectancy is not affected. There is temporal lobe calcification.

Angelman Syndrome

This was formerly called "happy puppet" syndrome (Figure 6.4 and Video 6.1, Angelman). The genetics are complex, and the disorder is not usually inherited. The facial appearance is characteristic, often permitting an instant diagnosis (see also Chapter 8, Movement Disorders). Typically, the child has:

- Red or blonde hair
- Frequent laughing and hand flapping
- Unsteadiness
- Seizures
- Micro- and brachycephaly
- Cognitive and speech impairment
- Rarer features include tongue-thrusting and fascination with water

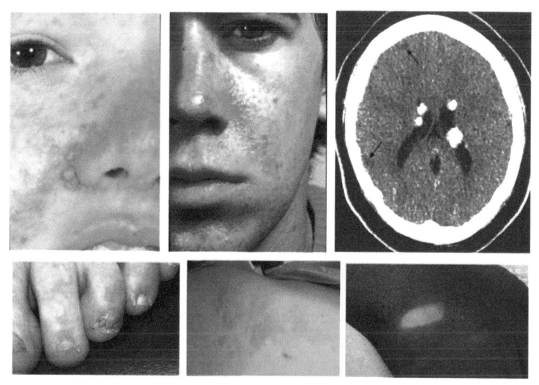

FIGURE 6.1: Tuberous sclerosis (TS). **Top left and top center**: Adenoma sebaceum. Note the subtle soft, cyst-like swellings particularly in the nasolabial groove. **Top right**: CT axial brain scan showing several calcified subependymal nodules. Cortical tubers (black arrows) appear as hypodense areas involving the cortex and subcortical region. **Bottom left**: Periungual fibromas. Note the adenoma sebaceum as well. **Bottom center**: Ash leaf spot and shagreen patch in TS. The shagreen patch is skin-colored and has raised edges. The ash-leaf spot is light in color and flat and shows up best in ultraviolet light. **Bottom right**: Ash-leaf macule in Afro-Caribbean subject. Top right image reproduced from Figure 94.3 in the chapter Tuberous Sclerosis, by S Pruthi. Oxford University Press. DOI:10.1093/med/9780199755325.003.0094. Bottom center image reproduced from Figure 48.23. Oxford University Press.

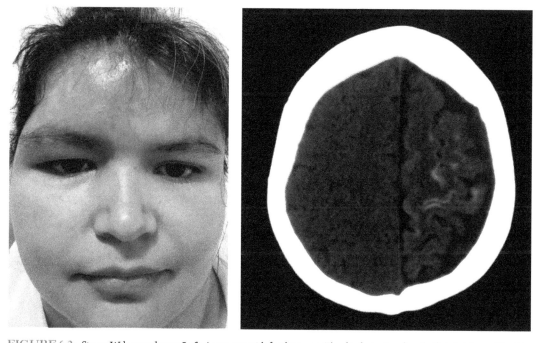

FIGURE 6.2: Sturge-Weber syndrome. **Left**: A teenager with focal seizures. The skin lesion involves the first divisions of the right trigeminal nerve. **Right**: Unenhanced axial brain CT scan demonstrating prominent subcortical white matter "tramline" calcification. Left image courtesy Jaime Toro, Bogota, Colombia. Right image courtesy Bart's Health Neuroimaging Department, London.

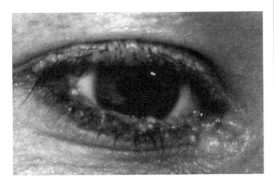
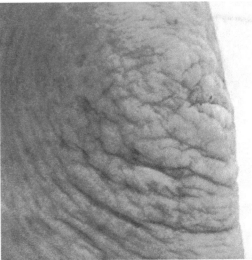

FIGURE 6.3: Lipoid proteinosis (Urbach-Wiethe disease) in a woman with epilepsy and amnestic deficit. **Left**: Beaded eyelid papules. **Right**: Hyperkeratosis with verrucous lesions on the extensor surfaces of the elbows. Reproduced with permission from Quirici and da Rocha (2013), Figure 1.

Rett Syndrome

This is an X-linked disorder due to mutation in the gene methyl CpG binding protein 2 (*MECP2*). The male form is usually fatal; hence the disorder affects girls (Figure 6.5 and Video 6.2, Rett). It is characterized by:

- Hyperventilation, breath-holding or sighing; mutism
- Stereotypies: hand wringing/rubbing and squeezing
- Seizures (affect 80%). Sometimes vacant spells occur that are due to brainstem disorder and may be confused with epilepsy.
- Dystonia affecting limbs and spine leading to contractures and kyphoscoliosis

Often it can be diagnosed instantly because of stereotyped behavior. It is sometimes misdiagnosed as autism spectrum disorder.

Note that a Rett-like clinical profile is associated with beta-propeller protein–associated neurodegeneration (Chapter 8).

Sotos Syndrome

This is a form of cerebral gigantism that arises by spontaneous mutation of the NSD1 gene. It should be recognizable at once by the facial appearances and height (Figure 6.6). Patients are unusually tall with a large dolichocephalic skull. It is associated with seizures and behavioral problems.

Linear Sebaceous Nevus Syndrome

The main features are a large linear birthmark (sebaceous nevus) on the face, scalp or neck, associated with seizures, cognitive impairment, agenesis of corpus callosum, agyria (see Figure 6.7).

HISTORY AND EXAMINATION

Epileptic auras are manifestations of brain epileptic overactivity and may indicate what part of the brain is abnormal. It is helpful to ask:

- "Can you tell when you are about to have a seizure?" or
- "Do you ever feel that you are about to have a seizure and then not have one?"

Patients with primary generalized epilepsy (and some focal seizures, particularly frontal) may have no warning; the first thing they know, they are on the ground with people standing around.

Following are some Handles that may help your diagnosis:

In general:

▶ Sudden onset and offset suggest a seizure.
▶ Gradual onset and offset suggests a faint.
▶ Rising epigastric aura favors epilepsy.
   In a true epileptic attack, there may be a strange, fear-like sensation ("butterflies") in the epigastric zone that ascends through the chest up to the neck just prior to

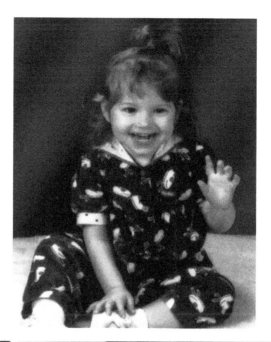

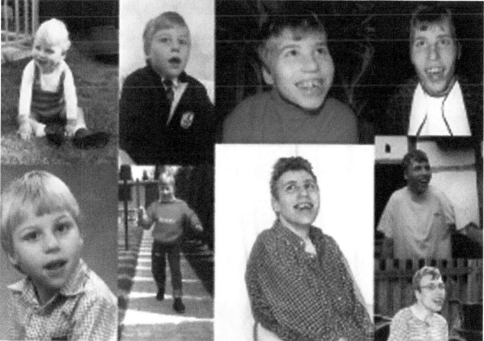

FIGURE 6.4: Angelman syndrome. **Top:** Happy appearance in a young girl. The hands are flapped frequently. Not all are blonde! **Bottom:** A male child at various stages of development. Top image reproduced with permission from Franz et al. (2000), Figure 1. Bottom image reproduced from Van Buggenhout and Fryns (2009), Figure 1.

impairment of consciousness. This is typical of a partial seizure.

In a simple faint, the sensation is more likely to stay in the epigastrium.

▶ In general, an epileptic aura produces *positive* symptoms, such as tingling, odd smell/taste, unusual noise, flashing lights, or pain lasting less than 5 seconds.

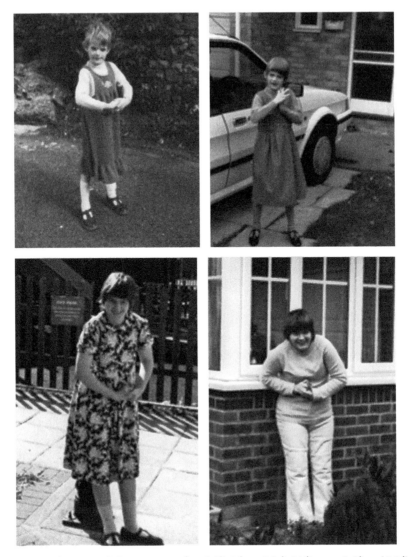

FIGURE 6.5: Rett syndrome. Serial photos at ages 7 (**top left**), 9 (**top right**), 24 (**bottom left**), and 26 (**bottom right**). Observe the hand-wringing position in all photos except top right. Also note microcephaly and progressive kyphosis. Images courtesy Anthony and Janet Best.

Negative symptoms like numbness, clumsiness, or heaviness lasting more than 5 seconds are probably not epileptic and more like transient ischemic attacks (TIAs). Main exception: amyloid spells (see Chapter 9, Stroke)

▶ Sudden falls forward in the elderly without loss of consciousness suggest a drop attack. The patient collapses without warning on to the knees or face, causing injury. The mechanism is probably sudden hypotonia due to brainstem ischemia.

▶ Involuntary laughing suggests gelastic epilepsy.
This is a rare form of seizure in which the patient laughs involuntarily; it is mirthless. In general:
  ○ If consciousness is retained, the cause is a hypothalamic hamartoma.
  ○ If consciousness is lost, the lesion is in the temporal or, rarely, frontal lobe.

▶ A complementary disorder is *dacrystic seizures* where the patient cries involuntarily, occasionally laughing as well. The lesion site

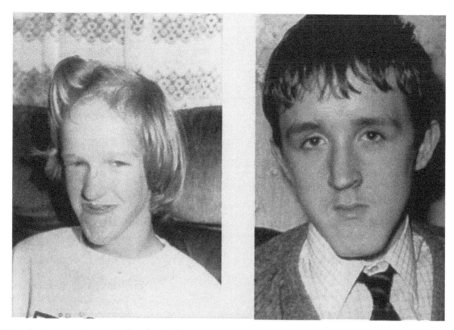

FIGURE 6.6: Sotos syndrome. Both individuals are tall and suffer from epilepsy. Note the narrow face, pointed chin, down-slanting palpebral fissures (right patient) and dolichocephaly (left subject). Reproduced with from: J C Agwu et al. (1999).

for dacrystic seizures is the same as gelastic attacks.

▶ Low-grade tumors present with seizures. High-grade tumors start with focal neurological signs, such as hemiplegia.

This is a useful general rule that probably relates to the speed of tumor growth. Also, the tumor prognosis is better when presentation is epileptic.

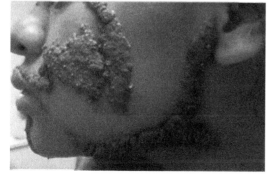

FIGURE 6.7: Linear sebaceous nevus syndrome. A 12-year-old female with extensive epidermal nevi, seizures, mental retardation present since birth. Reproduced with permission under Creative Commons BY-NC-ND license from: Boger LS et al. (2012).

▶ Visual hallucinations and occipital calcifications suggest celiac disease.

The patient presents with a variety of occipital seizures consisting of visual hallucinations (scenes, colored dots) and often no symptoms of bowel disorder. Occipital calcification (Figure 6.8) clinches the diagnosis. The teeth are sometimes mottled.

▶ Myoclonic jerks in a child or teenager at breakfast is likely juvenile myoclonic epilepsy (JME) (Video 6.3, JME)

Myoclonic jerks may happen throughout the day and when dropping off to sleep, but most are experienced during the early morning, when washing, brushing the teeth, or having breakfast. Patients experience generalized tonic-clonic or absence seizures as well.

▶ Olfactory or gustatory aura suggests a lesion in the anterior temporal lobe (amygdala).

It is regularly followed by a partial seizure that may generalize. Most adults with this history turn out to have a structural lesion, such as a glioma (Figure 6.9).

▶ *Posterior* shoulder dislocation is likely due to a seizure or electric shock injury.

Most shoulder dislocations are anterior. Apart from electric shock injury (which probably

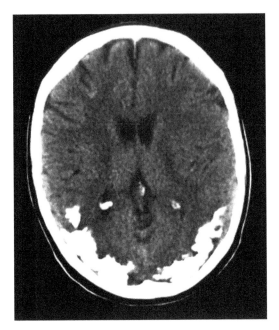

FIGURE 6.8: Celiac disease. Axial CT brain scan shows bilateral serpentine calcification in the parieto-occipital regions in a patient with confirmed celiac disease and occipital lobe seizures. The serpentine nature of calcification sometimes leads to a misdiagnosis of Sturge Weber syndrome. Reproduced with permission from Pfaender et al. (2004), Figure 1.

causes a convulsion), seizures are by far the major cause of posterior dislocation. The shoulder dislocates because of the impact of the fall out of bed or from strong muscle contractions around the shoulder, and may be bilateral. The usual history is that the patient wakes up from sleep on the floor with a painful shoulder (Figure 6.10). This history is strongly suggestive of a sleep-associated seizure, although attacks during wakefulness may also cause a posterior dislocation. Some patients withhold such information because they are reluctant to lose their driver's license.

▶ First seizure in a patient from Asia or South America is likely due to neurocysticercosis or TB.

The former is caused by the pork tapeworm, *Taenia solium*. CT or MRI is usually diagnostic and reveals single or multiple lesions (Figure 6.11). Some have calf hypertrophy due to intramuscular cysts; if not, there is focal calcification visible on plain X-ray. Cerebral TB is another possibility and may have very similar MRI appearances.

▶ Some anticonvulsants increase seizure frequency.

These include:

• *Sodium valproate.* This worsens Alper's syndrome, metabolic conditions such

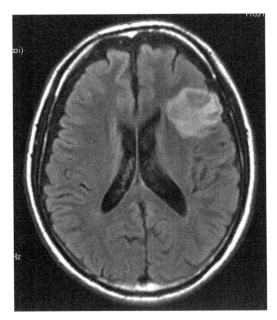

FIGURE 6.9: T2-weighted brain MRI from a patient who presented with olfactory hallucinations. These were caused by a large oligodendroglioma that involved the anterior pole of the left temporal lobe.

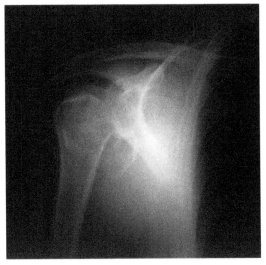

FIGURE 6.10: Posterior dislocation of the shoulder due to nocturnal seizure. Courtesy Ken Shauger.

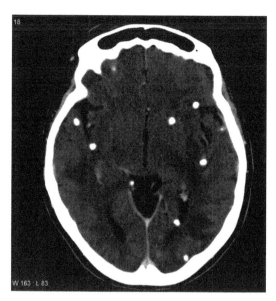

FIGURE 6.11: Post-contrast CT shows numerous calcified 3- to 7-mm lesions with surrounding edema characteristic of neurocysticercosis. MRI images may show a ring with central hyperintensity, which is the head of the tapeworm. Reproduced with permission from Dr. F Gaillard, Radiopedia, ID 7773.

as hyperglycinemia, and mitochondrial disorders. Alper's syndrome is caused by a mutation in the *POLG1* gene and affects infants and children. It is characterized by refractory seizures, mental retardation, spastic quadriplegia, blindness, deafness, and occipital lobe calcification.

- *Carbamazepine, phenytoin, and vigabatrin.* Any of these may increase the frequency of myoclonus or absence episodes in JME. Phenytoin may worsen myoclonus in *progressive myoclonus epilepsy*. Porphyria may worsen if the patient is taking hepatically metabolized drugs (e.g., carbamazepine or phenytoin).
- *Tiagabine.* This is probably the worst offender. It is a frequent cause of nonconvulsive status epilepticus.
- *Benzodiazepines.* These may precipitate tonic status in Lennox-Gastaut syndrome.
- *Sodium channel blocking agents* should be avoided in Dravet's syndrome (a sodium channelopathy), for example:
  o Phenytoin
  o Carbamazepine
  o Lamotrigine
  o Vigabatrin

▶ Episodes of spitting, coughing, vomiting, nose wiping, or water drinking are likely peri-ictal vegetative symptoms.
Typically, the patient wakes from sleep and displays automatisms followed by bouts of these behavior patterns for around 20 seconds. They are a feature of the actual seizure and not the aura (Kellinghaus et al. 2003), except for nose wiping, which is a postictal phenomenon.

▶ Apparent loss of consciousness with awareness of surroundings

This is typical of the following:

- Simple faint
- Nonepileptic attacks
- Cataplexy

There are two clues for cataplexy: (1) the history prior to the fall, characteristically a strong emotion or laughter; (2) the deep tendon reflexes and muscle tone are depressed. See Video 6.4, Cataplexy (courtesy Paul Reading). There is no loss of consciousness and weakness develops in a rostro-caudal fashion (i.e., from the face downward).

A cataplectic attack may occur during sex and is reported as a sudden collapse. There is no headache as in coital migraine.

▶ Blackout while shaving suggests a *hypersensitive carotid sinus*.
This is sometimes called "shaving syncope."

▶ Blackout on swallowing is *swallowing syncope*. This relates to vagal stimulation and consequent hypotension. It may be a situational faint (because of esophageal pain, etc.), cardiac arrhythmia (typically bradycardia due to vagal stimulation), or a sensitive carotid sinus.

▶ Falling episode while watching a video game points to:
  o Cataplexy or:
  o Photic-induced seizure. This happens because of rapidly alternating patterns that synchronize with EEG. rhythms.

The laughter or other emotion provoked by a humorous cartoon or video recording may induce a cataplectic attack. Consciousness is not lost, but often a "blackout" is reported. Without telemetering, such an episode can be subtle.

▶ Seizure at a night club. Think of
  o Photic-induced convulsion
  o Recreational drug exposure
  o Alcohol (withdrawal or excess)
  o Sleep deprivation (in epileptic)
▶ Lower lip trembling while reading followed by blackout suggests reading epilepsy.
▶ Seizure while taking a bath, shower, or swimming suggests water immersion epilepsy.
  This is a rare form of reflex epilepsy which may result in a complex partial attack or generalized from the outset. Two genetic loci have been identified, on chromosomes 10q and 4q.
▶ Musicogenic epilepsy
  This is another form of probable reflex epilepsy triggered by a passage of music or by playing a musical instrument. The focus is typically in the right temporal lobe.
▶ Sudden falls following loud noise suggests cataplexy, hyperekplexia, myotonia congenita, or startle epilepsy.

Hyperekplexia may be congenital or acquired and starts in infancy or childhood. The congenital variety of hyperekplexia is characterized by

  · Generalized stiffness
  · Exaggerated startle responses
  · Hypertrophic muscles

Most mutations involve glycine metabolism. The causes of acquired hyperekplexia include the following:

  · Stiff person syndrome
  · Progressive encephalomyelitis with rigidity and myoclonus (PERM)
  · Psychogenic disorders
  · Numerous poorly understood, culturally associated afflictions characterized by bizarre behavior, such as Latah (Malaysia and Indonesia), Jumping Frenchmen of Maine (Canada, Eastern USA), Goosey, Hyperstartlers (USA), Ragin' Cajuns (Louisiana)
▶ Acquired progressive dysphasia in children with sleep seizures is likely the Landau-Kefler syndrome.
  The child develops normally to start with and then experiences a gradually worsening, predominantly expressive dysphasia. There

may be generalized daytime seizures, but some only have seizure activity during sleep; thus, a sleep EEG recording is essential for the diagnosis.
▶ Eyelid myoclonus, eye closure-induced seizures, absences, photosensitivity starting in childhood is *Jeavon's syndrome* (Video 6.5, Jeavon's). Eyelid myoclonus is the Handle! It means rapid fluttering of the eyelids, sometimes associated with upward deviation of the eyeballs and neck extension. It can be confused with a tic or Tourette syndrome.
▶ Absence or myoclonic seizures self-induced by looking at sun through waving fanned-out fingers is the *sunflower syndrome*. Also, it may be induced by rapidly opening and closing the eyes, thus causing confusion with Jeavon's syndrome.
▶ Simian gait with mild ataxia and seizures suggests Dravet's syndrome See Video 6.6, Dravet (courtesy Professor Ingrid Scheffer).

This is a sodium channelopathy that presents in childhood with the following characteristics:

  · Refractory seizures often following pertussis vaccination
  · Aggravation of attacks with sodium channel-blocking anticonvulsants
  · Mildly ataxic "simian" gait
▶ Figure-of-eight head movement
  Such head movements are a feature of two rare forms of childhood epilepsy:
    o Rhombo-encephalo-synapsis (Video 6.7, RES) is a developmental disorder of the brainstem with absence of the cerebellar vermis and fusion of the cerebellar hemispheres.
    o Ohtahara syndrome is an autosomal dominant epileptic encephalopathy due to a mutation in the STXBP1 gene (Video 6.8, Ohtahara). The main features are refractory tonic seizures, encephalopathy, and a characteristic figure-of-eight head movement.

Guides to Localization

Epileptologists use the words *lateralization* and *localization* in a confusing but specific manner. *Lateralization* refers to one or other cerebral hemisphere. *Localization* refers to a particular region within a cerebral hemisphere.

▶ *Postictal weakness* (Todd's paralysis) implies a lesion in the cerebral hemisphere opposite the side of weakness. In general:

▶ Postictal weakness lasting more than 24 hours is caused by a structural defect such as a tumor.

▶ *Versive seizures.* Head and eye deviation while the patient is alert (i.e., simple partial seizure) indicates a focus in the contralateral motor cortex (i.e., opposite to the direction of head and eye movement). Versive head and eye movements that occur as the partial seizure becomes generalized only *lateralize* the defect to the contralateral hemisphere; it has no *localization* value.

▶ *Fencer's sign* (Figure 6.12). This is a form of asymmetric tonic limb posturing that may help localization. One arm is flexed at the elbow and abducted at the shoulder; the other arm is extended and abducted at the shoulder in the position of a fencer's stance. It suggests a lesion in the supplementary motor area opposite the extended arm.

▶ *Figure-of-four sign* (Figure 6.13, with permission from Kotagal et al. 2000). This is a variant of the fencer's sign and is characterized by one arm semi-flexed over the chest and

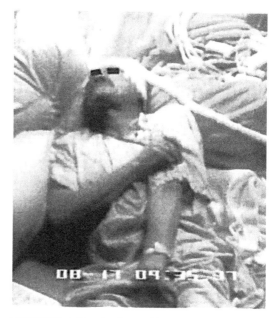

FIGURE 6.13: The figure-of-four sign. Note the flexed right arm and extended left arm, suggesting a focus in the right frontal or temporal lobe. Reproduced courtesy of Kotagal et al. (2000).

the other fully extended down the side of the trunk, resembling the shape of the number 4. The lesion is opposite the extended arm, and it is seen in temporal or frontal lobe disorders.

▶ Ictal pouting. See Figure 6.14 and Video 6.9, Ictal Pouting (courtesy Koc et al. 2017). This is also known as the *chapeau de gendarme* (Napoleonic policeman's hat). It is an expression of fear or disgust. In the attack, the mouth is turned down and the lips puckered for 5 seconds or more. It is a feature of frontal lobe epilepsy resulting from a lesion in the anterior cingulate cortex.

▶ *Spreading sensory symptoms usually stem from the opposite parietal lobe.*

Nonmigrating sensory symptoms only help *lateralize.* If a patient describes a tingling sensation, say, in one hand, that spreads up the arm and then into the ipsilateral lower limb, this *localizes* to the contralateral somatosensory cortex. There are two rare exceptions:

o Sensory symptoms may be reported with a contralateral medial frontal disorder. A lesion affecting the insula may evoke a sensation of someone grabbing the throat.

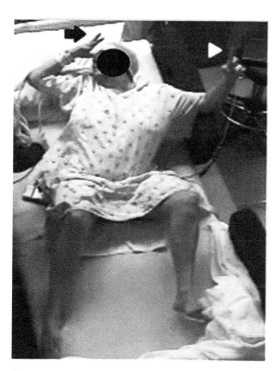

FIGURE 6.12: Fencer's sign.

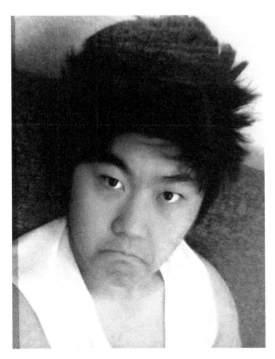

FIGURE 6.14: Ictal pouting, also known as the *chapeaux de gendarme* sign. It is an expression of fear or disgust. In the attack the mouth is turned down and lips puckered. It is a feature of frontal lobe epilepsy resulting from a lesion in the anterior cingulate cortex. Figure reproduced with permission from Hayakawa and Kubota (2018).

> o Bilateral sensory symptoms may occur with a lesion of the superior temporal gyrus.
> ▶ An aura of pain usually localizes to the opposite parietal lobe. Rarely, a thalamic focus will cause pain that is ipsilateral.
> ▶ Formed visual hallucinations indicate a seizure arising in the posterior temporal-parietal area.
> ▶ Musical auras usually localize to the nondominant superior temporal gyrus.

REFRACTORY SEIZURES

It is important to be aware of possible causes of refractory seizures. Nonepileptic attack disorders (NEADs) are frequently the reason, as discussed later. In status epilepticus, if there is a structural lesion, it often resides in the frontal lobe. The reason is that the frontothalamic connections have an important inhibitory/stabilizing effect, so that any process that disrupts this pathway—for example, a tumor,

hemorrhage, or leucotomy—increases the risk of status epilepticus.

> ▶ Seizures developing after pertussis vaccination may be due to Dravet syndrome.
> This disorder is caused by a mutation in the sodium channel gene, *SCN1A*. Usually, the convulsion is ascribed to vaccine-related encephalopathy, but it is likely that children with Dravet's syndrome are predisposed to seizures after vaccination, probably induced by fever. Note that aggravation of seizure frequency in Dravet's syndrome may occur with sodium-blocking medication, as listed previously. The gait is typical, displaying a slightly crouched stance with the knees semiflexed, but the gait is not markedly broad-based. (Video 6.6, Dravet). Occasionally patients with Dravet's syndrome are overlooked and present to adult neurologists.

Refractory Status Epilepticus

The more common explanations are as follows:

- Encephalitis
- Stroke, including cortical vein thrombosis and cerebral hemorrhage
- Hypoxia
- NEAD
- Valproate-induced hyperammonemic encephalopathy (see MRI in Figure 6.15)
> ▶ With refractory seizures, psychosis, and low blood sodium level, think of
> o Leucine-rich glioma inactivated-1 (LGI-1) antibody encephalitis
> o NMDA antibody encephalitis
> o Porphyria
> o Medication, such as carbamazepine
> ▶ Multiple unilateral facio-brachial dystonic seizures favor an LGI-1 channelopathy
> (See Video 6.10, Facio-Brachial-Dystonic Seizures.) Patients experience, on average, 50 attacks per day, and these may precede limbic encephalitis by several weeks. Disconcertingly, the routine EEG may be normal. LGI-1 channelopathy results in autoimmune encephalitis. Patients are usually male with low plasma sodium but no underlying cancer. Standard anticonvulsants are ineffective, but immunotherapy such

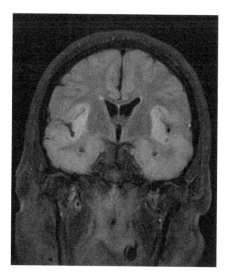 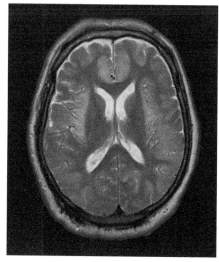

FIGURE 6.15: MRI images in a case of proven valproate encephalopathy with refractory seizures. There are diffuse, relatively symmetrical, cortical high T2 signals, with swelling and restricted diffusion within all lobes throughout both cerebral hemispheres, most marked within the limbic system and temporal poles. Notably, the basal ganglia are spared. Courtesy Bart's Health Neuroimaging Department, London.

as immunoglobulin or plasma exchange may help.

▶ Seizures, psychosis, language deterioration, stereotypy, catatonia, and dysautonomia suggests anti-NMDA receptor encephalitis. The EEG may show the extreme delta brush pattern (see Figure 6.18 and Video 6.11, NMDA). This is a subacute disorder. About 60% of women harbor ovarian teratoma or other neoplasia. Men with this disorder may have a testicular tumor.

▶ Stiff person, cerebellar ataxia, and seizures This combination likely relates to glutamate decarboxylase (GAD) antibodies. Many such individuals have small-cell lung cancer.

▶ Continual partial seizures in a young adult or child suggest epilepsia partialis continua (Video 6.12, EPC and Video 6.13, Rasmussen). This is a feature of the following:

○ Rasmussen encephalitis. This is associated with progressive hemiparesis and cognitive decline. Cause is unknown.

○ Channelopathies related to encephalitis with antibodies to LGI-1, NMDA receptors

○ Complex partial status

○ Ring chromosome 20 disorder. The diagnosis may be confirmed by a sleep EEG

that shows continual generalized theta activity and prolonged bilateral paroxysmal high-voltage slow waves with occasional spikes. The disorder is more like nonconvulsive status (see Figure 6.17, *top*).

○ Hypoglycemia, nonketotic hyperglycemia, hypocalcemia, hypomagnesemia

▶ Episodic ataxia or exercise-induced dyskinesia, anticonvulsant-refractory seizures, and very low cerebrospinal fluid (CSF) glucose suggests glucose transporter type 1 deficiency syndrome (De Vivo disease).

This is an autosomal dominant disorder caused by diminished activity of glucose transporter protein (GLUT1). Relief by a sugary drink is characteristic, whereas prolonged fasting may lead to status epilepticus. The CSF glucose is usually very low because of defective transport across the blood–brain barrier.

Note: Sometimes milder forms are misdiagnosed as refractory absence seizures resulting in preventable cognitive decline.

EEG Handles

Occasionally, the EEG reveals a highly characteristic pattern that allows you to make an instant diagnosis as follows (Figures 6.16–6.19):

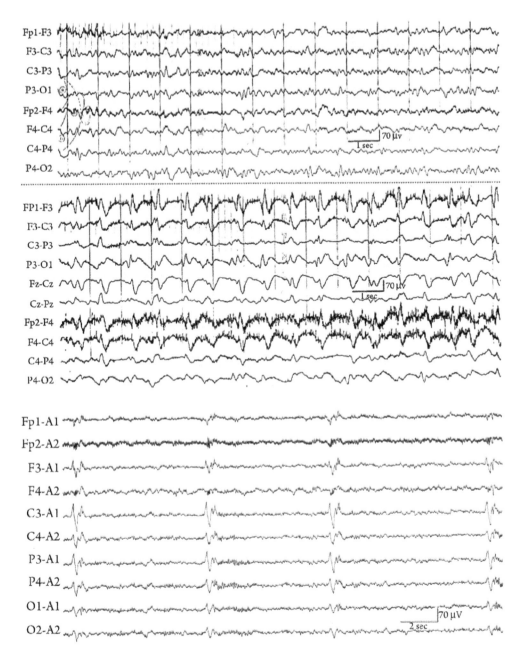

FIGURE 6.16: Characteristic EEG patterns. **Top pair:** A 69-year-old patient with Creutzfeldt-Jakob disease. The upper tracing initially showed only subtle periodic discharges or "clocking," that is, regular sharp waves occurring about once per second. The lower tracing obtained 2 weeks later showed very clear periodic discharges with a periodicity of 1.2 per second. **Bottom EEG:** Typical generalized periodic discharges lasting 1 to 2 seconds in a child with subacute sclerosing panencephalitis (SSPE). Reproduced from *Atlas of EEG, Seizure Semiology, and Management. Clinical EEG*, by KE Misulis, Figures 4-75 (left) and 4-79 (right). Oxford University Press. DOI:10.1093/med/9780199985906.003.0004.

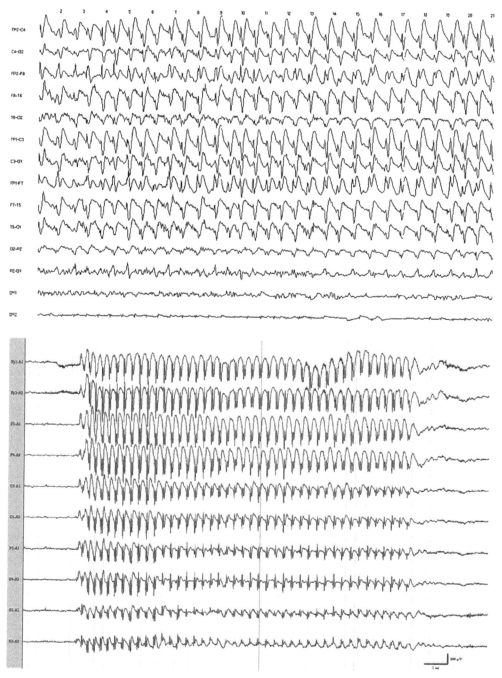

FIGURE 6.17: Characteristic EEG patterns. **Top**: Ring chromosome 20 disorder. "Interictal" EEG with continuous high-voltage 1.5 to 2 Hz spike and waves affecting mainly the frontal areas in a 12-year-old patient. Such activity is seen typically during sleep. **Bottom**: Absence seizure in a 9-year-old girl with spells of staring and unresponsiveness for 1 year. There is an abrupt-onset prolonged discharge of generalized 3Hz well-formed spike-and-wave activity. Top image reproduced with permission from Ville et al. (2006). Bottom image reproduced from *Atlas of EEG, Seizure Semiology, and Management*. Clinical EEG, by KE Misulis, Figure 4-95. Oxford University Press. DOI:10.1093/med/9780199985906.003.0004.

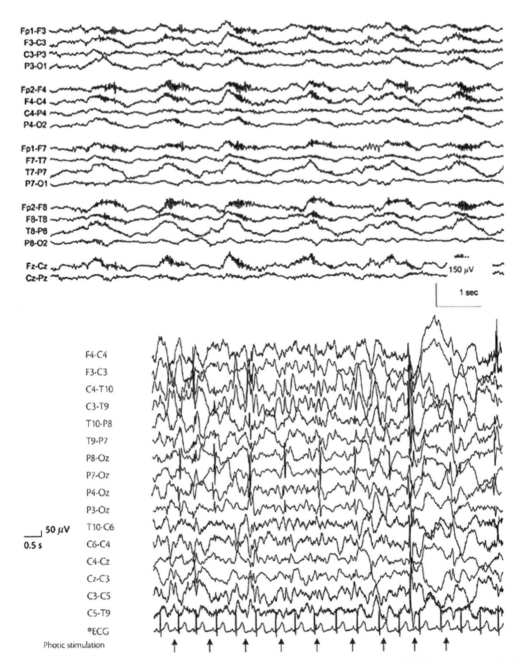

FIGURE 6.18: Characteristic EEG patterns. **Top**: Extreme delta brush sign from a man with NMDA receptor antibodies. There is delta frequency activity at 1 Hz with superimposed, mainly frontal bursts of rhythmic beta frequency activity. **Bottom**: Neuronal ceroid lipofuscinosis. Enhanced response posteriorly on EEG to photic stimulation suggestive of the late infantile form. Vertical arrows represent photic stimulation. Top image reproduced with permission from Schmitt et al. (2012), Figure 1. Bottom image reproduced from Figure 30.1 in the chapter Seizures and Related Disorders in Children, by H Cross. Oxford University Press. DOI:10.1093/med/9780198569381.003.0693.

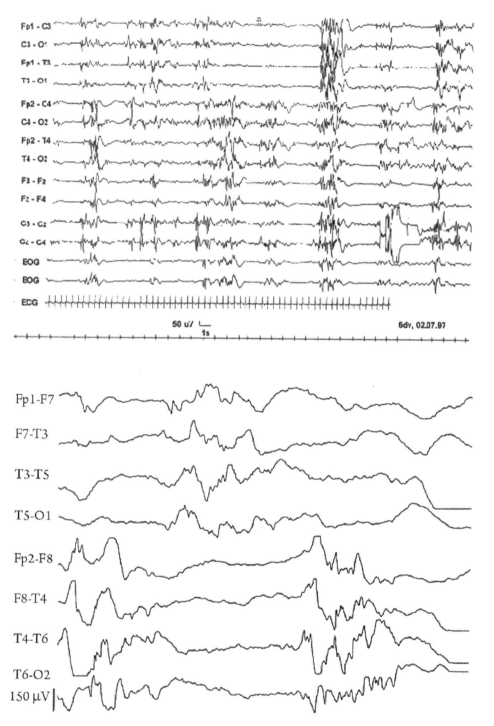

FIGURE 6.19: Top: Aicardi syndrome (myoclonic encephalopathy, agenesis of corpus callosum, and Swiss cheese retinopathy). The EEG shows burst suppression activity arising independently from either hemisphere because of corpus callosum agenesis, producing a "checkerboard" pattern. **Middle/Bottom:** Another EEG of Aicardi syndrome showing asynchronous firing. Top image Reproduced with permission from Costa et al. (2001), Figure 1. Middle/bottom images reproduced from *Atlas of EEG, Seizure Semiology, and Management.* Clinical EEG, by KE Misulis, Figure 4-123. Oxford University Press. DOI:10.1093/med/9780199985906.003.0004.

- Classic Creutzfeldt-Jacob disease (CJD; Figure 6 16, *top*).
  Note: If the EEG looks like an electrocardiogram (EKG), the diagnosis is CJD
- Subacute sclerosing panencephalitis (SSPE) (Figure 6.16, *bottom*)
- Ring chromosome 20 disorder (Figure 6.17, *top*)
- Absence seizures (Figure 6.17, bottom)
- NMDA receptor encephalitis (Figure 6.18, *top*)
- Neuronal ceroid lipofuscinoses (Figure 6.18, *bottom*)
- Aicardi syndrome (Figure 6.19)

NONEPILEPTIC ATTACK DISORDERS

The following are a series of Handles and Red Flags that may help you diagnose NEADs. Remember that some patients experience real *as well as* simulated episodes.

▶ Mattress on the floor sign (Figure 3.1)
  This occurs when a patient is admitted to a general hospital with epilepsy "so severe" that nursing staff feel that the patient has to be put on the floor for their own safety. NEADs are the most likely cause. Occasionally patients with simulated seizures become violent—often directed at their medical attendants. Later, they boast about how many people were required to "hold them down" in the attack. Note that some severe, institutionalized, genuine epileptics do have to be nursed on the floor.

▶ Slippers sign (Figure 3.2)
  Some patients with NEADs like wearing large animal-style slippers. Many carry teddy bears or similar cuddly toys into the clinic.

▶ Wearing dark glasses indoors
  Some patients use dark glasses indoors because of photophobia or dislike of fluorescent light, as in severe migraine. More often, this sign indicates a psychogenic condition.

▶ Convulsion on abrupt standing after hyperventilation
  This is probably a self-induced attack provoked by intense hyperventilation. It is sometimes called the "fainting lark" or "mess trick" to avoid school or work.

The following Handles, during or shortly after an attack, favor a nonepileptic attack:

▶ Blackout with eyes tightly shut
  In a genuine blackout, the eyes are characteristically open and staring with dilated unresponsive pupils. If the eyes happen to

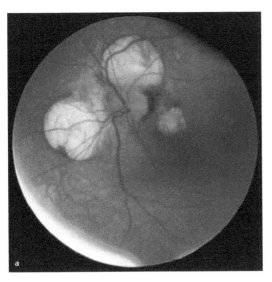
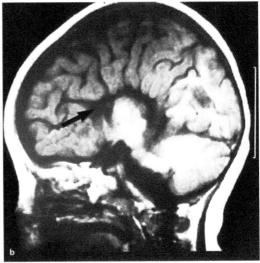

FIGURE 6.20: Left: Circumpapillary chorioretinal lacunae (Swiss cheese retinopathy) in a girl with Aicardi syndrome. **Right**: MRI changes that show marked hypoplasia of the corpus callosum (arrow). Figures reproduced with permission from *Clinical Neuro-ophthalmology*, eds. U Schiefer, H Wilhelm, W Hart, Figures 19.10a and 19.10b. Springer 2007.

be closed, there should be no difficulty in opening them. If resistance to eye opening is displayed, this will indicate a functional disorder.

▶ Conjugate gaze away from examiner
If the patient's eyes are deviated to look at the ground or mattress, it is worth rolling them over to the other side. In a genuine attack, the eyes will stay in the same direction; in a simulated episode the eyes will turn to face the floor or mattress again.

▶ Fast regular breathing
This is rare in a genuine epileptic attack but common in simulated episodes. Stertorous breathing is a feature of genuine attacks.

▶ Weeping and/or pain during after the attack
The patient may indicate severe pain when the examiner moves the patient's limbs gently. This is common in functional disorders but rare in the epileptic variety.

▶ Violent or thrashing movements sometimes directed at medical attendants

▶ Attack in the vicinity of medical staff (see Video 6.14, NEAD).

▶ "Epileptic" attack when EEG electrodes are being attached. This remarkable and frustrating sign is well known to epileptologists (Woollacott et al. 2010).

▶ Duration of motor activity ("convulsions") longer than 2 minutes

▶ Involuntary movements that wax and wane

▶ Seizures occurring with suggestion or intravenous saline

▶ Mirror sign. If a mirror is held in front of a patient whose eyes are open, he or she may focus on their reflection in the mirror.

▶ Awareness of surroundings during generalized convulsive movements

Munchausen's Syndrome

Also termed *factitious disorder imposed on self*; in this disorder, patients simulate a variety of illnesses including seizures.
Handles include:

▶ Multiple hospital visits for apparently serious/emergency illness in widely separated regions of a country

▶ Simulated seizures, chronic pain, weakness or coma.

▶ History of several invasive procedures (e.g., laparotomy, burr holes)

▶ Tendency to self-discharge from ward

▶ Dislike of being photographed

SLEEP-RELATED DISORDERS

This is a relatively new specialty of major importance. So often, a neurologist interviews a patient with some form of involuntary movement during sleep and the question is raised of sleep-related epilepsy. The patient is usually unable to give an account, and one must rely on the partner (if any) who may not have been particularly alert at the time of the episodes. Apart from sleep laboratories, the widespread availability of smartphones that have a video recording capability permits an earlier diagnosis.

Following are some useful Handles that should help clarify the nature of attacks.

▶ Generalized or focal myoclonic jerks, particularly on falling asleep are normal phenomena. They are often incorporated into dream narratives and associated with K complexes on EEG. If excessive or continuous, they suggest myoclonus epilepsy.

▶ Pelvic rocking, head banging, or thumb sucking on going to sleep suggests sleep–wake transition disorder.
It is benign and does not necessarily require treatment.

▶ Cycling or rocking movements during sleep
These are a feature of frontal lobe seizures which occur in any non-rapid eye movement (REM) sleep phase. See Video 6.15, FLE-1, and Video 6.16, FLE-2 (courtesy Paul Reading). In attacks, the patient appears awake, with eyes open, and frightened as in night terrors. Apart from cycling movements and rocking, there may be any of the following: paroxysms of choreoathetoid, ballistic, or dystonic movements; rapid on/off short seizures or clusters.

▶ Sudden awakening, especially with vocalization and fearful staring eyes, suggests a night terror.
The patient may leave the bed but typically cannot describe the nightmare. This happens in the first third of sleep; that is, during non-REM sleep. See Video 6.17, Night Terror (courtesy Matthew Walker). If a similar episode occurs in the second half of sleep and the eyes are closed, this is likely REM-sleep behavior disorder (RBD).

▶ Violent limb movement during sleep and vocalization with eyes shut is probably RBD.

The movements usually occur in the second half of the night, and the patient remains in bed with the eyes shut. They are found in:

o Cocaine addicts
o Parkinson's disease and its prodrome
o Multiple system atrophy (MSA)

RBD must be distinguished from sleep walking, in which the patient gets out of bed in the early part of the night during non-REM sleep. The eyes are open and nonviolent purposeful acts may be executed. See Video 6.18, RBD (courtesy Paul Reading).

▶ Frequent waking during night with jerking legs, particularly dorsiflexion of the ankle, is likely periodic limb movements of sleep.

They recur every 30–60 seconds, often waking the partner. See Video 6.19, PLM (courtesy Paul Reading).

▶ Rapid tremulous movement of thighs on lying down without necessarily being asleep is probably propriospinal myoclonus.

Typically, the movement starts in the thighs and moves up the body.

▶ *Expiratory* groaning in sleep is catathrenia. See Video 6.20, Catathrenia (courtesy G. Hagemann).

This occurs toward morning, mostly in REM sleep, and it is benign. Often it is confused with obstructive sleep apnea, but this is associated with *inspiratory* snoring.

▶ Noisy, high-pitched *inspiratory* stridor during sleep (and daytime) suggests multiple system atrophy (MSA). (see Video 6.21, MSA with Stridor).

The stridor is due to vibration of the vocal cords, which are adducted, obstructing air entry. It conveys a poor prognosis. The inspiratory snoring noise of patients with obstructive sleep apnea has a deeper pitch

▶ Excess daytime somnolence is related to the following:

• Obstructive sleep apnea
• Periodic limb movements of sleep (e.g., restless legs syndrome)
• Prodromal classic Parkinson's disease
• With confusion, behavioral disturbance, craving for sugar, and hypersexuality *in bouts* lasting several days; this is the Klein-Levine syndrome.

• With narcolepsy, ataxia, and deafness this is autosomal dominant cerebellar ataxia, deafness, and narcolepsy (ADCADN)

▶ Attacks of compulsive sleep during inappropriate situations (e.g., meals, standing, conversation) suggests narcolepsy. It may be triggered by sudden emotion or noise. See Video 6.22, Narcolepsy Fisherman (courtesy Paul Reading). Narcolepsy is associated with:

• Cataplexy
• Sleep paralysis
• Vivid dreams on falling off to sleep or wakening
• Poor sense of smell.
• Previously, the A/H1NI vaccine (Pandemrix) swine flu injection. This may develop because of molecular mimicry between hypocretin (Orexin) and a similar epitope on the 2009 influenza A strain that activates CD4-positive T cells against hypocretin (De la Herran-Arita et al. 2013).

▶ Parasomnias, sleep apnea, daytime somnolence, stridor, bulbar syndrome, and ataxia is the IgLON5 syndrome

Insomnias:

• Continual insomnia suggests thyrotoxicosis, bipolar affective disorder, severe anxiety state
• Reduced sleep duration, dream enactment, and parkinsonism is likely *fatal familial insomnia.*

In fatal familial insomnia, autonomic features and visual hallucinations may be prominent. There is loss of sleep spindles, delta waves, and persistent non-REM EEG activity. It is a prion disease now classified under the category "agrypnia excitata." This disorder includes delirium tremens and Morvan's syndrome. In Morvan's syndrome, there are fibrillary muscle twitches related to the underlying pathology, which is a potassium channelopathy.

• Familial migraine with advanced sleep phase disorder

(See also Chapter 5.) This is a newly discovered familial form of migraine associated with an advanced shift of the circadian rhythm. Characteristically, patients go to bed around 7 P.M. and wake at 4 A.M. It is due to a mutation in casein kinase 1 delta (CK1δ) (Brennan et al. 2013).

▶ Sleep paralysis

This is associated with the REM sleep phase and happens when falling asleep or wakening. There is generalized atonia and sometimes terrifying hallucinations. It is associated with narcolepsy and migraine.

SUMMARY

- Urinary incontinence is not uncommon in everyday faints.
- Urinary incontinence and tongue biting occur in nonepileptic attack disorders.
- Syncope and epilepsy may be present in the same patient.

Inspection

- Adenoma sebaceum, periungual fibromas, hypomelanotic macules, shagreen patches: *tuberous sclerosis*
- Port-wine stain on face with seizures: *Sturge-Weber syndrome*; also, mental retardation, vascular lesions in the meninges with tramline calcification on CT
- Young adult with beaded eyelid papules, hyperkeratosis, and verrucous lesions on the elbows: *lipoid proteinosis*
- Child with red or blonde hair, laughs frequently, flaps the hands, unsteady: *Angelman's syndrome*
- Girl with hyperventilation, breath-holding or sighing, stereotypies, seizures, mute, dystonia leading to contractures and kyphoscoliosis: *Rett syndrome*; similar features in *beta-propeller protein–associated neurodegeneration*
- Tall child/adult with seizures, narrow face, pointed jaw, palpebral fissures down-slanting, dolichocephaly: *Sotos syndrome*
- Large linear birthmark (sebaceous nevus) on the face, scalp or neck; seizures; cognitive impairment; agenesis of corpus callosum; agyria: *linear sebaceous nevus syndrome*

History and Examination

- Sudden onset and offset suggests a seizure.
- Gradual onset and offset suggests a faint.
- Rising epigastric aura: epilepsy. Stationary epigastric aura: syncope
- Epileptic aura produces positive symptoms. Migraine and TIAs are associated with negative symptoms. Main exception: amyloid spells

- Sudden falls forward in the elderly without loss of consciousness suggest a drop attack.
- Involuntary laughing attacks are gelastic epilepsy. Causes are hypothalamic hamartoma (consciousness retained) or temporal lobe lesion (consciousness impaired). Involuntary crying attacks are dacrystic seizures.
- Low-grade tumors present with seizures. High-grade tumors start with focal neurological signs.
- Visual hallucinations and occipital calcification: celiac disease
- Myoclonic jerks in child/teenager at breakfast suggests JME.
- Olfactory or gustatory aura suggests a lesion in the anterior temporal lobe (amygdala).
- Posterior shoulder dislocation suggests a generalized seizure or electric shock injury.
- First seizure in a patient from Asia or South America is likely neurocysticercosis or TB.
- Anticonvulsants that aggravate seizures: (1) sodium valproate: *Alper's syndrome*, metabolic or mitochondrial disorder; (2) carbamazepine, phenytoin, or vigabatrin may worsen JME, porphyria, or progressive myoclonic epilepsy; (3) tiagabine can worsen all types of epilepsy and cause nonconvulsive status; (4) benzodiazepines may precipitate tonic status in *Lennox-Gastaut syndrome*; (5) medication that acts on the sodium channel, for example, phenytoin, carbamazepine, lamotrigine, vigabatrin, may worsen *Dravet syndrome*.
- Bouts of spitting, coughing, vomiting, nose wiping, or water drinking: peri-ictal vegetative symptoms
- Apparent loss of consciousness with awareness of surroundings: syncope, NEADs, or cataplexy
- Blackout while shaving: hypersensitive carotid sinus
- Blackout on swallowing is swallowing syncope; causes are faint, cardiac arrhythmia or sensitive carotid sinus.
- Fall while watching video game: photic-induced seizure, cataplexy
- Seizure in a night club: photic-induced fit, recreational drugs or alcohol withdrawal or excess, sleep deprivation in epileptic
- Lower lip trembling while reading followed by blackout: reading epilepsy

- Seizure while taking a bath or shower or swimming suggests water immersion epilepsy.
- Musicogenic epilepsy: probable reflex epilepsy triggered by music
- Sudden falls following loud noise: cataplexy, hyperekplexia, myotonia congenita, startle epilepsy. Hyperekplexia may be due to *stiff person syndrome*, PERM, psychogenic disorders, culturally mediated episodes (e.g., Latah).
- Acquired progressive dysphasia in children with sleep seizures: *Landau- Kefler syndrome*
- Eyelid myoclonia, absences, photosensitivity starting in childhood is *Jeavon's syndrome*.
- Absence or myoclonic seizures self-induced by looking at sun through waving fanned-out fingers is the *sunflower syndrome*.
- Simian gait with mild ataxia and seizures suggests *Dravet syndrome*.
- *Figure-of-eight head movement* suggests rhombo-encephalo-synapsis or *Ohtahara syndrome*.

Guides to Localization
- Postictal weakness (Todd's paralysis). The lesion is in the cerebral hemisphere opposite the side of weakness. If weakness lasts more than 24 hours, then a structural cause is likely.
- Versive seizures: head and eye deviation while the patient is alert (i.e., simple partial seizure) indicates a focus in the contralateral motor cortex.
- *Fencer's sign*: lesion in the supplementary motor area opposite the extended arm
- *Figure-of-four*: lesion in the temporal or frontal lobe on the side opposite the extended arm
- Ictal pouting suggests lesion of anterior cingulate cortex.
- Spreading sensory symptoms usually stem from the opposite parietal lobe.
- Aura of pain usually localizes to the opposite parietal lobe, rarely ipsilateral thalamus.
- Bilateral sensory symptoms may occur with a lesion of the superior temporal gyrus.
- Sensation of someone grabbing the throat suggest a lesion of the insula.
- Formed visual hallucinations indicate a seizure arising in the posterior temporal-parietal area.
- Musical auras usually localize to the nondominant superior temporal gyrus.

Refractory Seizures
- After pertussis vaccination may be due to *Dravet syndrome.* They have typical gait and sensitivity to sodium channel blocker medication.
- Refractory status epilepticus: encephalitis, stroke (including cortical vein thrombosis and cerebral hemorrhage), hypoxia, NEAD, valproate hyperammonemic encephalopathy
- Psychosis and low blood sodium level: LGI-1 antibody encephalitis, NMDA antibody encephalitis, porphyria, medication (carbamazepine)
- Multiple unilateral facio-brachial dystonic seizures: LGI-1 channelopathy
- Seizures, psychosis, language deterioration, catatonia, and dysautonomia: NMDA receptor channelopathy.
- Ovarian teratoma or testicular tumor: EEG may show the extreme delta brush pattern.
- Stiff person, cerebellar ataxia, and seizures: gamma-aminobutyric acid (GABA) receptor antibody; small-cell lung cancer
- Continual partial seizures in young adult: *Rasmussen encephalitis*, channelopathies related to encephalitis with antibodies to LGI-1 or NMDA, complex partial status, ring chromosome 20 disorder, hypoglycemia, non-ketotic hyperglycemia, hypocalcemia, hypomagnesemia
- Episodic ataxia or exercise-induced dyskinesia, anticonvulsant-refractory seizures, and very low CSF glucose: *glucose transporter type 1 deficiency syndrome* (De Vivo syndrome)

EEG Handles
Characteristic patterns in:
▶ Classic Creutzfeldt-Jacob disease, subacute sclerosing panencephalitis (SSPE), ring chromosome 20 disorder, absence seizures, NMDA receptor encephalitis, neuronal ceroid lipofuscinoses, Aicardi syndrome (Swiss cheese retinopathy and hypoplasia of corpus callosum)

Nonepileptic Attacks
General
- Mattress on the floor sign
- Slippers and teddy bear signs
- Wearing dark glasses indoors

- Apparent partial or generalized seizure on abrupt standing after hyperventilation

During or After Attack

- Blackout with eyes tightly shut
- Conjugate gaze away from examiner
- Fast regular breathing
- Weeping and/or pain after attack
- Violent thrashing movements
- Attack in vicinity of medical staff
- "Epileptic" attack when EEG electrodes are being attached
- Duration of motor activity longer than 2 minutes
- Involuntary movements that wax and wane
- Seizures occurring with suggestion or intravenous saline
- Mirror sign
- Awareness of surroundings during generalized convulsive movements
- Multiple hospital visits for apparently serious/emergency illness in widely separated regions of a country suggests Munchausen's syndrome. Seizures common, burr holes, self-discharge, dislike photographs of themselves

Sleep-Related Disorders

- Generalized or focal myoclonic jerks, particularly on falling asleep, are normal phenomena.
- Pelvic rocking, head banging, or thumb sucking on going to sleep suggests sleep–wake transition disorder.
- Cycling movements during sleep: frontal lobe seizures
- Sudden awakening, especially with vocalization and fearful staring eyes: night terror
- Violent limb movements during sleep and vocalization with eyes shut: REM-sleep behavior disorder; occurs in cocaine addicts, Parkinson disease, and its prodrome; MSA
- Frequent waking during the night with jerking legs, particularly dorsiflexion of ankle, is likely periodic limb movements of sleep.
- Rapid tremulous movements of thighs on lying down but not necessarily asleep: propriospinal myoclonus
- *Expiratory* groaning in sleep is catathrenia.
- Noisy high-pitched *inspiratory* stridor during sleep (*and daytime*) suggests MSA.

Excess daytime somnolence causes:
- Obstructive sleep apnea
- Periodic limb movements of sleep (e.g., restless legs syndrome)
- Prodromal feature of classical Parkinson's disease
- With confusion, behavioral disturbance, craving for sugar, and hypersexuality *in bouts* lasting several days: *Klein-Levine syndrome*
  - Attacks of compulsive sleep during inappropriate situations (e.g., meals, standing, conversation) suggests narcolepsy. Associated with: cataplexy, sleep paralysis, vivid dreams on falling off to sleep or wakening, poor sense of smell, A/H1N1 flu vaccine for swine flu
  - Parasomnias, sleep apnea, daytime somnolence, stridor, bulbar syndrome and ataxia is the *IgLON5 syndrome*.

Insomnias:
- Continual insomnia suggests thyrotoxicosis, bipolar affective disorder, severe anxiety state
- Reduced sleep duration, dream enactment, and parkinsonism is likely fatal familial insomnia.
- Familial migraine with advanced sleep phase disorder. Patients go to bed at 7 P.M. and wake at 4 A.M. Mutation in casein kinase 1 delta

Sleep paralysis:
Happens when falling asleep or wakening. Associated with narcolepsy and migraine.

SUGGESTED READING

Agwu JC, Shaw NJ, Kirk J, Chapman S, Ravine D, Cole TR. Growth in Sotos syndrome. *Arch Dis Child.* 1999;80(4):339–342.

Boger LS, Awasthi S, Eisen DB. Sebaceous nevus syndrome: a case report of a child with nevus sebaceus, mental retardation, seizures, and mucosal and ocular abnormalities. *Dermatol Online J.* 2012 ;18(9).

Brennan KC, Bates EA, Shapiro RE, et al. Casein kinase idelta mutations in familial migraine and advanced sleep phase. *Sci Transl Med* 2013;5:183ra56.

Costa JC, Nunes ML, Fiori RM. [Seizures in the neonatal period]. *J Pediatr (Rio J).* 2001;77(Suppl 1):S115–S122.

De la Herran-Arita AK, Kornum BR, Mahlios J, et al. CD4+ T cell autoimmunity to hypocretin/orexin and cross-reactivity to a 2009 H1N1 influenza A epitope in narcolepsy. *Sci Transl Med.* 2013;5:216ra176.

Franz DN, Glauser TA, Tudor C, et al. Topiramate therapy of epilepsy associated with Angelman's syndrome. *Neurology*. 2000;54:1185–1188.

Hayakawa I, Kubota M. Ictal pouting: kabuki visage or chapeau de gendarme? [Published online ahead of print March 23, 2018]. *Pract Neurol*. doi:10.1136/practneurol-2017-001847.

Kellinghaus C, Loddenkemper T, Kotagal P. Ictal spitting: clinical and electroencephalographic features. *Epilepsia*. 2003;44:1064–1069.

Koc G, Bek S, Gokcil Z. Localization of ictal pouting in frontal lobe epilepsy: a case report. *Epilepsy Behav Case Rep*. 2017;8:27.

Kotagal P, Bleasel A, Geller E, Kankirawatana P, Moorjani BI, Rybicki L. Lateralizing value of asymmetric tonic limb posturing observed in secondarily generalized tonic–clonic seizures. *Epilepsia*. 2000;41(4):457–462.

Pfaender M, D'Souza WJ, Trost N, Litewka L, Paine M, Cook M. Visual disturbances representing occipital lobe epilepsy in patients with cerebral calcifications and celiac disease: a case series. *J Neurol Neurosurg Psychiatry*. 2004;75:1623–1625.

Quirici MB, da Rocha AJ. Teaching neuroimages: lipoid proteinosis (Urbach-Wiethe disease): typical findings in this rare genodermatosis. *Neurology*. 2013;80:e93.

Schmitt SE, Pargeon K, Frechette ES, Hirsch LJ, Dalmau J, Friedman D. Extreme delta brush: a unique EEG pattern in adults with anti-NMDA receptor encephalitis. *Neurology*. 2012;79:1094–1100.

Van Buggenhout G, Fryns JP. Angelman syndrome (AS, MIM 105830). *Eur J Hum Genet*. 2009;17:1367–1373.

Ville D, Kaminska A, Bahi-Buisson N, et al. Early pattern of epilepsy in the ring chromosome 20 syndrome. *Epilepsia*. 2006;47:543–549.

Woollacott IO, Scott C, Fish DR, Smith SM, Walker MC. When do psychogenic nonepileptic seizures occur on a video/EEG telemetry unit? *Epilepsy Behav*. 2010;17:228–235.

Chapter 7: Myopathy and Motor Neuron Disorders

MYOPATHY

Accurate identification of myopathy is not always easy at the bedside, and the advent of molecular diagnostic techniques has made it clear that a similar phenotype may have several genotypes; conversely, an identical genotype may be associated with multiple phenotypes. What follows are some of the traditional clues, most of which will need verification by further tests such as electromyogram (EMG), muscle biopsy, or genotyping.

Dystrophies

Take a look at Figure 7.1. There is only one diagnosis with such a characteristic facial appearance. Within minutes, you should have checked for myotonia and neck muscle strength and made the diagnosis: dystrophia myotonica. Corroborative details follow.

Dystrophia Myotonica Type 1

Dystrophia myotonica type 1 (DM1) is the most common muscular dystrophy. It is autosomal dominant and essentially a multisystem disorder caused by excess CTG trinucleotide repeats. Also view Video 7.1, DM1, which shows history and examination of two patients with DM1.

Following are some useful Handles.

Presentation

▶ Young adult with muscular stiffness, often worse in cold weather
▶ Predominantly distal weakness and poor grip due to weak long finger flexors.
▶ Excess daytime sleepiness. This relates to obstructive sleep apnea or nocturnal hypoventilation.

Examination

▶ Frontal baldness, thinning of the lower face, ptosis, open jaw, inverted smile, maloccluded teeth ("hatchet face"), and swan neck deformity (Figure 7.1)
▶ Myotonia after gripping or percussion of the thenar eminence. Myotonia *lessens*

with repeated contraction ("warm up"). In paramyotonia, the myotonia *worsens* with repetitive movement.

▶ Neck flexor weakness. This is mandatory for the diagnosis.
▶ Premature cataract (Christmas tree type, Figure 7.2). This results in referral to an eye clinic and may be the first suggestion of disease.
▶ The "shank sign" (Figure 7.3) refers to the appearance of the arm muscles when viewed from the rear (Pradhan 2007).
▶ Pectus excavatum.
▶ Electrocardiogram (EKG) may show cardiomyopathy or arrthymia. This confers risk of sudden death.
▶ Plain skull X-ray shows thickening of the calvarium, small pituitary fossa, large frontal sinuses, elongated mandible.
▶ Brain MRI may show increased signal intensity in the temporal poles that is sometimes misinterpreted as multiple sclerosis (MS) or small vessel disease (Figure 7.4).

Red Flags

◀ If the neck flexors are not weak, the diagnosis of classic DM1 is wrong.
◀ Absence of *clinical* myotonia makes the diagnosis of DM1 unlikely, but the myotonia can be subtle or even absent if the grip has become very weak. Evidence of *electrical* myotonia on EMG is vital in this context.
◀ Severe myotonia suggests nondystrophic myotonia such as Thomsen's disease (see later discussion).

There are three situations in which the diagnosis of DM1 may have been overlooked:

◀ A patient with apparent motor polyneuropathy, spinal muscular atrophy (SMA), or myasthenia gravis (MG) may have DM1. Always check for myotonia.

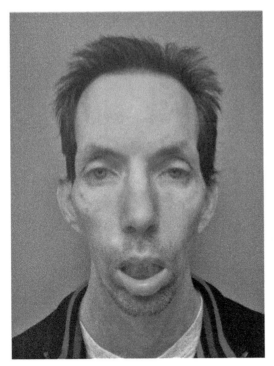

FIGURE 7.1: Dystrophia myotonica type 1 (DM1). **Left**: The classic features of DM1. There is frontal balding, temporalis muscle wasting, mild bilateral ptosis, and moderate perioral weakness with a fish-mouth appearance. **Right**: Woman with DM1 but the appearances are subtle. Note the mild ptosis, thin face, wasted temporal and neck muscles, and myopathic smile. Frontal balding was concealed by combing. Left image reproduced with permission from Wicklund (2013), Figure 2.10.

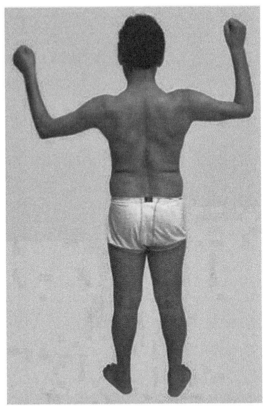

FIGURE 7.3: The "shank sign," where there is normal appearance of shoulder muscles but significant tapering distally because of wasting in the biceps, triceps, and distal forearm muscles (Pradhan 2007).

◀ Failure to resume spontaneous breathing after a general anesthetic

◀ In a mother who delivers a baby with congenital myotonic dystrophy (Figure 7.5)

The confinement may have been complicated by polyhydramnios due to imperfect swallowing of amniotic fluid by the weak fetus, delayed second stage of labor, and forceps delivery. The baby is floppy, feeds poorly, and suffers aspiration pneumonia. There is ptosis and a tented appearance of the upper lip. Often it is realized only then (i.e., after the baby is diagnosed) that the mother has DM1.

Severe myotonia is unusual in DM1 but typical of myotonia congenita (Thomsen's disease) where there is

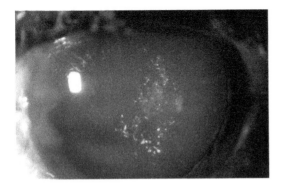

FIGURE 7.2: The Christmas tree cataract of Dystrophia myotonica type 1 (DM1). Reproduced from Figure 9.29 in the chapter Neuro-ophthalmology, by V Sundaram and J Elston. Oxford University Press. DOI:10.1093/med/9780199237593.003.0009.

▶ Muscle hypertrophy, with Hercules-like appearance (Figure 7.6, myotonia congenita)

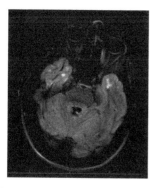
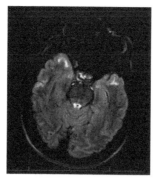
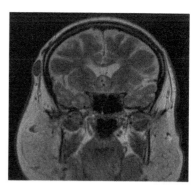

FIGURE 7.4: **Left and center**: Axial FLAIR MRI brain images from a 36-year-old woman with dystrophia myotonica type 1 (DM1). There is increased signal intensity in both temporal poles, sometimes misinterpreted as multiple sclerosis or small vessel disease. **Right**: Coronal MRI views from another patient with DM1 showing white matter changes in the anterior temporal region. Left image reproduced with permission from Wicklund (2013), Figure 2.11. Right image courtesy Bart's Health Neuroimaging Department, London.

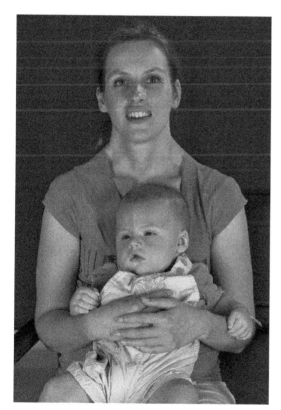

▶ Often startle myotonia
▶ Little or no weakness

Infants and children with apparent myotonia may have the very rare *Schwartz-Jampel syndrome* (Figure 7.7), in which there is

- Blepharophimosis
- Perioral tonic contractions
- Pursed lips, low-set ears

The apparent myotonia on EMG is due to bizarre repetitive discharges, not classic myotonia.

Note: Some newborns with myotonic discharges on EMG may have *infantile acid maltase deficiency (Pompe's disease) or myotonia congenita*.

FIGURE 7.5: This woman has adult-onset classical myotonic dystrophy type 1 with a medium expansion (200–700 CTG repeats) in the *DMPK* gene. Her son has congenital myotonic dystrophy type 1 with a large expansion (>700 CTG repeats). Note the son's tent-like mouth due to facial myopathy. Clinical myotonia does not occur, but myotonic discharges are seen on electromyogram (EMG). Reproduced from Figure 25.3 in the *Oxford Textbook of Neuromuscular Disorders*, The Myotonic Dystrophies, by C Turner and D Hilton-Jones. Oxford University Press. DOI:10.1093/med/9780199698073.003.0025.

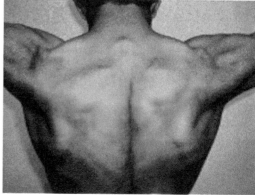

FIGURE 7.6: Myotonia congenita. Note the marked muscle hypertrophy. Reproduced with permission from Varkey and Varkey (2003).

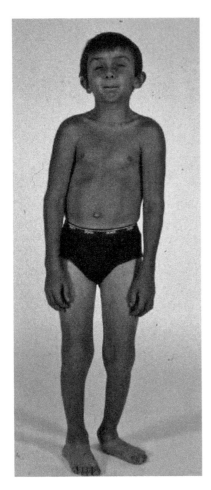

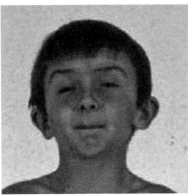

FIGURE 7.7: Schwartz-Jampel syndrome. There is blepharophimosis, pursed lips, low-set ears, and stiffness of facial expression. Note the bowing of the tibiae, valgus deformities of the ankles, and pes planus. Reproduced with permission from Ho et al. (2003)

Dystrophia Myotonica Type II

Also known as proximal myotonic myopathy (PROM), this variety is likewise autosomal dominant but much rarer. It is caused by mutations in the cellular nucleic acid–binding protein gene (*CNBP*), with the following characteristics:

- Later onset: middle age
- Muscle pain and stiffness
- Little *clinical* myotonia and sometimes only subtle *electrical* myotonia on EMG
- Weakness is mainly proximal.
- It should be considered in suspected DMI cases that have negative genetic testing.

Duchenne Muscular Dystrophy

Duchenne muscular dystrophy (DMD) is caused by mutations in the DMD gene on the X chromosome, predominantly affecting males but manifesting female carriers are recognized. The main features are as follows:

- Onset in boys, 2–5 years
- Toe walking, proximal limb, and neck flexor weakness
- Calf and tongue hypertrophy
- Waddling gait, excess lumbar lordosis
- Very high creatine kinase (CK)
- Gower's sign (Figure 7.8)
- Frequent cardiac involvement. Progressive cardiomyopathy may affect manifesting (female) carriers.

Red Flags

◀ If the CK is not very high (i.e., >10,000), the diagnosis is wrong.

◀ A boy with muscular dystrophy still walking after age 16 probably does not have the Duchenne variety unless he has responded well to steroids.

Consider the Becker variant or limb girdle muscular dystrophy (LGMD). In Duchenne dystrophy, transition to a wheelchair usually takes place before the age of 12 years.

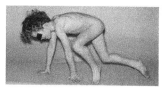
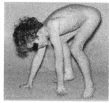
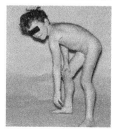
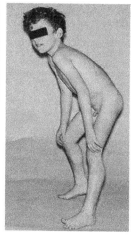

FIGURE 7.8: Gowers' maneuver. The patient "climbs up the legs" to get up from the sitting or lying position. Figures 663-666 reproduced with permission from *A Colour Atlas of Clinical Neurology*, 2nd ed., M Parsons. Mosby Year Book Europe. 1993.

Becker Muscular Dystrophy

This is an X-linked dystrophy, closely related genetically to DMD, that starts at a variable age but classically around the age of 12. These are the clinical features:

▶ Weakness commencing in the pelvic then shoulder girdle

▶ Calf enlargement and wasted lower pectoral muscles (Figure 7.9, *left* and *center*)

▶ The "valley sign" (Pradhan 2004). If the arms are abducted and viewed from the rear, this may reveal a deep groove because all muscles traversing the posterior axillary fold are wasted (Figure 7.9, *right*).

▶ Cramp and myoglobinuria or dilated cardiomyopathy. This may be the only feature even in previously asymptomatic adults.

▶ T-wave inversion on EKG, in keeping with cardiomyopathy

Note: Becker muscular dystrophy can mimic a metabolic myopathy.

Fascioscapulohumeral Muscular Dystrophy

Fascioscapulohumeral muscular dystrophy (FSHMD) is an autosomal dominant condition due to contraction of the D4Z4 macrosatellite repeat on chromosome 4 (i.e., *reduced* repeat number; see Video 7.2, FSH MD). Up to 30% cases arise *de novo* without any family history. The main Handles are as follows:

▶ Scapular winging, asymmetric limb-girdle weakness, and bilateral facial weakness

▶ Long-standing inability to whistle
Although the facial muscles may appear normal to standard tests, closer examination may reveal slight weakness of forceful eye closure and difficulty in pursing the lips, resulting in failure to whistle.

▶ Sleeping with eyes open

In the limbs, there are multiple clues to the diagnosis:

▶ Shoulder hump signs (Figure 7.10, *center*)

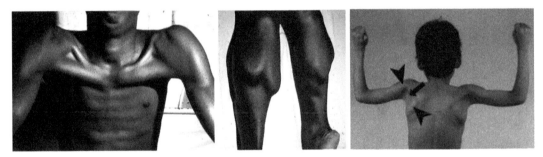

FIGURE 7.9: Becker muscular dystrophy. **Left**: Severe wasting of the lower pectoral muscles (pectoralis major) with preservation of pectoralis minor. **Center**: Marked calf pseudohypertrophy. **Right**: The valley sign (center arrow), characteristic of Becker dystrophy and some cases of Duchenne muscular dystrophy. There is slight enlargement of deltoid and infraspinatus (upper and lower arrows). Reproduced with permission from Pradhan (2004).

When the patient is asked to abduct the upper limbs, the scapulae elevate, producing a marked hump on either side of the neck, and, related to this:

▶ Multiple shoulder humps: the triple hump or poly-hill sign (Figure 7.10, *right*; Pradhan 2002)

When the arms are abducted and viewed from the rear, as in Figure 7.10 (*right*), there are multiple humps over the upper border of the shoulders.

▶ Shoulder shrugging is weak.

▶ Infraspinatus may be hypertrophied, and the scapulae appear small.

▶ Biceps and triceps are weak, but deltoid and brachioradialis are spared (Figure 7.10).

▶ The anterior axillary folds are reversed.

Wasting of the lower pectoral muscles leads to reversal of the anterior axillary folds (Figure 7.10, *center*).

▶ Recurrent shoulder dislocation due to shoulder instability

▶ High-stepping gait

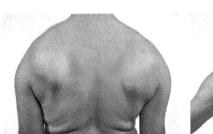
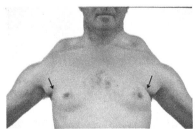
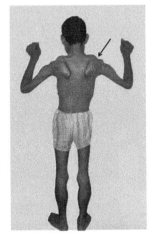

FIGURE 7.10: Facioscapulohumeral muscular dystrophy (FSHMD). **Left**: Marked downward-sloping shoulders and winging of scapulae even at rest. Note the characteristic lumbar lordosis. **Center**: When shoulder abduction is attempted the scapulae elevate because of serratus anterior weakness and abduction is incomplete. This is the "shoulder hump" sign that is typical of FSHMD. Note wasting of the upper pectoral, biceps, and triceps muscles but preservation of deltoid. Upper pectoral muscle atrophy leads to reversal of the anterior axillary folds (arrows), which point inward toward the neck instead of outward toward the shoulder. **Right**: When the arms are abducted and viewed from the rear there are multiple humps over the shoulders (arrow)—the poly-hill or triple-hump sign. Observe the scapular winging, small scapulae, preservation of deltoid bulk, and hypertrophy of infraspinatus. Reproduced with permission from Pradhan (2002), Figure 1.

This is to avoid catching the toes and results from weakness of ankle dorsiflexion; joint position sense is normal.

▶ Waddling gait, marked lordosis, and pot belly

▶ Beevor's sign (rostral movement of the umbilicus on attempted trunk flexion)
This results from weakness of the lower abdominal muscles. Apart from T10 spinal lesions, it is said to be pathognomonic of FSHMD (Shahrizaila and Wills 2005).

Other less well-established Handles are as follows:

▶ Camptocormia
Literally, this means "bent trunk" and happens most often in ankylosing spondylitis and parkinsonian syndromes (see Chapter 8, Movement Disorders). Back extensor muscle weakness in FSHMD results in forward flexion of the trunk; to compensate, most patients overextend the lumbar spine, giving rise to marked lordosis. See Video 7.3, Camptocormia FSH (courtesy K. Docherty). In some patients the back extensors fatigue, and they walk flexed at the hip. The spine becomes straight when supine. Camptocormia is recognized in other myopathies, thus it is not a specific feature of FSHMD; some clinicians argue that it is not true camptocormia.

▶ Occasionally, hearing loss and retinal vasculopathy are associated.

There are six Red Flags that should make you question a diagnosis of FSHMD:

◀ Absent shoulder hump sign
◀ Involvement of bulbar or extraocular muscles
◀ Neck muscle weakness
◀ Early respiratory involvement
◀ Weak brachioradialis muscle
◀ Weak iliopsoas or calf muscles in the absence of other lower limb weakness

Main Differentials for FSHMD

1. Other myopathies with scapular winging, such as
   a. LGMD (limb girdle muscular dystrophy) type 2A (calpainopathy) and types 2C–2F (sarcoglycanopathies)
   b. VCP-mutated distal myopathy (see later in this chapter)
2. Neuropathies such as neurogenic hereditary scapuloperoneal atrophy
3. Disorder of the long thoracic or accessory nerves. These are usually unilateral.
   a. The *long thoracic nerve* supplies serratus anterior to keep the inferior angle of the scapula applied to the chest wall. In patients with a long thoracic nerve lesion from, for example, acute brachial neuritis, the scapula elevates; but, unlike FSHMD, shoulder shrugging is strong because trapezius is spared.
   b. The *accessory nerve* supplies trapezius. Lesions of this nerve also result in scapular winging but no hump, as serratus anterior keeps the scapula low.

When the arms are abducted, there are hump signs on both sides in FSHMD and bilateral long thoracic nerve lesions. If there is scapular winging but no hump, the lesion is in the accessory nerve (see Table 7.1 and Figure 7.11).

Limb Girdle Muscular Dystrophy

LGMD is a term for a large group of more than 25 genetic disorders with a limb-girdle phenotype, only some of which have characteristic features. If the dystrophy is autosomal dominant, it is given a suffix of number 1 followed by a letter that indicates the chronology of discovery—thus LGMD1A is dominant and discovered first; number 2 indicates recessive inheritance.

TABLE 7.1: DIFFERENT PATTERNS IN THREE MAJOR CONDITIONS ASSOCIATED WITH SCAPULAR WINGING

Disorder	Shoulder hump sign	Weak shoulder shrugging
Facioscapulohumeral muscular dystrophy	+	+
Accessory nerve palsy	–	+
Long thoracic nerve palsy	+	–

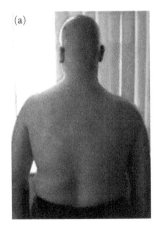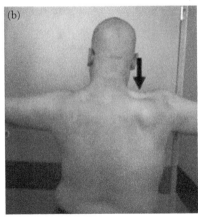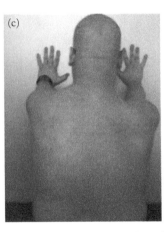

FIGURE 7.11:   Right scapular winging due to accessory nerve lesion resulting in weakness and wasting of trapezius (arrow). The shoulder is dropped as in (**A**). Note that the scapula does not elevate on abduction as it would in FSHMD, due to preservation of serratus anterior function, which keeps the scapula low (**B**). (**C**) shows unilateral scapular winging. Reproduced with permission from Tsivgoulis et al. (2012), Figures 1a–c.

Compared to the recessive varieties, all dominant forms of LGMD have the following characteristics:

- Extremely rare (<15% of all LGMD)
- Mildly elevated CK levels
- Later age of onset (typically >20 years)

The main features of LGMD are summarized in Table 7.2. See also Video 7.4, Rippling Muscle Disease (courtesy Martin Pucar).

Red Flags for LGMD

◀ Weak neck muscles
◀ Sensory neuropathy; autonomic or visceral dysfunction in the early phase of disease excludes LGMD
◀ Facial muscle involvement
◀ Early respiratory insufficiency

Additional Handles for muscle disorder with:

▶ *Calf hypertrophy.* There are six mutations associated with this: Dystrophin, Caveolin, Calpain, Sarcoglycan, Fukutin-related, and Anoctamin. Note: calf hypertrophy may be found in S1 radiculopathy, hypothyroidism, and cysticercosis infection of calf muscle.

▶ *CK greater than 10,000*: There are also six associated mutations: Dystrophin, Calpain, Sarcoglycan, Dysferlin, Fukutin-related, and Anoctamin
▶ *Macroglossia*: LGMD type C–F (sarcoglycanopathies), LGMD type 2I (Fukutin-associated), DMD, childhood-onset acid maltase deficiency, and mucopolysaccharidoses (e.g., Hunter's and Hurler's syndromes).
  Note that macroglossia may occur in amyloid neuropathy (associated with ageusia), acromegaly, and hypothyroidism.

Emery-Dreifuss Muscular Dystrophy

Emery-Dreifuss muscular dystrophy (EDMD) is a rare, distinctive phenotype that may be autosomal dominant or recessive, characterized by the following:

▶ Childhood onset of biceps, triceps, and ankle dorsiflexor weakness. Deltoid power is preserved.
▶ Contractures at elbows, ankles, and spine. This is a key finding (see Figure 7.12). Ankle contractures result in toe walking.
▶ Cardiac dysfunction. The somatic muscle CK is usually normal or slightly elevated.

TABLE 7.2: MAIN VARIETIES OF LIMB GIRDLE MUSCULAR DYSTROPHY (LGMD) AND THEIR CHARACTERISTIC FEATURES

LGMD type	Age of onset (years)	Mutant protein	Main muscles affected	Handles
1A	20–40	Myotilin	Proximal and distal	Rare. Nasal dysarthria and hypophonia, cardiac and respiratory involvement
1B	5–25	Lamin A or C	Proximal and distal	Early contractures like Emery-Dreifuss myopathy, cardiac and respiratory involvement
1C	5–25	Caveolin	Proximal or distal	Rare. Mounding/rippling muscles (Video 7.4, Rippling Muscle Disease). Calf hypertrophy. Cardiac involvement. Very high creatine kinase (CK)
1D	30–50	DNAJB6	Proximal	Rimmed vacuoles on biopsy
1E	15–50	Desmin	Proximal	Dilated cardiomyopathy
1F	<15 & >20	Transportin 3	Scapular and pelvic	Anticipation
1G	30–47	Not identified	Proximal and distal	Limited finger and toe flexion
Autosomal dominant	>40	Valosin-containing protein	Proximal and distal	IBM with Paget disease and frontotemporal dementia. Raised alkaline phosphatase
2A	5–25	Calpain	Proximal lower limb	Most common recessive type. Scapular winging, calf hypertrophy. Weak hip extension, knee flexion, and hip adduction. High CK. Rarely cardiac or respiratory involvement
2B	10–30	Dysferlin	Proximal and distal	Asian and Mediterranean dwellers. Some are athletic early in life. Unable to stand on toes. Extremely high CK. Rare cardiac/respiratory involvement. Muscle biopsy similar to that for polymyositis. Diamond on quadriceps sign (Figure 7.14).
2C-2F	3–20	Sarcoglycan	Proximal	North Africans and Brazilians. Cardiac and respiratory involvement. Scapular winging, calf and tongue hypertrophy, lumbar lordosis. Simulates FSHMD. High CK
2G	2–15	Telethonin	Proximal and distal	Brazilians. Cardiac involvement. Chair-bound at age 40
2H	5–30	TRIM32	Proximal	Hutterites of Manitoba, Canada
2I	1–40	Fukutin-related	Proximal lower limb and calf	Most from Northern Europe and Japan. Calf and tongue hypertrophy. Cardiac and respiratory involvement. Lumbar lordosis. High CK
2J	5–20	Titin	Proximal	Finnish
2L	20–50	Anoctamin 5	Proximal and distal	Northern Europe. Asymmetric quadriceps and biceps atrophy. Calf hypertrophy and high CK. No cardiac or respiratory involvement

Type 1 is dominant and usually late onset; type 2 is recessive and usually earlier onset. The letters after this number correspond to the sequence of discovery.

IBM, inclusion body myositis.

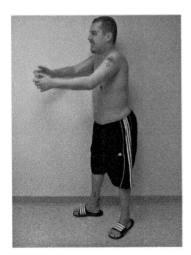
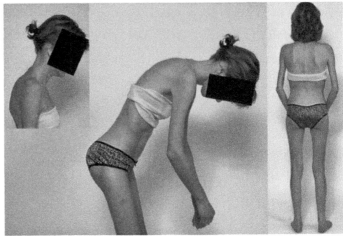

FIGURE 7.12: Emery-Dreifuss muscular dystrophy. **Left**: A 24-year-old man who from an early age developed prominent contractures of the elbows, spine, and ankles. The patient is maximally extending the elbows. He has ankle scars from Achilles tendon–lengthening surgeries at age 12 years for plantar flexor contractures. **Right**: A 10-year-old girl with diffuse muscle atrophy, elbow contractures, and limited ability to flex the neck and trunk. Genetic testing showed autosomal dominant EDMD due to lamin A/C mutation. Left image reproduced with permission from Wicklund (2013), Figure 2.22. Right image reproduced with permission from Ghosh and Milone (2014), Figure 1.

▶ Confusion with:
- ○ *LGMD type 1B* where there are also joint contractures
- ○ *Rigid spine syndrome,* an autosomal recessive congenital muscular dystrophy due to a mutation in *SEPN1,* where there are contractures of muscles at the paraspinal, elbow, and ankle joints. Facial and body appearance is characteristic. See Figure 7.13.

Oculopharyngeal Muscular Dystrophy
Oculopharyngeal muscular dystrophy (OPMD) is a GCN trinucleotide repeat disorder caused by mutations in the polyadenylate-binding protein 1 gene (*PABPN1*). Inheritance is usually autosomal dominant. Most patients come from Quebec (Canada), Israel, Argentina, or New Mexico. It commences in middle age with the following:

▶ Bilateral ptosis, frontalis overactivity with head extension to help overcome the ptosis (Figure 7.15.). This is followed by:
▶ Difficulty in upgaze without diplopia (progressive external ophthalmoplegia), then dysphagia

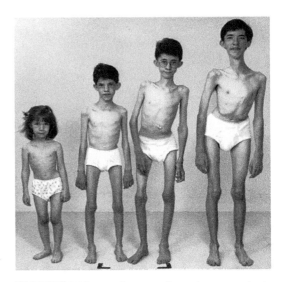

FIGURE 7.13.: Rigid spine syndrome due to mutation in SEPN1 in four sibs. There is central facial hypoplasia which is said to be characteristic. Note the spinal tilt in all but the second from left. There is marked limb and neck muscle wasting with hypotonia and moderate muscle contractures that may cause confusion with Emery-Dreifuss syndrome. Reproduced with permission from; Flanigan KM, et al. (2000).

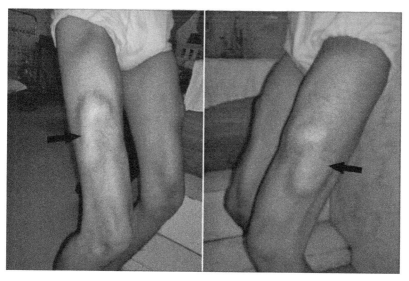

FIGURE 7.14.: Diamond on quads sign, characteristic of dysferlinopathy, either LGMD-2B or Myoshi distal myopathy. This sign is elicited by asking subjects to stand with knees slightly flexed. Reproduced with permission from S Pradhan (2008).

▶ Proximal lower limb weakness
▶ Finally, paresis of the proximal upper limbs, face, and tongue

The main differential diagnoses are

• Myasthenia gravis
• Mitochondrial myopathy

Further Myopathy Handles

▶ Quadriceps wasting is unusual in polymyositis but may be found in:
  ○ LGMD
  ○ Becker dystrophy
  ○ Inclusion body myositis (IBM)
  ○ Spinal muscular atrophy (SMA)

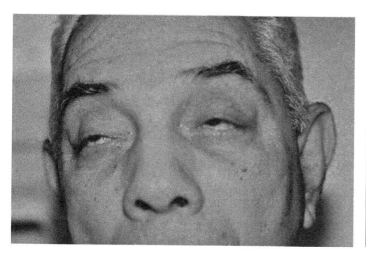
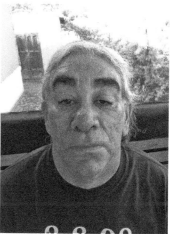

FIGURE 7.15: **Left**: Eye appearance in progressive external ophthalmoplegia. There is bilateral ptosis, facial weakness on both sides, but no diplopia. Note the use of frontalis to elevate the upper lids. **Right**: Similar appearances in someone with oculopharyngeal muscular dystrophy. Left image reproduced from Figure 13.8 in *Clinical Eye Atlas*, 2nd ed., D Gold and R Lewis. Oxford University Press. Right image reproduced with permission from Wicklund (2013), Figure 2.23.

▶ The neck is strong in LGMD but weak in similar conditions with proximal weakness, such as polymyositis and dermatomyositis.

▶ In polymyositis and dermatomyositis, respiratory involvement is later than in acid maltase deficiency and myotonic dystrophy.

▶ Hypertrophy of extensor digitorum brevis (EDB) supports limb girdle dystrophy. This sign is useful when trying to determine whether proximal weakness is due to myopathy or SMA. Hypertrophy, or at least preservation of EDB, favors limb girdle dystrophy (Figure 7.16), whereas wasting of EDB points to proximal SMA. Note that EDB is preserved in Udd distal myopathy.

▶ Patients with Kugelberg-Welander disease (SMA type III) sometimes display an atypical Gowers maneuver in which the legs are widely abducted on the floor, and the hands are then used to push up the trunk.

Dropped Head Sign

Some patients display marked weakness of neck extension, such that the head is continually slumped forward with the chin resting on the chest wall (Figure 7.17). It is usually part of a more generalized disorder, but it can be a presenting feature or part of camptocormia. The most common associations are amyotrophic lateral sclerosis (ALS) and parkinsonism. Several other causes are recognized, although many are based on single case reports.

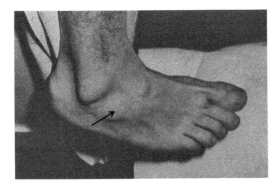

FIGURE 7.16: Hypertrophy of extensor digitorum brevis (arrow). Hypertrophy (or sparing) of extensor digitorum brevis (EDB) is a feature of limb girdle muscular dystrophy (LGMD) and Udd distal myopathy. If EDB is atrophic, this is a Red Flag for LGMD and suggests proximal spinal muscular atrophy, or Kugelberg-Welander disease (SMA type III). Figure courtesy CP Panayiotopoulos.

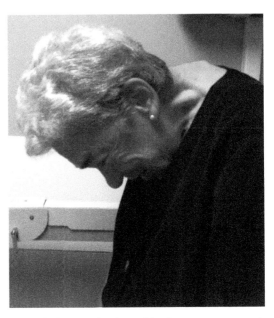

FIGURE 7.17: The dropped head sign in a patient with parkinsonism. The chin is resting on the chest. The main causes are extrapyramidal disease, motor neuron disorders, muscular dystrophies, inflammatory myopathies, and neuromuscular junction disorders.

Note: many begin with the letter M. Here are the main culprits

- Muscular dystrophies: mitochondrial, IBM, myotonic dystrophy, nemaline dystrophy, congenital muscular dystrophy due to LMNA mutation
- Inflammatory myopathies: polymyositis, isolated axial myopathy
- Neuromuscular junction disorder: MG, Lambert Eaton myasthenic syndrome (LEMS)
- Motor neuron disorders: ALS, SMA
- Extrapyramidal disorders: parkinsonism especially multiple system atrophy.
- Cervical dystonia

Note:

▶ In all but extrapyramidal disorders, neck tone is normal or reduced. In extrapyramidal conditions (e.g., progressive supranuclear palsy), neck rigidity may be so marked that it may be difficult to move the head passively into the neutral position.

NEUROMUSCULAR JUNCTION DISORDERS

Classic Myasthenia Gravis

The first step is to establish whether or not you are dealing with classic myasthenia gravis (MG); the presence of acetylcholine receptor antibodies (AchRA) will clinch the diagnosis in 85% cases. In purely ocular MG, the AchRA are usually negative. If there is doubt, then single-fiber EMG on weak muscles should show jitter and block (which is very sensitive but not specific) and decrement during 3 Hz supramaximal nerve stimulation.

Following are some Handles and Flags that may assist you in diagnosis while awaiting the more specific tests.

> ▶ *Jaw supporting sign.* This is highly typical of MG. Patients talk while supporting the underside of the jaw with one hand. This helps offset fatigue in the jaw muscles and prevents the head from dropping forward. Rarely, a similar phenomenon is seen in oromandibular dystonia or DM1. Unless supported, the jaw may sag and the mouth opens (Video 7.5 Myasthenia Gravis, and Figure 7.18).
> ▶ *Myasthenic snarl and triple-grooved tongue.* The snarl is a vertical smile that results from

weakness of the buccinator, which normally helps retract the mouth horizontally (see Figures 1.23, 7.19, and Video 7.5, Myasthenia Gravis). The triple-grooved tongue is a late sign, related to atrophy of the tongue muscles, but now it is rare, given effective therapy. It is commoner in muscle-specific tyrosine kinase (MuSK) myasthenia, where there is weakness and at times wasting of muscles innervated by the lower cranial nerves.

> ▶ *Isolated weakness of eye closure and opening with normal pupillary reactions* suggests classic MG. Conversely, *involvement* of pupillary reflexes excludes classic MG and most myopathies and favors congenital MG or LEMS.
> ▶ *Prolonged upgaze that results in progressive weakness of the upper lids* is characteristic of MG. If there is jerky downward movement of the upper lid, this is Cogan's sign and typical of MG.
> ▶ *Ice applied to the upper lid may improve the ptosis* (but not diplopia) of MG. Likewise, patients report improved swallowing with iced drinks. Similar improvement of dysphagia is seen in bulbar ALS.
> ▶ *Pseudo-internuclear ophthalmoplegia* happens because of intermittent fatigue in the medial and lateral rectus muscles. Differentiation

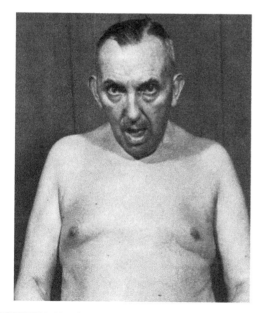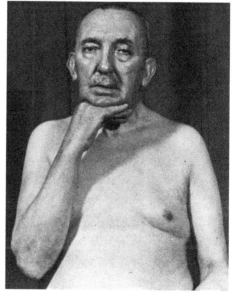

FIGURE 7.18: The jaw supporting sign of myasthenia gravis. **Left**: Note drooping of the neck and sagging jaw. **Right**: The patient uses his right hand to support weakness of both neck and jaw muscles as shown. Reproduced with permission from Figure 269 in *An Atlas of Clinical Neurology*, JD Spillane. Oxford University Press, 1968.

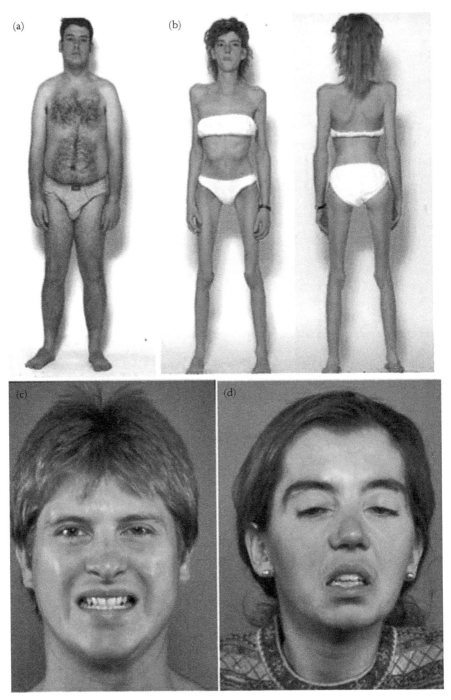

FIGURE 7.19: DOK7 congenital myasthenia in four patients (**A–D**) with variable phenotype. Patient A has mild weakness and atrophy of limb girdle muscles, and mild eyelid ptosis. Patient B has severe diffuse weakness and atrophy of limb and axial muscles. Patient C shows mild asymmetric ptosis whereas it is severe in patient D. Note the myasthenic snarl in patients C and D. Stridor, tongue wasting, and worsening by pyridostigmine are characteristic of DOK7 MG. Reproduced with permission from Selcen et al. (2008).

from demyelinating conditions is usually not a problem if fatigue of the extraocular muscles can be elicited.

▶ In general, *ptosis is asymmetric, even unilateral,* for long periods in MG. It may be the sole presenting symptom of the ocular variety. Make sure you do not misdiagnose for a pupil-sparing CN III palsy!

▶ The *pseudo plus-minus lid syndrome* is a variant of ocular MG, in which there is ptosis of one eye and lid retraction of the other (Bandini 2009). (See video link: https://www.youtube.com/results?search_query=pseudo+plus-minus+lid+syndrome. Alternatively, go to YouTube and type in "pseudo plus-minus lid syndrome.")

▶ *The head is tilted backward to improve vision under the drooped upper lids* and frontalis is often overactive to help keep the eyes open.

▶ *The lips are pursed to help keep the jaw closed.* This maneuver may also help with breathing.

▶ *Forward neck flexion is affected earlier and more severely than neck extension,* though both muscle groups are involved.

▶ *Fatigueable lower extremity weakness with negative AchRA favors congenital MG.*

Also note:

▶ *MG may be unmasked during recovery from a general anesthetic* (e.g., failure to resume spontaneous breathing after extubation).

▶ *Intercurrent infection may bring MG to light.* Similarly, myotonic dystrophy may be detected after surgery or infection.

▶ *A patient with MS with an apparent relapse may have developed MG.* The two conditions are associated.

▶ *A mother with MG or just AchRA without MG features may deliver a baby with arthrogryposis multiplex congenita* (AMC; Figure 7.20). This often fatal disorder is characterized by nonprogressive multiple joint contractures due to transplacental passage of maternal AchRA that reduce fetal movement. Thus, the baby may have both congenital/transient MG and AMC.

Red Flags for MG

◀ *Blepharospasm.* This can be mistaken for ocular myasthenia. In blepharospasm, there is difficulty opening the eyelids and no ophthalmoplegia.

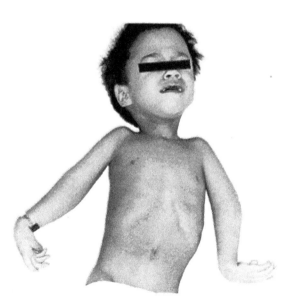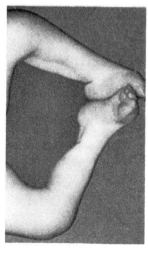

FIGURE 7.20: Arthrogryposis multiplex congenita (AMC). **Left**: Note the extended fusiform elbows and deformed hands. **Right**: The hips are flexed and externally rotated and there are fixed knee flexion and foot deformities. This may be associated with bulbar weakness due to congenital myasthenia gravis (MG), particularly resulting from a mutation in the *RAPSN* gene. The mother of a baby born with AMC may have myasthenia gravis (MG) and her baby might have both MG and AMC. AMC may have other causes (neurogenic or congenital myopathy), but the presence of AMC should prompt you to check the mother for MG. Reproduced with permission from Gibson and Urs (1970), Figures 3 and 4.

◀ *Apraxia of eyelid opening* can mimic ocular myasthenia. Here, patients can manually push up the eyelids and maintain them open, but the eyes cannot be opened voluntarily.

◀ *Involvement of pupillary reflexes* excludes classic MG and most myopathies. Congenital MG or LEMS is more likely.

◀ *Weakness and fatigue that worsens in hot weather* may lead to misdiagnosis of MS. Similar heat-sensitive symptoms are observed in MG and some peripheral neuropathies. As noted earlier, symptoms may improve with cold.

◀ *Apparent relapse of MG with fasciculation* may be due to cholinergic block. Currently, this is rare, but it used to happen with excess anticholinesterase medication such as pyridostigmine, resulting in depolarization block. A small dose of edrophonium given intravenously will aggravate cholinergic block transiently but improve a true myasthenic crisis.

◀ *The patient with rheumatoid arthritis who complains of fatigue* may have MG induced by penicillamine. Rarely, rheumatoid arthritis and primary MG coexist.

◀ Be alert for *MG in patients who have received aminoglycoside antibiotics*, particularly neomycin and streptomycin. Either drug may induce or aggravate MG.

◀ *Fluctuating lower cranial nerve weakness* could be tetanus. Cephalic tetanus is a rare variant, but it may trap the unwary clinician into a diagnosis of MG or brainstem vascular problem. To clarify the diagnosis:

  - Test mouth opening. The patient with tetanus may find this difficult because of jaw spasm (trismus).
  - Perform the spatula test. You examine the gag reflex as usual, expecting to find gagging, but in tetanus the spatula is bitten because of jaw spasm.
  - Look for other features of tetanus, such as marked autonomic instability (tachycardia and hypertension).

◀ Patients with negative acetylcholine receptor antibodies whose weakness is *aggravated* by pyridostigmine. This suggests late-presenting congenital MG, such as:

  - Slow channel syndrome
  - Acetylcholinesterase deficiency

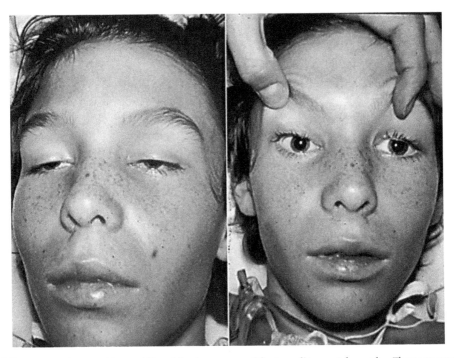

FIGURE 7.21: Botulism in a 14-year-old boy following compound fracture of his arm 5 days earlier. There was severe bulbar palsy followed by complete bilateral ophthalmoplegia with fixed dilated pupils. Reproduced from Wikipedia under Creative Commons Attribution License, from HL Fred, MD, and HA van Dijk.

- DOK7 variant
- COLQ-mutant myasthenic syndrome

Note: Pyridostigmine may also worsen *myotubular myopathy*, a disorder that resembles congenital MG. Use of an anticholinesterase inhibitor, such as pyridostigmine or neostigmine, will elevate acetylcholinesterase levels, causing depolarization block and increased weakness.

◀ *Subacute paralysis of all limbs and eye movements* could be due to botulism (Figure 7.21). You may be asked to see a patient who has become weak over the space of hours or days, and there is a question of MG. In botulism, you may observe:
  - Large pupils, unresponsive to light and accommodation
  - Paralysis of eye movement mimicking MG
  - Autonomic symptoms, particularly constipation

You should take a detailed dietary and trauma history.

Other Clues for Congenital Myasthenia Gravis

Although the onset of most congenital forms of MG is in infancy or childhood, some present in adulthood. The varying phenotype of the DOK7 variant is shown in Figure 7.19). Apart from aggravation of weakness by pyridostigmine as detailed previously, here are some further clues that might alert you to congenital myasthenia:

▶ Weakness of the thumb, neck extensors, and ankle dorsiflexors suggests the slow channel variant of congenital MG. This is the only one that is autosomal dominant; all others are recessive.
▶ Stridor, tongue wasting, and worsening by pyridostigmine are characteristic of the DOK7 mutation. Some respond to ephedrine or salbutamol.
▶ Ptosis with sparing of extraocular muscles if the defect is presynaptic (from choline acetyltransferase deficiency). Contrast this with acetylcholinesterase deficiency (synaptic), in which the extraocular muscles and pupillary light reflexes are involved.

Lambert Eaton Myasthenic Syndrome

LEMS is caused by antibodies to the presynaptic voltage-gated calcium channels present in the neuromuscular junction, autonomic nervous system, and cerebellum. Classically, it is associated with underlying lung cancer, but in the young adult this is less frequent and represents a primary autoimmune condition. Following are some Handles for LEMS.

History

▶ *Dry mouth, proximal weakness, and muscle fatigue on walking.* In its early stages, LEMS can be difficult to diagnose, especially when fatigue is not conspicuous and at rest there is no weakness. *The condition resembles a myopathy but the CK is normal.* There may be confusion with MS. The dry mouth, if not due to mundane causes like medication or mouth breathing, is a powerful clue suggesting autonomic nervous system involvement, which is frequent.
▶ *Other autonomic features*: impaired pupillary light reflexes, constipation, blurred vision, impaired sweating, orthostatic hypotension, and impotence

▶ *Fatiguing proximal weakness* with (usually) sparing of the extraocular muscles suggests LEMS or congenital MG. In typical MG, the extraocular muscles are nearly early always affected, but in LEMS they are usually spared.
▶ *Tingling in the face and upper limbs.* This may lead to misdiagnosis of panic disorder.

Examination

▶ *Reduced tendon reflexes*
▶ *Increased strength on prolonged muscle contraction.* Ask the patient to grasp your hand with sustained maximum force. The strength increases the longer the hand is clenched, indicating improvement in neuromuscular transmission.
▶ *Enhanced tendon reflex after contraction.* Test the biceps jerk before and after strong elbow contraction. After, say, 10 seconds, there may be a brisker response in LEMS compared to MG, where the reflex decreases.
▶ *Incrementing compound muscle action potential (CMAP) response to repetitive electrical nerve stimulation.* The combination of low-amplitude CMAPs on nerve conduction tests with a normal CK is an important diagnostic clue.

INFLAMMATORY MYOPATHIES

Chronic Polymyositis

The main Handles are as follows:

▶ *Slowly progressive symmetric weakness of proximal muscles, trunk, and, occasionally, bulbar muscles*
  Most dystrophies and spinal muscular atrophies will display some asymmetry at least until the late stages, but in polymyositis the weakness is highly symmetric from the start.
▶ *Neck flexion is always weak* in the established phase of disease.
▶ *Sparing of the extraocular muscles*
▶ *Preserved quadriceps power*
  Marked quadriceps weakness is unusual in polymyositis but common in IBM (Figure 7.22).
◀ Polymyositis is unlikely if the neck muscles are strong or quadriceps are weak.

Note: Recurrent polymyositis may simulate steroid-induced myopathy. In steroid myopathy, the EMG shows no fibrillation potentials, in contrast to polymyositis, and the CK is normal. In recurrent polymyositis, the CK is raised unless the disease is burned out. Steroid myopathy causes type II muscle fiber atrophy on biopsy, and there are no inflammatory cells.

Inclusion Body Myositis

See Video 7.6, IBM (courtesy Robert Pascuzzi MD). The main features are as follows:

▶ *Gradually progressive, sometimes familial myopathy* in a patient older than 50 years
▶ *Selective involvement of the thigh and forearm muscles* (Figure 7.22, *left*). This aspect may allow distinction from polymyositis.
▶ *Focal weakness of forearm finger flexors with poor grip and reduced finger dexterity.* IBM may be missed if forearm finger flexors are not tested specifically
▶ *Selective weakness of the long toe flexors, particularly flexor hallucis longus*, resulting in a continuously extended great toe. This is sometimes called the pseudo-Babinski sign (Figure 7.22, *right*). A superficially similar phenomenon occurs in:
  • Parkinsonian syndromes ("striatal toe sign")
  • Dystonia of the foot muscles (e.g., dopa-responsive dystonia)
  • Guillain-Barré syndrome (from selective weakness of flexor hallucis longus)
  • Multiple sclerosis (due to marked spasticity)
▶ Unexplained falls due to quadriceps weakness
▶ Unexplained dysphagia may predate limb weakness.
▶ If the EMG request form reads "possible myopathy" but the test suggests both myopathy and neuropathy, then think of IBM.

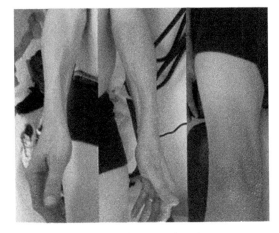 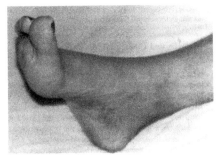

FIGURE 7.22: **Left**: Medial forearm and quadriceps wasting typical of inclusion body myositis (IBM). **Right**: The pseudo-Babinski sign in IBM. Left image reproduced with permission from Turner and Talbot (2013).

DYSTHYROID MYOPATHIES

Myxedema Myopathy

Patients have few specific muscle complaints, but there is generalized weakness, worse proximally, superimposed on classic signs of hypothyroidism. Here are some Handles:

▶ *Slow relaxing ankle jerks*
▶ *High CK*
▶ *Weak neck muscles*
▶ *Myoedema.* This means the formation of a small lump when the muscle belly is percussed.
▶ An adult with hypothyroidism, proximal weakness, pseudohypertrophy, and macroglossia has Hoffman syndrome. A similar disorder affects infants and children and is known as Kocher Debre Sémélaigne syndrome (infant Hercules).

Thyrotoxic Myopathy

In contrast to myxedema myopathy, patients with thyrotoxic myopathy have numerous muscular symptoms:

▶ *Proximal weakness.* Usually mild and not as severe as symptoms would suggest
▶ *Breathlessness*
▶ *Fasciculations*

Other features are:

▶ *Heat intolerance*
▶ *Normal or slightly raised CK*
▶ *Ophthalmopathy is infrequent*
▶ *Association with hypokalemic periodic paralysis and MG*
▶ *Atrial fibrillation*
◀ Exophthalmos with ptosis is a major Red Flag. It may indicate thyrotoxicosis with MG or a cavernous sinus problem (thrombosis or fistula).

PERIODIC PARALYSIS

▶ Episodes of generalized daytime weakness provoked by resting after exercise or eating food high in potassium suggest *hyperkalemic periodic paralysis.* There may be myotonia. During attacks, the serum potassium rises and the EKG T waves become tall.

▶ Episodes of generalized weakness starting in sleep, especially after a day of exercise or a large meal, suggest *hypokalemic periodic paralysis.* It may be clinically indistinguishable from thyrotoxic periodic paralysis.
   In attacks of either variety, weakness spares the face and breathing muscles. The tendon reflexes are depressed.
▶ Periodic paralysis with dysmorphic features and ventricular arrhythmias suggests *Andersen-Tawil syndrome.*
   This is a potassium channelopathy characterized by periodic paralysis, ventricular arrhythmias (long QT/QU interval), and developmental abnormalities (Figure 7.23).
▶ Eyes that stick shut after sneezing suggests *paramyotonia.*
   This is a sodium channelopathy in which myotonia or stiffness is provoked by cold weather or cold food or drink, typically ice cream. There is often paradoxical *worsening* of myotonia following repeated voluntary muscle contraction. Compare myotonic dystrophy and myotonia congenita where the stiffness is *lessened* by exercise.

MCARDLE'S SYNDROME

The main Handles are as follows:

▶ Calf or thigh muscle pain on exercise that the patient can walk through.
   This is a pathognomic feature called "second wind." The condition results from inability to metabolize muscle glycogen stores. Patients find the initial phase of exercise unpleasant as it is associated with severe fatigue, weakness, dyspnea, and muscle pain.
▶ Isometric muscle activities (e.g., squats) are impossible because they lead to a severe cramp known confusingly as a *contracture.*
   In McArdle's syndrome, *contracture* refers to a continual muscle spasm that may last for hours and not the muscle atrophy and fibrosis that result from muscle disuse.
▶ Myoglobinuria, often described as the color of tea or coke, is a well-recognized feature.
   Early diagnosis is important as there is a tendency to muscle fibrosis and permanent muscle weakness especially in the paraspinal and girdle muscles.

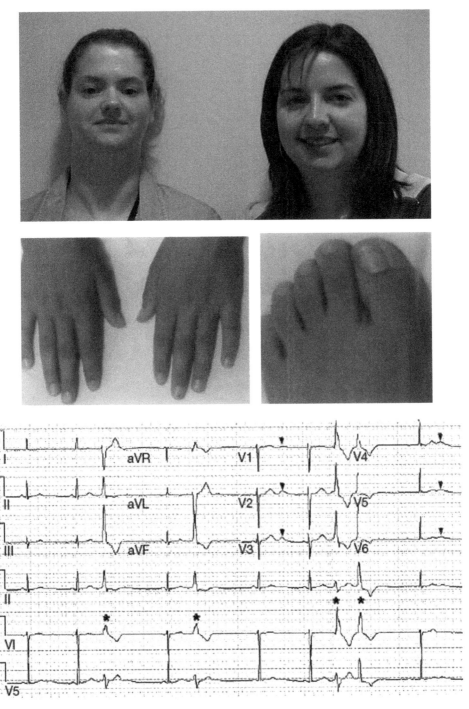

FIGURE 7.23: Andersen-Tawil syndrome (ATS). Periodic paralysis with ventricular arrhythmias. **Top:** A 29-year-old woman with ATS (left) alongside her healthy sister, aged 30. Note the typical facial appearance: hypertelorism; broad forehead; small palpebral fissures; fullness of the nasal base with bulbous tip; malar, maxillary, and mandibular hypoplasia; and thin upper lip. There is also a high-arched palate, mild facial asymmetry, and microcephaly. **Center:** Clinodactyly, shortened digits, and partial syndactyly of the second and third toes. **Bottom:** A 12-lead EKG, characteristic of Andersen-Tawil syndrome. There is a prolonged QU interval with a prominent U-wave (indicated by arrowheads) and ventricular ectopy (asterisks). Top image reproduced with permission from Yoon et al. (2006). Center image reproduced from Venance et al. (2006). Bottom image reproduced with permission from Garcia-Touchard et al. (2007).

Further Handles are as follows:

▷ Inability to run more than 100 yards but walking at a slow pace is normal
▷ In children, a misdiagnosis of growing pains is frequent and leads to delayed diagnosis.
▷ Muscle pain may be evoked by anger or sexual intercourse.
▷ Later risk of obesity, ischemic heart disease, and gout

Red Flags:

◁ Calf or thigh pain on exercise may simulate claudication.
◁ A normal CK excludes McArdle's syndrome; the CK is always high.

McArdle's syndrome mimics include the following:

- *Paramyotonia congenita.* This is an autosomal dominant channelopathy typified by paradoxical myotonia (i.e., worsening of myotonia with repetitive muscle contraction). As in McArdle's syndrome, some individuals experience the second-wind phenomenon and aggravation by cold temperature.
- *Becker dystrophy,* in which there is severe cramp and myoglobinuria

MITOCHONDRIAL MYOPATHIES

These are quite difficult to diagnose rapidly and intuitively because many seemingly unrelated parts of the body can be affected in addition to muscle—for example, brain (especially cerebellum), spinal cord, eye, peripheral nerves, endocrine system, heart, alimentary tract, and kidney. A typical presentation is

▷ Long-standing nonfatiguing ptosis with external ophthalmoplegia
  There is difficulty moving the eyes, with normal pupil responses but no diplopia. If this variety is present in isolation, it is termed *chronic progressive external ophthalmoplegia* (CPEO; Figure 7.15, *left*).
◁ Double vision. This is most unusual in CPEO.

Clues to alternative disorders are as follows:

▷ Fatiguing external eye muscles and diplopia suggest *ocular MG.*

▷ CPEO with difficulty swallowing points to *oculopharyngeal myopathy.*
▷ CPEO with combinations of retinitis pigmentosa, cerebellar ataxia, occasionally dystonia, cardiac abnormalities, short stature, and elevated CSF protein is likely *Kearns-Sayre syndrome* (Video 7.7, Kearns-Sayre). Added features begin with the letter *d*: dementia, deafness, diabetes, and dysphagia.
▷ A patient under 40 years with epilepsy, muscle weakness, stroke-like episodes (especially occipital infarcts) triggered by mitochondrial toxins (sodium valproate, metformin, statins) suggests the *MELAS syndrome* (mitochondrial encephalopathy, lactic acidosis, and stroke-like episodes).
  In the related *MERRF syndrome* (mitochondrial encephalopathy with ragged red fibers) there is often myoclonus, epilepsy, and ataxia. Muscle pain and weakness occur in MERRF, but these symptoms are often overshadowed by the other clinical manifestations.
▷ Proximal myopathy with CPEO, cyclical vomiting, and autonomic dysfunction suggests the *MNGIE syndrome*— mitochondrial neurogastrointestinal encephalopathy.

Disorders Mistaken for Mitochondrial Myopathies

- *Oculopharyngeal muscular dystrophy*: where there is CPEO and difficulty swallowing
- *MG*: with fatigability of extraocular muscles and eyelids
- *Thyrotoxic ophthalmopathy*: associated with exophthalmos, lid lag, and failure of convergence.

DISTAL MYOPATHIES

The number of possible causes for this rare, predominantly distal myopathy is ever expanding (Udd 2012). The main types and their associated Handles are given in Table 7.3.

Figure 7.24 shows some clues to the Laing syndrome.

MEDICATION-INDUCED MYOPATHIES

There are four categories of medication-induced myopathies (MIM), as listed next, with their main causes.

TABLE 7.3: CHARACTERISTICS OF THE MAIN DISTAL MYOPATHIES

Myopathy type	Age of onset and inheritance	Mutated gene	Main muscles affected	Handles
Welander	Late adult AD	TIA1	Long extensors of hands,. Feet later	Index finger weakness. Scandinavian descent
Udd (tibial muscular dystrophy)	Late adult AD	TTN	Asymmetric ankle dorsiflexion	Sparing of extensor digitorum brevis and hand muscles. Finnish descent
Markesbery-Griggs	Late adult AD	ZASP	Anterior leg then finger/wrist extensors	Cardiomyopathy in advanced cases. Central European descent
VCP-mutated distal myopathy	Late adult AD	VCP	Mimics limb girdle or scapuloperoneal dystrophies	Paget disease. Frontotemporal dementia. Raised ALP
Desminopathy	Early adult AR	Desmin	Distal leg	Cardiomyopathy or respiratory failure. Moderately raised creatine kinase (CK)
Laing	Childhood onset AD	MYH7	Weak ankle and toe dorsiflexion	Hanging big toe and dropped finger signs (Figure 7.24). Weak neck flexors
Nonaka	Early adult AR.	GNE	Ankle and toe dorsiflexors	Quads spared. CK moderately raised
Miyoshi	Young adult AR	Dysferlin	Calves, then distal leg and forearm Sometimes asymmetric.	Knee bobbing. Calf-head and thigh diamond signs (Figures 7.14 and 7.25). CK very high. Typically Japanese descent

AD, autosomal dominant; AR, autosomal recessive; ALP, alkaline phosphatase.

- Direct muscle toxicity:
  - Alcohol, cocaine, steroids
  - Statins. Apart from muscle cramp, which is a common isolated phenomenon, these drugs may cause a painful proximal necrotizing myositis that may progress rapidly despite drug withdrawal. CK levels are very high (e.g., >20,000), and there are usually antibodies to HMG-CoA reductase.

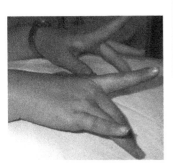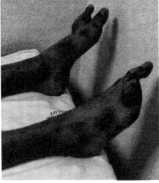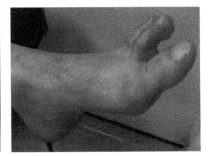

FIGURE 7.24: **Left**: A patient age 13 years with Laing dystrophy, attempting to extend the fingers fully; there is weakness and marked loss of extension of the third and fourth fingers. (2006). **Center**: The hanging big toe sign in a patient with Laing dystrophy. **Right**: Another example of the hanging great toe sign.   Left image reproduced with permission from Lamont et al. Center image reproduced with permission from Muelas et al. (2010). Right image courtesy Ros Quinlivan, London.

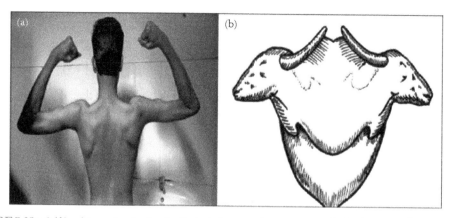

FIGURE 7.25: Calf-head sign on trophy showing the typical pattern of wasting in Miyoshi distal myopathy (a dysferlinopathy). Note the selective wasting of trapezius (producing the calf horn) and scapular muscles (supra- and infraspinatus). There is patchy enlargement of deltoid. Some have the diamond on quads sign (Figure 7.14). Reproduced with permission from Professor S Pradhan.

- o Mushroom poisoning
- o Antimalarials, vincristine, and colchicine. There may be a peripheral neuropathy as well. All cause vacuolar myopathy.
- o Zidovudine results in mitochondrial myopathy.
- Immunologically induced inflammatory myopathy:
  - o Penicillamine, procainamide
- Indirect muscle damage:
  - o Drug-induced coma (alcohol, cocaine) with subsequent ischemic muscle compression
  - o Medication-induced hypokalemia (e.g., diuretics, alcohol, laxatives); weakness may be periodic.
  - o Hyperthermia related to cocaine
  - o Neuroleptic malignant syndrome (NMS). There is fever, confusion, autonomic dysfunction (sweating, tachycardia, labile blood pressure), and marked extrapyramidal rigidity. It results from exposure to phenothiazines, haloperidol, *introduction/ withdrawal* of levodopa or dopamine agonists. Rigor causes rhabdomyolysis. The mechanism of NMS is acute dopamine receptor blockage.
  - o Malignant hyperthermia. This is due to an inherited susceptibility to general anesthetic agents, typically succinylcholine or halothane. There is high temperature, tachycardia, rapid breathing, and muscle

breakdown due to calcium release from muscle cells resulting in rigidity and metabolic acidosis. The CK is extremely high. Dantrolene is the best treatment.
- Direct muscle damage:
  - o Repeated injections of opiates (heroin or pentazocine) with muscle damage, indurated skin, and muscle contractures
  - o Inadvertent intra-arterial injections with ischemic muscle necrosis, livedo-like skin changes, or skin infarction (Nicolau syndrome)

The main clues to diagnosis obviously will come from the history if you are lucky.

Here are some Handles for medication-induced myopathy:

▶ Aggressive proximal myopathy with extremely high CK in a patient taking a statin is likely necrotizing myositis due to HMG-CoA reductase antibodies.

▶ Acute myopathy with delirium tremens, seizures, and metabolic problems is likely alcohol-related.

▶ In a drug addict, think of exposure to cocaine, heroin, or mushrooms.

▶ In patients with gout or cancer, colchicine or vincristine are the likely causes. Investigate for coexisting peripheral neuropathy.

▶ If the patient has AIDS, check for exposure to zidovudine.

- ▶ In patients with rheumatoid arthritis, penicillamine or glucocorticoids are likely culprits.
- ▶ In steroid-induced myopathy, the CK is normal, there are no fibrillations on EMG, and there is type II fiber atrophy on biopsy.
- ▶ In psychiatric patients, consider phenothiazine-related dystonia, serotonin syndrome, and neuroleptic malignant syndrome.
- ▶ Marked rigidity, hyperpyrexia, and dysautonomia after general anesthetic is malignant hyperthermia.

Miscellaneous Disorders
Myopathy with Deafness

There are just three categories:

- • Ehlers-Danlos syndrome
- • Mitochondrial disorders: Kearns-Sayre syndrome, atypical MELAS, myopathy, deafness and seizures due to mutation in tRNA-Ser gene
- • Congenital myopathy with diarrhea, zinc deficiency, and deafness (Levy-Yeboa syndrome, autosomal recessive)

Miscellaneous Handles in Myopathy

- ▶ Plantar flexion weaker than dorsiflexion strongly suggests dysferlin myopathy or distal hereditary motor neuropathy. Associated with knee-bopping sign.

In most neuropathies and myopathies, ankle *dorsiflexion* is weaker than plantar flexion, in part due to the greater bulk of the calf muscles. Paradoxically, in *Dysferlin myopathy* and *distal hereditary motor neuropathy*, plantar flexion is the weaker ankle movement. This causes *knee bobbing on standing* that is relieved by walking (Rossor et al. 2012). Comparable symptoms are found in the advanced stages of Charcot-Marie-Tooth disease when the initially preserved plantar flexors become weak (see Chapter 11, Peripheral Neuropathy, Figure 11. 40).

- ▶ Slowly progressive proximal weakness with difficulty breathing but not swallowing suggests *acid maltase deficiency*. Rarely, this presents with respiratory failure before limb weakness

Acid maltase deficiency is one of the glycogen storage disorders that may start in the teenage years and present as an adult to neurologists. The breathing difficulty is due to diaphragmatic weakness and is characteristically prominent on lying down but not so much on sitting or standing. EMG often shows myotonic discharges, but there is no clinical myotonia. Diagnosis is important given the availability of therapy with, for example, alglucosidase alfa (Lumizyme or Myozyme).

Infants may be affected and present as floppy babies. See Video 7.8, Pompe (courtesy Robert Pascuzzi, MD).

- ▶ Proximal myopathy with congenital pinpoint pupils is *Stormorken syndrome* (a tubular aggregate myopathy; see Figure 7.26).
- ▶ Exercise-induced deafness suggests a mitochondrial disorder.

MOTOR NEURON DISORDERS

Amyotrophic Lateral Sclerosis

The classic features of ALS when it begins in the upper limbs are

- ▶ Asymmetric hand weakness and wasting with fasciculation or cramp in unusual places.
  Many people get a cramp in the hamstring or calf muscles, notably after exercise or while recumbent, but in ALS, cramping may

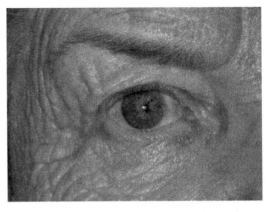

FIGURE 7.26: Small pupil sign in Stormorken syndrome. This is an autosomal dominant tubular aggregate myopathy characterized by thrombocytopenia, anemia, asplenia, and ichthyosis. Courtesy David Nicholl, Birmingham, UK.

be noted in the abdominal, back, or hand muscles. The patient may report abdominal cramp even when bending. Likewise, fasciculation is reported regularly by healthy people especially in the hands or calves after exercise, but it would be unusual in muscles of the forearm extensor compartment, abdominal wall, or back.

Here are some other Handles that might help clinch a diagnosis:

▶ Isolated dysarthria and/or dysphagia (usually with sialorrhea)
▶ Split hand sign

This is characteristic of ALS in its early stages (see Figure 7.27).
▶ Weak, wasted hand with brisk arm reflexes
This is the classic paradox. The lower motor neuron involvement causes hand weakness, wasting, and fasciculation. Depressed reflexes are expected, but they are brisk because of simultaneous upper motor neuron damage.
▶ Brisk leg reflexes, occasionally with downgoing plantars and preserved abdominal reflexes
This combination is characteristic; the reason for the absent Babinski response and preserved abdominal reflexes is not understood.

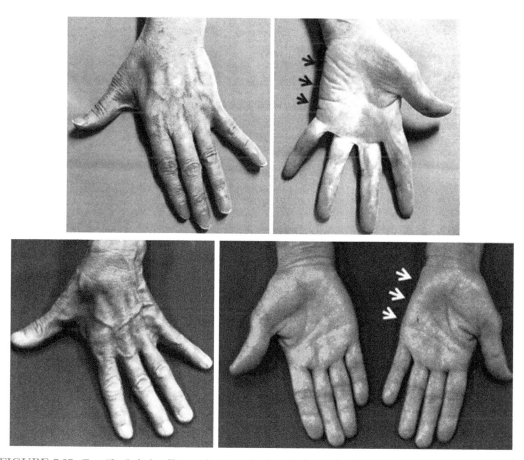

FIGURE 7.27: **Top**: The "split hand" sign of amyotrophic lateral sclerosis (ALS). It involves muscles we use frequently like the thumb and forefinger. There is wasting of the first dorsal interosseous (DIO) and thenar complex but sparing of the hypothenar muscles (arrows). Note that in ALS this sign becomes less reliable with progression of the disease to all intrinsic hand muscles. **Bottom**: Hand muscle atrophy in C8 radiculopathy. Note the marked atrophy of first dorsal interosseous as well as the hypothenar muscles (arrows). Split hand sign is also seen in brachial plexus lesions involving the lower trunk or medial cord and ulnar neuropathies due to weakness of the anterior interosseous muscles but sensory features are expected. Reproduced with permission from Eisen and Kuwabara (2012).

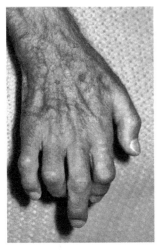
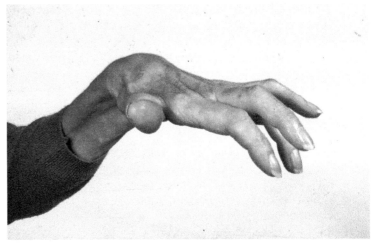

FIGURE 7.28: Amyotrophic lateral sclerosis (ALS). **Left**: Note the diffuse ("global") muscle wasting and uneven clawing of the fingers in this patient. If there is no sensory loss and the reflexes are brisk, then ALS is the most likely diagnosis. **Right**: Same patient, highlighting the dropped finger sign, indicating patchy weakness of the finger extensors.

▶ Painless neck weakness
This is nonspecific but very characteristic of ALS.
▶ Dropped finger sign (Figure 7.28)
Likewise, this is nonspecific but very typical of ALS. Other causes are as follows:
   ○ Cervical radiculopathy (Figure 7.29)
   ○ Syringomyelia
   ○ Neuralgic amyotrophy
   ○ Inclusion body myositis
   ○ Motor variant of chronic inflammatory demyelinating polyneuropathy
   ○ Laing distal muscular dystrophy (see Distal Myopathy section earlier)
   ○ Multifocal motor neuropathy with conduction block
▶ Patients with rheumatoid arthritis may have tendon rupture which could bear superficial resemblance to this sign.

Handles for Unusual Presentations of ALS

▶ *Unilateral painless foot drop*. This is a rare presentation of ALS in the early stages, often confused with a common peroneal nerve palsy or L4/L5 radiculopathy. There may be few sensory signs, and the diagnosis may not be made for several months unless a detailed EMG is undertaken.

▶ *Hemiparesis*. This is the Mills variant of ALS. There is increased tone and usually muscle wasting affecting the limbs just on one side.
▶ *Camptocormia*. This results from selective weakness of the trunk and sometimes neck muscles. See Chapter 8 (Movement Disorders) for further discussion.

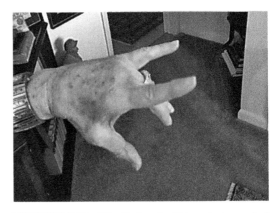

FIGURE 7.29: C7 radiculopathy. This patient was asked to extend the fingers. She had severe neck pain radiating into arm, digits, and medial to scapula. Scapular radiation is typical of a C7 root lesion. Another sign of C7 radiculopathy is an *inability to snap the fingers* (Swift's sign) due to weakness of flexor digitorum superficialis (sublimis) which has heavy C7 innervation.

▶ *Respiratory failure.* Selective involvement of the diaphragm is a rare early feature. Late-onset acid maltase deficiency needs consideration, as it may present with respiratory problems. The clue is sparing of swallowing, whereas swallowing is usually affected at the same time in ALS.

▶ *Pure spastic paraparesis with gradual progression* suggests primary lateral sclerosis (PLS), the least common variety of ALS. Initially, there are just upper motor neuron signs in the lower limbs with little weakness. After about 3 years, lower motor neuron signs appear.

Note:

▶ Bladder involvement is common in PLS, but it would be a major Red Flag in classic ALS.

ALS Mimics
FASIC Syndrome

FASIC stands for fasciculation anxiety syndrome in clinicians. This occurs frequently in doctors and medical students who worry excessively about ALS. There is no cramp, weakness, or wasting. Most have no serious cause, and a diagnosis of benign fasciculation is presumed.

Syringomyelia

This may have superficial resemblance to ALS, but the arm reflexes are depressed and there is nearly always sensory loss. Early in the disease, sensory signs may not be conspicuous but often start along the ulnar border of the hand and forearm.

The old saying is: *"If the arm reflexes are not depressed it is not syringomyelia."*

Thus, any brisk arm reflex would count against a diagnosis of syringomyelia.

Cervical Spondylotic Myeloradiculopathy

This can mimic ALS in the arms as root compression causes the lower motor neuron component and cord compression/ischemia will produce the upper motor neuron aspect. Neck discomfort is usually conspicuous in spondylosis, particularly if the patient has pain or limitation on lateral flexion of the neck.

▶ Sometimes the nerve roots are tender if palpated under or behind the sternomastoid muscle.

▶ Spurling's test, when positive, is reliable. For this procedure, the head is turned to the affected side while applying downward pressure on the vertex. If positive, there is pain radiating in the direction of the corresponding dermatome.

Cramp-Fasciculation Syndrome

Fasciculations and cramps in multiple areas without weakness or wasting suggest this disorder. In the related condition, *Isaac's syndrome*, a potassium channelopathy, there is generalized myokymia associated with cramp and increased sweating.

Man-in-a-Barrel Syndrome

See also Chapter 9 (Stroke). Here, both arms dangle lifelessly by the sides (Figure 7.31). This occurs mostly in spinal muscular atrophies or progressive

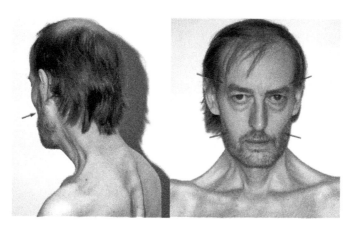

FIGURE 7.30: Facial onset sensory and motor neuronopathy. This shows the masseter and temporalis wasting in someone with facial onset sensory and motor neuronopathy (FOSMN) 10 years after onset. The neck is wasted and weak. Reproduced with permission from Broad and Leigh (2015).

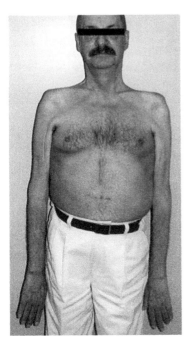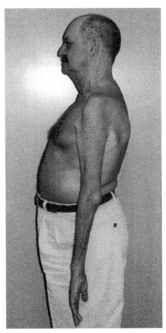

FIGURE 7.31: **Left**: A 59-year-old man with weakness and wasting of both arms 7 years after his initial symptoms. Note the neurogenic "man in the barrel" phenotype causing the arms to hang down flaccidly. **Right**: Severe neurogenic atrophy is shown throughout the arm and shoulder girdle. This is a selective form of spinal muscular atrophy. Reproduced with permission from Katz et al. (1999), Figure 1.

muscle atrophy variants, but it may also develop in the following:

- Bilateral borderzone infarcts of the frontoparietal cortex
- Anterior spinal artery territory spinal infarct. See Figure 7.30 and Video 7.9, Man-in-the-Barrel (courtesy Flanagan et al. 2014).
- Posttraumatic cervical myelopathy
- Severe neuropathies (e.g., Guillain-Barré syndrome)
- Radiculopathies, including bilateral lesions of the brachial plexus

Physical examination will reveal different patterns according to the involvement of upper or lower motor neurons and sensory system.

▶ Sensory impairment in the face that spreads into the arms and upper trunk followed by bulbar and upper limb lower motor neurone signs is facial onset sensory and motor neuronopathy (FOSMN). Ageusia is an early feature.

Hirayama Syndrome or Monomelic Motor Neuron Disease

This is a benign disorder of teenagers and young adults, mostly male and Indian, but described first in Japan. It is well-recognized in the Western world. The condition evolves slowly over 2–5 years with weakness and wasting from purely lower motor neuron involvement in just one extremity, usually the arm. Brachioradialis is relatively spared. There are no sensory signs. Rarely, the thigh muscles are affected in isolation. Occasionally, the sympathetic nervous system is involved, with sweating, cold hands, or hair loss.

Thus:

▶ A young male with gradually progressive lower motor neuron weakness affecting just one arm probably has Hirayama syndrome.

MRI Signs in ALS

There are three intriguing MRI signs in ALS:

1. *Snake-eye sign on cervical spine MRI* (Figure 7.32). This consists of abnormal symmetric signal coming from the anterior horn in some patients with ALS. It is not specific for ALS;

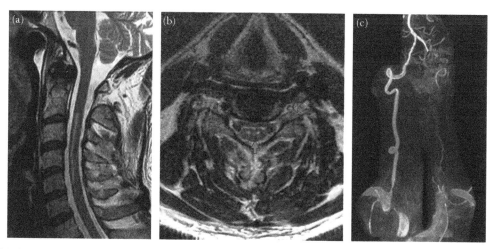

FIGURE 7.32: MRI of anterior spinal artery infarct in a patient with the phospholipid antibody syndrome. Sagittal T2-weighted images demonstrate a pencil-like hyperintensity in the anterior spinal cord (**A**) and axial images show a snake-eye pattern (**B**, arrow) and absence of the left vertebral artery flow void (**B**, arrowheads). Magnetic resonance angiography shows an occluded left vertebral artery (**C**). Reproduced with permission from Flanagan, McKeon, & Weinshenker (2014), Figure 1.

it has been described in anterior spinal artery territory spinal cord infarction. See Figure 7.33.

2. *Bright tongue sign* (Figure 7.34). This is a characteristic sign of ALS, though nonspecific. It is described also in Pompe's syndrome (acid maltase deficiency). It results from denervation of the tongue with replacement by fatty tissue and is seen best on T1-weighted images.

3. *The wine-glass sign* (Figure 7.35)

Red Flags for ALS

◀ Lack of progression

Fluctuation in disability is permitted, but if there is no overall progression then ALS is the wrong diagnosis.

◀ Lack of upper motor neuron signs

You should consider a motor neuropathy, hereditary spastic paraplegia, radiculopathy, SMA variant, IBM, or even myotonic dystrophy.

◀ Ruptured long head of biceps

Following strenuous exertion or tendon inflammation, as in rheumatoid arthritis, the biceps muscle tendon may be pulled out from the supraglenoid tubercle and the entire muscle bunches up toward its origin. If unilateral, such cases have been erroneously diagnosed as monomelic motor neuron disease (Figure 7.36).

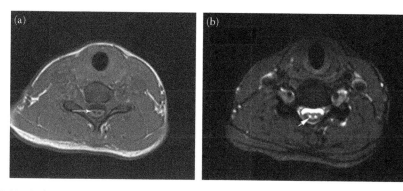

FIGURE 7.33: Snake-eye sign. MRI cervical spine (**A**) MRI cervical spine axial T1-weighted sequence shows symmetric hypointense signals (arrow) in the anterior horn. (**B**) MRI cervical spine axial T2-weighted sequence shows symmetric hyperintense signals (arrow) in the anterior horn. Reproduced with permission from Sharma et al. (2013).

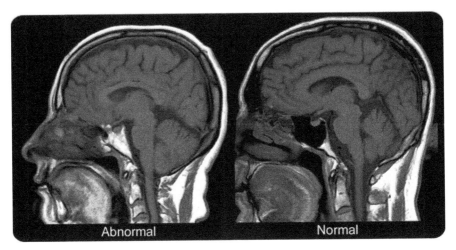

Abnormal   Normal

FIGURE 7.34: Bright tongue sign. Sagittal T1 MRI of the brain shows abnormal diffuse T1 hyperintensity of the tongue musculature (**left**). A normal tongue is shown on the **right**. Reproduced with permission from Fox and Cohen (2012).

◀ Sensory loss
Although detailed neurophysiological or pathological examination may show sensory fiber involvement, routine clinical examination will reveal either no or very mild sensory defects in classic ALS. Sensory *symptoms* such as tingling and discomfort in the upper limbs occur in some rapidly progressive cases, but anything beyond mild objective sensory signs should alert the physician to alternative conditions. The main exception is:

◀ *Paraneoplastic motor neuron disease*, where there may be a superimposed neuropathy.

◀ Diplopia or cerebellar ataxia
The cranial nerves controlling eye movement are involved only in extremely long-term survivors of ALS who are on respiratory support, and disorder of the cerebellum or its connections is not recognized. If your patient with suspected ALS reports diplopia or has cerebellar signs, think again!

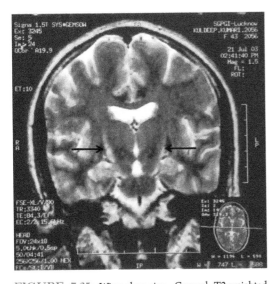

FIGURE 7.35: Wine-glass sign. Coronal T2-weighted image showing bilateral symmetrical hyperintensity along the corticospinal tracts (black arrows) forming a wine-glass appearance. This is seen occasionally in amyotrophic lateral sclerosis (ALS) but it is not specific. Reproduced with permission from Pradhan et al. (2006).

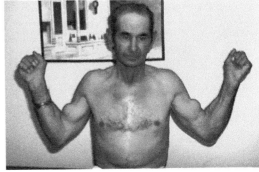

FIGURE 7.36: Bilateral rupture producing "Popeye" arms. The long head of biceps that arises from the supraglenoid tubercle has ruptured at its origin on both sides. The short heads are unaffected so that some elbow flexion is possible. If unilateral, it may be confused with monomelic motor neuron disease.

◀ ALS with behavioral manifestations and parkinsonian features

This is atypical for classic ALS and favors the syndrome of frontotemporal dementia due to mutations in chromosome 9 (C9ORF72) or the FUS (fused in sarcoma) gene, on chromosome 16.

◀ Pressure sores

In most bedbound patients, pressure sores develop rapidly unless nursing care is excellent, but ALS patients appear resistant to this complication. As pointed out originally by Charcot, this probably relates to the unimpaired sensation that triggers weight-shifting whenever discomfort is felt.

◀ Bladder disorder

This is very infrequent. It may relate to preservation of Onuf's nucleus, located in the sacral segment of the spinal cord. The main exception is primary lateral sclerosis (see earlier discussion).

◀ Absent reflexes in the upper limbs

This would be a very unusual pattern for ALS and raises the possibility of peripheral neuropathy, IBM, brachial plexopathy, or syringomyelia. Usually, sensory examination or EMG will resolve any doubt.

BULBAR PALSIES

Amyotrophic Lateral Sclerosis

There are two overlapping varieties of bulbar presentation in ALS with differing emphasis but equally poor survival of about 2 years. In *progressive bulbar palsy*, the features are predominantly lower motor neuron, with the three *d*'s: dysarthria, dysphagia, and dysphonia. Inspection of the tongue usually clinches the diagnosis, as it is wasted and fasciculating. The other variety, *pseudobulbar palsy*, involves predominantly the upper motor neurons and produces the same three *d*'s, but the jaw jerk is brisk and there is emotional lability. These two classic varieties are often indistinguishable. Some clinicians deny the existence of two separate categories; it is probably a question of emphasis. Thus:

▶ Progressive dysarthria, dysphagia, and dysphonia with fasciculating tongue suggest the progressive bulbar palsy variant of ALS.

▶ Progressive dysarthria, dysphagia, and dysphonia with no tongue fasciculation, brisk jaw jerk, and emotional lability suggest the pseudobulbar palsy variant of ALS.

Kennedy Syndrome

See Figure 7.37 and Video 7.10, Kennedy (courtesy Robert Pascuzzi, MD).

Kennedy syndrome (X-linked bulbospinal neuronopathy) is a disorder only affecting males and caused by a trinucleotide repeat in the androgen receptor gene resulting in androgen insensitivity. The main features are as follows:

- Difficulty in swallowing with tongue fasciculation
- Slow progression over 5 years or more, initially raising the possibility of bulbar ALS

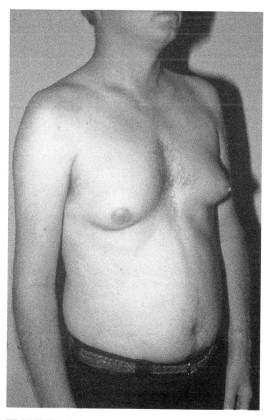

FIGURE 7.37: Kennedy syndrome (X-linked bulbospinal neuronopathy). This shows marked gynecomastia. Additional clues are chin fasciculations, essential-type tremor, absent reflexes, and testicular atrophy. Courtesy Robert Pascuzzi, MD.

- Arm tremor similar to essential tremor
- Chin fasciculation (allegedly pathognomic)
- Small testes and gynecomastia
- Depressed deep tendon reflexes on account of lower motor neuron involvement
- Down-going plantar responses, as the corticospinal tracts are spared.
- Rarely, Brugada syndrome (diagnosed on EKG)

Thus:

▶ Slowly progressive bulbar palsy in an adult male with arm tremor and chin fasciculation suggests Kennedy syndrome.

Other causes of gynecomastia and weakness in males: Kennedy Syndrome; myofibrillar myopathy; thyrotoxic hypokalemic periodic paralysis; use of anabolic steroids.

Adult Onset Hexosaminidase A Deficiency

▶ Bulbar palsy, motor neuropathy, and cerebellar ataxia in a teenager or adult suggest hexosaminidase A deficiency (Tay-Sachs disease). See Video 7.11, Hex A.

This rare combination is common in Ashkenazi Jews, and it is one of the GM2 gangliosidoses. Other features may include dystonia, choreoathetosis, and pyramidal signs. Visual evoked potentials are delayed, a feature which may result in misdiagnosis of MS.

The condition may be confused also with:

- Early-onset ALS
- Spinal muscular atrophy

Progressive Bulbar Palsy and Sensorineural Deafness

There are two major causes:

- Brown-Violetta-Van Laere (VL) syndrome. Onset is in childhood.
- Madras motor neuron disease. Onset is in young adults.

Fazio-Londe syndrome is probably the same disorder as VL. A useful confirmatory test for VL is the blood pyridoxine level, which is raised. This is now an important condition not to be missed, as it can be treated with high doses of riboflavin.

The Madras variant of ALS commences in teenagers (usually Indian) and pursues a relatively benign course. There is deafness, optic atrophy, and marked tongue wasting but relatively fewer upper motor neuron signs.

HEREDITARY SPASTIC PARAPLEGIAS

Hereditary spastic paraplegia (HSP) is included in the discussion here because it has similarity to ALS and a comparable prevalence. It is a group of mostly autosomal dominant paraplegias (70–80%), for which there are more than 60 known mutations. Recessive, X-linked, and mitochondrial varieties are recognized, but many are apparently sporadic. About half of the dominant forms are due to a mutation in the *SPG4* gene that codes for spastin. It is a "pure" form that affects teenagers and young adults, with the following features:

▶ Slowly progressive stiff-legged gait in the presence of little weakness and no sensory signs. Inspection of the shoes will show that the front of the sole is scuffed. The limbs are spastic with brisk reflexes.

▶ Easily obtained Babinski responses, echoing primary progressive MS, which is the main differential diagnosis, along with ALS.

▶ There are few upper motor neuron signs in the upper limbs; bladder function is little affected and the cranial nerves not at all.

▶ There may be cognitive decline and hand tremor but no sensory involvement.

▶ Patients often continue working until normal retirement age.

▶ MRI often shows atrophy of the corpus callosum.

◀ HSP may be confused with:
   o Dopa-responsive dystonia (DRD). The gait is similar in both conditions. In DRD but not HSP, there is variability, with more severe symptoms during the afternoon and evening.
   o Congenital diplegia and congenital spastic paraplegia, but neither tend to progress.

Features of the more common *autosomal dominant* forms are given in Table 7.4. The reader should refer to textbooks and reviews for details on the rare recessive and mitochondrial varieties of HSP.

▶ Progressive spastic paraplegia with small hyperpigmented macular lesions suggests the Kjellin syndrome (SPG15). See Figure 7.38.

TABLE 7.4: SUMMARY OF SOME OF THE MAIN FORMS OF AUTOSOMAL DOMINANT HEREDITARY SPASTIC PARAPLEGIA (HSP)

Disease	Protein	Key Clinical features
SPG3A, 6, and 8	Atlastin/NIOA1/Strumpellin	Pure HSP. Atlastin mutation is main cause of early-onset form
SPG4	Spastin	Pure HSP. Most frequent type. Variable age of onset. Rarely cognitive decline, neuropathy or hand tremor
SPG9	Unknown	Complicated. Cataract, motor neuropathy, gastroesophageal reflux
SPG10	Kinesin family member 5A	Pure or complicated. Early onset. Distal amyotrophy (Silver syndrome)
SPG12 and 13	Reticulon 2/heat shock protein 1	Pure early/adult onset
SPG17, 38, and 41	Seipin/unknown/unknown	Complicated. Amyotrophy of hand muscles (Silver syndrome)
SPG29	Unknown	Complicated: neonatal hyperbilirubinemia, deafness, persistent vomiting from hiatus hernia
SPG33 and 37	Protrudin/unknown	Pure
SPG35	FAHN	Movement disorder, leukodystrophy, thin corpus callosum. Bristle hair.
SPG36	Unknown	Early adult onset with polyneuropathy

Adapted from Faber et al. (2014).

This is an autosomal *recessive* variety of HSP (SPG15). Patients present with the following:

- Progressive spastic paraplegia
- Amyotrophy
- Learning difficulty
- Maculopathy
- ▶ Progressive spastic paraplegia with bristle hair and exotropia is likely SPG 35 (Figure 7.39).

This is an autosomal recessive form of SPG. There is a mutation in the gene coding for fatty acid hydroxylase-associated neurodegeneration (FAHN). There is a mixed movement disorder sometimes with leukodystrophy and a thin corpus callosum. The presence of bristle hair may be a useful Handle. The only other conditions with this phenomenon are Menkes disease "steely hair" and giant axonal neuropathy "kinky hair."

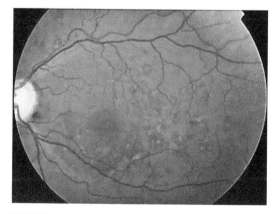

FIGURE 7.38: Kjellin syndrome. This shows small hyperpigmented lesions 0.1–0.2 disk diameters throughout the macula which are highly characteristic of this disorder. Reproduced with permission from Nowak et al. (2014).

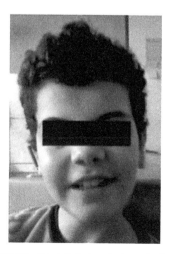

FIGURE 7.39: Bristle hair sign which may be diagnostic of SPG35. Reproduced with permission from Rattay et al. (2016).

SUMMARY

Myopathy

Dystrophia Myotonica Type 1

- Presentation: autosomal dominant; young adult with muscular stiffness, worse in cold weather, predominantly distal weakness and poor grip; excess daytime sleepiness
- Examination: frontal baldness, thinning of the lower face, ptosis, open jaw, inverted smile, maloccluded teeth ("hatchet face"), and swan neck deformity; myotonia lessens with repeated contraction; neck flexor weakness; Christmas tree cataract; shank sign, pectus excavatum, cardiomyopathy
- Abnormal plain skull X-ray: thickened calvarium, small pituitary fossa, large frontal sinuses, elongated mandible
- MRI: increased signal intensity in temporal poles

Red Flags

- If the neck muscles are not weak, the diagnosis is wrong.
- Absence of myotonia makes the diagnosis unlikely, but may be absent if grip has become very weak.
- Severe myotonia is unusual in DM1 but typical of myotonia congenita.

Late identification of DM1:

- A patient with apparent motor polyneuropathy, SMA, or MG may have DM1.
- Failure to resume spontaneous breathing after a general anesthetic
- In a mother who delivers a baby with congenital myotonic dystrophy
- Features of myotonia congenita (Thomsen's disease): muscle hypertrophy, with Hercules-like appearance; startle myotonia; little or no weakness
- Infants and children with apparent myotonia may have Schwartz-Jampel syndrome.
  - Features: blepharophimosis, perioral tonic contractions, pursed lips, low-set ears
- Newborns with myotonic discharges on EMG may have infantile acid maltase deficiency or myotonia congenita.

Dystrophia Myotonica Type II

- Presents in middle age with muscle pain, stiffness, and little myotonia
- Mainly proximal weakness

Duchenne Muscular Dystrophy

- X-linked recessive, male child, onset aged 2–5 years with a waddling gait and lumbar lordosis
- Toe walking, proximal limb and neck flexor weakness, calf and tongue hypertrophy
- Frequent cardiac involvement; very high CK and Gower's sign

Red Flags

- Normal or slightly raised CK
- Still walking after age 16 years (unless responding to steroids)

Becker Muscular Dystrophy

- X-linked recessive; onset in boys around the age of 12 years
- Pelvic then shoulder weakness; calf enlargement and wasted lower pectorals
- Valley sign: cramp, myoglobinuria or dilated cardiomyopathy may be the presenting feature.
- T-wave inversion on EKG
- Can mimic a metabolic myopathy.

Facioscapulohumeral Muscular Dystrophy

- Autosomal dominant. Scapular winging, asymmetric limb-girdle weakness and bilateral facial weakness; long-standing inability to whistle
- Sleeping with eyes open
- Shoulder hump signs, weakness of shoulder shrugging; triple hump or poly-hill sign
- Infraspinatus hypertrophied and scapulae appear small; biceps and triceps are weak, deltoid and brachioradialis are spared, reversal of the anterior axillary folds, recurrent shoulder dislocations
- High-stepping waddling gait due to weak ankle dorsiflexion, marked lordosis, and pot belly; Beevor's sign
- Occasionally: camptocormia, hearing loss, and retinal vasculopathy

Red Flags

- Absent shoulder hump sign. Involvement of bulbar or extraocular muscles, neck muscle weakness, early respiratory involvement; weak brachioradialis muscle; weak iliopsoas or calf muscles in the absence of other lower limb weakness

Differential Diagnosis for FSHMD
- LGMD type 2A (calpainopathy), types 2C-F (sarcoglycanopathies); VCP-mutated distal myopathy
- Neurogenic hereditary scapuloperoneal atrophy, long thoracic or accessory nerve lesions

Differential Diagnosis for Scapular Winging
- Other myopathies with scapular winging, such as LGMD type 2A (calpainopathy) and types 2C-2F (sarcoglycanopathies); VCP-mutated distal myopathy
- Accessory nerve lesion: no hump but weak shrugs
- Long thoracic nerve lesion: hump but shrugs strong and rarely bilateral

Limb Girdle Muscular Dystrophy
Compared to the recessive types, autosomal dominant forms are rarer and have mildly elevated CK levels and later onset (>20 years). For LGMD phenotypes, learn Table 7.2!

Red Flags for LGMD
◀ Weak neck muscles, sensory neuropathy, autonomic or visceral dysfunction in the early phase; facial muscle involvement and early respiratory insufficiency

Associations of muscle disorder with:

- *Calf hypertrophy*. Mutations in Dystrophin, Caveolin; Calpain; Sarcoglycan; Fukutin-related, and Anoctamin. Calf hypertrophy may be found in S1 radiculopathy, hypothyroidism, and cysticercosis infection of calf muscle.
- *CK greater than 10,000*: Dystrophin, Calpain, Dysferlin, Sarcoglycan, Fukutin-related, and Anoctamin
- *Macroglossia*. LGMD types C–F (sarcoglycanopathies), LGMD type 2I (Fukutin-associated), DMD. Macroglossia occurs in amyloid neuropathy (associated with ageusia), acromegaly, and hypothyroidism.

Emery-Dreifuss Muscular Dystrophy
- Childhood onset of weakness in biceps, triceps, and ankle dorsiflexors
- Contractures at elbows, ankles, and spine causing toe walking
- Cardiac dysfunction. Normal or slightly elevated CK; confusion with LGMD type 1B or rigid spine syndrome

Oculopharyngeal Muscular Dystrophy
- GCN trinucleotide repeat disorder, usually autosomal dominant
- Middle-age-onset ptosis with frontalis overactivity head extension, followed by difficulty in upgaze without diplopia, then dysphagia
- Proximal lower limb weakness; finally, paresis of the proximal upper limbs, face, and tongue

The main differential diagnoses:

- MG, mitochondrial myopathy

Further Myopathy Handles
- Quadriceps wasting is unusual in polymyositis but may be found in LGMD, Becker dystrophy, IBM, and SMA.
- The neck is strong in LGMD but weak in similar conditions with proximal weakness, such as polymyositis and dermatomyositis.
- Respiratory involvement is later in polymyositis and dermatomyositis than in acid maltase deficiency and myotonic dystrophy.
- Hypertrophy/preservation of extensor digitorum brevis (EDB) supports limb girdle dystrophy rather than SMA (type III), where it is atrophic. Preservation of EDB is seen in Udd distal myopathy.
- Atypical Gowers maneuver in Kugelberg-Welander disease (SMA type III)

Dropped Head Sign
- Muscular dystrophies: Inflammatory myopathies, neuromuscular junction disorder, motor neuron disorders, extrapyramidal disorders (parkinsonism, especially MSA).
- In all but extrapyramidal disorders, neck tone is normal or reduced. In extrapyramidal conditions, neck rigidity may be prevent passive head movement.

Neuromuscular Junction Disorders
Myasthenia Gravis

- Jaw supporting sign; myasthenic snarl and triple-grooved tongue
- Isolated weakness of eye closure and opening with normal pupillary reactions confirms classic MG. Involvement of pupillary reflexes excludes classic MG and most myopathies and favors congenital MG or LEMS.
- Prolonged upgaze that results in progressive weakness of the upper lids is characteristic of MG. Ice pack test; improved swallowing with iced drinks. Also seen in ALS.
- Pseudo-internuclear ophthalmoplegia. Ptosis is asymmetric, even unilateral for long periods. The pseudo plus-minus lid syndrome: ptosis of one eye and lid retraction of the other
- Head tilted backward and lips pursed. Overactivity of frontalis to keep eyes open. The lips are pursed to keep the jaw closed; weak neck flexion before neck extension.
- Fatigueable lower limb weakness with negative AchRA favors congenital MG.
- MG may be unmasked during recovery from general anesthetic or intercurrent infection. A patient with MS with apparent relapse may have developed MG.
- A mother with MG or just AchRA without MG features may deliver a baby with AMC. The baby might have both MG and AMC.

Red Flags for Myasthenia Gravis

- Blepharospasm; this can be mistaken for ocular myasthenia.
- Apraxia of eyelid opening can mimic ocular myasthenia.
- Involvement of pupillary reflexes excludes classic MG and most myopathies. Congenital MG or LEMS is more likely.
- Weakness and fatigue that worsen in hot weather may lead to misdiagnosis of MS. Excessive facial fasciculation in MG
- Apparent relapse of MG rarely may be due to cholinergic block.
- The patient with rheumatoid arthritis who complains of fatigue may have MG induced by penicillamine.
- Be alert for MG in patients who have received aminoglycoside antibiotics.

- Fluctuating lower cranial nerve weakness could be tetanus. Examine mouth opening and do spatula test.
- Negative acetylcholine receptor antibodies with weakness aggravated by pyridostigmine: slow channel syndrome, acetylcholinesterase deficiency, DOK7 variant, COLQ-mutant myasthenic syndrome, myotubular myopathy
- Subacute paralysis of all limbs and eye movements may be due to botulism.

Other Clues for Congenital Myasthenia Gravis

- Weakness of the thumb, neck extensors, and ankle dorsiflexors: slow channel variant of congenital MG It is autosomal dominant; all others are recessive.
- Stridor, tongue wasting, and worsening by pyridostigmine: *DOK7* mutation; some respond to ephedrine or salbutamol.
- Ptosis with sparing of extraocular muscles if the defect is presynaptic (due to choline acetyltransferase deficiency)

Lambert-Eaton Myasthenic Syndrome

- Dry mouth, proximal weakness, and muscle fatigue on walking
- Resembles a myopathy but the CK is normal
- Autonomic features. FATIGUING proximal weakness with (usually) sparing of the extraocular muscles favors LEMS or congenital MG.
- Tingling in the face and extremities may lead to misdiagnosis of panic disorder.

Examination

- Reduced tendon reflexes. Increasing grip strength on prolonged maximal hand gripping
- Enhanced tendon reflex after contraction suggests LEMS. Reduction of reflexes favors MG.
- Incrementing CMAP response to repetitive electrical muscle stimulation; combination of low-amplitude CMAPs on nerve conduction tests with a normal CK supports LEMS.

Inflammatory Myopathies
Chronic Polymyositis

- Slowly progressive symmetric weakness of proximal muscles, trunk, and occasionally

bulbar muscles. Neck flexion always weak in established phase
- Sparing of the extraocular muscles
- Preserved quadriceps power
- Recurrent polymyositis may simulate steroid-induced myopathy.

Red Flags
- Strong neck muscles or weak quadriceps

Inclusion Body Myositis
- Gradually progressive, sometimes familial myopathy in patient older than 50 years
- Selective involvement of the thigh and forearm finger flexor muscles
- Continuously extended great toe (pseudo-Babinski sign)
- Unexplained falls due to quadriceps weakness
- Unexplained dysphagia may predate limb weakness.
- If the EMG request form reads "possible myopathy" but the test shows features of neuropathy and myopathy, then IBM is likely.

Dysthyroid Myopathies
Myxedematous
- Slow relaxing ankle jerks; high CK; weak neck muscles; myoedema
- Hoffman syndrome, Kocher Debre Semelaigne syndrome

Thyrotoxic
- Mild proximal weakness, breathlessness, fasciculation, atrial fibrillation
- Heat intolerance, normal or slightly raised CK; ophthalmopathy is infrequent.
- Association with hypokalemic periodic paralysis and MG
o Exophthalmos with ptosis is a major Red Flag.

Periodic Paralysis
- *Hyperkalemic*: episodes of generalized daytime weakness provoked by resting after exercise or food high in potassium. May be myotonia. During the attack, the serum potassium rises and the EKG T waves become tall.
- *Hypokalemic*: episodes of generalized weakness, starting in sleep, especially after a day of exercise or a large meal; indistinguishable from thyrotoxic periodic paralysis.

- In attacks of either variety, face and breathing muscles are spared. Tendon reflexes are depressed.
- Periodic paralysis with dysmorphic features and ventricular arrhythmias suggests Andersen-Tawil syndrome.
- Eyes that stick shut after sneezing is likely *paramyotonia*.

McArdle's Syndrome
- Calf pain on exercise that the patient can walk through (second wind)
- Inability to run more than 100 yards or perform squats but able to walk at a slow pace
- Misdiagnosis of growing pains in children; muscle pain may be evoked by anger or sex.
- Myoglobinuria; later risk of obesity, ischemic heart disease, and gout

Red Flags
o Calf or thigh pain on exercise may simulate claudication. A normal CK excludes McArdle's syndrome.
o McArdle's syndrome mimics paramyotonia congenita and Becker dystrophy.

Mitochondrial Myopathies
- Long-standing nonfatiguing ptosis with external ophthalmoplegia
- Diplopia is a Red Flag.
- Fatiguing external eye muscles and diplopia suggest ocular MG.
- CPEO with difficulty swallowing favors oculopharyngeal myopathy.
- Kearns-Sayre syndrome, MELAS, MNGIE syndrome

Disorders Mistaken for Mitochondrial Myopathies
- Oculopharyngeal muscular dystrophy, MG, thyrotoxic ophthalmopathy

Distal Myopathies

- Learn Table 7.3.

Medication-Induced Myopathies
- Aggressive proximal myopathy with extremely high CK in a patient taking a statin is

likely necrotizing myositis due to HMG-CoA reductase antibodies.

- Acute myopathy complicated by delirium tremens, seizures, and numerous metabolic problems: alcohol-related
- In a drug addict: exposure to cocaine, heroin, or mushrooms
- If the patient has gout or cancer: colchicine or vincristine. Check for peripheral neuropathy.
- If patient has AIDS: zidovudine
- In a patient with rheumatoid arthritis: penicillamine or glucocorticoids. If steroid-induced, EMG shows no fibrillations and CK is normal; type II fiber atrophy on biopsy
- In a psychiatric patient: phenothiazine-related dystonia, serotonin syndrome, and neuroleptic malignant syndrome
- Marked rigidity, hyperpyrexia, and dysautonomia after general anesthetic is malignant hyperthermia.

Myopathy with Deafness
- Ehlers-Danlos syndrome. Mitochondrial disorders: Kearns-Sayre syndrome, atypical MELAS. Myopathy, deafness, and seizures due to mutation in *tRNA-Ser* gene. Congenital myopathy with diarrhea, zinc deficiency, and deafness is the Levy-Yeboa syndrome.

Other Myopathy Handles
- Plantar flexion weaker than dorsiflexion: dysferlin (Miyoshi) myopathy or distal hereditary motor neuropathy; knee bopping sign
- Slowly progressive proximal weakness with difficulty breathing but not swallowing suggests adult-onset acid maltase deficiency.
- Proximal myopathy with congenital pinpoint pupils is Stormorken syndrome.
- Exercise-induced deafness suggests a mitochondrial disorder.

Motor Neuron Disorders
Amyotrophic Lateral Sclerosis
- Asymmetric weakness/wasting, fasciculation, and cramp in unusual sites

- Isolated dysarthria and/or dysphagia; split hand sign; weak, wasted hand with brisk arm reflexes
- Brisk leg reflexes, occasionally with downgoing plantars and preserved abdominal reflexes; painless neck weakness
- Dropped finger sign. Also seen in cervical radiculopathy, syringomyelia, neuralgic amyotrophy, IBM, motor variant of CIDP, Laing distal muscular dystrophy, multifocal motor neuropathy with conduction block

Unusual Presentations of ALS
- Unilateral painless foot drop, hemiparesis, camptocormia, respiratory failure
- Pure spastic paraparesis with gradual progression: primary lateral sclerosis

Note: Bladder involvement is common in primary lateral sclerosis (PLS) but very rare in classic ALS.

ALS Mimics
- FASIC syndrome, syringomyelia, cervical spondylotic myeloradiculopathy
- Cramp fasciculation syndrome, generalized myokymia, cramp, and hyperhidrosis: Isaac's syndrome.
- Man-in-a-barrel syndrome: also seen in bilateral border zone infarcts of the frontoparietal cortex, posttraumatic cervical myelopathy, severe neuropathies (e.g., Guillain-Barré syndrome), radiculopathies and bilateral brachial plexus lesions, anterior spinal artery thrombosis, posttraumatic cervical myelopathy, severe neuropathies (e.g., Guillain-Barre syndrome)
- Facial onset sensory impairment that spreads to arms and upper trunk with bulbar and upper limb lower motor neurone signs: FOSMN
- Young male with gradually progressive lower motor neuron weakness affecting just one arm: Hirayama disease

MRI Signs
- Snake-eye sign in spinal cord, bright tongue sign on sagittal MRI brain, wineglass sign in the pyramidal tracts

Red Flags for ALS

- Lack of progression or lack of upper motor neuron signs. Unilateral rupture of the long head of biceps may simulate monomelic motor neuron disease.
- Significant sensory loss, diplopia, or cerebellar ataxia. Behavioral manifestations, dementia, or parkinsonian features.
- Pressure sores, early bladder problems, absent reflexes in the upper limbs

Bulbar Palsies
In ALS

- Progressive dysarthria, dysphagia, and dysphonia with fasciculating tongue: progressive bulbar palsy
- Progressive dysarthria, dysphagia, and dysphonia with no tongue fasciculation, brisk jaw jerk, and emotional lability: pseudobulbar palsy
- Most bulbar palsies in ALS are a mixture of the two varieties.

Other Bulbar Palsies

- Slowly progressive bulbar palsy in adult male with arm tremor and chin fasciculation suggests Kennedy syndrome. Other features: small testes, gynecomastia, depressed deep tendon reflexes, and downgoing plantar responses
- Bulbar palsy, motor neuropathy, and cerebellar ataxia in a teenager or young adult favors hexosaminidase A deficiency. Visual evoked potentials are delayed.
- Progressive bulbar palsy and sensorineural deafness: VL syndrome; Fazio-Londe syndrome is probably the same disorder as VL. Childhood onset; raised pyridoxine level; responds to riboflavin. Madras motor neuron disease: young adult onset with optic atrophy

Hereditary Spastic Paraplegia (HSP; Classic Form)

- Young adult: slowly progressive stiff-legged gait; little weakness and no sensory signs, easily obtained Babinski responses
- Upper limb tone, reflexes, and bladder are little affected and the cranial nerves not at all.

- Sometimes cognitive decline and hand tremor but no sensory involvement
- Patients often continue working until normal retirement age.
- MRI: atrophy of the corpus callosum

Mimics

- Gait of HSP similar to dopa-responsive dystonia but there is diurnal variability with more symptoms in the afternoon.
- Congenital diplegia and congenital spastic paraplegia, but neither progress

Rare recessive forms of SPG:

- Progressive spastic paraplegia, small hyperpigmented macular lesions: Kjellin syndrome (SPG15)
- Progressive spastic paraplegia with bristle hair and exotropia: SPG 35 (FAHN)

HSP Dominant Variants

- Learn Table 7.4.

SUGGESTED READING

Bandini F. Pseudo plus-minus lid syndrome. *Arch Neurol.* 2009;66:668–669.

Broad R, Leigh PN. Recognising facial onset sensory motor neuronopathy syndrome: insight from six new cases. *Pract Neurol.* 2015;15(4):293–297.

Eisen A, Kuwabara S. The split hand syndrome in amyotrophic lateral sclerosis. *J Neurol Neurosurg Psychiatry.* 2012;83:399–403.

Faber I, Servelhere KR, Martinez AR, Dabreu A, Lopes-Cendes I, Franca MC Jr. Clinical features and management of hereditary spastic paraplegia. *Arq Neuropsiquiatr.* 2014;72:219–226.

Flanagan EP, McKeon A, Weinshenker BG. Anterior spinal artery infarction causing man-in-the-barrel syndrome. *Neurol Clin Pract.* 2014;4(3):268–269.

Flanigan KM, Kerr L, Bromberg MB, et al. Congenital muscular dystrophy with rigid spine syndrome: a clinical, pathological, radiological, and genetic study. *Ann Neurol.* 2000;47(2):152–161.

Fox MD, Cohen AB. "Bright tongue sign" in ALS. *Neurology.* 2012;79:1520.

Garcia-Touchard A, Somers VK, Kara T, et al. Ventricular ectopy during REM sleep: implications for nocturnal sudden cardiac death. *Nat Clin Pract Cardiovasc Med.* 2007;4:284–288.

Ghosh PS, Milone M. Clinical reasoning: a 38-year-old woman with childhood-onset weakness. *Neurology.* 2014;83:e81–e84.

Gibson DA, Urs NDK. Arthrogryposis multiplex congenita. *J Bone Joint Surg.* 1970;52:483–493.

Ho NC, Sandusky S, Madike V, Francomano CA, Dalakas MC. Clinico-pathogenetic findings and management of chondrodystrophic myotonia (Schwartz-Jampel syndrome): a case report. *BMC Neurol.* 2003;3:3.

Katz JS, Wolfe GI, Andersson PB, et al. Brachial amyotrophic diplegia: a slowly progressive motor neuron disorder. *Neurology.* 1999;53:1071–1076.

Lamont PJ, Udd B, Mastaglia FL, et al. Laing early onset distal myopathy: slow myosin defect with variable abnormalities on muscle biopsy. *J Neurol Neurosurg Psychiatry.* 2006;77:208–215.

Muelas N, Hackman P, Luque H, et al. *MYH7* gene tail mutation causing myopathic profiles beyond Laing distal myopathy. *Neurology.* 2010;75:732–741.

Nowak VA, Bremner F, Massey L, et al. Kjellin syndrome: hereditary spastic paraplegia with pathognomonic macular appearance. *Pract Neurol.* 2014;14:278–279.

Pradhan S. Poly-Hill sign in facioscapulohumeral dystrophy. *Muscle Nerve.* 2002;25:754–755.

Pradhan S. Valley sign in Becker muscular dystrophy and outliers of Duchenne and Becker muscular dystrophy. *Neurol India.* 2004;52:203–205.

Pradhan S. Shank sign in myotonic dystrophy type-1 (DM-1). *J Clin Neurosci.* 2007;14:27–32.

Pradhan S, Yadav R, Mishra VN, Aurangabadkar K, Sawlani V. Amyotrophic lateral sclerosis with predominant pyramidal signs—early diagnosis by magnetic resonance imaging. *Magn Reson Imaging.* 2006;24:173–179.

Pradhan S. Diamond on quadriceps: A frequent sign in dysferlinopathy. *Neurology.* ;70(4):322-.

Rattay TW, Söhn AS, Karle KN, et al. Bristle hair may point to hereditary spastic paraplegia type Spg35/Fahn: 696. *Mov Disord.* 2016;31:S227.

Rossor AM, Murphy S, Reilly MM. Knee bobbing in Charcot-Marie-Tooth disease. *Pract Neurol.* 2012;12:182–183.

Selcen D, Milone M, Shen XM, et al. Dok-7 myasthenia: phenotypic and molecular genetic studies in 16 patients. *Ann Neurol.* 2008;64:71–87.

Shahrizaila N, Wills AJ. Significance of Beevor's sign in facioscapulohumeral dystrophy and other neuromuscular diseases. *J Neurol Neurosurg Psychiatry.* 2005;76:869–870.

Sharma S, Murgai A, Nair PP, Ramesh A. Teaching neuroimages: snake eyes appearance in MRI in patient with ALS. *Neurology.* 2013;81:e29.

Tsivgoulis G, Vadikolias K, Courcoutsakis N, Heliopoulos I, Stamboulis E, Piperidou C. Teaching neuroimages: differential diagnosis of scapular winging. *Neurology.* 2012;78:e109.

Turner MR, Talbot K. Mimics and chameleons in motor neurone disease. *Pract Neurol* 2013;13:153–164.

Udd B. Distal myopathies—new genetic entities expand diagnostic challenge. *Neuromuscul Disord* 2012;22:5–12.

Varkey B, Varkey L. Muscle hypertrophy in myotonia congenita. *J Neurol Neurosurg Psychiatry.* 2003;74:338.

Venance SL, Cannon SC, Fialho D, et al. The primary periodic paralyses: diagnosis, pathogenesis and treatment. *Brain.* 2006;129:8–17.

Wicklund MP. The muscular dystrophies. *Continuum (Minneap Minn).* 2013;19:1535–1570.

Yoon G, Quitania L, Kramer JH, Fu YH, Miller BL, Ptacek LJ. Andersen-Tawil syndrome: definition of a neurocognitive phenotype. *Neurology.* 2006;66:1703–1710.

Chapter 8: Movement Disorders

There are probably more Handles and Red Flags in the domain of movement disorders than any other branch of neurology. Many have not been verified by rigorous clinical studies, systematic imaging, or pathological confirmation, thus particular care is needed.

PARKINSON'S DISEASE

The experienced neurologist is able to identify the characteristic slowing of bodily movement within seconds. When a patient walks into the office displaying reduction of arm swing, *en bloc* movements, lack of facial expression, decreased blink rate, seborrhea, and slightly stooped posture, the neurologist makes a diagnosis of parkinsonism with ease (Figure 8.1). In early Parkinson's disease (PD) the signs can be subtle and may be missed unless looked for carefully. There are, of course, several causes of parkinsonism apart from classic PD. What follows is a description of Handles and Flags that suggest parkinsonism. The exact variety of disease usually requires more thought; we offer help in that direction as well.

Handles and Red Flags in the History
Prodromal/Early Features

Most patients with classic PD describe a variety of non-motor symptoms before onset of the classic symptoms: namely, tremor, rigidity, and akinesia. These include impaired sense of smell, rapid eye movement (REM) sleep behavior disorder (RBD), constipation, weight gain, and depression.

▶ *Impaired sense of smell* is a very common prodromal sign of PD

At least 80% patients with classic PD will have some impairment and, of these, half are anosmic; the rest are microsomic. Information is rarely volunteered, but when the patient is asked about it, the complaint may go back several years before the onset of classic symptoms. Only 40% patients with smell impairment are aware of it, so testing is mandatory using commercially available identification tests. Smell impairment occurs with normal aging and is not *specific* for PD

but it is *characteristic.* Less severe impairment is found in multiple system atrophy (MSA), but there is little impairment in progressive supranuclear palsy (PSP), corticobasal syndrome (CBS), and none in essential tremor. These differences can aid diagnosis

▶ *RBD suggests a synucleinopathy such as MSA, dementia with Lewy bodies (DLB), or classic PD*

During REM sleep (typically 4 A.M.), patients seem awake, but the eyes are closed, and they appear to act out their dreams, which are often violent (Video 6. 18, RBD). The individual usually stays in bed, unlike sleep walkers, who get up and experience their attack in non-REM sleep.

During Established Disease Phase

▶ *Repeated stopping of a self-winding watch*
Some watches depend on arm movement to keep the mainspring wound or battery charged. With little or no arm movement, the watch stops. This sign is sometimes called "Marsden's sign," after the late David Marsden.

▶ *Carpal tunnel syndrome followed by tremor or stiffness*
Here the process is somewhat similar to the Marsden sign. The reduced mobility of one arm leads to wrist edema, which tends to unmask a borderline carpal tunnel syndrome. The underlying problem of PD may come to light only after surgery to release the median nerve.

▶ *Deterioration of handwriting*
Only the more astute patient notices this, as it is such a gradual process. Over several years, the handwriting becomes smaller and less legible (Figure 8.2 and Video 8.1, Micrographia). It tends to be increasingly sloped (either up or down) toward the right side of the page in a right-handed person. Adolf Hitler probably had PD; knowledge of time-related change in handwriting was used by

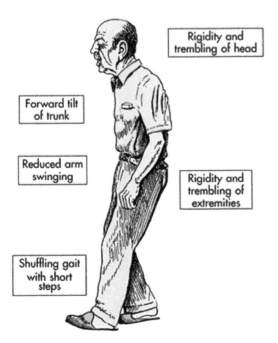

Rigidity and trembling of head

Forward tilt of trunk

Reduced arm swinging

Rigidity and trembling of extremities

Shuffling gait with short steps

FIGURE 8.1: The major features of Parkinson's disease. Reproduced from http://healthmeup.com/news-healthy-living/mental-health-what-is-parkinsons-disease/21495.

graphologists to determine (correctly) that some diaries attributed to Hitler were fake (see video link: www.youtube.com/watch?v=0w3nsAaOpq4).

▶ *Difficulty swimming in a straight line*
The asymmetric bradykinesia and muscle rigidity (which is characteristic) occasionally makes it difficult for the patient to swim in a straight line. Not many swimmers with PD make a complete circle, as there is rarely enough space in a pool, but swimming in designated lanes may cause a problem.

▶ *Unexplained frozen shoulder or back pain*
Watch for the patient who presents with a frozen shoulder, especially when there is no obvious reason for this, such as a prior fall or injury. The shoulder joint is one of the most common regions to be affected in PD, and motor symptoms may be inconspicuous. It is the bradykinesia and muscle rigidity that promote the shoulder joint problem. Cervical spondylosis often coexists, and the nuchal rigidity of PD will aggravate this. The same principle applies

to *low back pain*, which in retrospect may turn out to be the first symptom of PD.

• Watch out for *polymyalgia rheumatica*. It causes pain and stiffness in the shoulder and/or pelvic girdles, and may simulate parkinsonism.

▶ *Inability to talk and walk heralds the onset of falls.*
The likely reason is that during walking, the patient has to focus all attention on their gait. Talking, including cell phone use, likely diverts attention away from walking and increases the liability to fall.

▶ *Chest or abdominal pain that mystifies the cardiologist and gastroenterologist is likely an "off" phenomenon or intercostal muscle dystonia.*
This situation happens in patients receiving levodopa for PD. The pain may improve with levodopa treatment and is likely an "off" phenomenon (like breathlessness; see later discussion).

▶ *Difficulty walking but not cycling is characteristic of PD.*
The reason for this is poorly understood, but, in the basal ganglia, cycling suppresses the beta activity that is thought to be responsible for gait freezing. Patients who can hardly walk may be able to run, ride a bicycle, or roller-skate (see Video 8.2, PD Cycling).

▶ *Paradoxical kinesis*
This refers to the chair-bound patient with PD who suddenly gets up and bolts out of a room when exposed to a threatening stimulus (e.g., fire, thunderstorm, child in distress). It suggests that the motor circuits are intact and that strong emotional influence can override, at least transiently, a "brake" on the motor system.

▶ *Walking backward easier than forward*
This happens in:
  ○ Truncal or lower limb dystonia (Video 8.3, Tardive Dystonia)
  ○ Dopa-responsive dystonia (DRD; see earlier discussion)
  ○ Hysteria. See video link (note that there are two reports, the second of which shows recovery: www.youtube.com/watch?v=cnsNgOuTazM).
  ○ Patients with PD or spastic paraplegia
In the presence of rigidity or spasticity, there is often difficulty dorsiflexing the ankle

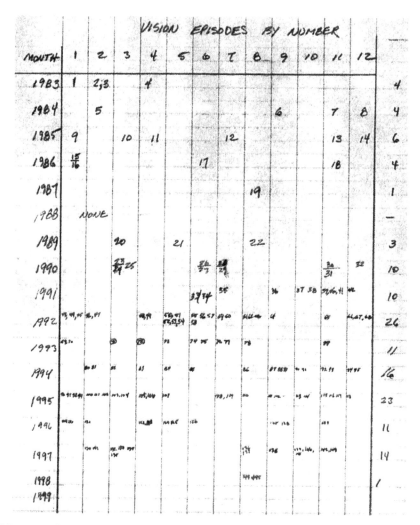

FIGURE 8.2: Patient diary recording the number of migrainous visual episodes experienced over a 15-year period. Between 1991 and 1993, the handwriting becomes progressively smaller. Note that an association between migraine and Parkinson's disease has been described recently. Reproduced from Counihan & Barbano (2000).

when walking forward. Upon walking backward, the toe of the foot may be dragged, and some individuals find walking easier in this manner.

▶ *Levodopa-induced dyskinesias suggests classic PD.*
This is a good indicator of presynaptic dopamine deficiency (Video 8.4, Levodopa Dyskinesia), although it may occur in other types of parkinsonism, notably MSA (facial dystonia; see Video 8.5, MSA Dystonia).

Red Flags in the History

◀ *Early severe orthostatic drop in blood pressure with severe constipation suggests MSA.*

◀ *Early cognitive impairment, hallucinations in the absence of medications, and medication sensitivity (due neuropsychiatric side effects) favors DLB.* Some believe there is a person nearby and keep looking over their shoulder—so-called *extracampine hallucinations.*

◀ *Falls in early stage of disease* Falling *early* in the course of parkinsonism is a Red Flag and suggests a diagnosis other than classic PD, such as PSP and MSA. In the *established* phase of PD, righting reflexes are significantly impaired, and falling automatically places the patient in Hoehn and Yahr stage 3/5.

◀ Marked asymmetry and cortical findings such as apraxia or cortical sensory loss favors CBS.

◀ Supranuclear gaze palsy (SNGP; especially downward) points to progressive supranuclear palsy

◀ *Breathlessness from classic PD is unusual.*

The main explanations are as follows:

- "Off-stage" difficulty breathing is related to tightness of the chest wall muscles or anxiety.
- Conversely, levodopa-induced dyskinesia may lead to irregular breathing.
- If the patient is on an ergot-containing dopamine agonist (cabergoline or pergolide but not lisuride), there is a small risk of breathlessness because of cardiac valve fibrosis, heart failure, and pulmonary fibrosis. In most countries, these drugs have been withdrawn from the market, so this is rare.
- Irregular breathing and stridor (often nocturnal) are important features of MSA (Video 8.6, Stridor).

Note: hypoventilation is a feature of Perry syndrome (early-onset parkinsonism and depression).

◀ PD and seizures may co-exist slightly more frequently than chance alone, but, in general, it is a major Red Flag for classic PD. Apart from structural lesions and rapidly progressive conditions such as Creutzfeldt-Jacob disease, you should consider:
  - Frontotemporal dementia
  - Adult-onset Gaucher's disease
  - Hypoparathyroidism with or without cerebral calcifications. See Video 8.7, Hypoparathyroid (courtesy L. Prashanth). This patient did not benefit from levodopa but made a good response to vitamin D and calcium supplements.
  - *POLG* mutations
  - Niemann Pick disease type C
◀ *Child or young adult with parkinsonism and oculogyric crises (OGC) will not have classic PD.* The likely causes are:
  - Reaction to medication—typically phenothiazine and other neuroleptics (Video 8.8, OGC).
  - Postencephalitic parkinsonism. This used to be the main cause of OGC but now it is rare.

Note:

- Patients with Tourette syndrome jerk the eyes in one direction briefly, but this is not a true OGC, where the ocular deviation is more sustained.

Related are the following:

◀ *A child or young adult with OGC and fluctuating dystonia or, rarely, parkinsonism, likely has* DRD, Segawa disease, DYT5. The underlying defect is in GTP cyclohydrolase 1.

Other features are as follows:

- Symptoms worsen later in the day.
- Dystonic features with a tendency to invert the feet or scuff the toes, sometimes mislabeled club foot. May be improved by walking backward.
- Misdiagnosis for cerebral palsy, infantile hemiplegia, or hereditary spastic paraplegia
- These patients may initially present with paroxysmal exertional dyskinesia (see later discussion).

Rarer causes of fluctuating dystonia with OGC are the following:

- Tyrosine hydroxylase deficiency
- Sepiapterin reductase deficiency; see Video 8.9, Sepi (courtesy Dr. G. M. Wali). Note: excess sleepiness is a feature of this disorder.
- Aromatic l-amino decarboxylase deficiency (AADC). Such patients may have paroxysms of worsening, and some develop prominent autonomic disturbances; see Video 8.10, AADC (courtesy Dr. K. Bhatia).
- Dopamine transporter deficiency syndrome
- Kufor-Rakeb disease. There is parkinsonism, SNGP, and OGC but no fluctuation of the movement disorder.

Handles and Red Flags on Examination

▶ *Re-emergent tremor on maintaining arms outstretched is characteristic of PD.* The tremor of PD is seen predominantly at rest and is lessened by voluntary movement. Patients soon discover this.

- If the tremor becomes embarrassing, they grip a nearby object (furniture or their walking cane) to damp it down.
- It is not uncommon for patients to report tremor while holding a newspaper or tray. This is not always ET but could be the re-emergent tremor of PD. On formal examination, it is sometimes recorded (incorrectly) that tremor is absent with the arms outstretched, often because of a rushed assessment. If the arms are held out for, say, 15 seconds, the tremor sometimes reappears—hence the name "re-emergent tremor," a useful confirmatory Handle for PD (Video 8.11, Re-emergent Tremor).

▶ In severe ET, rest tremor may be witnessed, but:
  - It persists and is usually worse during movement.
  - There is no latent period between assuming a new posture and the emergence of tremor.

It is good practice to observe the patient walking, as this activity often brings out rest tremor and, indeed, other involuntary movement, such as chorea or dystonia (Video 8.12, Walking).

▶ *Fatigue on repeated movement is typical of classic PD.*
  This phenomenon is tested by asking the patient to oppose the thumb and index finger repeatedly. The patient should be encouraged to make *large and fast movements*, otherwise the uninitiated clinician may be misled by rapid movements of small amplitude. A healthy person can perform this 10 times easily. In PD, the speed of finger movement slows, there are arrests of ongoing movements on one or both sides, and the magnitude of excursion diminishes (Video 8.13, Bradykinesia). In asymmetric parkinsonism, it is important to test one hand at a time to avoid synchronization (entrainment) of the affected hand by the normal hand.

▶ rapid small-excursion opposition of thumb and index finger *without* fatigue suggests PSP.
▶ *Mirror movements are frequent in PD.*
  They are usually overlooked. They may be elicited when performing repetitive movement of one hand, such as touching the tips of each finger in sequence. Provided the other hand is at rest, it may copy involuntarily the movement of the other hand.
  Mirror movements are also associated with:
    ○ Kallman's syndrome
    ○ Klippel-Feil anomaly (Video 8.14, Mirror Klippel-Feil).

Red Flags on Examination

◀ *Early camptocormia.* If camptocormia develops *early* in suspected classic disease, the diagnosis is wrong, but it is seen in advanced PD. Consider MSA (Video 8.15, Camptocormia Pisa MSA). Literally, *camptocormia* means "bent trunk." True camptocormia is shown in Figure 8.3. Usually, it is relieved by lying down and has to be distinguished from fixed kyphosis due to spinal abnormalities such as ankylosing spondylitis.
  Camptocormia occurs in the following:
    - Parkinsonism (e.g., MSA)
    - "Off"-period phenomenon in PD (Video 8.16, Camptocormia Off-State)
    - End-stage classic PD
    - Myopathies (e.g., facioscapulohumeral muscular dystrophy, idiopathic axial myopathy)
    - Axial dystonia
    - Psychogenic disorder
    - Drug reactions
◀ Strictly unilateral rest tremor that remains unilateral for more than 3 years is atypical and raises the question of a structural cause or CBS.
◀ Pisa syndrome (pleurothotonus) is a type of dystonia that results in sustained lateral flexion of the trunk. It is associated with the following:
    ○ Multiple system atrophy
    ○ After antipsychotic drug treatment, both typical and atypical antipsychotic agents.
    ○ It can be a manifestation of acute or tardive dystonia (Video 8.17, Pisa sign, and Video 8.18, Tardive Dystonia Pisa).
    ○ In Alzheimer's disease, patients receiving the anticholinesterase, donepezil (Aricept)

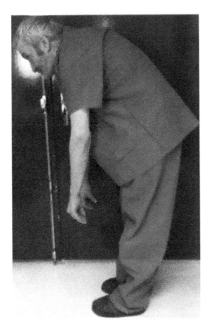

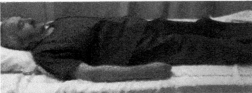

FIGURE 8.3: Camptocormia. In true camptocormia the bent spine can be straightened by lying flat, unlike that of fixed kyphosis which cannot. Reproduced with permission from Lenoir et al. (2010), Figure 1.

- o Neurodegeneration with brain iron accumulation (NBIA; see later in this chapter).
- o Brown-Sequard syndrome (rare) (Video 8.19, Brown-Sequard Pisa)
- o Spinal cord infection (rare)

Therefore:

◀ Reconsider the diagnosis of classic PD if there is sustained lateral flexion of the trunk suggesting Pisa syndrome *early* in the disease course.

◀ *A patient with head tremor probably does not have classic PD.* This is likely ET. Note that isolated head tremor in the absence of hand tremor favors tremulous cervical dystonia (Video 8.20, Cervical Dystonia).

◀ *Irregular rest tremor associated with an extended thumb.* This suggests that the tremor is dystonic and not due to classic PD, where the

tremor has a "pill-rolling" characteristic. If a dopamine transporter scan is undertaken, it is usually normal, hence the name SWEDD—scans without evidence of dopaminergic deficit. Individuals who have an unusual rest tremor with SWEDD are a heterogeneous group and may have dystonic, psychogenic, or ET, or perhaps a disorder that awaits full characterization (Video 8.21, Dystonic Tremor).

◀ *A patient with alleged PD who is chair-bound within 5 years of onset does not have classic PD.* There is no such thing as "malignant" classic PD as it never progresses so fast. You should think instead of PSP, MSA, and frontotemporal dementia.

◀ *Disproportionate anterocollis within 5 years of symptom onset.* The chin rests on the chest but there is no trunk flexion, as in camptocormia. It may be an "off" phenomenon in classic PD (Video 8.22, Anterocollis Off-On), but in most cases this is not PD. Instead consider:
- o Side effect of dopamine agonists. It reverses on their withdrawal
- o MSA
- o Dropped head syndrome due to neuromuscular disease, for example, polymyositis, amyotrophic lateral sclerosis (ALS), myasthenia, dystrophia myotonica (DM1). See Chapter 7 and Figure 8.4.

▶ Note that in all these alternatives, the neck is not stiff, but it is in MSA and especially in PSP.

◀ *Apparent PD with symmetric rigidity but no tremor.* In classic PD, there is usually some degree of limb muscle asymmetry right until the terminal phase of illness. In symmetric disease, think of PSP, MSA, or fronto-temporal lobar degeneration.

◀ *Lower body parkinsonism.* In this variety, the patient walks with a shuffling, hesitant gait but there is little to find wrong above the waist. There is often difficulty setting off from the standing position—so-called *gait ignition failure.* Such patients are usually elderly arteriopaths with multiple ischemic lesions affecting, in particular, the deep white matter and basal ganglia (Figure 8.5 and Video 8.23, Lower Body PD).

◀ *Early gait freezing.* In early classic PD, the gait disturbance is mild with just slight reduction of arm swing on one side and no gait hesitancy. Gradually, this progresses to gait

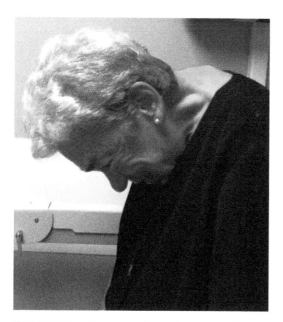

FIGURE 8.4: Dropped head in parkinsonism. If this sign appears within the first 5 years of suspected classic Parkinson's disease, then the diagnosis is wrong. You should consider variants such as multiple system atrophy (MSA). A similar posture occurs in muscular disease such as polymyositis, myasthenia gravis, axial myopathy, and amyotrophic lateral sclerosis.

freezing that can be disabling, particularly when passing through a doorway or crossing a road (Video 8.24, PD Gait, and Video 8.25, Gait Freezing). Early gait freezing is a Red Flag for classic PD. Think of PSP.

◀ *Apparent classic PD with normal sense of smell.* At least 80% of PD patients have some degree of smell-sense impairment. If olfaction is normal *on testing*, then consider:
  ○ Essential tremor
  ○ Vascular parkinsonism
  ○ Corticobasal syndrome
  ○ Progressive supranuclear palsy
  ○ MSA (some patients)
◀ *Parkinsonism in a <u>current</u> smoker is unlikely to be classic PD.* In a smoker, the ease of quitting smoking correlates with the onset of PD. Most patients with classic PD are lifelong nonsmokers. Instead, consider vascular PD, MSA, or PSP.
◀ *Parkinsonism with cataracts.* This rare combination should make you think of the following:
  ○ Hypoparathyroidism and pseudohypoparathyroidism
  ○ Fahr's syndrome
  ○ Galactosemia; adults may develop tremor, dystonia, and parkinsonism (Rubio-Agusti et al. 2013).
  ○ Mitochondrial disorders, including *POLG* mutations
  ○ Wilson's disease (sunflower cataract); see Figure 2.36.
  ○ Cerebrotendinous xanthomatosis (CTX). The best Handle for CTX is inspection of the Achilles or other tendons—knee or hands. There should be visible or palpable lumps on them (Figure 8.6, *left*). MRI of

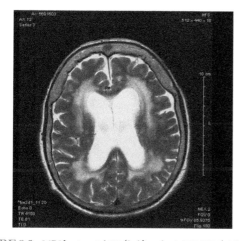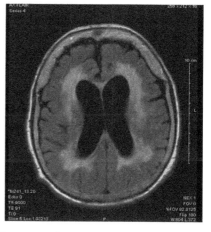

FIGURE 8.5: MRI brain axial T2 (**left**) and axial FLAIR (**right**) sequences depicting extensive periventricular white matter changes and central atrophy in vascular parkinsonism.

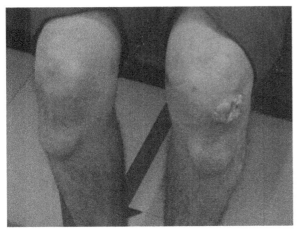 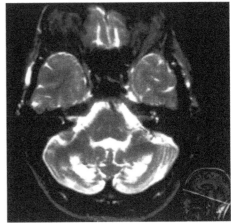

FIGURE 8.6: **Left**: Multiple xanthomas on the patella tendons. **Right**: T2-weighted brain axial MRI of a 39-year-old male with classic CTX showing symmetric lesions in the cerebellar white matter. Left image courtesy Dr. GM Wali. Right image reproduced with permission from Verrips et al. (1999).

the ankle may help with the diagnosis, and MRI of the brain shows increased signal in the dentate nuclei (Figure 8.6, *right*).

- o Patients with classic dystrophia myotonica (DM1) suffer premature cataract (Christmas tree pattern). Also, the face is often expressionless, which may lead to misdiagnosis of parkinsonism. Very rarely, levodopa-responsive parkinsonism or an MSA-like picture is associated with DM1.

◀ *Parkinsonism with progressive external ophthalmoplegia (PEO) is probably due to POLG or TWINKLE mutations.*

These are nuclear-derived genes important in mitochondrial DNA repair. Look for the following:

- Deafness
- Cerebellar signs
- Levodopa sensitivity with marked dyskinesia
- Marked sensory neuropathy
- Anosmia

Note that in some patients who express the *POLG* mutation there is

- Supranuclear gaze palsy instead of PEO, resulting in confusion with PSP
- Parkinsonism but no PEO; the presence of a sensory neuropathy may clinch the diagnosis of POLG mutation (Video 8.26, POLG).

◀ *Parkinsonian gait with dementia and incontinence suggests normal-pressure hydrocephalus (NPH).*

Not every patient has all three features, but certainly two of three would merit further investigation. The gait problem is really an apraxia rather than akinesia; the patient is unsure where to place the feet.

Note:

- In NPH, the third ventricle may be enlarged, but in cerebral atrophy from aging, the lower portion of the third ventricle is not dilated (Figure 8.7).
- The callosal angle is sharper in NPH but flatter in cerebral atrophy.
- *Adult polyglucosan body disease* may resemble NPH. Features include:
  - o Early severe urinary/bowel incontinence
  - o Parkinsonism
  - o Polyneuropathy
  - o Diagnosis is confirmed by sural nerve biopsy or gene testing.

◀ *Parkinsonism with patchy skin/iris depigmentation, susceptibility to infection, and giant white cell inclusions suggests Chediak-Higashi syndrome* (Figures 8.8 and 8.9).

Depigmentation of the iris and fundus with prolonged bleeding time are occasional features. Other neurological findings include dementia, peripheral neuropathy,

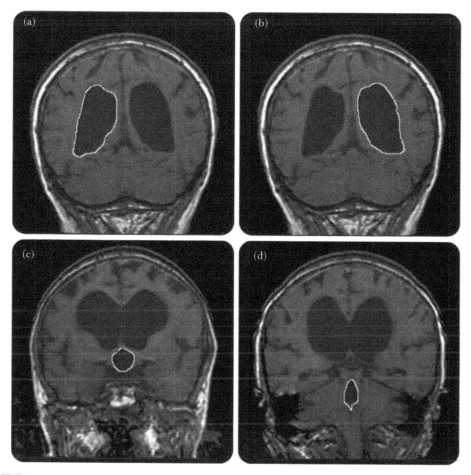

FIGURE 8.7: Normal-pressure hydrocephalus with areas of interest highlighted. Note the marked distension of the lateral ventricles with relatively little sulcal shrinkage. (**A**) Right lateral ventricle. (**B**) Left lateral ventricle. (**C**) Third ventricle. (**D**) Fourth ventricle. Reproduced with permission from Lenfeldt et al. (2012).

and cerebellar ataxia. See Video 8.27, Chediak-Higashi (courtesy Bettina Balint).

◀ *A Jewish patient with parkinsonism and pingueculae may have late-onset Gaucher's disease type 1* (Figure 8.10). Be aware that pingueculae develop with normal aging. Check for horizontal SNGP, enlargement of liver and spleen, and thrombocytopenia.

◀ *Parkinsonism and dystonia most frequently involving the jaw and the neck in a person of Filipino descent favors X-linked dystonia parkinsonism (DYT3; Lubag). It is seen occasionally in non-Filipinos.* See Video 8.28, Lubag (courtesy Alberto Espay).

◀ *Parkinsonism with orofacial dyskinesia in the absence of levodopa suggests parkinsonism induced by dopamine-blocking agents.*

◀ *Parkinsonism with a family history of dementia may be frontotemporal lobar degeneration (FTLD; a taupathy).*

◀ *Parkinsonism of rapid onset may be due to the following:*
  ○ Dopamine-blocking agents
  ○ Illicit drugs (MPTP, manganese, or methcathinone)
  ○ Prion disease
  ○ Central nervous system (CNS) lymphoma or CNS infections (bacterial, fungal, postencephalitic)
  ○ Rapid-onset dystonia parkinsonism (DYT12; see Table 8.2)
  ○ Vascular parkinsonism
  ○ Psychogenic parkinsonism (Video 8.25, Freezing).

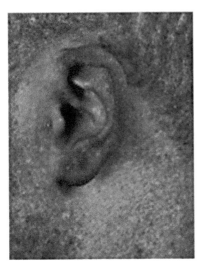 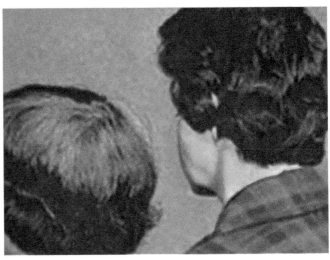

FIGURE 8.8: Chediak-Higashi syndrome. **Left**: African American patient with pigment dilution of the skin around the left ear. There may be iris or fundus depigmentation as well. **Right**: Note the silvery shine to the hair on the daughter's hair on the left. Left image reprinted from Bhambhani et al. (2013). Right image from *Genetic Skin Disorders*, 2nd ed., Disorders of the Dermis, by V Sybert. Oxford University Press. DOI: 10.1093/med/9780195397666.001.0001.

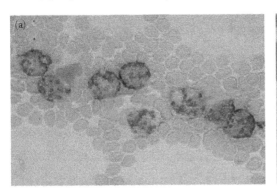 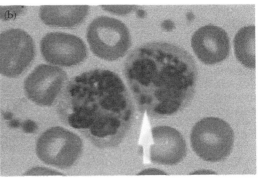

FIGURE 8.9: Chediak-Higashi syndrome. Light micrographs of leukocytes in peripheral blood smears. **Left**: Neutrophils containing numerous giant granules in the cytoplasm that stained markedly with peroxidase. **Right**: Higher magnification of the Leishman staining with arrow pointing to two giant granules in the cytoplasm of a neutrophil. Reproduced with permission from Silveira-Moriyama et al. (2004).

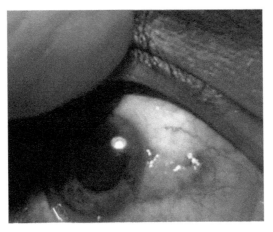

FIGURE 8.10: A pingueculum in the conjunctiva of a patient with type 1 Gaucher's disease. They start on the nasal side and may be multiple. Biopsy of this lipid deposit may clinch the diagnosis. Rarely, Gaucher's disease may present in adult life with parkinsonism. Reproduced with permission from eyerounds.org.

○ Subacute parkinsonism and cognitive difficulties may be due to dural arteriovenous fistula. Severe akinesia may occur. It is important to recognize this as it is treatable. See Video 8.29 Dural Fistula (courtesy of Pankaj Aggarwal).

◀ *Parkinsonism in a patient with HIV favors CNS opportunistic infection or HIV encephalopathy.*

◀ *Parkinsonism in a boxer or a retired athlete is likely chronic traumatic encephalopathy. The most famous example of this is the late world champion heavyweight boxer, Muhammad Ali.*

◀ *Parkinsonism with cleft lip and/or palate, conotruncal heart defects, ear anomalies, and characteristic facial features likely is DiGeorge syndrome (22q11.2 deletion syndrome, Figure 8.11)*

◀ *Unexplained worsening of tremor (rest and postural) in PD suggests onset of thyrotoxicosis.*

Other Mimics of Classic Parkinson's Disease

◀ Drug-induced parkinsonism (DIP): The clinical picture may be indistinguishable from PD. It can be caused by

· Most antipsychotics, typical and atypical apart from clozapine

· Dopamine depleters (reserpine, tetrabenazine)
· Antiemetics (metoclopramide, phenothiazines)
· Calcium channel blockers (flunarizine, cinnarizine)

If the parkinsonism does not resolve after 6 months of stopping medication, consider underlying PD. Here a DAT scan and smell testing are helpful.

▶ DAT scan and smell tests are both normal in drug-induced PD but both are abnormal in typical PD.

PROGRESSIVE SUPRANUCLEAR PALSY

PSP, also known as the Steele–Richardson syndrome, has the following features in the classic form (Richardson variant):

▶ *Supranuclear abnormalities of vertical gaze (usually downward) (Video 8.30, PSP Eye) with relatively rapid, progressive gait disorder, falls (typically backward), and difficulty looking downward*

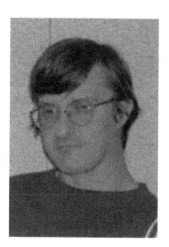 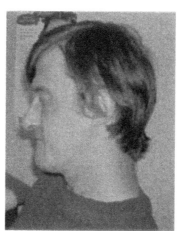 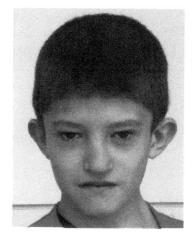

FIGURE 8.11: Di George syndrome. **Left and center**: 42-year-old male. Note the bulbous nasal tip, small ear with attached lobule, flat cheeks, and prognathism on the lateral view. Boy aged 11 years. Note short forehead, hooded eyelids, up-slanting palpebral fissures, flat cheeks, bulbous nasal tip with hypoplastic alae nasi, thin upper lip and protuberant ears. Left and center images reproduced with permission from Zaleski et al. (2009). Right image reproduced with permission from Bassett et al. (2011).

Additional features may include

- Cognitive decline and apathy
- Square-wave jerks; common but not specific.
- Progressive symmetric mainly axial rigidity with little or no tremor
- Poor response to levodopa with absence of levodopa-induced dyskinesia even at high dosage
- Photophobia; this is absent in corticobasal syndrome and may be helpful to distinguish the two conditions.

Apart from the typical variety as just discussed, many other phenotypes are documented with underlying PSP pathology. These include the following:

- PSP-parkinsonism (PSP-P). This is characterized by rest tremor, asymmetry, slower progression, and some response to levodopa, causing confusion with PD.
- Progressive nonfluent aphasia
- Pure akinesia
- Primary progressive gait freezing
- Corticobasal syndrome

Not surprisingly, autopsy studies show that diagnostic errors are common—in about 25% of cases.

To help diagnose classic PSP, you should pay particular attention to the face. This may reveal the following features:

▶ *Abnormal facial expression, deep naso-labial groove and the "procerus" sign.*
   As shown in Figure 8.12, the facial expression may be that of surprise, anxiety, or

mask-like. This is typical of PSP, probably because of facial dystonia. There is no such groove in classic PD.

The procerus sign refers to vertical wrinkles over the glabella that appear in normal people when angry. The procerus sign is a misnomer, as the vertical wrinkling is performed by the corrugator muscle, not procerus. Dystonia of the upper face often results in a startled expression. Patients have widened palpebral fissures and infrequent blinking ("reptilian stare"). This bears a superficial resemblance to thyrotoxicosis, but in Graves's ophthalmopathy there is proptosis and occasionally redness of the eyes.

Other Handles for PSP include the following:

▶ *Slow vertical saccades*
   In the early stages of PSP, before there is restriction of vertical eye movement, slow saccadic velocity may be observed, although the range of movement is normal. This is best demonstrated by using an optokinetic drum and rotating it upward. The normal corrective downward saccades may be absent and the eyes may drift upward.
▶ *Difficulty testing vestibulo-ocular reflexes* (VOR; doll's head eye movement)
   In the early phase of PSP, voluntary vertical gaze is impaired to pursuit, but there is preservation of vertical eye movement on VOR. This is tested by holding the sides of the patient's head, which the examiner flexes and extends while the patient fixes on the examiner's face (Video 8.30, PSP

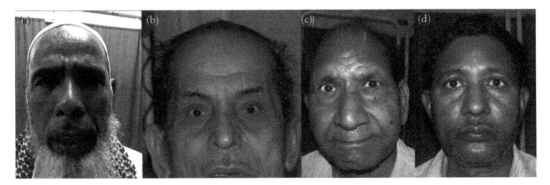

FIGURE 8.12: The varied faces of progressive supranuclear palsy (PSP) patients. (**A**) Procerus sign or vertical wrinkling of the forehead. (**B**) Surprised look. (**C**) Anxious look with chin dystonia. (**D**) Mask face. Note the deep nasolabial fold in all but D. Reproduced with permission from Batla et al. (2010).

eye). The test is often difficult because of marked neck muscle rigidity that prevents the clinician from moving the head fully up and down. In late stages, Bell's phenomenon and VOR may be absent.

▶ *Round the houses sign*
Here, the patient is asked to follow a target up and down with the eyes. Instead of moving the eyes straight up and down, the excursion takes a curved pathway toward the temporal side.

▶ *Applause sign*
The patient is asked to clap three times. In PSP, there is difficulty in stopping, and clapping continues for several seconds. This is characteristic but not specific for PSP and has been described in CBD and MSA (Video 8.31, Applause).

▶ *Fast micrographia*
Handwriting is small, in keeping with rigidity, but patients write rapidly as if unable to stop—the equivalent of festinant gait (Video 8.32, Fast Micrographia).

▶ *Rocket sign*
When the patient is asked to stand up from a chair, this is performed unusually rapidly and without caution, despite the high risk of falling.

▶ *Difficulty walking downstairs or reading*
The difficulty with downgaze is responsible for both of these features that may be reported by the more observant patient.

▶ *Trunk hyperextension with tendency to fall backward*
On standing, there is passive hyperextension of the trunk muscles—the opposite of the classic PD stance, which is slightly flexed. In PSP, falls in all directions are frequent, but backward falls are typical.

▶ Turning "en bloc"
On turning, the whole body is moved as a single unit, without the normal rotation at waist level, thus reflecting axial rigidity. This is characteristic but not specific for PSP and may be found in lower body parkinsonism from vascular disease, NPH, and advanced PD.

▶ *Palilalia, pseudobulbar affect, and stereotypies*
These symptoms are not seen in typical PD and point toward PSP (Video 8.33, Palilalia, and Video 8.34, Pseudobulbar Affect).

PSP Look-Alikes

The clinical picture of PSP, especially SNGP, may occur in:

- Corticobasal syndrome
- Dementia with Lewy bodies (DLB)
- Multiple system atrophy (MSA); rare
- Frontotemporal lobar degeneration (FTLD)
- Perry syndrome (respiratory depression, psychiatric problems, and parkinsonism)

In younger individuals, SNGP, either vertical or horizontal, may occur in the following:

- Niemann Pick type C (vertical; greater on downgaze); see Video 8.35, Niemann Pick C (courtesy David Zee).
- Kufor Rakeb syndrome (vertical)
- Gaucher's disease (horizontal; Video 8.36, Gaucher Disease)
- *POLG* mutations
- Cerebrotendinous xanthomatosis (CTX)
- CADASIL (cerebral autosomal dominant arteriopathy with subcortical infarcts and leukoencephalopathy)
- Spinocerebellar atrophies: SCA2 and SCA3 (see Chapter 12)

Here are some Handles to help distinguish these chameleons:

▶ *Familial PSP pattern with dominant inheritance suggests FTLD.*
▶ *PSP plus ALS picture suggests the C9ORF72 mutation.*
▶ *SNGP with early dementia and hallucinations suggests DLB.*
▶ *Dysautonomia and SNGP suggests MSA.*
▶ *History of neonatal jaundice and SNGP (chiefly downgaze) is diagnostic of Niemann Pick type C. Some have cataplexy.*
▶ *Supranuclear gaze palsy plus parkinsonism, psychiatric problems, and respiratory depression indicates Perry syndrome.*

Causes of a secondary PSP-like picture include multiple lacunar infarctions and aortic aneurysm repair surgery. The mechanism of the latter is unclear. Rapidly progressive PSP may be caused by:

- Neoplasms: lymphoma or gliomatosis cerebri
- Paraneoplastic process such as anti-MA2 encephalitis

MRI brain imaging may help distinguish PSP from MSA and from multiple lacunar infarcts.

MULTIPLE SYSTEM ATROPHY

There are two major varieties of MSA:

- MSA-P, in which akinesia and rigidity predominate. This comprises (80%) of MSA cases.
- MSA-C, where there is mainly cerebellar ataxia (20%). This type is commoner among Japanese.

Both varieties display progressive parkinsonism with dysautonomia that affects principally the bladder, orthostatic blood pressure control, and bowel. Usually the parkinsonian and autonomic features are detectable easily, but the dysautonomia may occur 2–3 years after the motor features, or there may be just dysautonomia initially, without motor features.

▶ Pure autonomic failure is a synucleinopathy with autonomic failure and hyposmia but no motor features.

Handles for MSA-P

▶ *Unexplained urinary retention/incontinence, severe constipation, or severe sexual dysfunction in a middle-aged or elderly person*
You may be referred this sort of patient from gynecology, urology, or gastroenterology units.

▶ *Unexplained postural hypotension or fainting episodes in a middle-aged or elderly person*
A geriatrician or cardiologist may have diagnosed postural hypotension but cannot explain why. Typically, there are overlooked parkinsonian features that allow you to clinch the diagnosis of MSA. Note that, on standing, there is minimal or no tachycardia to compensate for postural hypotension, a confirmatory sign of autonomic dysfunction.

▶ *Middle-aged or elderly person with unexplained cold hands*
This is a characteristic sign of MSA that reflects poor autonomic regulation of peripheral circulation. Complaint of cold feet is common among the elderly, but cold hands in the absence of Raynaud's phenomenon should alert you to the possibility of MSA. The reduction of body movement in parkinsonism aggravates the liability to cold extremities.

▶ *Early anteroflexion of the neck, camptocormia, or Pisa syndrome with parkinsonism* (Video 8.15, Camptocormia MSA)

▶ *Parkinsonism with dystonic facial contractions while receiving levodopa* (Video 8.5, MSA Dystonia)
In essence, this is a form of levodopa-induced dystonia that involves the face, in keeping with MSA.

▶ *Parkinsonism with marked stridor, typically inspiratory* (Video 8.6, Stridor)
This is very characteristic of MSA, resulting from laryngeal abductor paralysis (Bannister et al. 1981) or dystonia of the thyro-aretynoid muscles. Some patients develop an intermittent high-pitched voice.

▶ *Parkinsonism with jerky rest tremor.*
This is essentially a form of myoclonic tremor (mini-poly myoclonus) and suggestive of MSA. It may be induced by palmar stimulation. The same phenomenon is seen in CBS and late Alzheimer's disease

▶ *Hot cross bun sign on axial MRI of pons*
This is a characteristic MRI finding that relates to degeneration of fibers that cross the pons as they interconnect the cerebellar hemispheres (Figure 8.13). This sign is not specific for MSA and may occur in spinocerebellar ataxias (SCA).

How to Distinguish Early MSA-P from PD

- Tremor of MSA is jerky and irregular.
- Dysautonomia is more severe.
- Response to levodopa is incomplete and unsustained.
- Cardiac MIBG scan (a marker for norepinephrine) is normal in MSA (Figure 8.14) but abnormal in PD (Video 8.37, parkinsonism and Fluctuating Blood Pressure). In the video, the MIBG scan was abnormal in keeping with PD, and a pheochromocytoma was found coincidentally in the left adrenal gland that explained the intermittent hypertension.

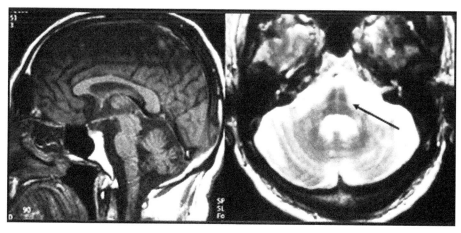

FIGURE 8.13: Sagittal and axial T2-weighted MRI views showing pontocerebellar atrophy and the hot cross bun sign in the pons (arrow).

How to Distinguish Essential Tremor from Early MSA-C

- The tremor of essential tremor is rhythmic and sinusoidal; it is jerkier and irregular in MSA.

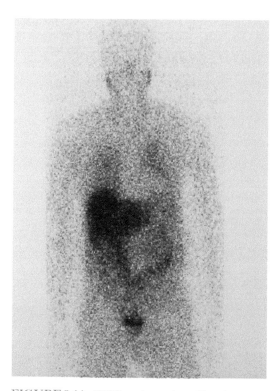

FIGURE 8.14: MIBG scan in a patient with parkinsonism and fluctuating blood pressure. It shows absent cardiac uptake, consistent with a diagnosis of Parkinson's disease.

- There are autonomic features in MSA, such as postural hypotension and bladder disorder.
- The gait is unsteady in MSA-C but normal in most cases of essential tremor.
- Head and voice tremor is a feature of essential tremor but not MSA.
- History in essential tremor is longer. A family history and alcohol responsiveness is frequent in essential tremor but rarely in MSA.
- ▶ *An elderly male with cerebellar tremor, ataxic gait, parkinsonism, cognitive decline, and dysautonomia likely has the fragile X–associated tremor ataxia syndrome (FXTAS)*
  FXTAS is caused by a premutation (i.e., trinucleotide repeat expansion) in the fragile X gene. It mimics MSA-C. (See Video 8.38, FXTAS.)
- ◀ *Occasionally a mild form of FXTAS affects a woman.*

How to Distinguish FXTAS from MSA-C

- Premature ovarian failure may be present in females with manifesting FXTAS.
- The dysautonomia in FXTAS is not as severe.
- Suspicion of FXTAS should be raised if the family history supports X-linked recessive inheritance—for example (1) an affected father has a healthy daughter whose son is intellectually disabled, or (2) an affected mother has an intellectually disabled son.
- Middle cerebellar peduncle (MCP) hyperintensity sign on MRI is typical of FXTAS (Figure 8.15), but it is not specific and may be seen occasionally in MSA-C with

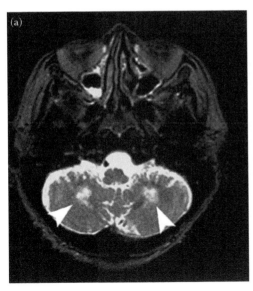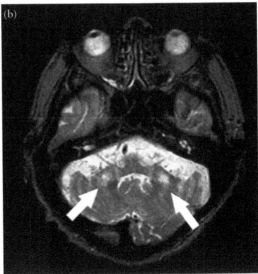

FIGURE 8.15: Fragile X tremor ataxia syndrome. Axial T2-weighted images demonstrate symmetrical bilateral hyperintense lesions in the cerebellar white matter (**A**, arrowheads) and middle cerebellar peduncles (**B**, arrows). Reproduced with permission from Goncalves et al. (2007), Figure 1.

or without a hot cross bun sign. Other causes of the MCP hyperintensity sign include the following:

o Metabolic disorder: Wilson's disease, liver cirrhosis, hypoglycemia
o Vascular disease: posterior reversible encephalopathy syndrome, hypertensive encephalopathy
o Demyelination and inflammatory disease: multiple sclerosis (MS), adrenoleukodystrophy, ADEM, Behçet's disease
o Some spino-cerebellar ataxias
o Alexander disease
o Neoplasms (Okamoto et al. 2003)

Remember that female carriers of the gene may develop abnormal neurological findings such as tremor, ataxia, and parkinsonism.

CORTICOBASAL SYNDROME

Classic corticobasal degeneration CBD was thought to have a typical and easily diagnosable clinical picture. Patients who had asymmetric motor features with apraxia, parkinsonism, and alien limb phenomenon were presumed to have the classic pathology of CBD—neuronal achromasia and corticostrionigral degeneration. It then became clear that this clinical picture may result from diverse pathologies including but not limited to the classic neuronal achromasia. In some studies, the pathological hallmark of CBD (neuronal achromasia) is found in less than one-third of clinically diagnosed CBD, thus it is safer to implement the term *corticobasal syndrome* (CBS) and to be cautious about the underlying pathology.

The core features of CBS are:

- Parkinsonism
- Dystonia
- Ideomotor apraxia
- Myoclonus (Video 8.39, CBS)
- Cognitive decline is a late feature.

Despite this, many patients with CBD pathology are seen in dementia clinics, which attests to the difficulty of making a clinical diagnosis.

With these caveats, here are some of the traditional diagnostic Handles.

▶ *Alien limb/hand phenomenon*
This well-known sign consists of involuntary purposeful movement of either arm. The arm may repeatedly and abruptly flex to clutch the throat. The unaffected arm may be used to prevent the alien limb from causing damage. If the alien limb phenomenon develops acutely, over minutes, then this is likely due to a parietal vascular lesion. A rapidly evolving alien

limb—over months—is likely a prion disorder such as Creutzfeldt-Jacob disease. The late British comedian Peter Sellers simulated a post-stroke alien limb in the movie "Dr. Strangelove," which is well worth watching. A clip of the simulated alien arm sequence is shown in the video link: https://youtu.be/zZct-itCwPE

▷ *"My hand does not obey me"* or *"my feet feel foreign."*
Patients who say this usually have CBS. It is a feature of the alien limb phenomenon.

▷ *A jerky useless arm or leg due to myoclonus and apraxia is highly characteristic of CBS.*

▷ *Marked asymmetry of signs.* CBS is the most asymmetric of the major parkinsonian syndromes.

▷ *CBS may begin with isolated orofacial apraxia* (Video 8.40, Orofacial Apraxia). Some present with isolated gait apraxia.

Hereditary diffuse leukoencephalopathy with axonal spheroids (HDLS)

This has a CBS-like presentation with extensive white matter changes on brain MRI (Figure 8.16). It is a rare autosomal dominant disorder due to a mutation in the colony stimulating factor 1 receptor gene. Patients have a complex picture including dementia and

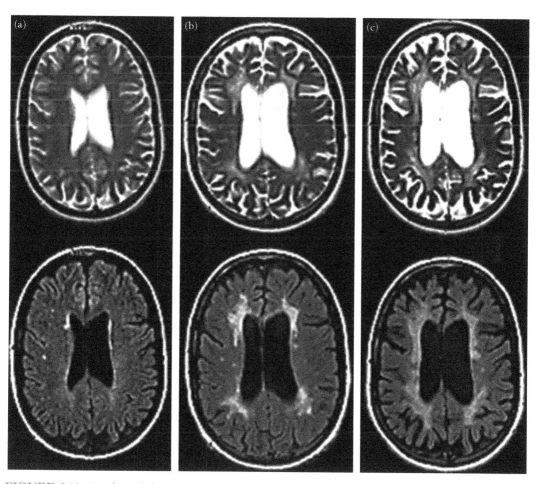

FIGURE 8.16: Hereditary diffuse leukoencephalopathy with axonal spheroids. Sequential MRI study of the proband. **Upper row**: T2-weighed images; **lower row**: FLAIR images. (**A**) Pre-symptomatic images (age 29 years) show subtle right-predominant frontal white matter signal changes. (**B**) Symptomatic images (age 36 years) show significant patchy and confluent bifrontal and biparietal periventricular white matter lesions, with moderate cortical and subcortical atrophy. (**C**) Symptomatic images (age 37 years) show severe symmetric confluent bifrontal and biparietal white matter lesions, with marked cortical and subcortical atrophy. Reproduced with permission from Van Gerpen et al. (2008), Figure 2.

parkinsonism. The white matter changes on MRI may cause confusion with MS.

Other conditions that may simulate CBS and may have an alien limb syndrome (see Figure 8.17) are as follows:

- Frontotemporal dementia
- PSP

- Perry syndrome
- Prion disease, for example, Creutzfeldt-Jacob disease, especially if rapidly evolving
- MS
- Vascular lesions: parietal infarct/hemorrhage and bilateral subdural hematomas
- Posterior reversible encephalopathy syndrome

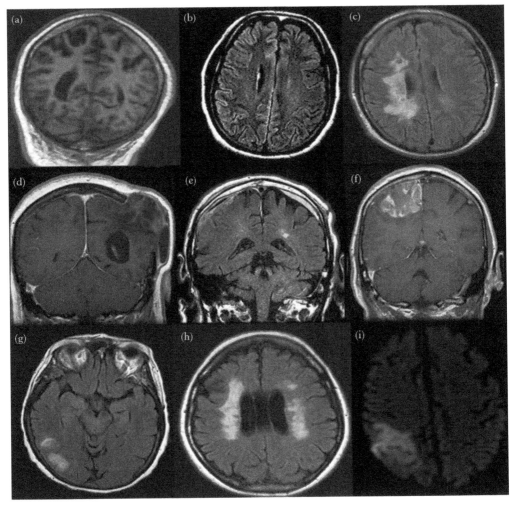

FIGURE 8.17: MRI changes associated with alien limb from various etiologies. The cases are described from top to bottom, from left to right. (a) coronal T1 MRI demonstrating right parietal atrophy attributed to corticobasal syndrome. (b) Axial T2-weighted FLAIR sequence showing right hemispheric cortical ribboning associated with Creutzfeld-Jacob disease. (c) T2-weighted FLAIR sequence showing a large demyelinating lesion in the right posterior corona radiata in a demyelinating disorder not otherwise specified. (d) Coronal T1-weighted sequence with prominent left parietal hemorrhage. (e) Coronal T2-weighted FLAIR sequence demonstrating bilateral subdural hematomata with subarachnoid hemorrhage and associated cortical irritation of the right parietal lobe. (f) Coronal gadolinium-enhanced T1-weighted sequence showing a right parietal tumor. (g) Axial FLAIR image demonstrating characteristic changes of the posterior reversible encephalopathy syndrome. (h) Axial FLAIR sequence demonstrating bilateral corona radiata abnormalities in hereditary diffuse leukodystrophy with axonal spheroids. (i) axial diffusion-weighted image demonstrating a right parietal infarct. In all cases, the alien limb was contralateral to the afflicted parietal lobe. Reproduced with permission from Graff-Radford et al. (2013), Figure 2.

- Parietal lobe tumors
- Familial Alzheimer's disease due to presenilin 1 mutation
- Rarely, stiff limb syndrome may be confused with CBS. See Video 8.41 Stiff Limb (courtesy Balint et al. 2014). There is reduced facial expression and slow finger movements and a striatal toe sign on left. Also, stiffness and posturing of the left leg is seen with knee extension and plantar flexion when walking and settle at rest.
- Other reported CBS mimics are autoimmune encephalopathies and vasculitis.

CHOREA

Chorea is characterized by random, nonrepetitive, semi-purposeful movements flowing from one body part to the other (Video 8.42, Sydenham Chorea). Chorea may be sporadic or inherited. Signs of chorea include the following:

- Tongue sign (an inability to keep the tongue protruded due to motor impersistence)
- Milkmaid grip (due to waxing and waning of maintained grip). Sometimes asterixis may result in intermittent waning of grip.
- Pendular knee jerks (due to hypotonia)
- Hung-up jerks, which are due to a choreic jerk superimposed on a tendon jerk (Video 8.42, Sydenham Chorea)
- Macrographia (Figure 8.18)
- Hypotonia, causing extension of the fingers at metacarpophalangeal joint when splayed out
- Wilson's sign. If the arms are elevated vertically, the affected side(s) hyperpronate so that the palm faces outward.

Chorea may involve the facio-bucco-lingual area, affect half the body (hemichorea), or be generalized. *Ballism* refers to severe flailing movements affecting proximal muscles. It may be present in half the body (hemiballism) or both sides (bi-ballism) (Video 8.43, Ballism).

Inherited choreas include Huntington's disease (HD), Huntington disease-like conditions (HDL), neuroacanthocytosis, SCAs, and dentato-rubro-pallido-luysian atrophy (DRPLA).

Huntington's Disease and Related Conditions

This is an autosomal dominant condition due increased number of CAG trinucleotide repeats of the huntingtin gene on chromosome 4p. The main features are progressive chorea, imbalance, depression, personality change, and subcortical dementia with onset around middle age (Video 8.44, HD). Often patients are adopted, and a family history is not available. Imaging shows atrophy of the caudate nuclei and occasionally abnormal signal in the putamina (Figure 8.19).

Handles for Diagnosis of HD

Following are some Handles that would point to a diagnosis of HD:

- *Generalized choreic movements, especially in an adopted adult*
- *Akinetic rigid syndrome in an adopted child suggests the Westphal variant of HD*; see Video 8.45, Westphal (courtesy Jim Carroll).
- Early oculomotor disturbances, such as impaired smooth pursuit (which may be present in pre-manifest HD) and delayed initiation of saccades
- *A family history of:*
  - Dementia
  - Suicide, particularly in a young akinetic rigid individual whose father had committed suicide

The trinucleotide repeat is more unstable when inherited from the father, suggesting genetic imprinting, and it is associated with earlier age of onset.

- A negative family history does *not* rule out HD.
- *An ill-kempt patient with chorea; strong body odor*
- *Chorea with early gait and balance problems* (Video 8.44 HD, second patient)
- *Chorea with prominent behavioral problems or a change in personality*
- *Prolonged but reversible chorea after cocaine abuse suggests an HD gene carrier.*

Red Flags

There are several Red Flags that should make you reconsider the diagnosis of HD (Martino et al. 2013).

23/1/91

"MINER ALIVE AFTER 45 DAYS IN THE
OUT BACK WITHOUT FOOD"
A MAN FOUND BY CHANCE IN THE QLD
OUTBACK HAS TOLD POLICE HE ATE NOTHING
FOR 45 DAYS. HE SURVIVED ONLY ON
WATER.

⊢—⊣
1 cm

FRI THE FIRST OF
NOVEMBER. 1991.
READY SET GO FOR
SHOW SHOW TIME
IS ON ALL DOING
OR C WITH VISITORS ALL
POURING IN FROM ALL
OVER AUSTRALIA
IT IS THE SHOW ARE
IT A LITTLE SHOW
...
FIND IN C COUNTRY

FIGURE 8.18: Handwriting from a patient with Huntington's disease, showing the development of macrographia from previous normal handwriting (**top** figure). Reproduced with permission from Phillips et al. (1994), Figure 1.

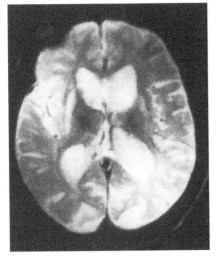 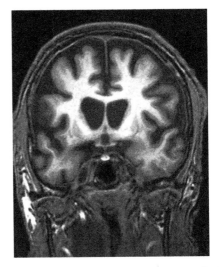

FIGURE 8.19: Huntington's disease. **Left**: A 67-year-old patient with a 23-year history of HD. **Right**: T1-weighted coronal MRI showing severe atrophy of the caudate head and cerebral cortex. Reproduced with permission from Radiopedia. Dr. Frank Gaillard, ID 8052.

◄ *Ethnicity*

If there is autosomal dominant inheritance leading you to suspect HD and your patient is born in

- *Africa*: think of Huntington disease-like 2 (HDL2). This may be clinically indistinguishable from HD, but it is due to a CTG repeat rather than a CAG repeat as found in classic HD (Video 8.46, HDL2).
- *Japan*: consider DRPLA. Ataxia is a prominent feature.
- *Cumbria* (NW England): this may be a neuroferritinopathy. The blood ferritin level is low.

◄ *Selective or predominant facio-bucco-linguo-masticatory (FBLM) movements.*

See Video 8.47, Neuroacanthocytosis. In HD, the chorea is widespread.

Selective involvement of the mouth, tongue, and jaw muscles suggests:

- Tardive dyskinesia (common) or
- Neuroacanthocytosis (rare)

The two main varieties of neuroacanthocytosis are

- Chorea-acanthocytosis
- McLeod's syndrome

In **chorea-acanthocytosis** (autosomal recessive) the main Handles are:

▶ *Tongue protrusion,* often while eating resulting in ejection of food (feeding dystonia). Note: ejection of food occurs also in the Lesch-Nyhan syndrome.

▶ *Lip/tongue biting, vocal tics*

▶ *Head drop and involuntary head-banging on furniture*

▶ *Recurrent belching and vocalizations*

▶ *Seizures*

▶ *Peripheral neuropathy sometimes leading to muscle wasting.*

▶ *Rubber-man gait.* See Video 8.48, Rubber-man C-A (reproduced with permission from Merwick Á et al.).

Acanthocytes are not always detected, but the erythrocyte chorein level is low or absent in CA and there is a mutation in the *ChAc* gene.

In the **McLeod's syndrome** (X-linked) the Handles are:

▶ *Vocalization but no tongue protrusion or lip biting*

▶ *Skeletal and cardiac muscle involvement with proximal myopathy, raised creatine kinase (CK), or cardiomyopathy*

▶ *Risk of sudden death from arrhythmia*

▶ *Absence of Kx antigen and reduction in Kell antigen due to mutation in the XK gene. If this is not identified prior to a blood transfusion, then severe hemolysis will result.*

Thus, chorea with:

▶ *Absent reflexes suggest neuropathy and a diagnosis of chorea-acanthocytosis or Friedreich's ataxia.*

▶ *Tongue protrusion or ejection of food or hand banging is likely chorea-acanthocytosis.*

▶ *Raised CK favors chorea-acanthocytosis or McLeod's syndrome.*

▶ *Severe transfusion reaction points to McLeod's syndrome.*

▶ *Sudden head drops are characteristic of but not specific for neuroacanthocytosis.*

FBLM dystonic movements and juvenile parkinsonism

This favors one of the following:

▶ *Pantothenate kinase–associated neurodegeneration (PKAN), also known as NBIA type 1 (NBIA1) and Hallervorden-Spatz disease (see Table 8.1).*

▶ *HARP syndrome (hypoprebetalipoproteinemia, acanthocytosis, retinitis pigmentosa, and pallidal degeneration). This is allelic with PKAN.*

Features include:

- Prominent dystonia
- Parkinsonism
- Pyramidal signs
- No seizures, cardiac problems, or CK elevation

Genetic testing for the *PANK2* mutation is the best way to diagnose PKAN. The MRI may show the "eye of a tiger" sign (Figure 8.20 and Video 8.49).

TABLE 8.1: SUMMARY OF MAIN FEATURES OF NEURODEGENERATION WITH BRAIN IRON ACCUMULATION (NBIA)

Disease name	Alternate names	Inheritance and mutation	Onset	Features	Red flags
PKAN (pantothenate kinase–associated neurodegeneration)	NBIA1; Hallervorden-Spatz syndrome HARP syndrome is allelic	AR. PANK2	Childhood–early adult	*Dystonic tongue protrusion*, parkinsonism, chorea, occasional *acanthocytes*, normal CK, cognitive decline, retinitis pigmentosa. Common in Dominicans. *Eye of tiger sign on MRI* (Video 8.49, PANK)	Seizures Raised CK Cardiomyopathy
PLAN (PLA2G6-associated neurodegeneration)	NBIA2 PARK14 Seitelberger disease	AR PLA2G6	Childhood–early adult	Levodopa-responsive parkinsonism with dyskinesia, dystonia, progressive motor and intellectual disability, truncal hypotonia, cerebellar ataxia, pyramidal signs. *Optic atrophy and developmental regression* in early-onset form (INAD). Cerebellar atrophy on MRI.	
Neuroferritinopathy	NBIA3	AD FTL (ferritin light polypeptide)	Middle age	Slowly progressive chorea, orofacial dystonia, *tongue protrusion*, choking and frontalis overactivity. Most come from NW England. *Low ferritin.* Resembles Huntington's disease. MRI may show cavitation in putamina	Acanthocytes
MPAN (mitochondrial membrane-associated neurodegeneration)	NBIA4	AR. C19orf12	Childhood–early adult	Dysarthria and ataxia, then spastic paraparesis, dystonia and parkinsonism, motor neuropathy, *optic atrophy,* cognitive decline, and psychiatric disorder	
BPAN (beta-propeller protein-associated neurodegeneration) SENDA	NBIA5	XLR WDR4S	Childhood–early adult	*Predominantly women.* Early deficits often static for years. Progressive dystonia and parkinsonism. Seizures. Stereotypies mimicking Rett syndrome. Cognitive decline. Sleep disorder. Levodopa responsive, with severe dyskinesias. *Halo sign in substantia nigra* (Figure 8.26)	Normal early development

Disease	Inheritance/Gene	Onset	Features
Kufor-Rakeb disease	PARK9 AR ATP13A2	Teenage	Parkinsonism, pyramidal signs, *supranuclear upgaze palsy, oculogyric crises*, lip tremor, and mini-myoclonus. Levodopa responsive. MRI maybe normal
Aceruloplasminemia	AR CP	Middle age	*Macular degeneration, diabetes*, dementia, face and neck dystonia blepharospasm, tremor. *Ceruloplasmin and copper levels low. Ferritin high; serum iron low. Abnormal liver and pancreas on MRI*
FAHN (fatty acid hydroxylase-associated neurodegeneration)	SPG3S AR FA2H	Childhood	Spastic paraparesis, leg dystonia, falls, *optic atrophy*, cerebellar atrophy and leukodystrophy.
Woodhouse-Sakati syndrome	AR. DCAF17	Teenage	*Hypogonadism, alopecia, diabetes mellitus*, intellectual disability, *deafness,* choreoathetosis and dystonia

Some of the more useful distinguishing features are in italics.

AR, autosomal recessive; AD, autosomal dominant; CK, creatine kinase; HARP, hypoprebetalipoproteinemia, acanthocytosis, retinitis pigmentosa, and pallidal degeneration; MRI, magnetic resonance imaging; NBIA, neurodegeneration with brain iron accumulation; XLR, sex-linked recessive.

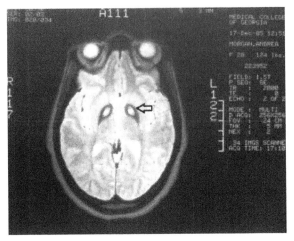 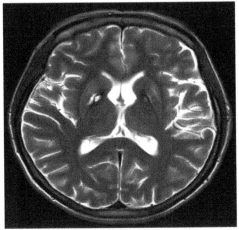

FIGURE 8.20: **Left:** MRI (T2 sequence) to show iron deposits and a central hyperintensity reflecting gliosis in the pallidum. Arrow points to the "eye-of-the-tiger." **Right:** MRI (T2 sequence) in neuroferritinopathy. There is again an "eye of the tiger" sign but it is less conspicuous than in the left picture.

▶ *Wilson's disease* (see later discussion)
▶ *Lesch-Nyhan syndrome*

Note: In an older person isolated FBLD, especially dystonic, may be of unknown cause (e.g., Meige syndrome).

◀ *Ataxia*
   If there is dystonia or chorea with prominent ataxia and you are considering HD, then think again. Consider SCA 17 (SCA17/HDL4), DRPLA, and SCA2
◀ *Seizures*
   In adult-onset HD, the presence of seizures constitutes a major Red Flag. Epilepsy only occurs in the juvenile variety of HD. You should explore the possibility of one of the following instead:
   ○ SCA17/HDL4
   ○ Chorea-acanthocytosis and McLeod's syndrome
   ○ DRPLA
   ○ Huntington's disease-like 1 (HDL1). This is an autosomal dominant prion disorder with more rapid progression than classic HD, where life expectancy is around 15 years from onset. Major psychiatric disorders, such as mania, are common.
   ○ The most common genetic phenocopy of HD is the C9ORF72 mutation.

Benign Hereditary Chorea

Benign hereditary chorea (BHC) is a benign autosomal dominant condition resulting from a mutation in the NKX2-1 gene located on chromosome 14q13 that encodes thyroid transcription factor-1. The main features are as follows:

• Chorea and sometimes myoclonus or dystonia appearing early in life
• Associated with hypothyroidism due to underdevelopment of thyroid gland
• No caudate atrophy on MRI
• Short stature
• Pulmonary fibrosis
• No intellectual deterioration

Nonprogressive and may improve with age

Adenyl Cyclase 5 Mutation

This autosomal dominant condition is due to a mutation in the adenyl cyclase 5 gene (ADCY 5) on chromosome 3q21; see Video 8.50 ADCY-5; (courtesy Pankaj Aggarwal). This gene is involved in the synthesis of cAMP. The phenotypic spectrum is diverse but may be confused with BHC. Clinical features include the following:

• Early-onset chorea with some progression
• Paroxysmal dyskinesia during sleep and eventual dystonia

- Hypotonia
- Facial myoclonic movements; see Video 8.50 ADCY-5
- Intact intellect, despite marked motor problems

Acquired Chorea

Chorea may be due to a wide range of acquired conditions, such as metabolic disorders, medication, and vascular or autoimmune causes.

Here are some useful Handles for acquired chorea:

▶ *In a young person, consider Sydenham's chorea* (Video 8.42, Sydenham Chorea). Note that chorea is often delayed when other signs of rheumatic fever, such as arthritis and carditis, have resolved.

▶ *Oral contraceptives may reactivate chorea* if there is a history of Sydenham's chorea. The same is true of chorea gravidarum that recurs during pregnancy. Rarely, chorea gravidarum occurs (Video 8.51, Chorea Gravidarum).

▶ *In a woman with migraine and repeated miscarriages, think of the phospholipid antibody syndrome* (Hughes syndrome).

▶ *History of recurrent vomiting and stupor as a child followed by progressive chorea and dementia suggests organic aciduria,* such as propionic acidemia (Video 8.52, Propionic Aciduria).

▶ *Chorea in an adult with arthralgia and skin rash may be lupus chorea.* Sometimes it is the presenting manifestation of lupus, and it is associated with phospholipid antibodies.

▶ *Drug-induced chorea may be due to dopamine-blocking agents.* Frequently the orofacial area is involved, but generalized chorea is recognized. In someone treated for seizures, the usual cause is phenytoin toxicity. In a patient with preexisting brain disease (e.g., structural lesions or HIV encephalopathy), chorea may develop even when the plasma levels of phenytoin are within the therapeutic range (Video 8.53, Phenytoin).

▶ *In a diabetic, hemi- or generalized chorea or ballism may result from basal ganglia damage in nonketotic hyperglycemia* (Video 8.54, Nonketotic Hyperglycemia). It is sometimes called "diabetic striatopathy." Non-contrast CT brain scan may show punctate hyperintensity. An unenhanced T1-weighted MRI scan may display markedly increased signal confined to the basal ganglia (Figure 8.21).

▶ *In elderly women, chorea may be the presenting manifestation of diabetes.*

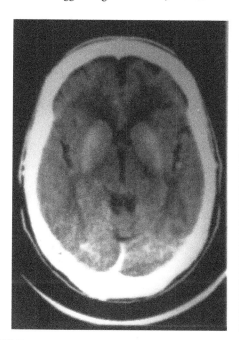 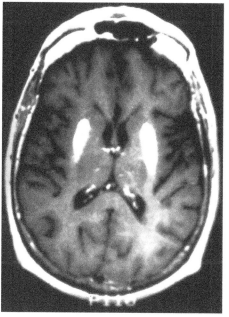

FIGURE 8.21: Nonketotic hyperglycemia associated with generalized chorea and ballism. **Left:** A non-enhanced CT brain scan shows increased attenuation confined to the basal ganglia. **Right:** T1-weighted MRI performed 3 days later shows increased signal consistent with methemoglobin secondary to petechial hemorrhage.

▶ *Chorea may be a complication of thyrotoxicosis* (Video 8.55 Thyrotoxic Chorea), digoxin toxicity (Video 8.56, Digoxin), or paraneoplastic disorders (Video 8.57, Paraneoplastic Chorea).

▶ *Chorea following major heart surgery favors post-pump chorea.*

▶ *Chorea in a patient with psychiatric problems suggests tardive dyskinesia.*

Hemichorea (see next section) is often due to a vascular lesion, but widespread lacunes may result in generalized chorea.

HEMIBALLISM AND HEMICHOREA

Hemiballism refers to violent flinging movements involving one-half of the body, with or without facial involvement. It is often accompanied by distal choreic movements. Hemiballism may be self-limiting or may evolve into hemichorea or hemidystonia.

Causes are:

- Lacunar infarction or hemorrhage in the contralateral basal ganglia; contrary to the usual teaching, the lesion is more often seen in the caudate or putamen rather than subthalamic nucleus (STN). Hemiballism may herald a major stroke due to basilar artery occlusion.
- Diabetic striatopathy
- Tumors: primary or metastatic; abscess involving the STN
- Head trauma
- Toxoplasmosis in an immunocompromised patient such as HIV
- Bi-ballism may be caused by diabetic striatopathy, phenytoin intoxication, or widespread cancer

WILSON'S DISEASE

This disorder of copper transport results in copper deposition in multiple organs, particularly the liver, cornea, and basal ganglia. Wilson's disease is a great mimic—beware! One can never be faulted for considering Wilson's disease in a young person with virtually any movement disorder. Wilson's disease presents to psychiatrists, gastroenterologists, endocrinologists, and gynecologists, as well as neurologists. Usually the movement disorder is mixed. Those who present with tremor may be confused with MS, PD, or ET. Remember:

- Presentation may be late, even in the seventh decade.
- The blood copper and ceruloplasmin levels are *both* low. The blood copper is reduced because the standard test measures total copper level, which is depressed because of deficiency in ceruloplasmin, the copper-binding carrier protein. The free (non-ceruloplasmin bound) copper is elevated.

Handles and Flags for Wilson's Disease

▶ *Dystonic vacuous smile* (Video 8.58, Wilson's disease smile)

▶ *Various tremors but typically the proximal, "wing-beating" tremor;* see Video 8.59, Wilson's Disease Tremor (courtesy Stewart Factor)

▶ *Parkinsonism in a young person*

▶ *Ataxia. Pure ataxia may develop in the absence of the other abnormal movements* (Video 8.60, Wilson's Disease Ataxia).

▶ *Chorea*

◀ *Pyramidal signs are uncommon.*

▶ *A patient with any movement disorder whose blue eyes turn brown likely has Wilson's disease.*

This happens because of copper deposition in the outer cornea that spreads progressively toward the center. Note that the process starts typically as a small crescent in the upper corneal sector at 12 o'clock and may be missed if you do not elevate the upper lid and ask the patient to look down. Next is the lower sector at 6 o'clock, and finally a complete ring is formed (Figure 8.22). In a brown-eyed person, the ring is difficult to see, but it appears gray rather than brown. See Chapter 2, Figure 2.36, for additional photographs, including the sunflower cataract. A similar iris color change occurs in Fuchs heterochromic iridocyclitis and following use of prostaglandin-blocking eye drops for glaucoma.

▶ *Dystonia with low platelet count is strongly suggestive of Wilson's disease.* May also occur in Niemann Pick type C.

The low platelet count in Wilson's disease is due to cirrhosis of the liver with portal hypertension and secondary hypersplenism. The blood ferritin level may be elevated. Note that *dystonia with polycythemia suggests hypermanganesemia.*

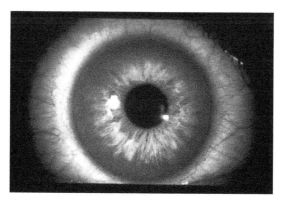

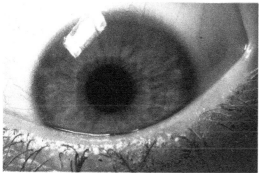
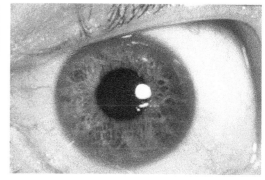

FIGURE 8.22: **Left**: Keyser-Fleischer ring in an 18-year-old woman with psychosis and a mixed movement disorder (see also Video 8.61, WD Mixed). **Center**: Complete Keyser-Fleischer ring in a 25-year-old woman who was thought to have multiple sclerosis. She had a rest tremor (not cerebellar) in keeping with mild parkinsonism. **Right**: A more advanced ring in a 35-year-old male. From Wikipedia, under CCAL.

▶ Blue nails (*azure lunula*). See Figure 1.1g. This is rare but worth checking.

▶ *Kayser-Fleischer rings may be absent to simple inspection.* They may be visible on slit-lamp examination, but even this can be negative in definite neurological Wilson's disease. Note: Eye movements are often said to be normal, but careful examination suggests otherwise. See Video 8.61, which shows mixed movement in a patient with Wilson's disease and macro square-wave jerks that improved following treatment.

▶ *There may be presentation with psychiatric problems and movement disorders in the absence of neuroleptics.*

▶ *Secondary amenorrhea is a rare presenting feature.*

Note: MRI brain scan is nearly always abnormal when there are neurological problems (Figure 8.23).

TREMOR

This is defined as rhythmic oscillation of a body part. Measurement of tremor frequency may be diagnostically useful. You can assess with a watch or smartphone app. These are the main frequency bands:

- Orthostatic tremor: 16–18 Hz
- Physiological tremor and ET: 7–12 Hz
- PD rest tremor: 4–6 Hz
- Palatal tremor and Holmes/rubral tremor: 1–4 Hz

Tremor Handles

▶ *Discomfort on standing that improves on walking is likely orthostatic tremor.*
Here are some clues for orthostatic tremor:
  ○ Patients dislike standing still in a line (queue) and may overbalance when washing their face or hair in a sink (Video 8.62, Primary Orthostatic Tremor). Be

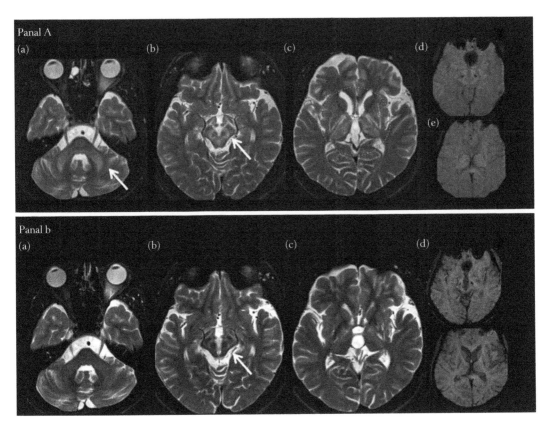

FIGURE 8.23: Serial MRI scans of a 22-year-old patient with Wilson's disease after 16 years of irregular treatment, demonstrating typical MRI changes associated with Wilson's disease and change in MRI abnormalities with supervised de-coppering. **Panel A**: MRI scan at age 22 years. Axial T2 MRI brain scan through (**a**) pons, (**b**) midbrain, and (**c**) basal ganglia, showing symmetrical hyperintensities in middle cerebellar peduncles, brainstem, striatum, globus pallidus, and thalami. In the mid-brain (**b**), the hyperintense signal of the white matter tracts shows the gray matter in relief. The midbrain therefore resembles the "face of the panda" (arrow) with the substantia nigra, red nucleus, and periaqueductal gray matter reminiscent of the ears, eyes, and mouth, respectively, of the panda. Axial susceptibility-weighted imaging (SWI) through the midbrain (**d**) and basal ganglia (**e**) show minimal susceptibility in the corpus striatum. **Panel B**: Follow-up MRI scan taken after 13 months of supervised de-coppering and substantial recovery of neurological disability. Compared to the initial scan in panel A, axial T2-weighted MRI images through the (**a**) pons, (**b**) midbrain, and (**c**) basal ganglia show regression in hyperintense signal and atrophy of cerebellum, brainstem, striatum, globus pallidus, and thalami. Axial SWI through the midbrain (**d**) and basal ganglia (**e**) show increased susceptibility and atrophy of the corpus striatum.   Reproduced with permission from Aggarwal and Bhatt (2014), Figure 1.

aware that leg discomfort on standing is seen in dysferlin myopathy and advanced Charcot-Marie-Tooth disease because of calf muscle weakness (see Chapter 11). In lumbar canal stenosis, standing is uncomfortable (postural claudication) and likewise in some patients with parkinsonism or restless legs syndrome (RLS). Trunk and upper limbs may be involved.

o Orthostatic tremor can be diagnosed with the patient standing by placing your hands on the thighs to feel the tremulous movements or by listening over the patella with a stethoscope. A helicopter-like sound may be heard at a typical frequency of 16 Hz (Video 8.62).

o It is improved when standing in a swimming pool.

o It may be of lower frequency and associated with PD.

▶ *Irregular rest tremor with an extended thumb or finger is likely dystonic tremor.*

This may be confused with PD (Video 8.21, Dystonic Tremor). Functional imaging is normal and the scans are termed SWEDDs (scans without evidence of dopaminergic deficit).

▶ *Tremor that improves with alcohol is likely essential tremor* (Video 8.63, essential tremor Alcohol-Responsive).

▶ *Tall male with tremor*
Think of chromosomal aneuploidy such as the XXYY syndrome. Patients have developmental delay, hypogonadism, epilepsy, and autism spectrum disorder. Other causes are Klinefelter's syndrome (XXY genotype) and Jacob syndrome (XYY) See Video 8.64.

▶ *Short stature in male or female with tremor*
  o Mitochondrial disease (e.g., Kearns-Sayre syndrome)
  o Pseudo-hypoparathyroidism
  o SCA-17 (with large number of repeats) and SCA 12
  o Coffin-Lowry syndrome associated with hyperekplexia
  o Cockayne syndrome

Note: Tremor associated with cerebellar, midbrain, and thalamic lesions may be delayed and known as Holmes, midbrain, or rubral tremor. The movement is typically unilateral, slow (2–4 Hz), of high amplitude, present at rest, enhanced by sustained posture, and markedly aggravated by goal-directed movements.

See Video 8.65, Holmes Tremor, and Video 8.66, Outflow Tremor, respectively, and Figure 8.24.

▶ *Action tremor in a patient with chronic obstructive pulmonary disease may be due to beta 2-stimulating drugs such as salbutamol.*

▶ *Action tremor in a psychiatric patient is usually drug-related, particularly lithium and sodium valproate.*

▶ *Tremor of sudden onset favors psychogenic etiology.*
Other features of this tremor variety are detailed later. Note that drugs such as beta-adrenergic stimulants or acute anxiety may worsen existing ET that is misinterpreted to be sudden in onset and of psychogenic origin.

▶ *Acute stroke affecting the thalamus or subthalamus can cause focal asterixis that may be confused with tremor.*

▶ *Isolated head tremor is rare in ET and suggests dystonic tremor as in CD* (Video 8.20, Cervical Dystonia).

▶ *Proximal tremor (wing-beating) suggests Wilson's disease.* See Video 8.59.

◀ Proximal tremor may be simulated by repeated shoulder dislocation; see Video 8.67 (courtesy Roongraj Bhidayasiri). Note: this subject has *bilateral* shoulder dislocations.

▶ *Tremor with weight loss or heat intolerance suggests thyrotoxicosis.*

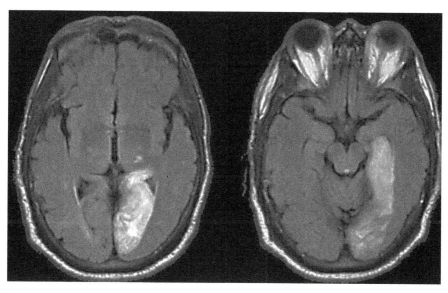

FIGURE 8.24: Patient with delayed Holmes tremor following posterior cerebral artery infarction involving posterior thalamus on the left side (see also Video 8.65, Holmes Tremor).

▶ A jerky tremor with a family history suggests familial cortical tremor. See Video 8.68.

▶ Tremor in a diabetic may relate to hypoglycemia.

▶ Tremor in an alcoholic may be due to delirium tremens or alcohol withdrawal.

Red Flags for Tremor

◀ *Tremor with no rigidity and a good sense of smell*
This association probably rules out classic PD and favors essential or dystonic tremor. Most patients with classic PD have a poor sense of smell, whereas it is usually normal in ET.

◀ *Apparent ET with seizures suggests familial cortical myoclonic tremor with epilepsy* (Regragui et al. 2006).
It is autosomal dominant or recessive and associated with a jerky postural tremor and seizures. There are giant somatosensory-evoked potentials; see Video 8.68, Familial Cortical Tremor (courtesy Steven Frucht).

◀ *Jerky rest tremor is likely myoclonus.* Causes include MSA, CBS, and occasionally DLBD.

◀ *Apparent ET in man with an intellectually disabled grandson (through his daughter) or a woman with a cognitively impaired son implies FXTAS.* The first example points to a male carrier of the FXTAS premutation and the second a manifesting female carrier. In men, tremor onset is late and there may be cognitive impairment (Video 8.38, FXTAS).
Women may experience premature menopause related to ovarian dysfunction.

NEURODEGENERATION WITH BRAIN IRON ACCUMULATION

Abnormalities in brain iron metabolism with excess iron levels are associated with several neurodegenerative diseases. MRI has facilitated the detection of brain iron accumulation (Figure 8.25). The nomenclature is confusing and changes frequently; see review by Schneider et al. (2012). The main categories are shown in Table 8.1.

TICS

Tics are repetitive short, jerky movements usually affecting the craniocervical region. Occasionally, they are more prolonged (dystonic tics; see Video 8.69, Dystonic Tics). They are common in children and teenagers but gradually decrease with time. The most important clinical Handles for their diagnosis are:

▶ *A premonitory sensation builds up before the tic.*
▶ *This sensation is relieved by execution of the tic.*
▶ *Improvement with concentration* (Video 8.70, Tourette syndrome)

Primary Tics

These may be inherited or sporadic and present as simple and chronic motor tics or Tourette syndrome.
If there is a family history of tic disorder, think of:

- Tourette syndrome
- Chorea-acanthocytosis
- Huntington's disease

Handles for Tourette Syndrome

▶ Multiple motor and vocal tics
▶ Onset before age 18 years
▶ Fluctuation: tics are worse when inactive and become less when focused on a given task.
▶ Tic activity increased by anxiety and stress.
▶ Tics can be suppressed temporarily.
▶ Associated with attention-deficit hyperactivity disorder and obsessive-compulsive disorder

Functional Tics

- Do not fluctuate
- Patient remembers date of onset

Secondary Tics (Tourettism)

These may be caused by

- Dopamine stimulants (levodopa) or dopamine-blocking drugs (e.g., phenothiazines), often with delayed onset after drug initiation or withdrawal—so-called *tardive Tourettism*
- Encephalitis
- Creutzfeldt-Jakob disease
- Sydenham's chorea
- Head trauma
- Stroke

Adult-Onset Tics

These tics may be late-presenting Tourette syndrome or secondary tics, as detailed earlier.
Note:

▶ *Tics with peripheral neuropathy favor CA.*

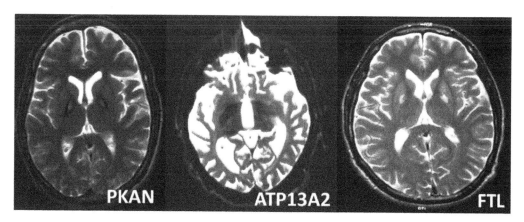

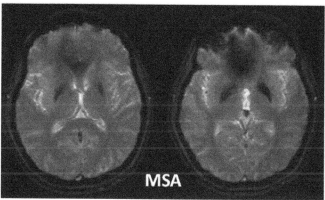

FIGURE 8.25: **Top**: Examples of brain MRI in neurodegeneration with brain iron accumulation (NBIA) disorders. **Left**: Pantothenate kinase–associated neurodegeneration (PKAN). There is a classic eye-of the-tiger sign. **Center**: Kufor-Rakeb disease due to ATP13A2 mutation. There is iron accumulation in the putamen and caudate. **Right**: Neuroferritinopathy due to FTL mutations. This shows iron deposition in the basal ganglia, with possible thalamic involvement. **Bottom**: MRI in multiple system atrophy (MSA), where iron accumulation characteristically affects the posterolateral putamina, rather than the globus pallidus, as seen in the NBIA disorders. Reproduced with permission from Schneider et al. (2012).

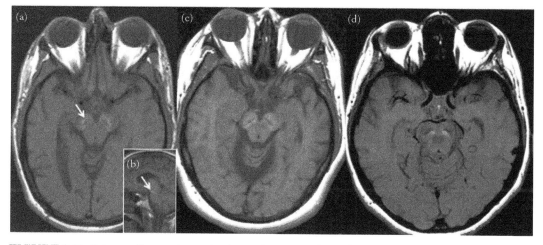

FIGURE 8.26: Beta-propeller protein-associated neurodegeneration (BPAN). MRI sequences show the halo sign in the substantia nigra (arrow), which is unique to BPAN. On T1-weighted axial imaging, substantia nigra shows a halo of hyperintense signal surrounding a thin linear region of hypointense signal on 1.5 T (**A** and sagittal view in **B** and **C**) and 3.0 T (**D**) field strength scanners. Reproduced with permission from Hayflick et al. (2013), Figure 1.

▶ *Tourette patients with severe and frequent dystonic tics of the head who develop limb weakness* may have developed:
  ○ Spondylotic cervical myelopathy with quadriparesis or:
  ○ Cervical artery dissection and stroke

RESTLESS LEGS SYNDROME AND PERIODIC MOVEMENTS OF SLEEP

RLS predominates in women. It is characterized by an irresistible urge to move the legs. Patients find it hard to describe (Video 8.71, Restless Legs).

Many individuals with RLS have a separate but related condition, periodic leg movements of sleep (PLMS). The bed partner frequently complains of being awakened by the kicking movements. In PLMS, the main movement is abrupt dorsiflexion of the ankle, but knee and hip flexion may occur, and occasionally arm muscles will jerk. In RLS, there are a variety of vague but strong sensory symptoms, typically, an irresistible urge to move that is relieved temporarily by repositioning the leg. Background causes of RLS are found rarely, but here are some:

- Iron deficiency
- Pregnancy
- Renal failure
- Peripheral neuropathy, as in diabetic polyneuropathy but not diabetes per se
◀ Neck and facial involvement does not occur in RLS.

Handles for RLS and PLMS

▶ *There is restlessness, worse in the evening, on sitting or lying down, relieved by walking.*
▶ *A worn carpet patch in front of the chair* where the patient's feet rest
▶ *A couple who have to sleep in separate beds.* Other reasons are obstructive sleep apnea and REM sleep behavior disorder.
▶ *RLS, especially in males, may be secondary to iron deficiency* from gastrointestinal bleeding, especially bowel cancer. Always check the blood count and ferritin level in RLS.
▶ *Difficulty falling asleep that worsens with hypnotics.* Most antidepressants and antihistamines (e.g., diphenhydramine) aggravate RLS (Video 8.72, Severe Restless Legs).
▶ Aggravation by alcohol, vigorous exercise in the evening, and pregnancy

Note the following related Handle:

▶ *Slow involuntary flexion/extension movements of the toes with burning/dull ache in the legs is the syndrome of painful legs and moving toes.* The disorder can usually be recognized instantly. One or both sides are affected. Identical toe movements may occur without pain, known as "painless legs–moving toes"; see Video 8.73, PLMT (courtesy Francesca Morgante), and a similar condition affects the upper limbs: "painful arms–moving fingers" (Video 8.74, Painful Arms). The pathophysiology of PLMT and its variants is not understood well.

DYSTONIA

Dystonia is characterized by sustained or intermittent muscle contractions causing abnormal, often repetitive, movements, postures, or both (see Table 8.2). Dystonic movements are typically patterned and twisting and may be tremulous. Dystonia is often made worse while moving another body part (overflow phenomenon). Many conditions that are associated with dystonia have already been discussed in this chapter.

Traditionally, it is classified as follows:

- Primary dystonia (genetic or sporadic)
- Dystonia plus, as in myoclonus dystonia
- Secondary dystonia in the aftermath of known insult
- Dystonia in heredodegenerative diseases

The primary dystonias can be focal or generalized. Patients with primary dystonias have no other neurological findings apart from tremor. The primary dystonias generally begin as action dystonia that may progress to dystonia at rest or contractures. Secondary dystonias and heredodegenerative disease often begin at rest and have features other than dystonia, such as dementia, ataxia, and spasticity. Following are some Handles:

▶ *Dystonia of rapid onset suggests*
  ○ Drug-induced
  ○ Psychogenic (Video 8.75, Psychogenic Dystonia)
  ○ Rapid-onset dystonia-parkinsonism (DYT12)
▶ *Fluctuating dystonia worse in afternoons is* DRD: DYT5.

Symbol	Gene and usual inheritance	Locus	Handles
DYT1	TOR1A AD	9q34	Childhood onset torsion dystonia. Ashkenazi Jews. Gradual generalization over 5 years
DYT2	HPCA AR	1p35	Childhood onset with slowly progressive dystonia starting in limbs then neck
DYT3	TAF1 XLR	Xq13.1	X-linked dystonia-parkinsonism (Lubag). Most from Panay in Philippines
DYT4	TUBB4 AD	19p13.3	Whispering (laryngeal) dysphonia. Onset age 10–30 years. Spread to neck and limbs. Hobby-horse gait. Repeated tongue protrusions.
DYT5	GCH1 AD	14q22.2	Dopamine-responsive dystonia. Onset 5–8 years. Symptoms worse in afternoon onward and after exercise. Often misdiagnosed as cerebral palsy/hemiplegia. Club foot and toe walking.
DYT5b	TH AR	11p15.5	Dopamine-responsive dystonia
DYT6	THAP1 AD	8p11.21	Starts in head and neck then spreads to arms and larynx
DYT7	Not known AD	18p?	Primary focal cervical dystonia, blepharospasm and writer's cramp. Rarely generalizes.
DYT8	MR1 AD	2q35	Paroxysmal nonkinesigenic dyskinesia. Trunk flexion and facial grimacing. Episodes lasting minutes–hours. Precipitated by fatigue, caffeine, and alcohol but not exercise.
DYT9	SLC2A1 AD	1p34.2	Childhood onset. Paroxysmal choreoathetosis, spasticity, or ataxia. Synonymous with DYT18.
DYT10	PRRT2 AD	16p11.2	Paroxysmal kinesigenic dyskinesia. Onset under 20 years. Precipitation by sudden movement or startle. Last 30–60 seconds up to 100 times per day. Dramatic response to anticonvulsants.
DYT11	SGCE AD	7q21.3	Myoclonic dystonia. Alcohol-responsive jerks involving arms and trunk.
DYT12	ATP1A3 AD	19q12	Rapid onset dystonia-parkinsonism or alternating hemiplegia of childhood
DYT13	Unknown. AD	1p36.32	Mild, cranio-cervical/upper limb dystonia in one Italian family. Onset in teenage years.
DYT14	GCH1 AD or AR	14q22.2	Childhood onset, dopa-responsive dystonia, with or without hyperphenylalaninemia. Pes cavus, club foot.
DYT15	Unknown AD	18p11	Myoclonus dystonia in Canadian family. Alcohol-responsive. Childhood onset
DYT16	PRKRA AR	2q31.2	Young onset dystonia-parkinsonism. Neck extension frequent.
DYT17	Unknown AR	20p11.2	One family from Lebanon. Started in teenage years with cervical dystonia then generalized.
DYT18	SLC2A1 AD	1p34.2	Paroxysmal exercise-induced dyskinesia due to glutamate 1 deficiency. Childhood onset. Triggered by fasting. Some have seizures. Very low spinal fluid glucose
DYT19	Probably PRRT2 AD	16q13	Episodic kinesigenic dyskinesia/choreoathetosis type 2. Probably synonymous with DYT10
DYT20	Unknown AD	2q31	Paroxysmal nonkinesigenic dyskinesia 2. Single Canadian family.
DYT21	Unknown AD	2q14.3	Adult-onset pure torsion dystonia
DYT23	CACNA1B AD	9q34.3	Adult-onset cervical dystonia. Arrhythmias and panic attacks in some.
DYT24	ANO3 AD	11p14.3	Cranio-cervical dystonia with prominent head tremor.

- *Dystonia with oculogyric crises—see previous discussion under "Oculogyric Crises"*
- *Dystonia–parkinsonism in a man of Philippine descent suggests Lubag.*
- *Autosomal dominant dystonia in a young Ashkenazi Jew beginning in the lower limbs is likely primary torsion dystonia.*
  A mutation in the *DYT1* gene results in a defective protein, Torsin A (Video 8.76, DYT1).
- *Autosomal dominant, adult-onset craniocervical dystonia that spreads to the limbs sometimes with dysphonia is likely DYT6 dystonia.*
  A mutation in the *DYT6* gene results in a defective protein, THAP.
- *Abrupt-onset dystonia especially in the craniocervical region suggests rapid-onset dystonia parkinsonism (RDP; DYT12 dystonia).*
  There are bulbar features. Patients may deteriorate slowly or display stuttering progression with attacks precipitated by fever.

Mutation in the *DYT12* gene (ATP1A3) is associated with alternating hemiplegia of childhood.
The same genetic defect causes cerebellar ataxia, pes cavus, optic atrophy and sensorineural hearing loss (CAPOS) syndrome

- *Foot dystonia after minor injury is probably psychogenic* (Video 8.77, Psychogenic Foot Dystonia).
- *Foot dystonia in a diabetic is likely stiff limb syndrome. This is a variant of stiff person syndrome (SPS).*
  The diagnosis is confirmed by electromyelogram (EMG) of the back muscles, which shows ongoing motor unit activity resembling voluntary activity. There is also a high titer of antibodies to glutamic acid decarboxylase (Video 8.78, Stiff Person and Video 8.41, Stiff Limb).
- *Stiff legs with horizontal lumbar creases is SPS.*
  It is associated with extensor spasms of the lumbar spine (Figure 8.27).

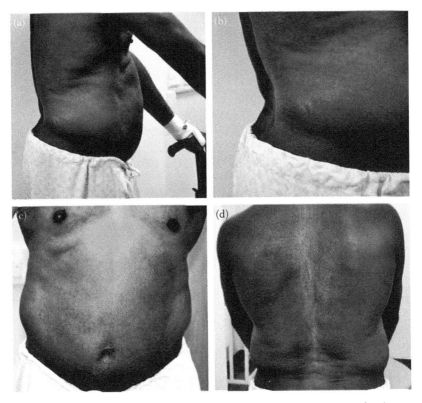

FIGURE 8.27: Postural abnormalities and examination findings in stiff person syndrome. **A** and **B** show increased lumbar lordosis. (**C**) shows coexistent contraction of abdominal muscles. (**D**) Note the skin creases in the lumbar region of the back, in keeping with exaggerated lordosis. Reproduced with permission from Hadavi et al. (2011), Figure 1.

- *Stiff person with hyperekplexia, weight loss, gastrointestinal disturbance, cognitive impairment suggest a PERM variant (progressive encephalomyelitis with rigidity and myoclonus) due to DPPX antibodies.*
- *Dystonia with jerky movements improved by alcohol suggests myoclonus dystonia.*
  The likely cause is a mutation in the sarcoglycan gene (Video 8.79, Myoclonus Dystonia). Often there is a psychiatric history and alcohol dependence.
- *Involuntary head rotation improved by one finger is cervical dystonia.*
  The finger or hand is placed on the opposite chin to correct head turning. It is remarkable that light pressure is so effective at centralizing the head. The phenomenon is called "geste antagoniste" by the French and "sensory trick" by American neurologists (Figure 8.28 and Video 8.80, Sensory Trick). This phenomenon is not limited to CD and may be seen in other dystonias (Video 8.81, Segmental Dystonia Toothpick).
- *Dystonia triggered by prolonged exercise is likely paroxysmal exertional dyskinesia.*
  - If the CSF glucose is low, this is diagnostic of GLUT-1 deficiency (DeVivo disease). See Video 8.82, Glut 1 deficiency.
  - Also consider *DRD*, or young-onset parkinsonism due to *Parkin disease.* In Parkin disease there is unsteadiness, worse in the *morning* and before meals. Conversely, the unsteadiness of DRD is worse in the *afternoon.*
- *Dystonia and ataxia in a patient with downgaze palsy is likely Niemann-Pick disease type C* (Video 8.35, Niemann Pick C).
- *Dystonia in a patient with horizontal gaze palsy is probably Gaucher's disease.* There may be myoclonus, enlargement of the liver and spleen, and pingueculae (Figure 8.10) Blood count may show a low platelet level.
- *Dystonia with SNGP, seizures, and recurrent encephalopathy may be thiamine transporter deficiency* (Ortigoza-Escobar et al. 2014).
  The MRI is highly abnormal. The condition is important to identify as it can be treated successfully with thiamine (Figure 8.29).
- *Truncal or cervical dystonia with purely extensor posturing is likely tardive dystonia* (Video 8.3, Tardive Dystonia and Video 8.83, TD Neck Extension). Prominent neck extension is also described in DYT 16 (PRKRA mutation)
- Dystonia and orofacial dyskinesia is probably tardive dystonia.
- *Dystonia with pontine facial sensory loss suggests CLIPPERS syndrome* (See Chapter 4, Demyelination). Occasionally there is parkinsonism.

Cervical Dystonia
Cervical dystonia is the most common form of adult-onset focal dystonia. It is often termed *torticollis,* but that refers to rotational movement, whereas CD may result in torticollis, laterocollis, and retrocollis. Dystonia is only one of the causes of abnormal neck position. Cervical dystonia often begins gradually, and there are jerky or slower movements, tremors, and frequently a sensory trick. (Video 8.80, cervical dystonia Sensory Trick).
- *Abrupt onset of a fixed neck posture suggests non-dystonic torticollis.*

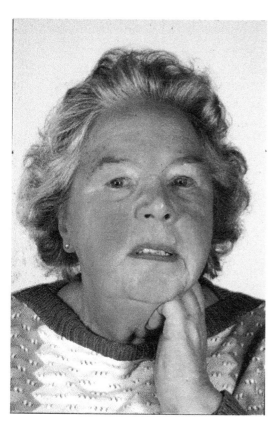

FIGURE 8.28: Cervical dystonia showing the geste antagoniste or sensory trick used to overcome the head turn. There was marked hypertrophy of the right sternomastoid muscle in keeping with this variety of dystonia.

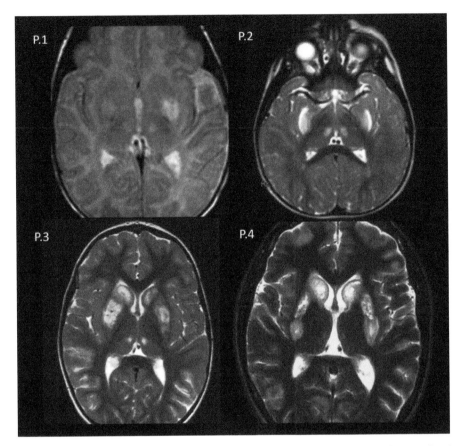

FIGURE 8.29: MRI axial T2 images in four patients (P.1–P.4) with thiamine transporter deficiency. This shows bilateral symmetric involvement of the putamina and medial thalamic nuclei. The head of the caudate is involved in all but Patient 1. Reproduced under the terms of the Creative Commons Attribution License from Ortigoza-Escobar, Serrano, Molero, Oyarzabal, Rebollo, Muchart, Artuch, Rodriguez-Pombo, and Perez-Duenas (2014), Figure 1.

There is no sensory trick. The causes are as follows:

- Congenital wry neck (Figure 8.30)
- Atlanto-axial dislocation; see Video 8.84, Atlanto-axial (courtesy Cindy Comella)
- Acute cervical disc prolapse
- Acute infections: cervical lymphadenitis, retropharyngeal abscess
- Cephalic tetanus; see Video 8.85, Tetanus (courtesy Beom S. Jeon)
- Trochlear nerve palsy; see Video 8.86, Bielschowsky Sign (courtesy Michael Rivner)
- Muscle fibrosis following surgical trauma or radiation

Several disorders may be confused with dystonia on the basis of abnormal posture. Disorders that simulate dystonia (pseudo-dystonia) include:

- Bent spine, camptocormia, scoliosis
- Dupuytren's contracture
- Trigger finger

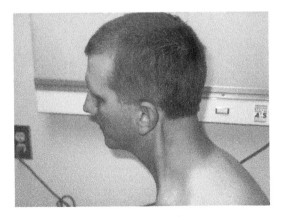

FIGURE 8.30: Congenital wry neck.

- Tetany
- Orthopedic and rheumatological conditions causing joint deformities
- Sandifer syndrome: a disorder during childhood in which there are abnormal neck postures related to gastric reflux; see Video 8.87 (courtesy Francesca Morgante)
- Deafferentation (pseudoathetosis). (See Video 4.1)
- Isaac syndrome (see Chapter 7, Myopathy and Motor Neuron Disorders)
- Satoyoshi syndrome. This is characterized by alopecia, diarrhea, cramps, and fixed postures (see Figure 8.37).
- Hemi-masticatory spasm. This affects the jaw muscles on one side, similar to hemifacial spasm.

Lesch-Nyhan Syndrome

The main clues for this rare X-linked disorder are the following:

▶ *Male with chorea and dystonic movements since childhood*; see Video 8.88, Lesch-Nyhan (courtesy L. N. Ghosh)

▶ *Self-injury or mutilation* (Figure 8.31); poking a finger in the eye

▶ *Fencer's posture due to dystonic spasm.* Similar to that seen in partial seizures.

▶ *Handcuffs or similar restraints to prevent self-harm*

▶ History of urate stones or gout

▶ Megaloblastic anemia

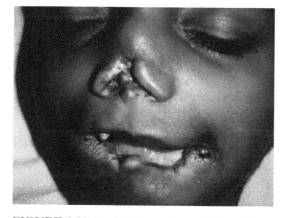

FIGURE 8.31: Lesch-Nyhan syndrome. Self-mutilation is typical of this disorder. Reproduced from Figure 1 with permission by Maramattom (2005).

CHARACTERISTIC GAIT DISORDERS

▶ Dancing or bobbing gait is likely the crack dance of a cocaine addict.

This usually accompanies a "high" induced by cocaine (see YouTube video link: http://www.youtube.com/watch?v=c1Wg0erGQNI) and related to excess brain levels of noradrenaline, dopamine, and serotonin. A variety of movement disorders occur among cocaine addicts, including dystonia, parkinsonism, and chorea.

▶ Hobby horse gait suggests DYT4 syndrome.

This is a primary dystonia due to *TUBB4a* mutation. The disorder causes a whispering dysphonia that may become generalized with a characteristic hobby-horse gait, as seen on Video 8.89, Hobby-Horse Gait (courtesy Robert Wilcox). A mutation in *TUBB4* gene also results in hypomyelination, atrophy of basal ganglia and cerebellum (H-ABC) syndrome.

▶ Walking on tip-toe is likely the cock-gait of manganese poisoning or manganese transporter mutation.

It is highly characteristic; see Video 8.90, Cock-Walk Gait (courtesy Orlando Barsottini). Distinguish this from toe-walking, where there is slight plantar flexion/inversion and the toes are dragged across the floor. Excess manganese exposure is seen in the following:

○ Drug abuse such as ephedrone (due to potassium permanganate used in preparation)

○ Exposure at the workplace (e.g., miners, welders, and smelters)

○ Liver cirrhosis

○ Hyperalimentation

○ Hereditary hemorrhagic telangiectasia (due to arteriovenous shunting)

○ Manganese transporter receptor mutation. Note that there is no exogenous excess of manganese. There may be cirrhosis of the liver and polycythemia. To verify the diagnosis, apart from measurement of blood manganese, the MRI scan shows a characteristic high signal in the globus pallidus and occasionally other basal ganglia and the pituitary gland on a T1-weighted sequence

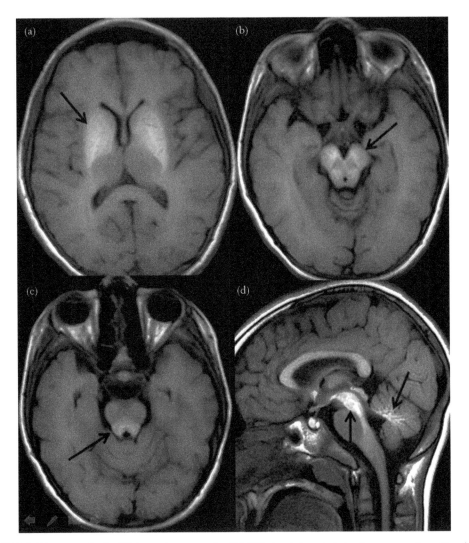

FIGURE 8.32: T1-weighted MRI shows the increased pallidal T1 signal characteristic of manganese deposition (arrow). In addition, there is an increased signal in other basal ganglia the pituitary gland and brainstem.   Courtesy Orlando Barsottini.

(Figure 8.32). The same abnormalities are seen in other causes of manganism

Toe Walking Without Ataxia

Consider the following:

▶ *Lower limb dystonia (especially dopamine-responsive dystonia)*
▶ *Hereditary spastic paraplegia*
▶ *Autism spectrum disorder*
▶ *Angelman syndrome (formerly "happy-puppet" syndrome; see Figure 8.33 and Video 6.1, Angelman.* In the classic form the child has the following:
   ○ Occasionally a prancing gait

   ○ Red or blonde hair (usually). Laughs frequently and flaps the hands
   ○ Seizures
   ○ Microcephaly and speech impairment
   ○ Tongue thrusting and a fascination with water.
   ○ Cri du chat syndrome is somewhat similar.
▶ *Duchenne muscular dystrophy*

PAROXYSMAL DYSKINESIAS

This heterogeneous group of disorders is characterized by sudden abnormal involuntary movements superimposed on normal motor behavior. The abnormal movements comprise the following either

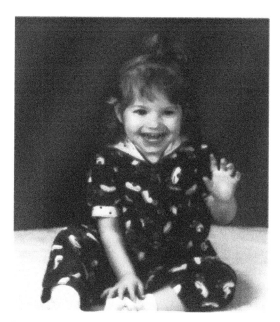

FIGURE 8.33: Angelman's syndrome. Note her happy face. Not all are blondes! The hands are flapped frequently. Reproduced with permission from Franz et al. (2000).

singly or in combination: ballism, dystonia, chorea, and athetosis.

There are five varieties. Note that *kinesigenic* means "induced by movement."

Paroxysmal Kinesigenic Dyskinesia (PKD)

See Video 8.91, PKD (courtesy Cindy Comella). These are the main features:

- *Age under 20 years*
- *Precipitated by sudden movement or startle*
- *Short duration and frequent, from 30–60 seconds, up to 100 times per day*
- *No pain or loss of consciousness*
- *Dramatic response to low-dose anticonvulsants*
- *Normal interictal examination in primary cases*

Paroxysmal Nonkinesigenic Dyskinesia (PNKD)

See Video 8.92, PNKD.

- *Occurs at rest*
- *Precipitated by fatigue, coffee, and alcohol*
- *Episodes last minutes to hours but attacks are not as frequent as PKD.*
- *Poor response to anticonvulsants*

Paroxysmal Exertion-Induced Dyskinesia (PED)

See Video 8.93, PED.

- *Occurs with prolonged exercise, instead of sudden movements* (Video 8.93, PED)
- *Familial or sporadic of unknown cause*
- *Associated with dopa-responsive dystonia or young-onset PD, such as Parkin mutation*
- *Associated with GLUT-1 deficiency; see Video 8.82, GLUT-1 Deficiency (courtesy Katya Koshet)*

Paroxysmal Hypnogenic Dyskinesia (PHD)

Most cases of "dystonic" episodes during sleep are due to nocturnal frontal lobe epilepsy. Daytime attacks with loss of consciousness are also recognized. Rarely, PHD may represent a paroxysmal dyskinesia.

- *Associated with insulinoma, therefore important to identify*
- *Night time attacks occur in patients with ADCY 5 mutation*
- *Patients with GABA-T mutation have attacks accompanied by drowsiness*

Secondary Paroxysmal Dyskinesia

Most cases are due to demyelinating disease (Video 8.94, Demyelinating). They are also called *tonic spasms* and often precipitated by brief hyperventilation.

Rarely, this type is associated with the following:

- *Stroke: usually a lacune in the putamen (Video 8.95, Stroke PKD); transient ischemic attack (TIA) may manifest as a paroxysmal dystonia. In some the distal field of the carotid artery involves the basal ganglia, and these attacks may herald a stroke (Hess et al. 1991).*
- *Basal ganglia calcification often with hypoparathyroidism*
- *Hypoglycemia*
- *Head trauma (Video 8.96, Head trauma PKD)*
- *Very often psychogenic disorders (Video 8.97, Psychogenic PKD)*

Handles for Paroxysmal Dyskinesias

▶ *Onset in childhood is more likely primary, sporadic, or inherited.*
   ○ *Onset in adulthood is more likely secondary.*

o *Pain during paroxysmal dyskinesia or pre-cipitation by brief hyperventilation suggests secondary paroxysmal dyskinesia due to demyelinating disease* (tonic spasms; Video 8.94, Demyelinating), trauma (Video 8.96, Head Trauma PKD), or functional disorder.

▶ *Precipitated by coffee and alcohol suggests paroxysmal nonkinesigenic dyskinesia. Older age onset favors vascular paroxysmal dyskinesia—TIA or a stroke* (Video 8.95, Stroke PKD).

▶ In a diabetic patient, paroxysmal dyskinesia may indicate hypoglycemia.

▶ *Paroxysmal dyskinesia precipitated by standing is likely orthostatic paroxysmal dystonia* due to severe bilateral carotid disease (Video 8.98, Orthostatic PD) (Sethi et al. 2002).

▶ *Unusual precipitants such as vibration, touch, or bright light, point to psychogenic paroxysmal dyskinesia* (Video 8.97, Psychogenic PKD).

▶ *Clusters of paroxysmal dyskinesia in early morning hours with polyneuropathy suggest insulinoma.*

STEREOTYPIES

A *stereotypy* is a repetitive or ritualistic movement, posture, or utterance. The movements may be simple, as in body rocking, or complex, such as self-caressing, crossing and uncrossing of legs, and marching on the spot. Unlike tics, there is no buildup of inner tension that is relieved subsequently by movement.

Causes of stereotypies include the following:

- Autism spectrum disorder
- A child, usually female, with stereotypic episodes of leg-crossing, rocking, and no distress is probably self-stimulating for pleasure.
- Intellectual disability
- Psychosis (Video 8.99, Schizophrenia)
- Catatonia (Video 8.100, Catatonia)
- N-methyl-D-aspartate (NMDA) receptor antibody–mediated encephalitis. This important condition is treatable once recognized. The majority of those affected are women who develop psychiatric problems, encephalopathy, seizures, stereotypies, and autonomic disturbances. Most have an underlying ovarian teratoma (Video 8.101, NMDA). In adult males, the underlying tumor is usually a testicular teratoma. The disorder may also occur in children after an infection; see Video 8.102, Postinfectious NMDA (courtesy

Jeff Blackie). The movement disorders seen in NMDAR encephalitis is often complex ranging from stereotypy to dystonia and bizarre posturing reminiscent of catatonia.

MISCELLANEOUS HANDLES FOR MOVEMENT DISORDERS

▶ *Lentiform fork sign*
This is a recently reported MRI feature that may be detected on axial fluid-attenuated inversion recovery (FLAIR) sequences. It has been associated with fluctuating parkinsonism and uremia (Fabiani et al. 2013), but the underlying feature is probably metabolic acidosis (Figure 8.34).

▶ *Basal ganglia calcification*
This is sometimes found by chance in healthy people and confined usually to the pallidum. In general, MRI is not useful for imaging calcification and may cause more confusion than guidance. If it is more widespread and associated with mild parkinsonism, it is usually called *Fahr's syndrome* (Figure 8.35). Other causes include the following:

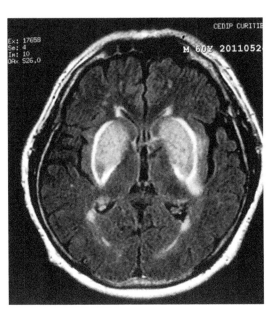

FIGURE 8.34: Lentiform fork sign seen on axial MRI FLAIR sequence. Here it was associated with fluctuating, reversible parkinsonism in a patient with uremic encephalopathy. Reproduced from Fabiani, Teive, and Munhoz (2013).

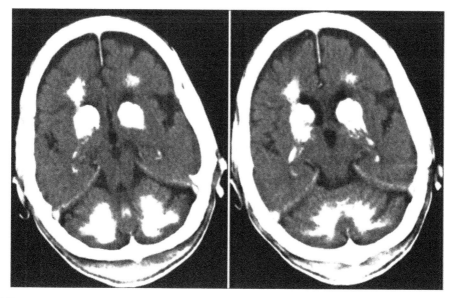

FIGURE 8.35: Fahr's syndrome. Unenhanced CT scan at the level of midbrain showing multiple bilaterally symmetrical calcified lesions in the basal ganglia, thalami, and white matter of cerebellar hemispheres.

- o Hypoparathyroidism and pseudo-hypoparathyroidism
- o Metabolic and infectious disorders
- o Cockayne syndrome, tuberous sclerosis, and Down syndrome
- o Mitochondrial disease
▶ *Repeated tongue protrusion*
This feature is found in:
- o Tardive dyskinesia/dystonia (most common)
- o Chorea-acanthocytosis
- o Angelman's syndrome
- o Lesch-Nyhan syndrome
- o NBIA1
- o Whispering dysphonia (Video 8.89, Hobby-Horse Gait).
- o Chorea and any severe cerebellar condition

The protrusion in tardive dyskinesia is not tremulous. Compare this to the "trombone tongue," which is tremulous and a classic sign of tertiary syphilis.

▶ *Child who adopts strange postures of head and trunk after eating*
This is Sandifer's syndrome and it responds to treatment for gastroesophageal reflux. It very rarely occurs in adults; see Video 8.87, Sandifer (courtesy Francesca Morgante).
▶ *Psychotic patient with dystonic movements*

The major causes are as follows:
- o Tardive dystonia
- o Wilson's disease
- o Recreational drug abuse, including use of ephedrone (especially in Eastern Europe and Russia)
▶ *Child with head tremors*
There are two main possibilities:
- o Spasmus nutans
This is a 3–4 Hz head movement of infants, in either vertical or horizontal planes, in association with a head tilt. There may be a shimmering-type pendular nystagmus and amblyopia. It is usually benign, with onset in the first year of life, resolving before the age of 8 years. Rarely, it signals a tumor of the anterior visual pathway; thus, imaging is essential; see Video 8.103, Spasmus Nutans (courtesy David Zee).
- o Another rhythmic movement affecting the head in children is *bobble-head doll syndrome* (due to an arachnoid cyst in the third ventricular area (Figure 8.36 and Video 8.104, Bobble Head)
▶ *Girl with galactorrhea*
If the condition is not related to medication or sarcoidosis, the likely diagnosis is *tyrosine hydroxylase deficiency*. The blood prolactin level will be raised.

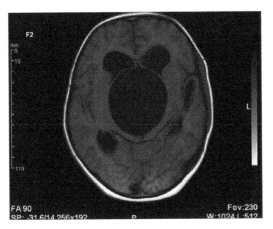

FIGURE 8.36: Bobble-head doll syndrome. T1-weighted axial MRI brain scan showing a cystic lesion in the suprasellar region causing obstructive hydrocephalus. Reproduced with permission from Reddy, Gafoor, Suresh, and Prasad (2014), Figure 1.

Handles for Abnormal Head Movement

▶ *Horizontal rhythmical tremor: ET but always in association with hand tremor*

▶ *Vertical rhythmical tremor: dystonia or titubation*

▶ *Jerky head movement in any direction: cervical dystonia*

▶ *Slow nodding head movement: Nodding disease. Found mainly in Africa (Sudan and Uganda)*

▶ *Doll-like*: bobble-head doll syndrome. See Video 8.104, Bobble-Head, and Figure 8.36. The movements are multidirectional, hence the name, but mostly in the vertical plane. The syndrome is associated with large cystic lesions of the third ventricle region.

▶ *Rocking: self-stimulation in autism*

▶ *Spasmus nutans (see preceding section)*

▶ *Figure-of-eight head movement* (see Chapter 6: Video 6.7, RES and video 6.8 Ohtahara).

This unusual but characteristic head movement is seen in two main disorders: Ohtahara syndrome (usually caused by mutation in STXBP1 gene) and rhombo-encephalo-synapsis (developmental). The head is moved involuntarily in a figure-of-eight. There is always epilepsy and developmental delay.

PSYCHOGENIC/ FUNCTIONAL MOVEMENT DISORDERS

See also discussion in Chapter 3. This is a dangerous area for the novice clinician. Do not forget that until some 50 years ago cervical dystonia and blepharospasm were labeled "psychogenic" by many experts, and it was commonplace for psychiatrists to care for these patients. Pioneering studies by the late David Marsden made it clear that many cases of apparent psychogenic movement were forms of dystonia.

It is often said that a diagnosis of psychogenic movement disorder should be made only by a doctor over the age of 40 in a patient under the age of 40!

Following is a summary of some of the major Handles.

Handles in History

▶ *Abrupt onset—at least according to the patient, who appears to cope well*

▶ *Excessively concerned family members. More than three present in consulting room.*

▶ *The overfriendly patient*

▶ *Over-idolization of the physician followed by rapid devaluation*

▶ *Junior doctors express extreme urgency to see patient.*

▶ *Static course with spontaneous remissions*

▶ *History of psychiatric disorders or multiple somatizations*

▶ *Employed in the health professions*

▶ *Pending litigation or compensation*

▶ Young age and history of childhood abuse

Handles on Examination

▶ *Use of dark glasses indoors* (Video 8.97, Psychogenic PKD)

▶ *Adult clutching a teddy bear*

▶ *Wearing bunny or large animal slippers*; inappropriate undergarments

▶ *Effortful or sighing response* during neurologic examination ("huffing and puffing" sign)

▶ *Adult living with parents.*

▶ *Entrainment* (i.e., synchronization) of tremor

To elicit this, ask patients to make a rhythmical movement with their normal hand. The frequency of the normal side will synchronize with the "abnormal" side. Sometimes the abnormal tremor disappears.

▶ *Ability to trigger or relieve the abnormal movements* with unusual or nonphysiological interventions (e.g., trigger points of the body, tuning fork, tendon jerk elicitation)

▶ *Photosensitivity* (Video 8.97, Psychogenic PKD)

▶ *Pauses in tremor.* If there is, for example, a unilateral postural tremor, it is helpful to distract the patient's attention with another task. Thus, while the arms are outstretched, ask the patient to perform the finger–nose test with the normal side. This may result in reduction of the tremor while the test of coordination is in progress. Alternatively, ask the patient to perform simple mental arithmetic with the arms at rest or outstretched, and, once more, there may be improvement in the tremor. Note that, with movement or muscle contraction, the tremor of genuine PD may stop briefly.

▶ *Variability.* The tremor frequency and amplitude change according to the level of attention perceived by the patient.

▶ *Spread of movement.* If the affected body part is restrained, the tremor spreads elsewhere (Video 8.105, Psychogenic Spread).

▶ *False and painful weakness*

▶ *False sensory complaints*

▶ *Self-inflected injuries*

▶ *Deliberate slowness of movements* (Video 8.106, Psychogenic Slow)

▶ *Functional disability out of proportion to examination findings*

▶ *Abnormal movements that are bizarre, variable, multiple, or difficult to classify* (Video 8.107, Psychogenic multiple)

▶ *The weak leg is lifted up* when getting off couch in genuine weakness.

Therapeutic Responses

▶ *Unresponsive to appropriate medications*

▶ *Response to placebos*

▶ *Remission with psychotherapy*

MYOCLONUS

Myoclonus refers to rapid muscle jerks, either irregular or rhythmic, but they are always simple.

- It is caused by sudden muscle contraction (positive myoclonus) or brief lapses of contraction (negative myoclonus).
- It only affects voluntary muscle.
- Precipitation is by a stimulus (visual, tactile, auditory or movement), which distinguishes myoclonus form a choreic jerk or a tic.

Following are some Handles:

▶ *Myoclonus plus renal failure suggests the action myoclonus renal failure syndrome.*

▶ *Myoclonus with ataxia is likely a mitochondrial disorder, celiac disease, or Prickle1 mutation.*

▶ *Myoclonus with seizures*
  ○ Neuronal ceroid lipofuscinoses (Batten's disease)
  ○ Unverricht-Lundberg syndrome (Baltic myoclonus)
  ○ Sialidosis type 1
  ○ Lafora body disease
  ○ Mitochondrial disease such as MERRF (myoclonus epilepsy and ragged red fibers)
  ○ DRPLA (dentato-rubro-pallido-luysian atrophy; see earlier discussion)
  ○ North Sea progressive myoclonus epilepsy

▶ *Myoclonus with opsoclonus.* This may be paraneoplastic or postinfectious (Video 8.108, Opsoclonus-Myoclonus). Other causes include HIV and toxic/metabolic insults. Also seen in NMDAR encephalitis.

▶ *Hung-up jerks suggests subacute sclerosing panencephalitis;* see Video 8.109, SSPE (courtesy Manoj Goyal and Vivek Lal). There may be chronic chorio-retinitis and optic atrophy

▶ Facial myoclonus, hypotonia, and paroxysmal dyskinesia induced by drowsiness suggests the ADCY 5 mutation.

▶ Rapidly progressive myoclonus with dementia suggests Creutzfeldt-Jakob disease

▶ Slowly progressive dementia with myoclonus suggests Alzheimer's disease.

▶ Myoclonus plus parkinsonism suggests MSA or CBS.

▶ Action and intention myoclonus plus falls due to negative myoclonus after anoxic brain damage (usually respiratory arrest) is posthypoxic myoclonus (Lance Adams syndrome). This is often diagnosed erroneously as psychogenic (Video 8.110).

▶ Repetitive cortical myoclonus in a single body part (mostly face and hand) is epilepsia partialis continua (EPC).

▶ In EPC, the surface EEG can be normal and may disappear during sleep (see Video 6.12, EPC).

▶ Multifocal myoclonus (positive and negative) suggests a toxic metabolic encephalopathy. Note: Focal myoclonus includes palatal myoclonus (tremor) and spinal myoclonus.

▶ Essential (isolated) palatal tremor is nearly always functional.

▶ Propriospinal myoclonus is often functional in origin.

CHECKLIST FOR MOVEMENT DISORDERS WITH

1. Hematological Disorder

This is a rare combination, but the following Handles may be helpful

▶ *Anemia*
If due to iron deficiency think of RLS. Megaloblastic anemia occurs in Lesch-Nyhan syndrome. Vitamin B_{12} deficiency usually associated with megaloblasts causes sensory dystonia (pseudoathetosis).

▶ *Low platelet count and dystonia is likely Wilson's disease or Niemann-Pick type C.*

▶ *Polycythemia and dystonia in a child, sometimes with "cock-walk" gait, suggests manganesemia (manganese transporter receptor mutation).*

▶ *Acanthocytes with:*
  o Tics, sudden episodes of head flexion, or facio-bucco-linguo-masticatory movement suggest neuroacanthocytosis.
  o Chorea favors chorea-acanthocytosis or McLeod's syndrome.
  o Early-onset parkinsonism suggests HARP (hypo-prebetalipoproteinemia, acanthocytes, and retinitis pigmentosa). Note that HARP is allelic with NBIA1.
  o Ataxia is abeta-lipoproteinemia.

▶ *Prolonged bleeding time, giant white cell inclusions, parkinsonism, and depigmented skin or iris favors the Chediak-Higashi syndrome* (Figure 8.9 and Video 8.27, Chediak-Higashi).

▶ *Hemolysis:* GLUT-1 deficiency, which may be associated with paroxysmal exertional dyskinesia. Wilson's disease. Phosphoglycerate kinase deficiency is associated with fluctuating parkinsonism.

▶ *Pancytopenia:* Niemann-Pick type C and Gaucher's disease (often with hepatosplenomegaly)

▶ *Abnormal blood ferritin:* high serum ferritin and iron suggests aceruloplasminemia. Low ferritin favors neuroferritinopathy.

▶ *Copper.* Low blood copper and ceruloplasmin with high urine copper suggests Wilson's disease.

2. Optic Atrophy

▶ *PLA2G6-associated neurodegeneration (PLAN), mitochondrial membrane-associated neurodegeneration (MPAN), and fatty acid hydroxylase-associated neurodegeneration (FAHN)*

▶ *Aceruloplasminemia*

3. Retinitis Pigmentosa

▶ *With anosmia: Refsum's disease*

▶ *With cerebellar signs:*
  o SCA7 (spinocerebellar atrophy type 7)
  o AVED (ataxia with vitamin E deficiency)
  o PHARC (polyneuropathy, hearing loss, ataxia, retinitis pigmentosa, and cataract)
  o Abetalipoproteinemia (Bassen-Kornzweig syndrome)
  o Joubert's syndrome and Kearns-Sayre syndrome

▶ *With predominant dystonia:*
  o PKAN (pantothenate kinase–associated neurodegeneration)
  o HARP (hypoprebetalipoproteinemia, acanthocytosis, retinitis pigmentosa, and pallidal degeneration)
  o Mitochondrial disease: NARP (neuropathy, ataxia, and retinitis pigmentosa)

4. Deafness

▶ *Mitochondrial diseases,* including deafness-dystonia-optic neuronopathy syndrome (Mohr Tranebjaerg syndrome)

▶ *Superficial siderosis;* also have ataxia, myelopathy and anosmia.

▶ *Kernicterus*. Diagnosis may be delayed until childhood.
▶ *DRPLA*
▶ *Niemann-Pick disease type C*
▶ *Woodhouse-Sakati syndrome (Figure 8.38)*

5. Diabetes Mellitus

▶ *Hyperglycemic chorea*
▶ *Stiff person syndrome (with GAD antibodies)*
▶ *Aceruloplasminemia*
▶ *Woodhouse-Sakati syndrome*
▶ *Satoyoshi syndrome (Figure 8.37)*

6. Diarrhea

▶ *Satoyoshi syndrome*
▶ *Cerebrotendinous xanthomatosis*
▶ *AVED*
▶ *Whipple's disease*
▶ *Refsum's disease*
▶ *DPPX antibody syndrome*

7. Ovarian Dysfunction or Amenorrhea

▶ *Fragile X syndrome in females*, with premature ovarian failure
▶ *Wilson's disease:* secondary amenorrhea
▶ *Ovarian cancer:* with opsoclonus myoclonus syndrome and ataxia
▶ *POLG mutation:* primary gonadal failure
▶ *NMDA receptor encephalitis with ovarian teratoma*
▶ *Patients with psychogenic movement disorders may have undergone oophorectomy.*

8. Dysautonomia

▶ *Multiple system atrophy*
▶ *Fragile-X tremor ataxia syndrome*
▶ *Aromatic l-amino acid decarboxylase deficiency (AADC)*. This is one cause of dopamine-responsive dystonia.
▶ *Diffuse Lewy body disease*
▶ *PD*
▶ *Pure autonomic failure*
▶ *Neuroleptic malignant syndrome, malignant hyperthermia*
▶ *NMDA receptor antibody–mediated encephalitis*

9. Respiratory Problems

▶ *PD as levodopa wears off and MSA (laryngeal stridor)*
▶ *Tardive dyskinesia*

▶ *Leigh's disease (dystonia and ataxia)*
▶ *Perry syndrome (hypoventilation and parkinsonism)*
▶ *Chronic obstructive pulmonary disease with asterixis and drop attacks*
▶ *Psychogenic*
▶ *Rett syndrome*

10. Oculomotor apraxia

▶ *Ataxia telangiectasia (AT)*
▶ *AT-like disorder*
▶ *AOA 1 and 2*

11. Alopecia

▶ *Satoyoshi syndrome*: childhood-onset muscle spasms, fixed postures, alopecia, diarrhea, and amenorrhea (Figure 8.37)
▶ *Woodhouse-Sakati syndrome* (hypogonadism, alopecia, diabetes mellitus, deafness, intellectual disability, and extrapyramidal signs) (Figure 8.38)
▶ *Systemic lupus erythematosus*
▶ *CARASIL (cerebral autosomal recessive arteriopathy with subcortical infarcts and leukoencephalopathy)*. See Figure 9.30.

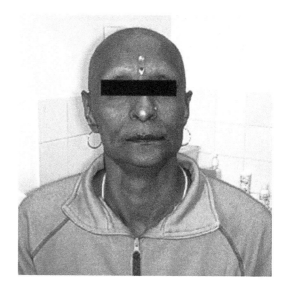

FIGURE 8.37: Patient with Satoyoshi syndrome showing alopecia affecting the hair and eyebrows. The patient experienced painful muscle spasms, diarrhea, and dry eyes and mouth. Reproduced with permission from Asherson et al. (2008) License: 3455910949958.

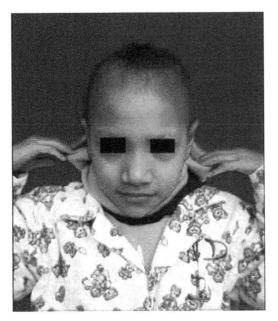

FIGURE 8.38: Woodhouse-Sakati syndrome in an 11-year-old girl. Reproduced from Aranda et al. (2008).

This is the recessive variant of CADASIL. Apart from alopecia there is dementia, lumbar spondylosis, and extrapyramidal signs.

12. Supranuclear Gaze Palsy
In a Young Person
▶ *Niemann-Pick disease type C.* There is vertical gaze palsy, mainly for downgaze. Apart from cerebellar signs there are also seizures, cataplexy, limb dystonia, and deafness. Platelet count may be low.
▶ *Gaucher's disease.* Adult onset with parkinsonism. Gaze palsy is horizontal.
▶ *Thiamine transporter deficiency.* A treatable disorder that causes generalized dystonia and seizures.
▶ *Spinocerebellar ataxia type 2 (SCA 2)*

In an Older Person
▶ *Progressive supranuclear palsy*
▶ *Corticobasal syndrome*
▶ *Multiple system atrophy*
▶ *Dementia with Lewy bodies*
▶ *Vascular disease with multiple lacunes resulting in supranuclear gaze palsy and parkinsonism*
▶ *Frontotemporal dementia syndromes*
▶ *Perry syndrome*

▶ *Paraneoplastic (anti MA 2 encephalitis)*
▶ *Infiltrative disorders such as primary CNS lymphoma or gliomatosis cerebri*

In Either Young or Old
▶ *Creutzfeldt-Jacob disease*
▶ *Kufor-Rakeb syndrome*
▶ *Wernicke's encephalopathy*; cute onset with ataxia
▶ *SCA 2*
▶ *POLG mutation*

13. Alcohol Responsiveness
Some patients discover that their involuntary movement is lessened by drinking alcohol in modest amounts. The two main conditions are:

▶ *Essential tremor*
▶ *Myoclonus dystonia with "lightning jerks"*

SUMMARY

Parkinson's Disease

Handles in History
▶ Prodromal/early features: impaired sense of smell, RBD, weight gain, constipation and depression. Repeated stopping of a self-winding watch. Unexplained frozen shoulder or low back pain.
▶ Proximal pain and stiffness may be polymyalgia rheumatica
▶ Carpal tunnel syndrome followed by tremor or stiffness
▶ Progressive deterioration of handwriting
▶ Difficulty swimming in a straight line
▶ Unable to talk and walk simultaneously heralds onset of falls.
▶ Chest or abdominal pain while receiving levodopa that mystifies the cardiologist and gastroenterologist. "Off" phenomenon or intercostal dystonia.
▶ Difficulty walking but not cycling
▶ Paradoxical kinesis
▶ Walking backward easier than forward
▶ Levodopa-induced dyskinesias usually indicate classic PD pathology, occasionally MSA.

Red Flags in History
◀ Early severe orthostatic drop in blood pressure and severe constipation: MSA

◄ Early cognitive impairment, hallucinations, and medication sensitivity: Lewy body disease (extracampine hallucinations)

◄ Falls in early stage of disease: PSP or MSA

◄ Marked asymmetry, apraxia or sensory loss: CBS

◄ Supranuclear gaze palsy: PSP

◄ Unexplained breathlessness in treated patients: off-stage phenomenon, dopa-induced dyskinesia, ergot dopamine agonist. Stridor suggests MSA. Hypoventilation: Perry's syndrome

◄ Parkinsonism and seizures. Causes: structural lesions, Creutzfeld-Jacob disease, frontotemporal dementia, adult Gaucher's disease, hypoparathyroidism with or without cerebral calcifications, *POLG* mutations, Niemann Pick disease type C

◄ Child or young adult with parkinsonism and OGC does not have classic PD. Think of phenothiazine reaction, post-encephalitic PD, Tourette syndrome, dopa-responsive dystonia, tyrosine hydroxylase deficiency, sepiapterin reductase deficiency, aromatic l-amino acid decarboxylase deficiency, dopamine transporter deficiency syndrome, Kufor-Rakeb disease.

Handles and Red Flags on Examination

▶ Re-emergent tremor, fatigue on repeated movement, rapid small-excursion opposition of thumb and index finger *without* fatigue suggests PSP; mirror movements.

◄ Camptocormia in advanced stage (Red Flag if in early phase)

Red Flags on Examination

◄ Early-onset camptocormia may signify MSA, off-period stage, myopathy, axial dystonia, psychogenic, drug reaction

◄ Strictly unilateral rest tremor that remains unilateral for more than 3 years may be dystonic tremor.

◄ Pisa syndrome

◄ A patient with head tremor probably does not have classic PD.

◄ Irregular rest tremor affecting mainly an extended thumb: dystonic tremor (SWEDD)

◄ A patient with alleged PD who is chair-bound within 5 years of onset does not have classic PD. More likely it is PSP or MSA.

◄ Disproportionate antecollis within 5 years of symptom onset is more likely "off" phenomenon, dopamine agonist withdrawal, dropped head syndrome, PSP, or MSA. Can be due to myopathy, ALS, or myasthenia.

◄ Apparent PD with symmetric rigidity but no tremor: PSP or MSA

◄ Lower body parkinsonism: gait ignition failure; usually vascular parkinsonism

◄ Early gait freezing may be PSP or vascular parkinsonism.

◄ Apparent classic PD with normal smell sense: consider essential tremor, vascular parkinsonism, corticobasal syndrome, progressive supranuclear palsy, MSA.

◄ Parkinsonism in a current smoker is unlikely to be classic PD.

◄ Parkinsonism with cataracts: hypoparathyroidism and pseudohypoparathyroidism, Fahr's syndrome, galactosemia (in children), mitochondrial disorder, Wilson's disease (sunflower cataract), cerebrotendinous xanthomatosis, dystrophia myotonica

◄ Parkinsonism with progressive external ophthalmoplegia: *POLG* or *TWINKLE* mutations

◄ Parkinsonian gait with dementia and incontinence: normal-pressure hydrocephalus, adult polyglucosan body disease (with polyneuropathy)

◄ Parkinsonism with patchy skin/iris depigmentation, susceptibility to infection and giant white cell inclusions: Chediak-Higashi syndrome

◄ Jewish patient with parkinsonism and pingueculae: Gaucher's disease type 1

◄ Parkinsonism with fainting early in the disease course

◄ Parkinsonism with hallucinations and delusions in the absence of dopaminergic drugs: dementia with Lewy bodies.

◄ Parkinsonism and orofacial dystonia in a person of Filipino descent: X-linked dystonia parkinsonism (DYT3, Lubag)

◄ Parkinsonism with orofacial dyskinesia in the absence of levodopa suggests parkinsonism induced by dopamine-blocking agents.

◄ Parkinsonism with a family fistory of dementia may be frontotemporal lobar degeneration (a taupathy).

◄ Parkinsonism of rapid onset: dopamine-blocking agents, illicit drugs (MPTP, manganese, or methcathinone), prion disease, CNS lymphoma or CNS infections, rapid-onset dystonia parkinsonism (DYT12), vascular and psychogenic parkinsonism

◀ Subacute parkinsonism and cognitive impairment: dural arteriovenous fistula.
◀ Parkinsonism in a patient with HIV favors CNS opportunistic infection or HIV encephalopathy.
◀ Parkinsonism in a boxer or a retired athlete is chronic traumatic encephalopathy.
◀ Parkinsonism in a patient with cleft lip and/or palate, conotruncal heart defects, ear anomalies, and characteristic facial features such as a prominent nasal bridge: DiGeorge syndrome (22q11 deletion syndrome)
◀ Unexplained worsening of tremor (rest and postural) in PD suggests onset of thyrotoxicosis.
◀ Mimics of classic PD: drug-induced: all phenothiazines, sodium valproate, most antipsychotics, dopamine depleters, antiemetics (metoclopramide, levosulpiride), calcium channel blockers (flunarizine, cinnarizine)

Progressive Supranuclear Palsy
Main Features

- Supranuclear abnormalities of vertical gaze (usually downward) Relatively rapid, progressive gait disorder, falls (typically backward) and difficulty looking downward
- Cognitive decline and apathy; square-wave jerks. Common but not specific
- Progressive symmetric mainly axial rigidity with little or no tremor
- Poor response to levodopa; no levodopa-induced dyskinesia
- Spontaneous arm levitation; photophobia

Other PSP Phenotypes:
- PSP-parkinsonism: progressive nonfluent aphasia, pure akinesia, primary progressive gait freezing.
- Pure akinesia: Corticobasal syndrome.

Other Features of Classic PSP: Facial expressions: surprise, anxiety, or mask-like; deep nasal-labial groove (absent in classic PD); procerus (corrugator) sign; slow vertical saccades. Difficulty testing vestibulo-ocular reflexes; round the houses sign. Applause sign. Fast micrographia. Rocket sign. Difficulty with walking downstairs or reading. Trunk hyperextension with tendency to fall backwards;

turning "en bloc." Palilalia, pseudobulbar affect, and stereotypies. Photophobia. Stereotypy with skin erosion

PSP Look-Alikes

- Supranuclear gaze palsy (SNGP) occurs in corticobasal syndrome, dementia with Lewy bodies, MSA, frontotemporal lobar degeneration, and Perry syndrome.
- In younger individuals, SNGP is found in Niemann Pick disease type C, Kufor Rakeb syndrome (vertical), Gaucher's disease (horizontal), *POLG* mutations, CTX, CADASIL, SCA2, and SCA3.

More Handles to help distinguish these varieties:

▶ Familial PSP pattern with dominant inheritance suggests FTLD.
▶ PSP plus amyotrophic lateral sclerosis picture suggests the *C9ORF72* mutation.
▶ Supranuclear gaze palsy with early dementia and hallucinations suggests DLB.
▶ Dysautonomia and SNGP suggest MSA.
▶ History of neonatal jaundice and SNGP is diagnostic of Niemann Pick type C. Some have cataplexy.
▶ Supranuclear gaze palsy plus parkinsonism, psychiatric problems, and respiratory depression indicates Perry's syndrome.
▶ Secondary PSP-like picture includes multiple lacunar infarctions and aortic aneurysm repair surgery.
▶ Rapidly progressive PSP causes: neoplasms (lymphoma or gliomatosis cerebri); paraneoplastic process (e.g., anti-MA2 encephalitis)

Multiple System Atrophy Type P
Main Handles

▶ Unexplained urinary retention/incontinence, severe constipation, or severe sexual dysfunction in a middle-aged or elderly person
▶ Unexplained postural hypotension or fainting episodes in a middle-aged or elderly person
▶ Middle-aged or elderly person with cold hands

- Early anteroflexion of the neck, camptocormia, or Pisa syndrome with parkinsonism
- Parkinsonism with dystonic facial contractions while receiving levodopa
- Parkinsonism with marked stridor, typically inspiratory
- Parkinsonism with jerky rest tremor
- Hot cross bun sign on axial MRI of pons

How to Distinguish
1. Early MSA-P from PD

- Tremor of MSA is jerky and irregular. Dysautonomia is more severe. Response to levodopa is incomplete and unsustained with frequent occurrence of facial dystonia. Cardiac MIBG scan is normal in MSA but abnormal in PD.

2. Essential Tremor from Early MSA Type C (MSA-C)

- Tremor of essential tremor is rhythmic and sinusoidal; it is jerkier and irregular in MSA. There are autonomic features in MSA, such as postural hypotension and bladder disorder. Gait is unsteady in MSA-C but normal in most cases of essential tremor. Head and voice tremor is a feature of essential tremor but not MSA. History longer in essential tremor. Family history and alcohol responsiveness are seen in essential tremor but not in MSA.
- An elderly male with cerebellar tremor, ataxic gait, parkinsonism, cognitive decline, and dysautonomia likely has the *fragile X–associated tremor ataxia syndrome (FXTAS)*. Occasionally a mild form of FXTAS affects a woman.

3. FXTAS from MSA-C

- Premature ovarian failure may be present in females with manifesting FXTAS. Less severe dysautonomia in FXTAS. Family history in keeping with X-linked inheritance. Middle cerebellar peduncle hyperintensity sign on MRI is typical of FXTAS but not specific.

Corticobasal Syndrome
Core features: parkinsonism, dystonia, ideomotor apraxia, myoclonus, cognitive decline late feature

Main Handles
- Alien limb/hand phenomenon
- "My hand does not obey me"; "My feet feel foreign"
- A jerky, useless arm or leg due to myoclonus and apraxia
- CBS is the most asymmetric of the major parkinsonian syndromes.
- May begin with isolated orofacial apraxia
- CBS-like presentation with extensive white matter changes on MRI brain suggests hereditary diffuse leukoencephalopathy with axonal spheroids.

Corticobasal Syndrome Mimics
Frontotemporal dementia, PSP, Perry syndrome, prion disease, MS, vascular lesions: parietal infarct/hemorrhage and bilateral subdural hematomas, PRES, parietal lobe tumors, and familial Alzheimer's disease due to presenilin 1 mutation. Stiff limb syndrome. Autoimmune encephalopathies and vasculitis

Chorea
Main Features
- Tongue sign, milkmaid grip, pendular knee jerks, hung-up jerks, macrographia. Hypotonia with extension of fingers at metacarpophalangeal joint. Wilson's sign.

Huntington's Disease and Related Conditions
Handles for HD
- Choreic movements, especially in an adopted adult
- Akinetic rigid syndrome in an adopted child suggests the Westphal variant of HD.
- Early oculomotor disturbances
- Family history of dementia; premature death from suicide
- A negative family history does not rule out HD.
- Ill-kempt patient with chorea
- Chorea with early gait and balance problems
- Chorea with prominent behavioral problems or a change in personality
- Prolonged but reversible chorea after cocaine abuse suggests an HD gene carrier.

Red Flags for HD
- Ethnicity: Africa: HDL2; Japanese: DRPLA; Cumbria (England): neuroferritinopathy

◄ Selective facio-bucco-linguo-masticatory movements (FBLM) suggest neuroacanthocytosis (chorea-acanthocytosis and McLeod's syndrome) and tardive dyskinesia

◄ In **chorea-acanthocytosis** there is tongue protrusion resulting in ejection of food, lip biting, vocal tics, head drop and involuntary head-banging on furniture, recurrent belching, seizures, and sometimes peripheral neuropathy.

◄ In the **McLeod's syndrome (X-linked)**: vocalizations but no tongue protrusion or lip biting; skeletal and cardiac muscle involvement with proximal myopathy, raised CK, or cardiomyopathy; risk of sudden death from arrhythmia; absence of Kx antigen and reduction in Kell antigen due to mutation in the XK gene. Risk of severe hemolysis if not identified before transfusion.

Red Flags for Chorea with:

◄ Absent reflexes suggest neuropathy and diagnosis of chorea-acanthocytosis or Friedreich's ataxia.

◄ Tongue protrusion or ejection of food or head banging: chorea-acanthocytosis

◄ Raised CK: chorea-acanthocytosis, McLeod's syndrome

◄ Severe transfusion reaction: McLeod's syndrome

◄ Sudden head drops: neuroacanthocytosis

◄ FBLM dystonic movements and juvenile parkinsonism: PKAN, Wilson's disease, Lesch-Nyhan syndrome, or Meige syndrome

◄ Ataxia: spinocerebellar ataxia type 17 (SCA17) and DRPLA.

◄ Seizures: SCA17, chorea-acanthocytosis, DRPLA, Huntington's disease-like 1 (HDL1)

Benign Hereditary Chorea. Autosomal dominant condition with chorea, sometimes myoclonus, or dystonia appearing early in life. Short stature, pulmonary fibrosis, no intellectual deterioration. Nonprogressive and may improve with age. Associated with hypothyroidism; no caudate atrophy on MRI.

Adenyl Cyclase 5 Mutation. Autosomal recessive. Mutation in the adenyl cyclase 5 gene (ADCY 5). May be confused with BHC. Features: early-onset chorea with some progression, paroxysmal dyskinesia during sleep and eventual dystonia, hypotonia, facial myoclonic movements, intellect intact.

Handles for Acquired Chorea

▶ Young person: Sydenham's chorea

▶ Chorea is often delayed when other signs of rheumatic fever such as arthritis and carditis have resolved.

▶ A woman receiving oral contraceptives often indicates reactivation of chorea if there is a history of Sydenham's chorea.

▶ A woman with migraine and repeated miscarriages suggests the phospholipid antibody syndrome.

▶ Recurrent vomiting and stupor as a child, followed by progressive chorea and dementia suggests organic aciduria, such as propionic acidemia.

▶ An adult with arthralgia and skin rash may have lupus chorea.

▶ Drug-induced chorea may be due to dopamine blocking agents.

▶ In someone treated for seizures, drug-induced chorea is likely, phenytoin usually.

▶ In a diabetic, hemi- or generalized chorea or ballism may result from basal ganglia damage from nonketotic hyperglycemia (diabetic striatopathy). Non-contrast CT brain may show punctate hyperintensity in basal ganglia.

▶ In elderly women, chorea may be the presenting manifestation of diabetes.

▶ Complication of thyrotoxicosis

▶ A patient treated for cardiac arrhythmia or congestive cardiac failure may have digoxin-induced chorea.

▶ Chorea in an adult with cancer: think of paraneoplastic chorea. It can be focal.

▶ Chorea following major heart surgery favors post-pump chorea.

▶ Chorea in a patient with psychiatric problems suggests tardive dyskinesia

HEMIBALLISM AND HEMICHOREA

• Violent flinging movements involving one half of the body: Causes: lacunar infarction or hemorrhage, diabetic striatopathy, tumors (primary or metastatic), abscess involving the STN, head trauma, toxoplasmosis in an immunocompromised patient such as HIV.

• Bi-ballism may be caused by diabetic striatopathy, phenytoin intoxication, or dissemination of cancer

Wilson's Disease
Main Features:

Dystonic vacuous smile. Various types of tremor; wing-beating tremor characteristic. Limb dystonia. Parkinsonism in young person. Isolated ataxia. Chorea.

Note:

- Presentation up to seventh decade
- Blood copper *and* ceruloplasmin levels are both low.
- Kayser-Fleischer rings are sometimes absent in definite neurological Wilson's disease.

Handles for Wilson's Disease:

▷ Pyramidal signs are uncommon.
▷ Patient with any movement disorder whose blue eyes turn brown
▷ Dystonia with low platelet count and raised ferritin
▷ Blue nails, secondary amenorrhea
▷ Presentation with psychiatric problems and movement disorders in the absence of neuroleptics
▷ Eye movements may be abnormal.
▷ MRI is nearly always abnormal when there are neurological problems.

Tremor Handles

▷ Orthostatic tremor: 16–18 Hz; physiological tremor and ET: 7–12 Hz; PD rest tremor: 4–6 Hz; palatal tremor and Holmes/rubral tremor: 1–3 Hz
▷ Discomfort on standing that improves on walking is likely orthostatic tremor. Patients dislike standing still in a line. Tremulous movements are palpable over the thighs. Tremor improves when standing in a swimming pool; associated with PD.
▷ Irregular rest tremor affecting mainly an extended thumb or finger: dystonic tremor (SWEDD)
▷ Tremor that improves with alcohol is likely essential tremor.
▷ Tall male with tremor: XXYY syndrome or Klinefelter syndrome (XXY genotype)
▷ Short stature with tremor: mitochondrial disease (e.g., Kearns-Sayre syndrome), pseudo-hypoparathyroidism, SCA-17,

SCA-12, Coffin-Lowry syndrome, Cockayne syndrome
▷ Tremor after thalamic, midbrain, and cerebellar outflow lesions is often delayed; called Holmes, midbrain, or rubral tremor.
▷ Action tremor in a patient with chronic obstructive pulmonary disease: drug-induced (e.g., beta 2-stimulating drugs [salbutamol])
▷ Action tremor in a psychiatric patient is usually drug-related, particularly lithium and sodium valproate.
▷ Tremor of sudden onset favors psychogenic tremor.
▷ Acute stroke affecting the thalamus or subthalamus can cause focal asterixis that may be confused with tremor.
▷ Isolated head tremor is rare in essential tremor and suggests dystonic tremor as in cervical dystonia
▷ Proximal tremor (wing-beating) suggests Wilson's disease. Note that proximal tremor may be simulated by repeated shoulder dislocation.
▷ Tremor with weight loss or heat intolerance suggests thyrotoxicosis.
▷ A jerky tremor with a family history suggests familial cortical tremor.
▷ Tremor in a diabetic may relate to hypoglycemia.
▷ Tremor in an alcoholic may be due to delirium tremens or alcohol withdrawal.

Red Flags for Tremor

◁ Tremor with no rigidity and good sense of smell is likely essential or dystonic tremor. Classic PD is unlikely.
◁ Apparent ET with seizures suggests familial cortical myoclonic tremor with epilepsy.
◁ Jerky rest tremor is likely myoclonus. Causes include MSA, CBS, and occasionally DLBD.
◁ Apparent essential tremor in man with an intellectually disabled grandson (through his daughter) or a woman with a cognitively impaired son implies FXTAS.

Neurodegeneration with Brain Iron Accumulation

- Learn Table 8.1.

Tics

Features: Premonitory sensation that builds up before the tic. Sensation is relieved with execution of the tic; improvement with concentration.

Primary Tics

These may be inherited or sporadic and present as simple and chronic motor tics or Tourette syndrome. If there is a family history of tic disorder think of: Tourette syndrome, chorea-acanthocytosis, Huntington's disease.

Handles for Tourette Syndrome

▶ Multiple motor and vocal tics, onset before age 18 years. Fluctuation: tics are worse when inactive, become less when focused on a given task. Tic activity increased by anxiety and stress. Tics can be suppressed temporarily. Associated with attention-deficit hyperactivity disorder and obsessive-compulsive disorder

▶ Functional tics: Do not fluctuate. Patient remembers date of onset

▶ Causes of secondary tics (Tourettism): Dopamine stimulants (levodopa) or dopamine-blocking drugs, encephalitis, Creutzfeldt-Jakob disease, Sydenham's chorea, head trauma, stroke

▶ Adult-onset tics: May be late-presenting Tourette syndrome or secondary tics

▶ Tics with peripheral neuropathy favor chorea-acanthocytosis

▶ Tourette patients with severe and frequent dystonic cervical tics may develop cervical myelopathy with quadriparesis or cervical artery dissection and stroke.

Restless Legs Syndrome (RLS) and Periodic Movements of Sleep (PLMS)

• In PLMS, the main movement is abrupt dorsiflexion of the ankle; occasionally the arm muscles will jerk.

RLS and PLMS Handles

▶ Affects mainly women. Irresistible urge to move the legs. Sensation difficult to describe. Restlessness, worse in the evening, on sitting or lying down, relieved by walking. A worn carpet patch in front of the chair where the patient's feet rest. A couple may have to sleep in separate beds. Difficulty falling asleep worsens with hypnotics.

▶ Associated with iron deficiency, pregnancy, renal failure

▶ Iron deficiency in males may signify bowel cancer.

▶ Note: Neck and facial involvement does not occur in RLS.

Painful Legs and Moving Toes

Features: Slow involuntary flexion/extension movements of the toes. One or both sides affected. Burning or dull ache in the legs. May be painless. Also: painful arms–moving fingers syndrome

Dystonia

Types: Primary dystonia (genetic or sporadic). Dystonia plus, as in myoclonus. dystonia. Secondary dystonia following known insult. Dystonia in heredodegenerative diseases

Handles for Dystonia

▶ Sudden or rapid onset: drug-induced, psychogenic; rapid-onset dystonia-parkinsonism (DYT12)

▶ Fluctuating dystonia worse in afternoons: DRD (DYT5)

▶ With oculogyric crises—see DRD

▶ Dystonia–parkinsonism in a man of Philippine descent: Lubag (DYT3)

▶ Dystonia beginning in the lower extremities of a young person, especially an Ashkenazi Jew, is primary torsion dystonia (DYT1).

▶ Autosomal dominant craniocervical dystonia in an adult that spreads to limbs: DYT6

▶ Rapid-onset dystonia, especially in the craniocervical region, suggests rapid-onset dystonia parkinsonism (RDP; DYT12). The same genetic defect causes CAPOS syndrome.

▶ Foot dystonia after minor injury: psychogenic.

▶ Foot dystonia in a diabetic: stiff limb syndrome. Confirm by EMG of the back muscles. High titer of antibodies to glutamic acid decarboxylase

▶ Stiff legs with horizontal lumbar crease: SPS with extensor spasms of the lumbar spine

▶ Stiff person with hyperekplexia, weight loss, gastrointestinal disturbance, and cognitive impairment suggest a PERM variant due to DPPX antibodies.

▶ Dystonia with jerky movements improved by alcohol is due to myoclonus-dystonia.

▶ Involuntary head rotation improved by one finger: geste antagoniste or sensory trick

▶ Dystonia triggered by prolonged exercise is likely paroxysmal exertional dyskinesia. Think of GLUT-1 deficiency, DRD, or young-onset parkinsonism due to PARK2 (Parkin mutation).

▶ With ataxia in a patient with supranuclear downgaze palsy: Niemann-Pick disease type C

▶ In patient with supranuclear horizontal gaze palsy: Gaucher's disease. There is often enlargement of the liver and spleen and pingueculae and low platelet count.

▶ With SNGP, seizures and recurrent encephalopathy may be thiamine transporter deficiency.

▶ Truncal or cervical dystonia with purely extensor posturing is likely tardive dystonia.

▶ With orofacial dyskinesia (mixed movement disorder), this is probably tardive dystonia.

▶ With pontine facial sensory loss suggests CLIPPERS syndrome.

Cervical Dystonia (CD)

· Begins gradually. May be jerky or slower movements, tremors, and frequently a sensory trick.

· Causes of non-dystonic cervical dystonia: congenital wry neck, atlanto-axial dislocation, acute cervical disc prolapse, acute infections, cephalic tetanus, trochlear nerve palsy, muscle fibrosis following surgical trauma or radiation.

· Abrupt onset of a fixed neck posture suggests non-dystonic torticollis.

Conditions that may be confused with dystonia: Bent spine, camptocormia, scoliosis. Dupuytren's contracture, trigger finger, tetany, orthopedic and rheumatological conditions causing joint deformities, Sandifer syndrome, deafferentation (pseudoathetosis), Isaac syndrome, Satoyoshi syndrome, hemi-masticatory spasm

Lesch-Nyhan Syndrome, Main Handles

▶ Male with chorea and dystonic movements since childhood

▶ Self-injury/mutilation; poking finger in the eyes

▶ Fencer's posture

▶ Handcuffs or other restraints to prevent self-harm

▶ History of urate stones or gout

▶ Megaloblastic anemia

Characteristic Gait Disorders

· Dancing/bobbing gait in cocaine addict: crack dance

· Hobby-horse gait: DYT4 syndrome

· Walking on tip-toe: due to manganese poisoning from ephedrone abuse or manganese transporter mutation, industrial exposure, liver cirrhosis Hyperalimentation. Cock-walk gait is characteristic.

· Toe walking without ataxia: dopamine-responsive dystonia, hereditary spastic paraplegia, autism spectrum disorder. Angelman's syndrome

Paroxysmal Dyskinesias

Types: Paroxysmal kinesigenic dyskinesia, paroxysmal nonkinesigenic, dyskinesia, paroxysmal exertion induced dyskinesias, paroxysmal hypnogenic dyskinesias, secondary paroxysmal dyskinesia. See main text for more detail.

Handles

▶ Onset in childhood is more likely primary, sporadic, or inherited.

▶ Onset in adulthood is probably secondary.

▶ Pain during paroxysmal dyskinesia or precipitation by brief hyperventilation suggests secondary paroxysmal dyskinesia due to demyelinating disease (tonic spasms), trauma, or functional disorder.

▶ Precipitated by coffee and alcohol suggests paroxysmal nondyskinesigenic dyskinesia.

▶ Older age onset favors vascular paroxysmal dyskinesia—TIA or a stroke.

▶ In a diabetic patient, paroxysmal dyskinesia may indicate hypoglycemia.

▶ Paroxysmal dyskinesia precipitated by standing is likely orthostatic paroxysmal dystonia due to severe bilateral carotid disease.

▶ Unusual precipitants such as vibration, touch, or bright light point to psychogenic paroxysmal dyskinesia.

▶ A girl with stereotypic episodes of leg crossing, rocking, and no distress is probably self-stimulating for pleasure.

▶ Clusters of paroxysmal dyskinesia in sleep with polyneuropathy suggests insulinoma.

Stereotypies

Causes: autism spectrum disorder, intellectual disability, psychosis; catatonia, NMDA receptor antibody–mediated encephalitis

Miscellaneous Handles

- ▶ *Lentiform fork sign:* fluctuating parkinsonism, uremia, metabolic acidosis
- ▶ *Basal ganglia calcification:* Fahr's syndrome, hypoparathyroidism, pseudo-hypoparathyroidism, metabolic and infectious disorders, Cockayne syndrome, tuberous sclerosis, Down syndrome, mitochondrial disease
- ▶ *Repeated tongue protrusion:* tardive dyskinesia/dystonia, CA, Angelman's syndrome, Lesch-Nyhan syndrome, NBIA1, trombone tongue of neurosyphilis, whispering dysphonia
- ▶ *Child adopting strange postures of the head and trunk after eating:* Sandifer's syndrome.
- ▶ *Psychotic patient with dystonic movements:* tardive dystonia, Wilson's disease, recreational drug abuse
- ▶ *Child with head tremor:* spasmus nutans.
- ▶ Nodding with photosensitivity and cystic lesions of third ventricle: bobble-head doll syndrome
- ▶ *Girl with galactorrhea.* If not related to medication or sarcoidosis, the likely diagnosis is tyrosine hydroxylase deficiency.
- ▶ *Figure-of-eight head movement.* Rhombo-encephalo-synapsis and Ohtahara syndrome and (Videos 6.5 and 6.6)

Handles for Abnormal Head Movement

- ▶ Horizontal rhythmical tremor: ET
- ▶ Vertical rhythmical tremor: PD or dystonia
- ▶ Jerky head movement in any direction: CD
- ▶ Slow nodding head movement: nodding disease (Africa)
- ▶ Doll-like: bobble-head doll syndrome
- ▶ Rocking: self-stimulation in autism
- ▶ Spasmus nutans
- ▶ *Figure–of-eight head movement:* rhombo-encephalo-synapsis and Ohtahara syndrome and (Videos 6.5 and 6.6)

Psychogenic/Functional Movement Disorders
History

- Abrupt onset—at least according to the patient, who appears to cope well
- Excessively concerned family members and friends; more than three present in consulting room
- The overfriendly patient
- Over-idolization of the physician followed by rapid devaluation
- Junior doctors express extreme urgency to see patient.
- Static course with spontaneous remissions
- History of psychiatric disorders or multiple somatizations
- Employed in the health professions
- Pending litigation or compensation
- Young age, history of childhood abuse

Examination

- Wearing dark glasses indoors, adult clutching a teddy bear, wearing bunny slippers or inappropriate undergarments
- Overly concerned family members, the overfriendly patient, effortful or sighing response during neurological examination, adult living with parents,
- Entrainment. Ability to trigger or relieve the abnormal movements with unusual or nonphysiological interventions
- Photosensitivity
- Pauses in tremor. Variability, spread of movement; if the affected body part is restrained the tremor spreads elsewhere.
- False and painful weakness. False sensory complaints. Self-inflected injuries
- Deliberate slowness of movements. Functional disability out of proportion to examination findings. Abnormal movements that are bizarre, variable, multiple, or difficult to classify
- *The weak leg is lifted up* when getting off couch in genuine weakness.

Therapeutic Responses

- Unresponsive to appropriate medications. Response to placebos. Remission with psychotherapy

Myoclonus
Handles for Association with:

- ▶ Renal failure suggests the action myoclonus renal failure syndrome.
- ▶ Ataxia is likely mitochondrial disorder, celiac disease, or Prickle1 mutation.
- ▶ Seizures: neuronal ceroid lipofuscinoses, Unverricht-Lundberg syndrome, sialidosis

type 1, Lafora body disease, mitochondrial disease such as MERRF, DRPLA, North Sea progressive myoclonus epilepsy

▶ Opsoclonus: paraneoplastic or postinfectious (HIV and toxic/metabolic insults); also seen in NMDAR encephalitis

▶ Hung-up jerks and chronic chorio-retinitis: subacute sclerosing panencephalitis

▶ Facial myoclonus, hypotonia, and paroxysmal dyskinesia induced by drowsiness is ADCY 5 mutation.

▶ Rapidly progressive myoclonus with dementia suggests Creutzfeldt-Jakob disease.

▶ Slowly progressive dementia with myoclonus suggests Alzheimer's disease.

▶ Myoclonus plus parkinsonism suggests MSA or CBS.

▶ Action and intention myoclonus plus falls due to negative myoclonus after anoxic brain damage (usually respiratory arrest) is posthypoxic myoclonus (Lance Adams syndrome).

▶ Repetitive cortical myoclonus in a single body part (mostly face and hand) is epilepsia partialis continua.

▶ In EPC, the surface EEG can be normal and may disappear during sleep.

▶ Multifocal myoclonus (positive and negative) suggests a toxic metabolic encephalopathy.

▶ Focal myoclonus includes palatal myoclonus (tremor) and spinal myoclonus.

▶ Essential (isolated) palatal tremor is nearly always functional.

▶ Propriospinal myoclonus is often functional in origin.

Checklist for Movement Disorders
See main text.

SUGGESTED READING

Aggarwal A, Bhatt M. The pragmatic treatment of Wilson's disease. *Move Disord Clin Pract*. 2014;1:14–23.

Aranda F, Chívez M, Quispe-Mauricio A, Caro A. Syndrome de Woodhouse Sakati. UNMSM. Facultad de Medicina; 2008, pp. 260–262.

Asherson RA, Giampaolo D, Strimling M. A case of adult-onset Satoyoshi syndrome with gastric ulceration and eosinophilic enteritis. *Nat Clin Pract Rheumatol*. 2008;4:439–444.

Balint B, Mahant N, Meinck HM, Fung V. Stiff limb syndrome mimicking corticobasal syndrome. *Mov Disord Clin Pract*. 2014;1(4):354–356.

Bannister R, Gibson W, Michaels L, Oppenheimer DR. Laryngeal abductor paralysis in multiple system atrophy. A report on three necropsied cases, with observations on the laryngeal muscles and the nuclei ambigui. *Brain*. 1981;104:351–368.

Bassett AS, McDonald-McGinn DM, Devriendt K, et al. Practical guidelines for managing patients with 22q11.2 deletion syndrome. *J Pediatr*. 2011;159(2):332–339.

Batla A, Nehru R, Vijay T. Vertical wrinkling of the forehead or Procerus sign in progressive supranuclear palsy. *J Neurol Sci*. 2010;298:148–149.

Bhambhani V, Introne WJ, Lungu C, Cullinane A, Toro C. Chediak-Higashi syndrome presenting as young-onset levodopa-responsive parkinsonism. *Mov Disord*. 2013;28:127–129.

Counihan TJ, Barbano RL. Progressive micrographia in a migraineur. *Neurology*. 2000;54:2107.

Fabiani G, Teive HA, Munhoz RP. Lentiform fork sign and fluctuating, reversible parkinsonism in a patient with uremic encephalopathy. *Mov Disord*. 2013;28:1053.

Franz DN, Glauser TA, Tudor C, Williams S. Topiramate therapy of epilepsy associated with Angelman's syndrome. *Neurology*. 2000;54:1185–1188.

Goncalves MRR, Capelli LP, Nitrini R, et al. Atypical clinical course of FXTAS: rapidly progressive dementia as the major symptom. *Neurology*. 2007;68:1864–1866.

Graff-Radford J, Rubin MN, Jones DT, et al. The alien limb phenomenon. *J Neurol*. 2013;260:1880–1888.

Hadavi S, Noyce AJ, Leslie RD, Giovannoni G. Stiff person syndrome. *Pract Neurol*. 2011;11:272–282.

Hayflick SJ, Kruer MC, Gregory A, et al. Beta-propeller protein-associated neurodegeneration: a new X-linked dominant disorder with brain iron accumulation. *Brain*. 2013;136:1708–1717.

Lenfeldt N, Hansson W, Larsson A, Birgander R, Eklund A, Malm J. Three-day CSF drainage barely reduces ventricular size in normal pressure hydrocephalus. *Neurology*. 2012;79:237–242.

Lenoir T, Guedj N, Boulu P, Guigui P, Benoist M. Camptocormia: the bent spine syndrome, an update. *Eur Spine J*. 2010;19:1229–1237.

Maramattom BV. Self-mutilation in the Lesch-Nyhan syndrome. *Neurology*. 2005;65:E25.

Martino D, Stamelou M, Bhatia KP. The differential diagnosis of Huntington's disease-like syndromes: 'Red Flags' for the clinician. *J Neurol Neurosurg Psychiatry*. 2013;84:650–656.

Merwick Á, Mok T, McNamara B, Parfrey NA, Moore H, Sweeney BJ, Hand CK, Ryan AM. Phenotypic Variation in a Caucasian Kindred with Chorea-Acanthocytosis. *Movement Disorders Clinical Practice*. 2015 Mar;2(1):86–9.

Okamoto K, Tokiguchi S, Furusawa T, et al. MR features of diseases involving bilateral middle cerebellar peduncles. *AJNR Am J Neuroradiol*. 2003;24:1946–1954.

Ortigoza-Escobar JD, Serrano M, Molero M, et al. Thiamine transporter-2 deficiency: outcome and treatment monitoring. *Orphanet J Rare Dis*. 2014;9:92.

Phillips JG, Bradshaw JL, Chiu E, Bradshaw JA. Characteristics of handwriting of patients with Huntington's disease. *Mov Disord.* 1994;9:521–530.

Reddy OJ, Gafoor JA, Suresh B, Prasad PO. Bobble head doll syndrome: a rare case report. *J Pediatr Neurosci.* 2014;9:175.

Regragui W, Gerdelat-Mas A, Simonetta-Moreau M. Cortical tremor (FCMTE: familial cortical myoclonic tremor with epilepsy). *Neurophysiol Clin.* 2006;36:345–349.

Rubio-Agusti I, Carecchio M, Bhatia KP, et al. Movement disorders in adult patients with classical galactosemia. *Mov Disord.* 2013;28:804–810.

Schneider SA, Hardy J, Bhatia KP. Syndromes of neurodegeneration with brain iron accumulation (NBIA): an update on clinical presentations, histological and genetic underpinnings, and treatment considerations. *Mov Disord.* 2012;27:42–53.

Sethi KD, Lee KH, Deuskar V, Hess DC. Orthostatic paroxysmal dystonia. *Mov Disord.* 2002;17:841–845.

Silveira-Moriyama L, Moriyama TS, Gabbi TV, Ranvaud R, Barbosa ER. Chediak-Higashi syndrome with parkinsonism. *Mov Disord.* 2004;19:472–475.

Van Gerpen JA, Wider C, Broderick DF, Dickson DW, Brown LA, Wszolek ZK. Insights into the dynamics of hereditary diffuse leukoencephalopathy with axonal spheroids. *Neurology.* 2008;71:925–929.

Verrips A, Nijeholt GJ, Barkhof F, et al. Spinal xanthomatosis: a variant of cerebrotendinous xanthomatosis. *Brain.* 1999;122(Pt 8):1589–1595.

Zaleski C, Bassett AS, Tam K, Shugar AL, Chow EW, McPherson E. The co-occurrence of early onset Parkinson's disease and 22q11.2 deletion syndrome. *Am J Med Genet A.* 2009;149A:525–528.

Chapter 9: Stroke

Stroke is the third leading cause of death and a major cause of disability in the developed world. There is now great interest given the opportunity to treat cerebral infarcts by antithrombotic agents or direct removal of clot, making accurate and swift diagnosis critical to the outcome. Time is Brain!

We have classified the information provided in this chapter according to history and major arterial, cortical, brainstem, and lacunar syndromes. Inevitably, there is overlap among them.

HISTORY

A large proportion of stroke patients have hypertension and receive hypotensive medication but it is usually treated inadequately. Even in young people with stroke, the most common causes are hypertension and diabetes; other etiologies, such as sickle cell disease, are more prevalent among young people than in the elderly.

▶ Recurrent nose bleeds and stroke in a young adult strongly suggest Osler-Weber-Rendu syndrome (hereditary hemorrhagic telangiectasia; Figure 9.1).

The nasal telangiectases cause epistaxis, usually in childhood and teenage years. There may be a history of intestinal bleeding as well. The strokes may be related to aneurysm, dural arteriovenous fistula, cavernomas, cerebral abscess, and arteriovenous malformations. Some patients have pulmonary vascular malformations that cause paradoxical embolism to the brain. Telangiectases are readily visible on the skin, particularly the lips and tongue.

▶ Abrupt onset of one arm clutching the other arm, throat, or other body part inappropriately is the *alien limb syndrome.*

Abrupt-onset alien limb is likely a vascular lesion of the corpus callosum or parietal lobe. See Chapter 8 and Figure 8.17.

▶ SMART syndrome (stroke-like migraine attacks after radiation therapy; see Figure 9.2

A few years after radiotherapy for brain tumor some patients develop headaches and hemiparesis for several weeks, raising the question of tumor recurrence. The weakness usually resolves spontaneously. The pathophysiology is poorly understood but bears similarities to that of PRES (posterior reversible encephalopathy syndrome).

Note: If headache is not conspicuous, the weakness could be due to internal carotid stenosis from delayed radiotherapy-induced intimal swelling with thrombosis.

▶ Stroke-like episodes triggered by metformin, sodium valproate, or statins suggest MELAS (the mitochondrial encephalomyopathy, lactic acidosis, and stroke-like episodes) (Figure 9.3).

All three drugs are potentially toxic to mitochondria.

▶ Alleged infantile hemiplegia may be *dopa-responsive dystonia.* This is both a Handle and Red Flag for teenagers and young adults who carry a label of infantile hemiplegia. If the weakness varies throughout the day, typically worse in the afternoon, then the correct diagnosis is likely to be dopa-responsive dystonia. This can be treated successfully with small doses of levodopa.

▶ Transient episodic memory loss following unaccustomed exertion, sexual intercourse, emotion, or cold exposure is *transient global amnesia* (TGA).

During the attack, patients appear alert, but they are muddled and ask the same questions repeatedly, often a few seconds apart, and because of their confusion, act inappropriately, appearing less or more active than customary. The incident lasts a few hours with complete loss of episodic memory. Most affected individuals experience a single event, and the risk of future

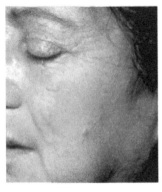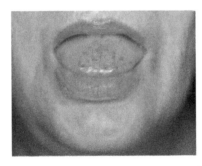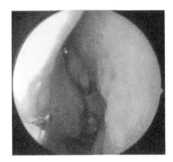

FIGURE 9.1: Hereditary hemorrhagic telangiectasia. **Left**: Characteristic tiny dilated vascular lesions on the cheek in middle-aged woman. **Center**: Red maculopapular lesions on the tongue and lower lip in a 55-year-old female with cerebral arteriovenous malformation. **Right**: Nasal endoscopy showing telangiectasias on the anterior septum and inferior turbinate in a 59-year-old male. Reproduced from Figure 13-45 in the chapter Capillary Malformations, Hyperkeratotic Stains, Telangiectasias, and Miscellaneous Vascular Blots, by JB Mulliken. Oxford University Press. DOI:10.1093/med/9780195145052.003.0013.

stroke is not increased although many present to stroke services. The underlying cause is debated, but there is an association with the following:

- o Migraine
- o Seizure activity (i.e., transient epileptic amnesia [TEA]). See Chapter 13 for more details.
- o Concussion

Table 9.1 summarizes the main differentiating aspects of TGA and TEA

▶ Persistent acute-onset global amnesia although rare, suggests thalamic or medial temporal lobe infarction (Figure 9.4).

Memory in patients with unilateral infarcts usually returns after 6 months, while amnesia persists when the thalamic or medial temporal lobe infarction is bilateral. Visual field abnormalities are often present in bilateral medial temporal lobe infarcts.

▶ Recurrent fluctuating episodes of weakness resulting in a complete stroke is the *capsular warning syndrome*.

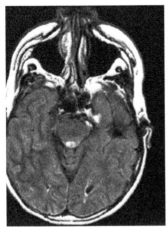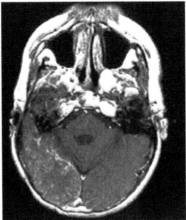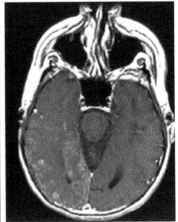

FIGURE 9.2: SMART syndrome (stroke-like migraine attacks after radiation therapy). MRI FLAIR (**left**) and T1 with gadolinium (**middle and right**) axial sequences performed during an episode when the patient developed left homonymous hemianopia, left hemisensory deficits, and moderate left hemiparesis with headache and photophobia without evidence of seizure activity on EEG. Note the extensive gyral thickening shown in the FLAIR sequences, involving the right temporal, parietal and occipital lobes, associated with contrast enhancement. Reproduced with permission from Pruitt et al. (2006), Figure 1.

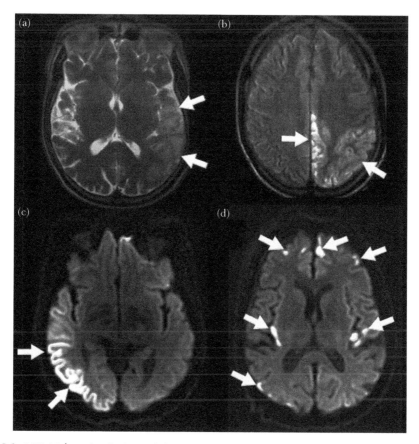

FIGURE 9.3: MELAS (mitochondrial encephalomyopathy, lactic acidosis, and stroke-like episodes syndrome). Cortical hyperintense signal on T2-weighted imaging during the first episode at age 24 (**A**), fluid-attenuated inversion recovery image during the second episode at age 25 (**B**), and diffusion-weighted imaging sequences during the last two episodes at age 33 (**C**, **D**). Arrows indicate abnormal areas. Reproduced from Allou et al. (2012).

TABLE 9.1: SUMMARY OF MAIN DIFFERENCES BETWEEN CLASSIC TGA, TGA DUE TO MIGRAINE, AND TEA

	Age and Gender	Attack Duration	Onset Time	Headache	EEG	Other Features
Classic TGA	50–80 years Equal gender prevalence	2–8 hours	Mornings	Occasional	Usually normal	Single event. Selective inability to encode new episodic memory. No semantic loss. Perseveration
TGA due to migraine	Middle-aged Female	2–24 hours	Any time of day	During attack	Intermittent slow-wave abnormalities	Attacks recur
TEA	Middle-aged Male	Less than 1 hour	On wakening	None	Sometimes epileptic discharges	Attacks recur. Global cognitive disturbance, including loss of semantic knowledge. Olfactory hallucinations

TEA, transient epileptic amnesia; TGA, transient global amnesia.

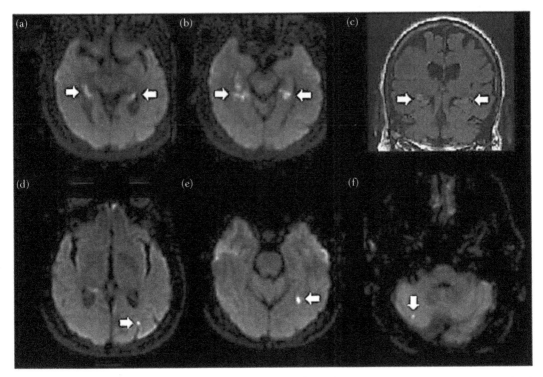

FIGURE 9.4: MRI (**A–F**) of a patient with several embolic infarcts (arrows) but mainly in both hippocampi associated with amnesia.

The hemiparesis is due to disease of a single penetrating artery that feeds the internal capsule. Attacks occur over 1–2 days. The frontal and temporal lobes are spared, thus there is no aphasia. It signals imminent cerebral infarction, hence the generally accepted need for rapid thrombolytic treatment.

▶ A single episode of weakness/visual failure lasting more than 1 hour is not a transient ischemic attack (TIA).

Typically, an embolic TIA lasts no more than 10 minutes and may be recurrent. A defect lasting over 1 hour is probably a completed infarct due to a major embolic event or lacune. The infarct is best seen on MRI as increased signal on diffusion-weighted imaging (DWI) sequences (Figure 9.5). The older classification allowed 24 hours for the maximum duration of a TIA. This is no longer accepted but has yet to be replaced.

▶ TIA induced by hyperventilation mainly in children is characteristic of *Moyamoya disease* (Kim et al. 2003).

Here, there is progressive stenosis of the major intracranial arteries (anterior circulation), and presumably the lowered CO_2 provoked by overbreathing causes further reduction of flow in the affected arteries. The deficit is typically hemiparesis, but the side of this may vary. This phenomenon may be seen when crying, blowing up a balloon, or playing a wind instrument, especially the harmonica. See MRI in Figure 9.6.

▶ Bouts of dystonia and weakness on either side, often starting during sleep, lasting minutes or days, is the alternating hemiplegia/hemidystonia syndrome of childhood. This is likely a form of *paroxysmal dystonia*.

Onset is in early childhood, but presentation in adolescence is recognized. There is a mutation in the gene coding for ATP1A3 and mutations in the same region explain the overlap with rapid-onset dystonia-parkinsonism (see Chapter 8, Movement Disorders). This is no longer considered a variety of migraine.

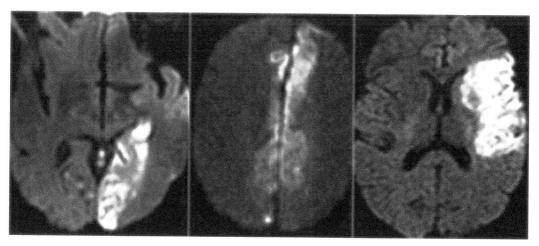

FIGURE 9.5: Axial MRI with diffusion-weighted imaging to show an infarct in the left middle cerebral artery territory.

▶ Hemiparesis after childbirth is usually caused by *cortical venous sinus thrombosis*.
This affects Afro-Caribbean and Asian women especially. Note: a routine CT brain scan may be normal in the first few days—a real trap for the unwary clinician. Other possible causes include the following:
   ○ Extracranial dissection from exertion during delivery
   ○ Cerebral hemorrhage
   ○ Postpartum vasculitis
   ○ Posterior reversible encephalopathy syndrome (PRES (Figure 9.7)
   ○ Reversible cerebral vasoconstrictor syndrome (RCVS)
   ○ Hemolysis, elevated liver enzymes, low platelet count (HELLP)
   ○ Functional disorder: common
The underlying mechanism for the PRES, RCVS, and HELLP syndromes is likely systemic hypertension secondary to eclampsia and thrombocytosis, which is prone to occur during the peripartum period.

▶ Stroke with contralateral elongated styloid process is the *Eagle syndrome* (Figure 9.8). When the neck is turned, the elongated styloid process kinks the carotid artery,

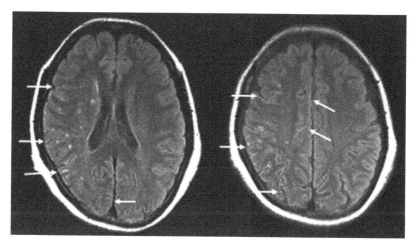

FIGURE 9.6: Unenhanced axial MRI FLAIR sequence in Moyamoya disease shows the "ivy sign" (arrows). The appearance resembles creeping ivy on a wall. It is due to leptomeningeal high signal along the cerebral sulci or on the brain surface. This was a 47-year-old woman with frequent transient left upper and lower limb weakness. Reproduced with permission from Mori et al. (2009).

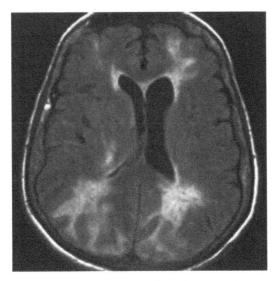

FIGURE 9.7: Posterior reversible encephalopathy syndrome (PRES). MRI axial FLAIR image demonstrates confluent juxtacortical and deep white matter T2 hyperintensity in frontal, posterior parietal, and occipital lobes that is characteristic of PRES. Reproduced with permission from Hamilton and Nesbit (2008).

causing occlusion or dissection. Patients may experience TIA or stroke with neck pain over the styloid process.

▶ Abrupt hemiplegia with dyspnea paradoxically relieved by lying down suggests a *left atrial myxoma* with emboli.

Major arterial emboli are serious risks of this condition. Other findings include the following:

○ Cardiac murmurs that vary with position
○ Paroxysmal arrhythmias
○ Raised erythrocyte sedimentation rate (ESR) and abnormal serum proteins

▶ Recurrent, stereotyped, spreading paresthesia, sometimes with weakness, lasting several minutes and simulating TIAs are likely due to *amyloid spells* or migraine.

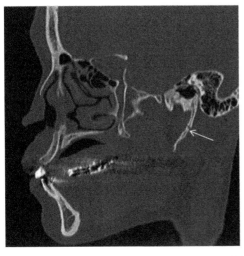
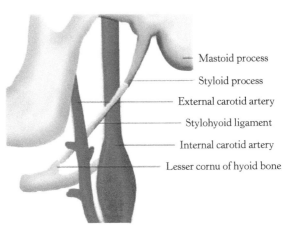

Mastoid process
Styloid process
External carotid artery
Stylohyoid ligament
Internal carotid artery
Lesser cornu of hyoid bone

FIGURE 9.8: Eagle syndrome. **Left:** Lateral CT of the skull shows elongated styloid process (white arrow). **Right:** The anatomical relationship between the long styloid process and the internal carotid artery. X-ray and drawing Reproduced with permission from Dr. Frank Gaillard, Radiopedia ID 7257.

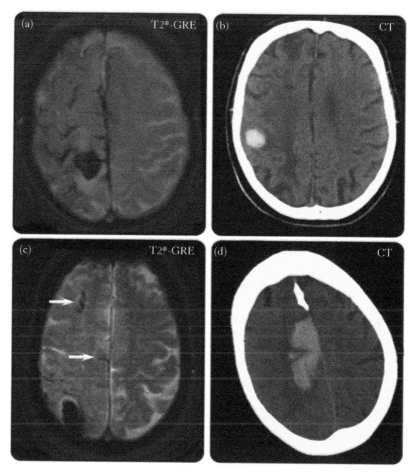

FIGURE 9.9: Cortical superficial siderosis and intracerebral hemorrhage (ICH). Subsequent ICH at (or close to) the site of pre-existing siderosis in two patients with superficial siderosis: female patient, aged 85 years; time interval between baseline imaging (**A**) and incident ICH (**B**): 19 months; and male patient, aged 80 years; time interval between baseline imaging (**C**) and incident ICH (**D**): 35 months. (**A, C**) Baseline MRI, T2*-weighted images. (**B, D**) Follow-up unenhanced CT scans. T2*-GRE = T2*-weighted gradient-recalled echo. Reproduced with permission from Charidimou et al. (2013), Figure 1.

Amyloid spells are reminiscent of a sensory seizure, which indeed is a possible mechanism in amyloid angiopathy, where there is focal irritation from hemorrhage-induced siderosis (Figure 9.9). Such episodes may also represent complicated (hemiplegic) migraine, but in this condition there is frequently headache, nausea, and photophobia. Clearly, use of blood thinners would be unwise if you suspected an amyloid spell.

◀ Some patients with amyloid spells presenting after the age of 60 years are thought to have migraine without headache. This can be a challenging diagnosis when there is a prior history of migraine with aura as a child or young adult.

◀ Positive phenomena are unusual in classic TIAs.

Distinguishing aspects of migraine, TIA, stroke, seizures, syncope, and amyloid spells are shown in Table 9.2.

Stroke Mimics

These are basically Red Flags. A patient who is seen acutely on account of alleged stroke may have one of the following:

◀ Postictal paresis (Todd's paresis)

TABLE 9.2: COMPARISON OF FEATURES IN MIGRAINE, TIA, STROKE, SEIZURES, SYNCOPE, AND AMYLOID SPELLS

Feature	Onset	Offset	Duration	Quality	Loss of Function/Comment
Migraine with aura	Gradual	Gradual	10–30 minutes	Positive, followed by negative	Usually none or temporary. Age at first attack <50 years. Headache *after* aura
TIA	Sudden	Gradual	Minutes. Less than 1 hour	Negative (loss of function), rarely stereotyped. Do not migrate	Temporary. Loss of consciousness rare. Age >50 years. Headache *during* attack
Stroke	Sudden	Ongoing	Long term	Negative	Permanent, incomplete recovery
Seizure	Sudden, recurrent	Sudden	Seconds. Rarely more than 2 minutes	Positive and stereotyped. May migrate	Todd's paresis. LOC. Lateral tongue biting, incontinence
Syncope	Gradual	Gradual	Seconds	Positive, e.g., blurred vision, muffled hearing	Rapid recovery
Amyloid spells	Gradual	Gradual	Minutes	Positive, sensory and stereotyped. May migrate	Usually none or temporary. May simulate complicated migraine

LOC, loss of consciousness; TIA, transient ischemic attack.

In general, if the Todd's paresis lasts more than 24 hours, then you are dealing with a structural lesion such as a tumor or stroke.

A hemorrhagic stroke is more likely to cause a seizure than is thromboembolism.

◄ Hypoglycemia
This is so easily forgotten. Thankfully, most paramedics check the blood glucose on the way to hospital. The diagnosis is more frequently unnoticed in hospital wards.

◄ Sepsis
Cerebral abscess in a patient with septicemia will induce a stroke (often associated with seizures). Sometimes this occurs from secondary infarction but you would need to be cautious about use of thrombolytic therapy. The correct diagnosis should be revealed by a brain scan.

◄ Hemiplegic migraine
Some patients have recurrent episodes of weakness and a positive family history of migraine.

◄ Psychogenic weakness
Clues for identifying functional disorders are given in several other chapters (see Chapter 3, Limbs and Trunk; Chapter 6, Epilepsy and Sleep; and Chapter 8, Movement Disorders).

◄ MELAS syndrome is associated with stroke-like episodes and occurs in patients with severe headaches resembling migraine.
Check medication history for consumption of metformin, sodium valproate, or statins.

FOCAL CORTICAL AND BRAINSTEM SYNDROMES

In the older literature, there were multiple guides for localizing an infarct or hemorrhage. With the advent of CT and MRI, most such pointers have been shown to be unreliable. We list some of the more robust indicators next.

▶ A homonymous field defect cannot be due to a single lesion in the frontal cortex.
This is basic applied anatomy. The optic radiation involves the parietal, occipital, and posterior temporal lobes only.
Localizing a face-sparing hemiparesis.
When the cranial nerves are normal it can be difficult to distinguish hemiparesis due to a cervical cord lesion from a hemiparesis due to an intracranial defect (cortical or brainstem). Here are two ways of separating out these possibilities:

▶ Shoulder shrugs
If there is no fatigue on repeated bilateral shoulder shrugging, the lesion is likely

spinal in origin; if there is fatigue, the lesion is intracranial.

▶ Jaw jerk

Hyperactive limb reflexes with a normal or underactive jaw jerk strongly suggest a spinal lesion. If the jaw jerk is brisk, the lesion is intracranial, above the mid-pons.

▶ Diplopia associated with a stroke usually indicates a pontine or midbrain lesion. There are three eponymous disorders associated with this:

▶ Third nerve palsy with contralateral hemiparesis is Weber syndrome, a disorder that results from a midbrain lesion on the same side as the CN III nerve deficit (Figure 9.10). The oculomotor nerve crosses medial to the peduncle, and the condition results usually from occlusion of a perforating branch of the basilar or posterior cerebral arteries. There may be a contralateral homonymous hemianopia if there is significant ischemia of the posterior cerebral artery (Figure 9.10).

▶ CN VI and VII cranial nerve lesion with contralateral hemiparesis and sensory impairment is Foville's or Millard-Gubler syndrome. It suggests a lesion of the ventral pons on the side of the cranial nerve deficits (Figure 9.11).

▶ Third-nerve palsy with contralateral ataxia and tremor is Benedikt's syndrome. This is due to a vascular lesion or tumor principally affecting the red nucleus, emerging third nerve fibers, medial lemniscus and substantia nigra (Figure 9.12).

◀ In a cortical stroke due to hemorrhage or a large infarct, CN VI nerve palsy on the side of the hemorrhage/infarct is likely a false localizing sign. The presence of marked swelling may result in a false localizing CN VI palsy on the side of the edema secondary to a tentorial pressure cone. For example, a right middle cerebral infarct will cause a left hemiparesis and right CN VI defect mimicking the Foville syndrome (although there is no CN VII deficit).

▶ Supranuclear paralysis of upgaze with fixed dilated pupils favors Parinaud's syndrome. This is due to a lesion of the dorsal midbrain (Figure 9.12 and Video 2.2, Supranuclear Paralysis of Upgaze). Usually it is caused by

- Pinealoma
- Hydrocephalus
- Vascular lesions in the dorsal midbrain

The difficulty with upgaze can be corrected by the doll's-head eye maneuver, in keeping with supranuclear gaze palsy; but if there is a progressively enlarging tumor (e.g., pinealoma), it can be replaced by a *nuclear* gaze palsy and absence of upgaze even with dolling. Retraction nystagmus is seen occasionally (see Video 2.2, Supranuclear Paralysis of Upgaze). There should be no diplopia.

▶ Sudden onset of ataxia, vomiting, and dysphagia favors Wallenberg syndrome (lateral medullary syndrome, Figure 9.13). It results from occlusion/dissection of a vertebral artery that produces occlusion of the posterior inferior cerebellar artery, which supplies the dorsolateral medulla. Other features are as follows:

- Headache
- Severe nystagmus
- Ipsilateral Horner's syndrome
- Ageusia
- Loss of pain and temperature on the ipsilateral face and contralateral body: the latter is the only contralateral feature.
- The patient leans toward the side of the lesion when trying to sit or stand because of truncal ataxia.
- Pyramidal tract is spared.
- Rarely, there is sudden complete inversion of vision.
- The full complement of features is shown in Figure 9.13.

▶ Inability to sneeze is a rare feature in the recovery phase of Wallenberg's syndrome. It is presumed that there is a sneezing center in the dorsolateral medulla. Occasionally, the onset of infarction is preceded by recurrent compulsive sneezing.

▶ Gradual onset of quadriparesis (sparing the face), dysarthria, hypoglossal palsy, nystagmus, and sometimes respiratory failure suggests *bilateral medial medullary infarction*. It is caused by thrombosis of a vertebral artery or one of the basilar artery perforating vessels to the medial medulla that supplies both pyramidal tracts, decussation of the medial menisci, medial longitudinal fasciculus, and the

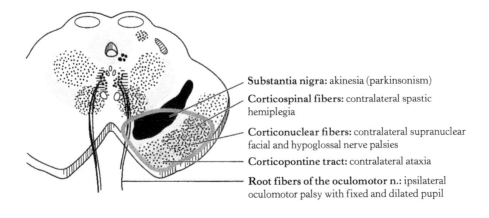

Substantia nigra: akinesia (parkinsonism)

Corticospinal fibers: contralateral spastic hemiplegia

Corticonuclear fibers: contralateral supranuclear facial and hypoglossal nerve palsies

Corticopontine tract: contralateral ataxia

Root fibers of the oculomotor n.: ipsilateral oculomotor palsy with fixed and dilated pupil

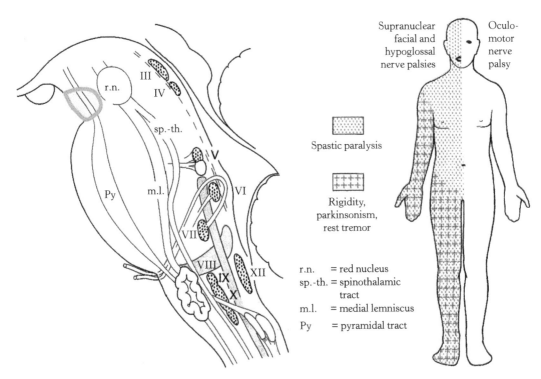

FIGURE 9.10: Weber's syndrome. This results from a lesion of the cerebral peduncle and it is a combination of oculomotor palsy due to emerging CN III nerve fibers, contralateral hemiparesis with facial and tongue weakness from damage of the cerebral peduncle, and contralateral homonymous hemianopia if the posterior cerebral artery is thrombosed. There is inconstant damage to the substantia nigra that results in contralateral parkinsonism. Reproduced with permission from *Duus' Topical Diagnosis in Neurology*, 5th ed., p. 156. Thieme, 2012.

hypoglossal nerve/nuclei (see Figure 9.13 for anatomy). MRI may reveal the "heart sign" (Figure 9.14). The disorder may be confused with (a) brainstem encephalitis; (b) Guillain-Barré syndrome, especially when the deep tendon reflexes

are depressed, as they may be early on in acute pyramidal lesions.

▶ Hemiparesis on the same side as a cortical lesion might be caused by Kernohan's notch. If there is a large space-occupying lesion (e.g., intracerebral hemorrhage, subdural

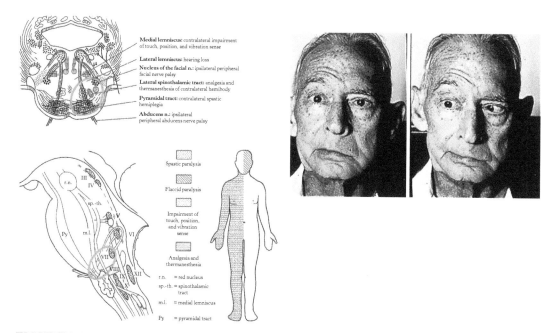

FIGURE 9.11: **Top and Center**: Anatomy of the Foville or Millard-Gubler syndrome. This results from a lesion in the caudal basis pontis and causes an ipsilateral CN VI and CN VII lesion with contralateral hemiparesis and sensory deficits. Reproduced with permission from *Duus' Topical Diagnosis in Neurology*, 5th ed., p. 151. Thieme, 2012. **Bottom**: Patient with a right CN VI and VII lesion due to Foville syndrome.

hematoma, or tumor) on the left side, the weakness may also be on the left side. This is a false localizing sign caused by swelling of the left cerebral hemisphere with uncal herniation through the tentorium cerebelli resulting in pressure on the opposite (right) cerebral peduncle, making an indentation called *Kernohan's notch* (Figure 9.15). Pressure on the right cerebral peduncle causes a left hemiparesis (i.e., on the same side as the lesion). Occasionally, there is pressure on the ipsilateral oculomotor nerve resulting in a CN III palsy and hemiparesis on the same side. Compare this with Weber's syndrome, where the CN III lesion is on the side opposite side the weakness.

◀ Weak arm on one side with weak leg on the other is usually due to a small vascular lesion at the caudal medulla affecting some of the decussating pyramidal fibers (Figure 9.16).

One-and-a-Half Syndrome

Absence of horizontal gaze except for abduction of one eye suggests the one-and-a half syndrome. See Video 9.1, One-and-a-Half (courtesy David Zee). The only horizontal pursuit movement is that achieved by the lateral rectus on one side. For example, if there is absence of *conjugate* gaze to the left, then, on attempted gaze to the right, only the right abducens muscle contracts and usually shows nystagmus. Characteristically, this results from a lesion in the right paramedian pontine reticular formation that impairs conjugate gaze to the right, as well as fibers in the medial longitudinal fasciculus destined for the right medial rectus complex of CN III. Thus, the only movement remaining is contraction of the right lateral rectus. Convergence is normal because this is a midbrain function (see Video 9.1). Most cases are due to pontine vascular lesions, but some result from multiple sclerosis (MS) (Figure 9.17).

MAJOR ARTERIAL SYNDROMES

Internal Carotid Artery Stenosis

As a very general rule:

▶ Patients with stroke related to internal carotid artery stenosis (ICAS) are normotensive and give a history of TIAs, whereas:

▶ Patients with hemorrhagic stroke are hypertensive and have not experienced prior TIAs.

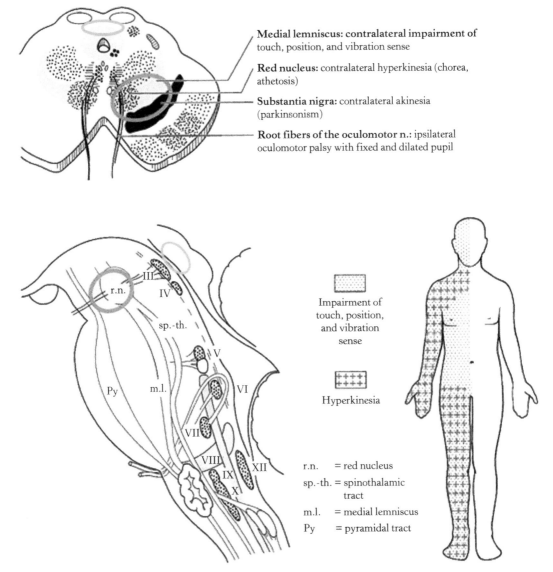

Medial lemniscus: contralateral impairment of touch, position, and vibration sense

Red nucleus: contralateral hyperkinesia (chorea, athetosis)

Substantia nigra: contralateral akinesia (parkinsonism)

Root fibers of the oculomotor n.: ipsilateral oculomotor palsy with fixed and dilated pupil

Impairment of touch, position, and vibration sense

Hyperkinesia

r.n.   = red nucleus
sp.-th. = spinothalamic tract
m.l.   = medial lemniscus
Py   = pyramidal tract

FIGURE 9.12: Midbrain lesions. Benedikt's syndrome (green circles and figure of a man) is caused by a lesion, usually vascular, that involves the red nucleus, emerging CN III fibers, substantia nigra, and medial lemniscus. It results in contralateral cerebellar tremor and sensory impairment, with an ipsilateral CN III lesion. There is often tremor at rest (Holmes or rubral tremor). In Parinaud's syndrome (blue rings), the defect is in the tectal plate region (dorsal mid-brain) where it damages the vertical gaze center. Examination findings are confined to conjugate eye movement and pupillary changes. Reproduced and modified with permission from *Duus' Topical Diagnosis in Neurology*, 5th ed., p. 155. Thieme, 2012.

Typically. TIAs due to ICAS represent emboli from an atheromatous plaque at the origin of the ICA or more proximally. There is no disturbance of *flow* unless the narrowing is severe; namely, more than 95% of the cross-sectional area.

The main blood supply to the eye is the ophthalmic artery, which is a branch of the ICA, but in healthy people there is a good collateral supply from the external carotid vessels (see Figure 2.27). Thus, ocular ischemia will develop only if there is poor flow

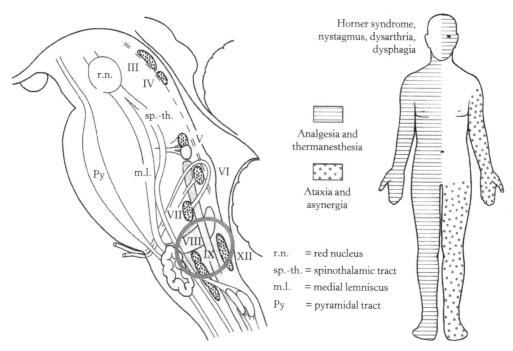

Inferior vestibular nucleus: nystagmus and tendency to fall to ipsilateral side

Dorsal nucleus of the vagus n.: tachycardia and dyspnea
Inferior cerebellar peduncle: ipsilateral ataxia and asynergia

Nucleus of the tractus solitarius: ageusia

Nucleus ambiguus: ipsilateral paresis of palate, larynx, and pharynx; hoarseness; dysphagia

Nucleus of the cochlear n.: hearing loss

Nucleus of the spinal tract of the trigeminal n.: ipsilateral analgesia and thermanesthesia of the face; absent corneal reflex

Central sympathetic pathway : Horner syndrome, hypohidrosis, ipsilateral facial vasodilatation

Anterior spinocerebellar tract: ataxia, ipsilateral hypotonia

Lateral spinothalamic tract: analgesia and thermanesthesia of contralateral hemibody

Central tegmental tract: palatal and pharyngeal myorhythmia

Reticular formation (respiratory center): singultus (hiccups)

Horner syndrome, nystagmus, dysarthria, dysphagia

Analgesia and thermanesthesia

Ataxia and asynergia

r.n.   = red nucleus
sp.-th. = spinothalamic tract
m.l.   = medial lemniscus
Py   = pyramidal tract

FIGURE 9.13: Wallenberg syndrome. Typically, this results from occlusion/dissection of a vertebral artery with damage to the dorsolateral medulla. It is rare to find all the features listed in the figure. Reproduced with permission from *Duus' Topical Diagnosis in Neurology*, 5th ed., p. 149. Thieme, 2012.

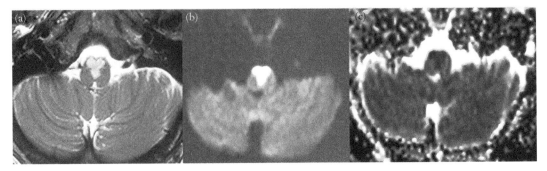

FIGURE 9.14: The heart sign of bilateral medial medullary infarction. (**a**) T2-weighted axial MRI brain image showing heart-shaped hyperintensity in ventral medulla. (**b**) Diffusion-weighted axial images showing restricted diffusion in the infarcted area. (**c**) Apparent diffusion coefficient (ADC) map showing low ADC in the affected medullary zone. Reproduced with permission from: Gupta et al. 2014.

in the internal *and* external carotid vessels—as in severe atheroma and vasculitis.

Following are some Handles that would alert you to the possibility of severe internal carotid narrowing.

▶ Transient monocular blindness on going outdoors

Typically, the patient walks out into sunshine or other situations where there is abrupt transition from subdued to bright light. There is dimming of vision in one eye rather than a shade or curtain effect. The mechanism of this is debated. Impaired regeneration of retinal pigments is one explanation, but apart from the glare experienced by patients with unilateral cataract, there are few other conditions that produce this characteristic symptom.

▶ Unilateral corneal arcus senilis

This sign (Figure 9.18) indicates more severe ischemia on the side with the absent or less obvious corneal arcus. The reason for this is not clear, but it is a useful sign to help identify the abnormal side.

▶ Unilateral ischemic or proliferative diabetic retinopathy

Both conditions suggest severe ipsilateral carotid stenosis associated with retinal ischemia. Some patients display more advanced cataract on the ischemic side.

▶ Unilateral rubeosis iridis

There are many local ocular diseases that cause rubeosis iridis (Figure 9.19), which literally means "red iris." The sign is caused by formation of new vessels in the iris (neovascularization). If local ocular causes

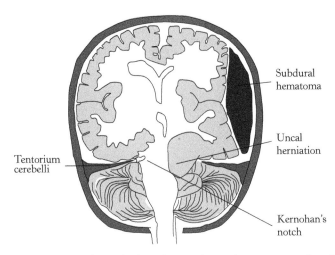

FIGURE 9.15: Simplified illustration of Kernohan's notch, secondary in this instance, to a large left subdural hematoma. This would produce a left hemiparesis. Reproduced with permission under the Creative Commons Attribution License, from Panikkath et al. (2013).

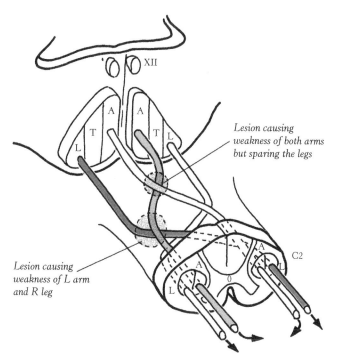

FIGURE 9.16: Anatomy of the lower medulla at the level of the corticospinal tract decussation. Rostral is in the upper part of the figure, caudal is in the lower part. Note that the leg fibers (red) cross slightly lower than the arm fibers (blue). Thus, a discrete lesion in the caudal left medulla (shaded circle) might result in weakness of the *left* arm and *right* leg as shown. Also, a lesion in the central decussation would cause weakness of both arms but spare the legs. Reproduced and modified with permission from *Neurological Differential Diagnosis*, 2nd ed., J Patten, Figure 11.5. Springer-Verlag, 1995.

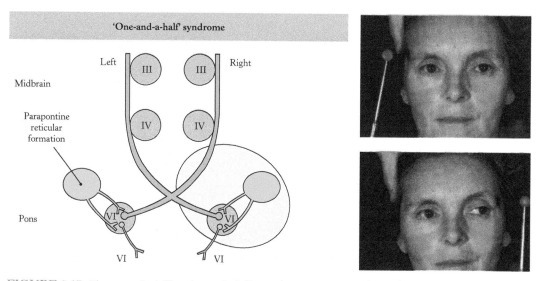

FIGURE 9.17: The one-and-a-half syndrome. **Left** (diagram): There is a lesion (yellow) affecting the right CN VI nucleus (pink/gray circle), adjacent paramedian pontine reticular formation (green) and fibers (blue) that cross to ascend in the medial longitudinal fasciculus (MLF) destined for the opposite medial rectus nucleus for contralateral adduction. Therefore, the only horizontal movement remaining is abduction of the left eye. **Right**: The patient cannot follow the red target to her right, i.e. right conjugate gaze palsy, nor can she adduct the left eye. The only horizontal movement possible is abduction of the left eye. Reproduced with permission from *Clinical Examination*, Figure 12.78, by O Epstein, GD Perkin, DP de Bono, and J Cookson. Gower Medical Publishing, 1992.

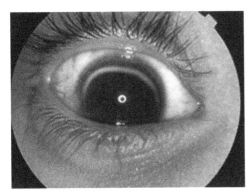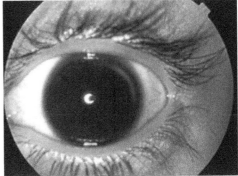

FIGURE 9.18: Unilateral corneal arcus. This suggests more severe carotid disease on the side with the smaller or absent arcus—here on the patient's left side. The eye with the poorer blood supply does not develop an arcus. Courtesy Dr. Irina Gout, Prince Charles Eye Unit, Windsor.

such as central retinal artery occlusion are excluded, then ipsilateral ICAS is a strong possibility because of severe ocular ischemia. Another mechanism for rubeosis is reversed blood flow in anastomotic channels of the *external* carotid artery via the facial artery and ciliary arteries to the carotid syphon. With a finger, it is sometimes possible to detect the presence of reduced pulsation in the facial artery either side of the nasal bridge or as it crosses the mandible, but we do not find this a particularly reliable Handle.

▶ Jerking leg (or arm) on standing
This is also known as "orthostatic limb shaking" or "limb-shaking TIAs." The typical patient describes involuntary jerking or dyskinesia of one leg and/or arm on the same side when standing, occasionally

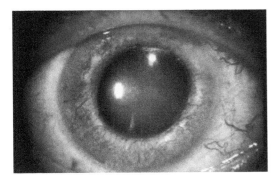

FIGURE 9.19: Rubeosis iridis. The photo shows neovascularization of the iris. This may be a sign of severe ipsilateral internal carotid insufficiency. Courtesy Dr. Irina Gout, Prince Charles Eye Unit, Windsor.

after coughing or exercise (see Video 8.98, Orthostatic PD). Rarely, an arm or both legs will shake. They are brief and recurrent and spare the face. It is an important sign because it can be confused with a focal seizure or with orthostatic tremor (if both legs are involved). The usual explanation is that perfusion along a severely narrowed ICA is sufficient when lying or sitting, but, on standing, gravity reduces internal carotid flow further. This affects the most distal carotid territory; namely, the terminal branches of the anterior cerebral artery that supply the leg area.

▶ Horner's syndrome and contralateral hemiparesis after a traffic accident is likely an ICA dissection.
  • Less often, the vertebral artery is affected. The hemiparesis is due to ICA stenosis/occlusion with ischemia in the middle cerebral artery territory. Horner's syndrome results from injury to the internal carotid arterial sheath that carries the sympathetic fibers to the pupil. It may be associated with pain around the eye or neck.
  • Pulsatile tinnitus
  • Ipsilateral hypoglossal nerve lesion. This occurs because of the proximity of CN XII to the carotid sheath

When the tongue is protruded, it deviates away from the hemiplegic side; the inexperienced clinician may diagnose a medullary lesion. The prognosis for ICA dissection with a Horner's syndrome is generally better than that for a vertebral dissection. Note

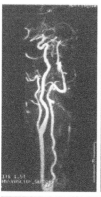
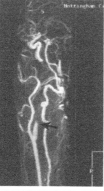
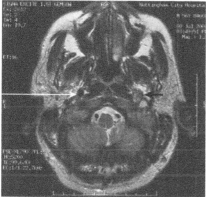
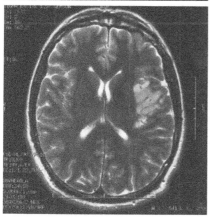

that the motor vehicle accident does not have to be severe—it could be a simple whiplash injury—and may have taken place several days previously.

▶ Recurrent bouts of coughing, vomiting, seizures, or tics (including Tourette syndrome) may cause arterial dissection.
These may produce cervical artery dissection because of repeated abrupt neck movement. The MRI may show the "crescent sign" from the presence of blood in the vessel wall (Figure 9.20).

POSTERIOR CIRCULATION ISCHEMIA

Following are some Handles for posterior circulation ischemia (PCI):

▶ Imbalance on looking upward
Imbalance in an elderly hypertensive person on looking upward suggests PCI. This is an alleged characteristic (some would say infamous) sign of PCI. Thus, a patient who is elderly and hypertensive looks up at a bird or plane in the sky and overbalances or even falls. It is sometimes called the "cathedral syndrome" when an elderly person looks up to admire an elegant cathedral roof and falls backward. Mirrors now fitted to most churches help to avoid this. One explanation for PCI is that it results from vertebral artery narrowing by neck osteophytes, with further narrowing provoked by neck movement.

This is likely to account for a minority of cases. Other causes are as follows:

· Benign paroxysmal positional vertigo
· Chiari type I syndrome, particularly in a younger patient (Figure 9.21); often this is associated with cough headache.
· Parkinsonism and related disorders
· Impaired joint position sense from polyneuropathies
▶ Stroke following head turn to one side is Bow Hunter's syndrome.
This syndrome results from usually temporary occlusion of a vertebral artery provoked by turning the head within the physiological range (Figure 9.22). The occluded artery

FIGURE 9.20: The crescent sign resulting from internal carotid dissection in a patient with aphasia and persisting left facial pain. **Top Left**: MR angiogram showing normal right carotid bifurcation. **Top Right**: MR angiogram showing tapering occlusion of left internal carotid artery (arrow). **Center**: T2-weighted MRI showing mural hematoma in left internal carotid artery (crescent sign, thick arrow). Note normal flow void of right internal carotid artery (thin arrow). **Bottom**: T2-weighted MRI showing small infarct in left insular cortex. Reproduced from Figure 1.3 in the chapter Is It a Stroke? by RJ Harwood, F Huwez, and D Good. Oxford University Press. DOI:10.1093/med/9780199558315.003.0001.

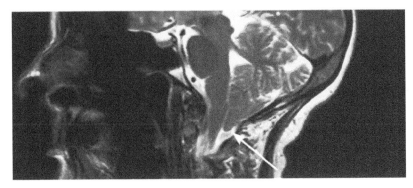

FIGURE 9.21: T2-weighted sagittal brain MRI of Chiari type I malformation. Arrow points to the tip of the cerebellar tonsils. Patients present with cough headache and ataxia, particularly on looking up. Reproduced from *Developmental and Genetic Disorders*, Figure 18–2 in the chapter Developmental and Genetic Disorders, by RW Baloh, V Honrubia, and KA Kerber. Oxford University Press. DOI:10.1093/med/9780195387834.003.0018.

is most often on the side opposite the direction of turning. Most cases involve the dominant (left) vertebral artery and are caused by osteophytes at C1 or C2 level. The symptoms are those of brainstem ischemia; namely, presyncope, paresis, and imbalance.

▶ TIAs following strenuous use one arm is likely the subclavian steal syndrome (Figure 9.23).

The stenosis has to be in the proximal subclavian artery, before the vertebral artery branch, and must be severe to provoke symptoms. Minor degrees of stenosis are usually asymptomatic. There is ischemic pain in the arm on the stenotic side with reduced radial pulse. Symptoms provoked by use of the relevant arm include transient blurred vision, ataxia, imbalance, and presyncope.

▶ Imbalance provoked by eating a large meal or standing up

This is another feature of PCI and probably relates to diversion of blood into the intestinal circulation when eating. A spinal dural fistula might also cause this—see Chapter 10.

▶ Ataxia with blindness (blind staggers)

The patient who is characteristically elderly and hypertensive reports episodes of bilateral visual loss and imbalance. The symptoms are basically a form of TIA affecting the

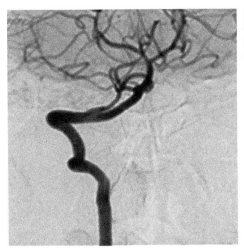
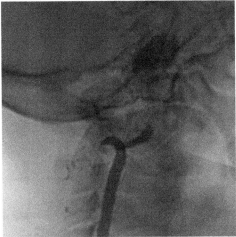

FIGURE 9.22: Bow Hunter's syndrome (stroke). **Left:** Normal right vertebral angiogram in a 50-year-old woman with the head in neutral position. **Right:** The right vertebral artery is occluded completely when the head is rotated to the left. Reproduced from Go et al. (2013), Figure 2.

- Atonic seizures; recall may be poor
- Cardiac arrhythmia, often with warning presyncopal symptoms
- Ménière's variant (otolith crisis)—as rare as hen's teeth

Locked-in Syndrome

▶ Quadriplegia with paralysis of all motor cranial nerves except for vertical eye movement and voluntary blinking is the locked-in syndrome.

The pupils react to light and consciousness is preserved, although patients are sometimes assumed (mistakenly) to be in a coma. The main causes are as follows:

- Anterior pontine thrombosis, hemorrhage, or tumor
- Fat embolus to the ventral pons resulting from major bone surgery or long bone fracture, with patent foramen ovale.
- Central pontine myelinolysis
- Neuromuscular disorder; myasthenia gravis or myotonic dystrophy following general anesthetic, which unmasks a latent disorder. The pupils are normal, but eye movements may be impaired in myasthenia gravis.
- Severe polyneuropathy (e.g., Guillain-Barré syndrome)
- Succinylcholine given without adequate anesthesia will induce complete paralysis of voluntary movement with no impairment of consciousness and normal pupillary reflexes, but all eye movements and blinks are paralyzed, so it is not a true locked-in state.

Note: If the patient is conscious, there will be a reactive alpha rhythm on EEG (Hawkes and Bryan-Smyth 1974).

HANDLES FOR CORTICAL SYNDROMES

▶ *Weakness of both arms dangling lifelessly by the side of the trunk suggests the "man-in-a-barrel" syndrome.* This may be associated with the following:
- Cortical borderzone (watershed) lesion (Figure 9.24). Typically the syndrome follows a major ischemic event such as cardiac arrest that causes border zone infarcts in the parietal overlap region between

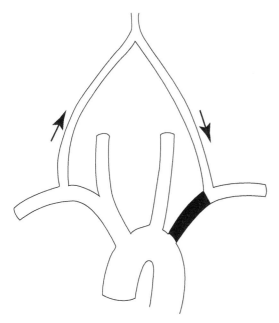

FIGURE 9.23: The subclavian steal syndrome. Severe stenosis in the proximal part of the left subclavian artery reduces flow to the left arm causing a "steal" of blood from the basilar and opposite vertebral arteries. The impaired basilar artery flow causes transient brain stem symptoms.

posterior circulation—chiefly the vestibular and visual pathways. The blindness results from reduced flow in the posterior cerebral arteries which supply the visual cortex. If you see a patient during an attack, check the pupils; they should react normally to light, in keeping with cortical blindness

▶ Drop attacks in the elderly mostly affect females and are usually unexplained. The patient falls to the ground without warning. Features include:
- Rapid recovery
- Knees bruised, face injured, and glasses, if worn, are damaged
- No loss of consciousness and good recall of event

The cause is presumably episodic ischemia in brainstem areas concerned with maintaining body tone, primarily the anterior cerebellum, vermis, and vestibular nuclei. Patients rarely develop a complete stroke, but they may have recurrent attacks. Less likely causes are the following:

- Carotid sinus syncope, induced by lateral head turning

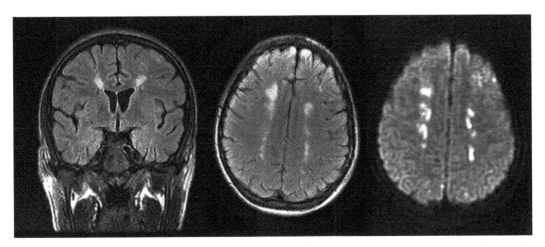

FIGURE 9.24: T2-weighted MRI scans that show bilateral typical linear infarcts in the border zone territory between the middle cerebral, anterior cerebral, and posterior cerebral arteries. This usually results from prolonged hypotension secondary to myocardial infarction.

the anterior and middle cerebral artery territories.

- Cervical myelopathy (Figure 9.25). A typical history relates to someone who walks with hands in their pockets, falls forward, cannot prevent a fall, and hits his head. The mechanism is either a spinal infarct or pressure from a disk.
- Slowly progressive varieties of amyotrophic lateral sclerosis or spinal muscular atrophy with extensive anterior horn cell loss in the cervical cord (see Figures 7.26 and 7.27):
- Severe neuropathies (e.g., Guillain-Barré syndrome) and radiculopathies
- Bilateral lesions of the brachial plexus

▶ *Patient who answers questions on behalf of person in the next bed has a right parietal lesion.* If a neighboring patient is asked to obey simple commands, such as "Close your eyes" or "Open your mouth," or is questioned about what he or she had for breakfast, the affected (adjacent) patient responds on behalf of the neighbor. This strange disorder is found predominantly in those with a right parietal stroke (Bogousslavsky and Regli 1988).

▶ *Recurrent strokes, hypertension, and pelvic rash (bathing trunk area)* (Figure 9.26, left) *suggest Fabry's syndrome.* It is a particularly important disorder to identify, given the availability of effective enzyme replacement treatment (e.g., Fabrazyme). Other features are as follows:

- Painful burning polyneuropathy

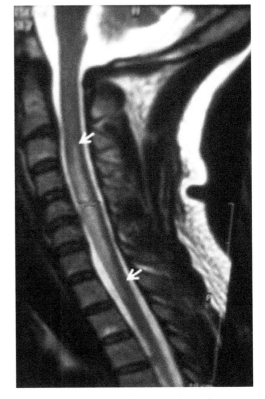

FIGURE 9.25: Man-in-a-barrel syndrome due to spinal infarct. T2-weighted MRI sagittal image. There is a longitudinally extensive high-intensity intramedullary lesion at C3–C8 (arrows) in keeping with acute cervical spinal cord infarction (red star). Reproduced from Antelo et al. (2013), Figure 1.

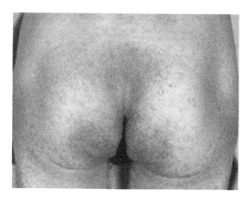 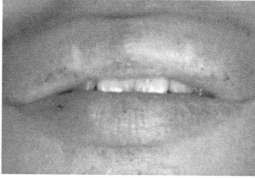

FIGURE 9.26: **Left**: The "bathing trunk" rash of Fabry's disease. **Right**: Small spot lesions on the lips. Both figures courtesy of Dr. GF Odland, Division of Dermatology, University of Washington. Reproduced from Figure 5.46 in the chapter Disorders of the Dermis, by V Sybert. Oxford University Press. DOI:10.1093/med/9780195397666.003.0005.

- Tortuous conjunctival or retinal vessels (Figure 1.16).
- Vortex keratopathy (Figure 11.19)
- Low-frequency deafness
- Impaired sweating
- Renal failure, restrictive cardiomyopathy
- Priapism

The rash may be inconspicuous and confined to the perineum or umbilicus. There may be small angiokeratomas on the lips (Figure 9.26, *right*). Note that heterozygous female carriers may have a mild form of the disease and present in middle age.

▶ *Headache, retinal infarcts, and deafness suggest Susac's syndrome* (Figures 9.27 and 9.28). This is a rare, presumed autoimmune disorder that affects mainly young adult women. Deafness is cochlear and involves principally the low frequencies. There may be cognitive problems, the most intriguing, allegedly characteristic, being the illusion that the person lives in a foreign country (www.standard.co.uk/news/the-woman-who-woke-up-thinking-she-was-french-7195089.html). The MRI brain scan shows punched-out infarcts on T1 sequences, mainly in the body of the corpus callosum, but on T2 sequences the lesions are like snowballs (Figure 9.28, *upper left*). The appearances can be confused with those of MS. There may be the "string of pearls" sign in the internal capsule area on DWI sequences (Figure 9.28, *lower left*).

▶ *Headache, hemiparesis, and seizures after carotid endarterectomy or stenting suggest the cerebral hyperperfusion syndrome.* It results from abrupt restoration of blood flow to an ischemic area where cerebral autoregulation is deficient because of long-standing ischemia. It usually takes place immediately after surgery but may be delayed up to 1 month. MRI shows extensive high T2 signal change and gyral swelling (Figure 9.29). Lowering of blood pressure is standard therapy.

▶ *Crossed-leg sign in the early phase after a stroke favors a better prognosis.* Those who cross their legs fare better than those who lie with both legs extended and uncrossed (Remi et al. 2011).

▶ *Herpes zoster followed by stroke suggests postviral cerebral angiitis.* This is a condition characterized by small- and medium-vessel inflammation.

The diagnosis of zoster-induced vasculitis may be overlooked if only the blood and cerebrospinal fluid (CSF) polymerase chain reaction (PCR) is undertaken. The correct test is for zoster immunoglobulins (IgM and IgG) in CSF.

▶ *Stroke in a patient with a history of migraine with aura suggests migrainous infarction.* It is well established that patients who experience migraine *with aura* are at higher risk of stroke (Lantz et al. 2017) Conversely, migraine may develop *as a result* of cerebral ischemia. Apart from migraine, other associations are as follows:

- CADASIL syndrome (cerebral autosomal dominant arteriopathy with subcortical

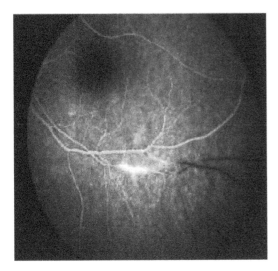

FIGURE 9.27: Fluorescein angiogram showing the characteristic hyperfluorescence proximal to the site of segmental arteriolar branch occlusion seen in Susac's retinopathy. Reproduced with permission from Plummer et al. (2005), Figure 1.

infarcts and leukoencephalopathy). Migraine is very common and always associated with aura. The clue to diagnosis is involvement of the anterior temporal lobes on MRI.

- o Moyamoya disease
- o Anti-phospholipid (Hughes) syndrome
- o MELAS (mitochondrial encephalopathy lactic acidosis and stroke-like episodes). Here there is limb muscle weakness, recurrent headache, seizures, and brief hemiparetic attacks
- o Fibromuscular dysplasia
- o Patent foramen ovale (controversial)
- ▶ *Autosomal recessive CADASIL-like syndrome with alopecia and lumbar spondylosis suggests the cerebral autosomal recessive arteriopathy with subcortical infarcts and leukoencephalopathy (CARASIL) syndrome.* See Figure 9.30. There is usually dementia and sometimes extrapyramidal features, such as rigidity.
- ▶ *Stroke with hemisensory loss that spares the trunk suggests that the lesion is cortical (parathalamic).* If there is impaired sensation over one side of the trunk, then the lesion is likely to be in the posterior thalamus (pulvinar) or its brainstem afferent pathways. Some maintain that loss of feeling over the axillary skin is a sign of a thalamic lesion.

The reason for this is that sensory fibers are packed close together in the thalamus or spinothalamic tracts, where they would be vulnerable to a small lesion. In the parietal cortex, the fibers are widely dispersed; thus a large defect would be required to damage trunk fibers, which have a relatively small cortical representation.

Note: Pulvinar lesions (posterior thalamus) are often associated with the thalamic pain syndrome and loss of taste.

- ▶ *Livedo reticularis and strokes suggest the Sneddon syndrome* (Figure 9.31). Phospholipid antibodies are present in the blood in about half the cases. The MRI may simulate MS.
  Other possible causes are:
  - o Polyarteritis
  - o Systemic lupus erythematosus
- ▶ *Starfish hand sign* (Figure 9.32) is a rare sequel of hemiplegia involving the caudate nucleus. It arises because of delayed dystonia affecting the hand muscles.
- ▶ *Sudden inversion of vision* is a rare feature of the following:
  - o Wallenberg's syndrome
  - o Thrombosis of the anterior inferior cerebellar artery
  - o Basilar migraine
  - o Lesions of the visual or parietal cortex
- ▶ *Vivid hallucinations ("peduncular hallucinosis"), cortical blindness, somnolence, paresis of vertical gaze, and all pupil reflexes without significant motor dysfunction suggest the top of the basilar syndrome.* Apart from cortical blindness and hallucinations, these symptoms are like those of a Percheron artery infarct This is a variably present branch of the first part of the posterior cerebral artery that supplies both paramedian thalamic regions and subthalamus (Figure 9.33).

HANDLES FOR LACUNAR SYNDROMES

- ▶ Complete hemiparesis including the face without aphasia, apraxia, agnosia, or field loss is the *pure motor hemiplegia syndrome.* This results from a lesion in the internal capsule, ventral pons, or, rarely, from a single medullary pyramidal lesion.

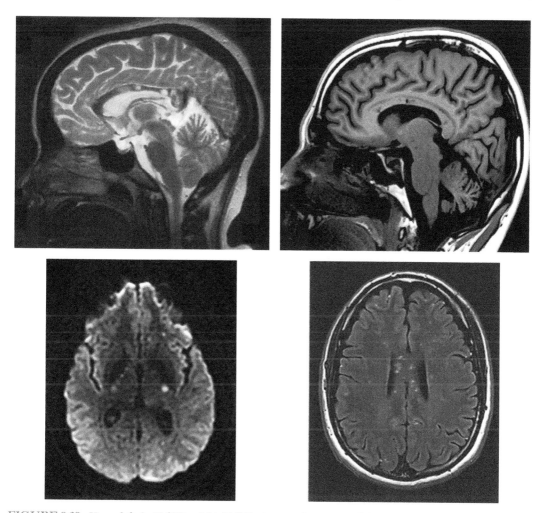

FIGURE 9.28: Upper left: Sagittal T2-weighted MRI brain scan of a woman with Susac's syndrome. This shows character-istic snowball-like lesions in the corpus callosum.

Upper right: Sagittal T1-weighted MRI brain scan of a person with Susac's syndrome. The lesions in the corpus callosum now appear as punched-out holes. **Lower left**: Axial DWI showing the "string of pearls" sign (four individual pearls) in the right internal capsule. These lesions correlate with spastic gait. **Lower right**: T1-weighted axial image that shows a similar "string of pearls" sign in the left internal capsule region. Upper left image reproduced with permission from Saenz et al. (2005), Figure 1. Upper right image courtesy Bart's Health Neuroimaging Department, London. Lower left image courtesy Dr. R Rennebohm. Lower right image courtesy Bart's Health Neuroimaging Department, London.

▶ Loss of feeling over the whole of one side of the body, including the face, axilla, and half of the trunk, with no aphasia, apraxia, agnosia, or field loss is the *pure hemisensory stroke syndrome*. It is due to a lacune in the main sensory nucleus of the thalamus (ventroposterior nucleus). A discrete le-sion in the ventroposterior *medial* thalamic nucleus just causes contralateral facial numbness.

▶ *Dysarthria–clumsy hand syndrome.* The syn-drome is self-explanatory and produces symptoms most obvious when the patient is writing.
It is due to a lesion in the paramedian mid-pons or posterior internal capsule on the side opposite the clumsy hand.

▶ Weakness and clumsiness in the same limb is the *ataxic hemiparesis syndrome*. It is charac-teristic of a lacune in the ventral pons, lower

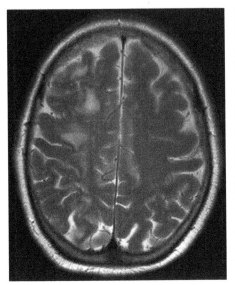 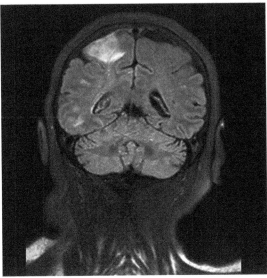

FIGURE 9.29: Cerebral hyperperfusion syndrome. Axial (**left**) and coronal (**right**) MR brain images. There is extensive right occipital and parietal high signal with mild right frontal cortical and subcortical high T2 signal with gyral swelling. This followed endarterectomy for 95% stenosis of the right carotid artery in a 68-year-old woman. Reproduced from Rafiq et al. (2014), Figure 2.

mid-brain, posterior internal capsule, or corona radiata.

It is not so useful in localization as the other lacunar syndromes, but the defect involves corticospinal and cerebellar fibers contralateral to the weak side. The presence of nystagmus favors a brainstem etiology.

HANDLES FOR HEMORRHAGIC DISORDERS

▶ *Subhyaloid hemorrhage* is a classic sign of subarachnoid hemorrhage (Terson syndrome) (Figure 9.34).

The hemorrhage can be subretinal, retinal, preretinal, or intravitreal. Its likely cause

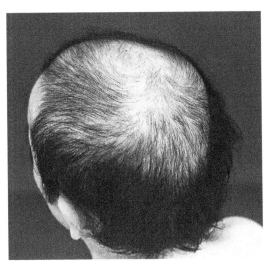

FIGURE 9.30: Diffuse baldness in a 33-year-old man with CARASIL (cerebral autosomal recessive arteriopathy with subcortical infarcts and leukoencephalopathy) syndrome. Reproduced with permission from Fukutake (2011).

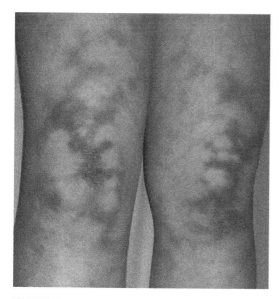

FIGURE 9.31: Livedo reticularis in Sneddon syndrome. Reproduced from Figure 20.4 in the chapter Vasculitis, by S Burge and D Wallis. Oxford University Press. DOI:10.1093/med/9780199558322.003.0020.

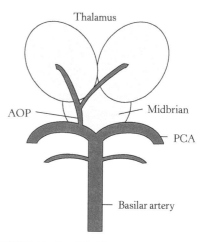

FIGURE 9.33: Simplified diagram of the blood supply to the paramedian thalamus. Normally this zone receives its own supply from the posterior cerebral artery (PCA). The artery of Percheron (AOP) is a variant in which a single branch from the proximal PCA supplies both thalami and sometimes the rostral midbrain. Thus, occlusion of AOP will result in bilateral thalamic ischemia. Reproduced under the Creative Commons Attribution License from Lee A et al. 2016.

is a rapid increase in intracranial pressure. A clue to the presence of subhyaloid hemorrhage is that *the hemorrhage may roll around as the patient changes position.*

▶ *Neck stiffness with negative Kernig's sign denotes raised intracranial pressure.* Neck stiffness with positive Kernig's sign favors meningeal irritation.

It is not widely recognized that raised intracranial pressure induces neck stiffness, probably from stretching of the meninges, and that it worsens with neck flexion. If you find neck stiffness and a positive Kernig's sign, this is good evidence of meningeal irritation from either infection or blood.

◀ *Stroke with rapid loss of consciousness* implies a sudden hemorrhage or basilar artery embolus. This can be due to subarachnoid hemorrhage or other causes of bleeding into the cerebral

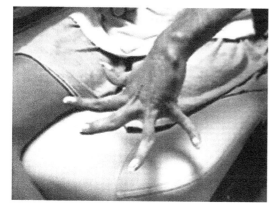

FIGURE 9.32: Starfish hand. This is a dystonic hand which in this instance, followed a right middle cerebral artery stroke involving the caudate nucleus. Reproduced from Ho et al. (2007).

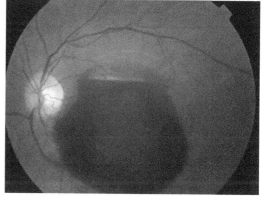

FIGURE 9.34: Subhyaloid hemorrhage, a sign of subarachnoid hemorrhage. This is called Terson's syndrome and is generally associated with a poor prognosis. The retinal changes associated with diabetes are similar. Courtesy Dr. Irina Gout, Prince Charles Eye Unit, Windsor.

hemisphere and especially brainstem. It is a major Red Flag.

▶ *Abrupt hemiplegia with head and eyes deviated to the side of weakness* suggests a cerebral hemorrhage in its early irritant phase.

Thus, a lesion in the left frontal area will induce a right hemiparesis and, on rare occasion, stimulate the left frontal eye fields that cause deviation of the head and eyes to the right, causing "wrong-way eyes." When the irritant effects of hemorrhage settle, the eyes will deviate away from the hemiparetic side, usually by the next day. A pontine infarct can also cause "wrong-way eyes," but in this case there is no head turn.

▶ Patient with distended abdomen and subarachnoid hemorrhage likely has polycystic kidneys. Patients with polycystic kidneys have increased risk (about 10%) of cerebral aneurysms and many experience subarachnoid hemorrhage.

CORTICAL SINUS THROMBOSIS (SAGITTAL OR LATERAL SINUSES)

This disorder is easily overlooked, as there may be few clinical signs. Following are some Handles and Flags.

History

- Postpartum period, especially in Afro-Caribbean and Asian women
- Dehydration (especially in marathon runners),excess alcohol
- Infection of ear or nasal sinuses
- Hemiparesis or paraparesis
- Focal seizures, particularly affecting the legs if there is sagittal sinus thrombosis
- Following any major surgery
- Clotting disorder (e.g., anti-phospholipid [Hughes] syndrome, protein C and S deficiency, blood dyscrasias) or underlying cancer, especially pancreatic
- Ulcerative colitis, Crohn's disease
- Use of any steroid medication, erythropoietin, heparin
- Following lumbar puncture

Physical Examination

- Drowsiness, headache, and vomiting
- Papilledema
- Neck pain made worse by head turning/tilting to either side but not by flexion

suggests cerebral or jugular vein thrombosis. It is likely caused by compression of the internal jugular veins on head turning or tilting, which elevates intracranial pressure. If the neck pain is made worse by neck *flexion* this suggests subarachnoid hemorrhage.

Imaging

▶ A routine CT brain scan may be normal in the first few days—but:

▶ Enhanced CT scan may show the empty delta sign. This is a triangular filling defect due to clot formation at the torcula (Figure 9.35).

Also note:

▶ Cerebral venous sinus thrombosis with dark urine, particularly in the morning, is diagnostic of paroxysmal nocturnal hemoglobinuria.

SUMMARY

History

- Recurrent nose bleeds and stroke in a young adult: Osler-Weber-Rendu syndrome

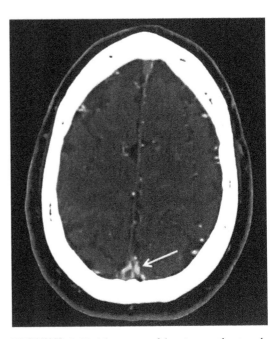

FIGURE 9.35: The empty delta sign at the torcula (arrow). Courtesy Radiopedia, case 1, Dr. Ayush Goel and Dr. Frank Gaillard.

- Abrupt onset of one arm clutching the other arm, throat, or other body part inappropriately: alien limb syndrome due to vascular lesion of corpus callosum or parietal lobes
- Stroke-like migraine attacks after radiation therapy: SMART syndrome or internal carotid stenosis from delayed radiotherapy-induced intimal swelling
- Stroke-like episodes triggered by metformin, sodium valproate, or statins: MELAS syndrome
- Alleged infantile hemiplegia may be dopamine-responsive dystonia.
- Transient loss of episodic memory following unaccustomed exertion, sex, emotion, or cold exposure is TGA. Also consider migraine, TEA, and concussion. Learn Table 9.1.
- Persistent acute-onset global amnesia suggests thalamic or medial temporal lobe infarction. Visual field defects present in the medial temporal lobe variety.
- Recurrent fluctuating episodes of weakness resulting in a complete stroke is the *capsular warning syndrome.*
- A single episode of weakness/visual failure lasting more than 1 hour is not a TIA.
- TIA induced by hyperventilation (mainly children) is characteristic of Moyamoya disease.
- Bouts of dystonia and weakness on either side, often starting during sleep, lasting minutes or days, is the alternating hemiplegia/hemidystonia syndrome of childhood.
- Hemiparesis after childbirth is usually cortical venous sinus thrombosis. Other causes: extracranial dissection, cerebral hemorrhage, postpartum vasculitis, PRES, RCVS, HELLP syndromes, and functional disorders
- Stroke with contralateral elongated styloid process is the Eagle syndrome.
- Abrupt hemiplegia with dyspnea relieved by lying down suggests a left atrial myxoma with emboli. Patients may also have cardiac murmurs that vary with position, paroxysmal arrhythmias, raised ESR, and abnormal serum proteins.
- Recurrent, stereotyped, spreading paresthesia, sometimes with weakness, lasting several minutes, simulating TIA is likely due to amyloid spells or migraine. Positive phenomena are unusual in classic TIAs.
- Amyloid spells may present after the age 60 as suspected migraine without headache.

Stroke Mimics
- Postictal paresis, hypoglycemia, sepsis, hemiplegic migraine, psychogenic disorders, MELAS
- A hemorrhagic stroke is more likely to cause a seizure than thromboembolism.

Focal Cortical and Brainstem Syndromes
- A homonymous field defect cannot be due to a single lesion in the frontal cortex.
- In face-sparing hemiparesis, check shoulder shrugs and the jaw jerk to determine whether the lesion is intracranial or spinal.
- Diplopia associated with a stroke usually indicates a pontine or midbrain lesion: CN III palsy with contralateral hemiparesis is Weber s syndrome. A CN VI and VII cranial nerve lesion with contralateral hemiparesis and sensory impairment is Foville's or Millard-Gubler syndrome. CN III nerve palsy with contralateral ataxia and tremor is Benedikt's syndrome.
- In a cortical stroke due to hemorrhage or a large infarct, CN VI palsy on the side of the hemorrhage/infarct is likely a false localizing sign.
- Supranuclear paralysis of upgaze with fixed dilated pupils is Parinaud's syndrome.
- Sudden-onset ataxia, vomiting, and dysphagia favors Wallenberg (lateral medullary) syndrome.
- Inability to sneeze is a rare feature in the recovery phase of Wallenberg's syndrome.
- Quadriparesis (sparing face), dysarthria, hypoglossal palsy, nystagmus, and sometimes respiratory failure suggests *bilateral medial medullary infarction.*
- Hemiparesis on the same side as a cortical lesion might be caused by Kernohan's notch.
- Weak arm on one side with weak leg on the other: vascular lesion at the caudal medulla affecting the decussating pyramidal fibers
- Absence of horizontal gaze except for abduction of one eye suggests the one-and-a half syndrome

Major Arterial Syndromes
Internal Carotid Artery Stenosis
When severe, there may be the following:

- Transient monocular blindness on going outdoors
- Unilateral corneal arcus senilis

- Unilateral ischemic or proliferative diabetic retinopathy
- Unilateral rubeosis iridis
- Jerking leg or arm on standing (orthostatic limb shaking)
- Horner's syndrome and contralateral hemiparesis after a traffic accident suggest dissection of the ICA. May be associated with pain around the eye or neck, pulsatile tinnitus, ipsilateral hypoglossal nerve lesion
- Recurrent bouts of coughing, vomiting, seizures, or severe tics (including Tourette syndrome) may produce cervical artery dissection as a result of repeated abrupt neck movement.
- MRI: "crescent sign" due to the presence of blood in the vessel wall

Posterior Circulation Ischemia

- Imbalance on looking upward: causes: posterior circulation ischemia; benign paroxysmal positional vertigo; Chiari syndrome in young patients, often with cough headache; parkinsonism and related disorders; impaired joint position sense from polyneuropathies
- Stroke following head turn to one side is Bow Hunter's syndrome.
- TIAs following strenuous use one arm: subclavian steal syndrome
- Imbalance provoked by eating a large meal or standing up. This also infers posterior circulation ischemia diversion of blood into the intestinal circulation. A spinal dural fistula might also cause this.
- Blind staggers: episodes of bilateral visual loss and imbalance due to PCI
- Drop attacks in the elderly mostly affect females and are usually unexplained. Other causes: carotid sinus syncope, atonic seizures, cardiac arrhythmia, Ménière's variant
- Quadriplegia with paralysis of all motor cranial nerves except for vertical eye movement and voluntary blinking is the locked-in syndrome. Main causes: anterior pontine thrombosis/hemorrhage/tumor, fat embolism following bone surgery, central pontine myelinolysis

Cortical Syndromes

- *Weakness of both arms dangling lifelessly by the side of the trunk suggests the "man-in-a-barrel" syndrome.*

- Patient who answers questions on behalf of person in next bed: *right parietal lesion*
- Recurrent strokes, hypertension, and pelvic rash (bathing trunk area): *Fabry's syndrome.* Heterozygous female carriers may have a mild form of the disease and present in middle age.
- Headache, retinal infarcts, and deafness: *Susac's syndrome.* Illusion that patient lives in a foreign country; punched-out infarcts on MRI of corpus callosum and "string of pearls" sign in the internal capsule area
- Headache, hemiparesis, and seizures after carotid endarterectomy or stenting: *cerebral hyperperfusion syndrome*
- Crossed leg sign in the early phase after stroke favors a better prognosis. Legs extended and uncrossed favor a worse prognosis.
- Herpes zoster followed by stroke: *postviral cerebral angiitis*
- Stroke with history of migrainous headache: migrainous infarct, *CADASIL, Moyamoya disease, anti-phospholipid syndrome, MELAS, and fibromuscular dysplasia, patent foramen ovale (possibly)*
- Migraine may develop *as a result* of cerebral ischemia.
- Autosomal recessive CADASIL-like syndrome with alopecia and lumbar spondylosis suggests *CARASIL syndrome.*
- Stroke with hemisensory loss that spares the trunk suggests a *cortical "parathalamic" lesion.* Involvement of trunk: *thalamic or brainstem lesion*
- Stroke with loss of feeling over the axilla suggests a *thalamic lesion.*
- *Pulvinar lesions* may cause a thalamic pain syndrome and loss of taste.
- Livedo reticularis and strokes: *Sneddon syndrome, polyarteritis, systemic lupus erythematosus*
- Starfish hand sign: caudate vascular lesion inducing dystonia
- Sudden inversion of vision; *Wallenberg's syndrome*, thrombosis of the anterior inferior cerebellar artery, basilar migraine, or lesions of the visual or parietal cortex
- Vivid hallucinations, cortical blindness, somnolence, paresis of vertical gaze, and all pupil reflexes without significant motor dysfunction: *top of the basilar syndrome.* Without

hallucinations and cortical blindness indicates Percheron artery infarct.

Lacunar Syndromes

- Complete hemiparesis including the face without aphasia, apraxia, agnosia, or field loss is the *pure motor hemiplegia syndrome*. The lesion is in the internal capsule, ventral pons, or rarely from a single medullary pyramidal lesion.
- Loss of feeling over the whole of one side of the body, including the face, axilla, and half of the trunk, with no aphasia, apraxia, agnosia, or field loss: *pure hemisensory stroke syndrome*. It is caused by a lacune in the main sensory nucleus of the thalamus.
- *Dysarthria–clumsy hand syndrome*: lesion is in the paramedian mid-pons or posterior internal capsule on the side opposite the clumsy hand.
- *Ataxic hemiparesis*: weakness and clumsiness in the same limb. Lacune in the ventral pons, lower midbrain, posterior internal capsule, or corona radiata

Hemorrhagic Disorders

- *Subhyaloid hemorrhage*: classic sign of subarachnoid hemorrhage (Terson syndrome)
- *Neck stiffness with negative Kernig's sign*: raised intracranial pressure
- *Neck stiffness with positive Kernig's sign*: meningeal irritation
- *Stroke with rapid loss of consciousness*: sudden hemorrhage or basilar artery embolus
- *Hemiplegia with head and eyes deviated to side of weakness*: cerebral hemorrhage in early irritative phase. A pontine infarct may cause "wrong-way eyes" but there is no head turning.
- Patient with distended abdomen and subarachnoid hemorrhage: polycystic kidneys

Cortical Sinus Thrombosis (Sagittal or Lateral Sinuses)
History

- Postpartum period; Dehydration (marathon runners), excess alcohol, infection of ear or nasal sinuses, hemi- or paraparesis, focal seizures, major surgery, clotting disorder, ulcerative colitis, Crohn's disease, medication, steroids, erythropoietin, heparin, lumbar puncture

Physical Examination
- Drowsiness, headache and vomiting, papilledema, neck pain made worse by head turning/tilting to either side but not by flexion

Imaging
A routine CT brain scan may be normal in the first few days. Enhanced CT scan may show the empty delta sign. Cerebral venous sinus thrombosis with dark urine, particularly in the morning, is diagnostic of paroxysmal nocturnal hemoglobinuria.

SUGGESTED READING

Allou T, Castelnovo G, Renard D. Teaching Neuro-Images: mitochondrial encephalopathy, lactic acidosis, and stroke-like episodes. *Neurology.* 2012;79:e125.

Antelo MGA, Facal TL, Sánchez TP, Facal MSL, Nazabal ER. Man-in-the-barrel. A case of cervical spinal cord infarction and review of the literature. *Open Neurol J.* 2013;7:7–10.

Bogousslavsky J, Regli F. Response-to-next-patient-stimulation: a right hemisphere syndrome. *Neurology.* 1988;38:1225–1227.

Charidimou A, Peeters AP, Jager R, et al. Cortical superficial siderosis and intracerebral hemorrhage risk in cerebral amyloid angiopathy. *Neurology.* 2013;81:1666–1673.

Fukutake T. Cerebral autosomal recessive arteriopathy with subcortical infarcts and leukoencephalopathy (CARASIL): from discovery to gene identification. *J Stroke Cerebrovasc Dis.* 2011;20:85–93.

Go G, Hwang SH, Park IS, Park H. Rotational vertebral artery compression: Bow hunter's syndrome. *J Korean Neurosurg Soc.* 2013;54:243–245.

Gupta A, Goyal MK, Vishnu VY, Ahuja CK, Khurana D, Lal V. Bilateral medial medullary infarction: the 'heart' reveals the diagnosis. *International Journal of Stroke.* 2014;9(4).

Hamilton BE, Nesbit GM. Delayed CSF enhancement in posterior reversible encephalopathy syndrome. *AJNR Am J Neuroradiol.* 2008;29:456–457.

Hawkes CH, Bryan-Smyth L. The electroencephalogram in the "locked-in" syndrome. *Neurology.* 1974;24:1015–1018.

Ho BK, Morgan JC, Sethi KD. "Starfish" hand. *Neurology.* 2007;69:115.

Kim HY, Chung CS, Lee J, Han DH, Lee KH. Hyperventilation-induced limb shaking TIA in Moyamoya disease. *Neurology.* 2003;60:137–139.

Lantz M, Sieurin J, Sjölander A, Waldenlind E, Sjöstrand C, Wirdefeldt K. Migraine and risk of stroke: a national population-based twin study. *Brain.* 2017;140(10):2653–2662.

Lee A, Moon HI, Kwon HK, Pyun SB. Clinical features of an artery of percheron infarction: a case report. *Brain Neurorehabil*. 2016;10(1). https://doi.org/10.12786/bn.2017.10.e2

Mori N, Mugikura S, Higano S, et al. The leptomeningeal "ivy sign" on fluid-attenuated inversion recovery MR imaging in Moyamoya disease: a sign of decreased cerebral vascular reserve? *Am J Neuroradiol*. 2009;30:930–935.

Panikkath R, Panikkath D, Lim SY, Nugent K. Kernohan's notch: a forgotten cause of hemiplegia—CT scans are useful in this diagnosis. *Case Rep Med*. 2013;2013:296874.

Plummer C, Rattray K, Donnan GA, Basilli S. An unusual disease presenting at an unusual age: Susac's syndrome. *J Clin Neurosci*. 2005;12:99–100.

Pruitt A, Dalmau J, Detre J, Alavi A, Rosenfeld MR. Episodic neurologic dysfunction with migraine and reversible imaging findings after radiation. *Neurology*. 2006;67:676–678.

Rafiq MK, Connolly D, Randall M, Blank C. Cerebral hyperperfusion syndrome. *Pract Neurol*. 2014;14:64–66.

Remi J, Pfefferkorn T, Owens RL, et al. The crossed leg sign indicates a favorable outcome after severe stroke. *Neurology*. 2011;77:1453–1456.

Saenz R, Quan AW, Magalhaes A, Kish K. MRI of Susac's syndrome. *AJR Am J Roentgenol*. 2005;184:1688–1690.

Chapter 10: Spinal Lesions and Cerebrospinal Fluid

Myelopathy refers to any lesion of the spinal cord, whether from within the cord (*intrinsic*) or from outside it (*extrinsic*). There are some general strategies that may help distinguish one from the other, although their use is somewhat fading, given the accuracy of MRI. Nonetheless, all neurologists should know these guides that remain reasonably robust Handles and may allow you to identify the site or type of lesion while waiting for a scan result.

HANDLES FOR LOCALIZATION

In general:

▶ Quadriparesis: lesion in the cervical cord
   Hemiparesis: lesion in the brain. Facial weakness, jaw jerk, and shoulder shrugs can help localize this further to either the brain or cervical cord (see discussion later in this chapter).
▶ *Useless hand syndrome*: the patient complains that one hand is useless, particularly for performing everyday skilled movements.
   The lesion is usually in the posterior columns at C2–C4 level and it is characteristic of multiple sclerosis (MS) (see Video 4.1). It can also occur in various forms of apraxia.
▶ Paraparesis with sacral sparing indicates an intrinsic spinal cord lesion.
   The anatomical explanation is that fibers for sacral sensation are located in the outer (superficial) region of the spinothalamic tract, so that a lesion in the central cord, such as an intrinsic tumor or syringomyelia, has to be quite large to reach these fibers. Conversely: Paraparesis without sacral sparing suggests an extrinsic lesion.
   The lesion will press on coccygeal and sacral fibers first because they are near the surface of the spinal cord. A useful mnemonic for the distribution of fibers in the spinothalamic tract is *ALS*, which stands for arm, leg, sacrum, in that order from

inside outward. Thus, patients with extrinsic lesions report gluteal numbness, often when they are sitting on the toilet. Urinary and fecal incontinence is common. Remember that the concentric loss of sensation is centered on the coccyx, not the anus.
▶ If you are not sure whether the lesion is intrinsic or extrinsic, go for extrinsic, as this is far more frequent.

The *upper limit of sensory loss* is an important sign, as it means that the lesion must be at least that high in the cord. In general, for unilateral lesions according to traditional precepts:

▶ The spinal cord defect is always above the upper sensory limit due to oblique crossing of the spinothalamic fibers.
   Thus, you need to subtract one to two spinal segments from a cervical sensory level, two to three spinal segments from a thoracic level, and three for a lumbar level. This concept was challenged by Nathan et al. (2001) on the basis of nociceptive stimulation experiments in patients with anterolateral cordotomy. It was concluded that spinothalamic fibers in fact cross horizontally, not obliquely. This observation awaits confirmation.

When progressing up the patient's trunk testing for pain sensation with a pin, the transition from reduced to normal pain appreciation may be gradual ("shaded") or quite abrupt. So here is another general rule:

▶ A gradual transition is typical of an intrinsic lesion; an abrupt change characterizes an extrinsic disorder.

The reason is that external pressure from, say, a disk or tumor, compresses the cord at the same vertebral level.

An intrinsic lesion will press on the spinothalamic tract from within, but it may take a few months of growth to affect all sensory fibers at that level.

Also note:

A spinal sensory level apparently at the upper third of the sternum is not helpful since C4, T2, T3, and T4 levels overlap there.

It is necessary to test the sensory loss in the fingers to be sure of the level in these cases. The "hot spots" (Chapter 3) are over the deltoid for C5, the thumb for C6, and the little finger for C8.

▶ Heavy weak leg on one side with numb or burning leg on the other is likely the *Brown-Sequard syndrome* (Figure 10.1)

This results from pressure on the corticospinal tract on the side of the lesion producing an ipsilateral weak leg. The same defect presses on the ascending spinothalamic tract, which has already crossed over,

thus impairing pain (and temperature) on the contralateral side. In the complete syndrome, the weak leg exhibits impaired joint position sense and vibration, and there is a sensory level to pain on the contralateral abdomen and ipsilateral dermatomal sensory loss at the level of the lesion. Presence of this syndrome favors extrinsic cord compression, but identical features may be found with intrinsic lesions such as MS or anterior spinal artery ischemia (Figure 10.3). Most Brown-Sequard lesions are partial or cross the midline of the cord, but because this pattern has relatively few causes it is important to recognize it.

▶ Test for a sensory deficit on the back as well as the front of the chest.

Some length-dependent neuropathies produce sensory impairment in the lower limbs that extends only onto the anterior chest wall in a so-called escutcheon pattern (like a shield), but the skin over the back is spared, resulting in confusion with the

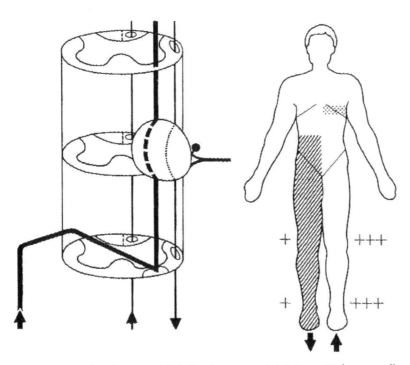

FIGURE 10.1: Brown-Sequard syndrome simplified. This shows an extrinsic lesion at T5 (e.g., neurofibroma) on the left that is damaging the descending left corticospinal tract, making the left leg weak and hyperreflexic. The same lesion is interrupting the ascending spinothalamic fibers, resulting in impaired pain appreciation on the right lower limb and abdomen. If the lesion affects the posterior columns there will be loss of vibration and joint position sense in the weak hyperreflexic left leg. There is a small area of radicular sensory impairment at T5 on the left due to pressure on the T5 nerve root at this level. Reproduced with permission from *A Color Atlas of Clinical Neurology*, 2nd ed., M Parsons, Figure 473. Wolfe Publishing, 1993.

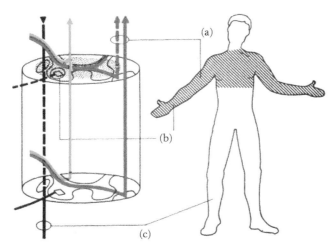

FIGURE 10.2: Syringomyelia. Shown here is the suspended sensory level of syringomyelia in the cervical cord. Follow the colored fibers from their entry into the cord at the bottom of the left figure. Fibers in the posterior columns for touch and joint position (green) are usually spared as they are peripheral to the centrally placed syrinx. Fibers in the spinothalamic tracts for pain and temperature (**a**, red) are damaged typically at the cervical and thoracic level, resulting in impaired pain and temperature over the cervical and upper thoracic segments (shaded gray on trunk). The hand wasting that is characteristic of syringomyelia is due to pressure on the anterior horn cells (**b**). The pyramidal tracts (**c**, black) are affected later and result in spastic paraparesis. Reproduced from *A Color Atlas of Clinical Neurology*, 2nd ed., M Parsons, Figure 457. Wolfe Publishing, 1993.

upper sensory level from cord compression. An upper boundary near the sternal notch is typical. Thus,

▶ An apparent sensory level on the anterior, but not posterior, chest wall may relate to a length-dependent polyneuropathy.
▶ Cape sensory loss ("suspended" sensory loss) suggests syringomyelia (Figure 10.2), paraneoplastic/traumatic lesions of the central cord, or porphyria (short fiber neuropathy).
  In syringomyelia and central cord lesions there is damage to the cervical spinothalamic tracts as they cross the central cord in the neck, resulting in dissociated sensory loss. This means there is impairment of pain and temperature but not joint position sense.
▶ Brisk knee jerks, depressed ankle jerks, and extensor plantars.
  This well-known combination has many causes, most of which are associated with myeloneuropathy (i.e., a mixture of upper and lower motor neuron pathology). Possible causes are as follows:
  ○ Subacute combined degeneration of the cord, amyotrophic lateral sclerosis

(ALS), widespread spinal spondylosis, syringomyelia, Friedreich's ataxia, taboparesis, copper deficiency, and neurofibromatosis
  ○ Rarer causes include HIV or human T-lymphotropic virus (HTLV-1)-related myeloneuropathy, spinal arteriovenous malformation, or dural fistula.
  ○ In men and rarely in women, adrenomyeloneuropathy, a disorder that affects the spinal cord and peripheral nerves
  ○ Sarcoidosis, when advanced, causes a polyneuropathy and there may be spinal cord involvement.

Also note:

▶ A completely normal sensory exam favors ALS.
▶ Reduced arm reflexes implicate cervical spondylosis and syringomyelia.
  Thus the saying: "If the arm reflexes are not reduced it's not a syrinx."
▶ Acute paraplegia with cutaneous sensory level but preserved joint position sense is most likely anterior spinal artery thrombosis.

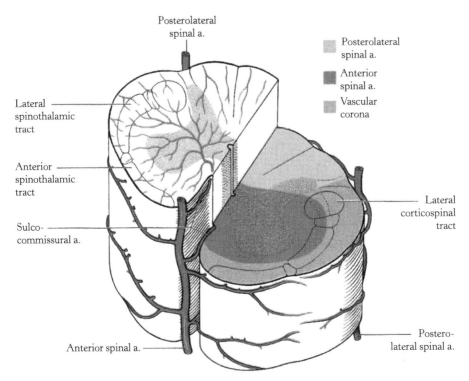

FIGURE 10.3: This shows the distribution of arterial blood supply to the spinal cord. Note that the single anterior spinal artery supplies the anterior two-thirds and the two posterolateral spinal arteries supply the posterior one third. There is a borderzone area between these two circulations. Reproduced with permission from *Duus' Topical Diagnosis in Neurology*, 5th ed., Figure 11.18, p. 282. Thieme, 2012.

This artery supplies the anterior two-thirds of the cord but the dorsal columns (that subserve joint position sense) are supplied by the posterior spinal artery, so that joint sense is spared (Figure 10.3). The patient is typically

- o Female elderly, diabetic, and/or hypertensive
- o Recently recovered from surgery with hypotensive episode from, for example, blood loss or myocardial ischemia

Anterior spinal artery thrombosis is a particular hazard after surgery to the abdominal aorta as the spinal arteries branch off from this vessel. The large artery of Adamkiewicz that arises between levels T8 and L1 is particularly susceptible to occlusion (sometimes following selective angiographic aortography), thus the defect is maximal at about T10. In ischemic myelopathy due to systemic hypotension the lesion is usually in the upper thoracic area (T1–T4), where the anterior spinal artery is farthest from its nearest feeding arterial supply. Thus:

▶ *Adamkiewicz artery occlusion* results in a level at T 10
▶ *Hypotension* causes a level at T1-4
▶ *Lumbar Lhermitte sign*
   Sometimes patients with lumbar spondylotic radiculopathy report shock-like sensations that shoot into the lower limbs on flexing or extending the lumbar spine. This develops because of nerve root irritation during lumbar spine movement. It is a useful sign that localizes to the lumbar area.
▶ The *shoulder-shrugging sign* is a useful way of deciding whether a face-sparing hemiparesis is of cranial or spinal origin.
   Hence the mnemonic: if **S**houlder **S**hrugs are **S**trong the lesion is **S**pinal. The reason is that an intracranial lesion will involve the pyramidal output to the accessory nerve, whereas this is less likely in a spinal disorder.
▶ *Brisk limb reflexes with a normal jaw jerk favors a cervical cord lesion.* If the jaw jerk is also brisk, the lesion must be above pontine level.

If all upper limb reflexes are brisk the lesion must be above that of the highest reflex, which is C5 and 6 (biceps jerk). The motor nucleus of CN V is in the pons, thus the lesion must be bilateral and above that level.

▶ *Myelopathy hand sign* (Souques sign)
This refers to passive abduction of the fifth finger when the arms are held out and pronated (see Figure 3.4). Adjacent fingers often abduct as well. It is essentially a sign of corticospinal tract disorder and not confined to the cervical cord.

▶ *Gradual-onset paraparesis with normal leg tone may be a cortical lesion.*
Clearly, a spinal cord lesion has to be excluded, but muscle tone is nearly always increased unless the lesion is acute, resulting in spinal shock. This lasts up to 6 weeks. Do not forget to scan the brain. A parasagittal meningioma has caught out so many neurologists. One clue in the history is the presence of focal seizures affecting the foot.

Note that:

▶ *Hydrocephalus produces greater leg than arm weakness and hyperreflexia.*
The explanation is that the corticospinal fibers for the lower extremities are stretched as they run around the enlarged ventricles from their origin parasagittally, whereas the hand and arm fibers go directly into the internal capsule.

▶ *Urinary urgency/incontinence about which the patient is unaware or unconcerned is characteristic of a frontal lobe lesion.*
Conversely, patients with spinal incontinence are embarrassed.

▶ *Back pain with a depressed ankle and knee jerk may have a mid- or upper lumbar canal lesion* such as tumor or abscess.
Most prolapsed lumbar disks affect the lower lumbar spine and spare the knee jerk.

▶ *Beware the patient with proximal leg weakness and depressed knee jerk.* If the ankle jerk is preserved this suggest a plexopathy such as Guillain-Barré syndrome. Most lumbar canal lesions affect the ankle jerk.

HANDLES THAT MIGHT LEAD TO A SPEEDY DIAGNOSIS

▶ *Acute paraplegia with mainly motor symptoms and signs favors compression* such as a prolapsed disk or tumor.
Conversely, acute paraparesis with predominant *sensory* symptoms and signs with relatively little weakness favors an inflammatory cause, such as MS or viral myelitis. One possible reason is that spinal motor fibers are more susceptible to pressure than sensory fibers, whereas sensory fibers appear to be more sensitive than motor fibers to inflammation.

▶ *Acute spontaneous paraplegia in an Asian or Afro-Caribbean patient suggests thalassemia major* (Figure 10.4).
This is due to enlargement of vertebrae from extramedullary hematopoiesis with clumps of hematopoietic tissue in the spinal canal to compensate for the anemia. This leads to cord compression, characteristically at the thoracic level.

▶ *Severe chest or back pain with leg weakness after strenuous exercise*
The main causes are as follows:
  ○ Dissection of the thoracic aorta. Pleural effusion or heart murmur are confirmatory signs.
  ○ Ruptured intervertebral, disk with compression of the spinal cord or cauda equina
  ○ Fibrocartilaginous emboli from the nucleus pulposus to the spinal cord
  ○ Syringomyelia (Figure 10.5). There may be worsening of symptoms after measures that increase intrathoracic pressure, such as exercise, repeated coughing and childbirth. It is thought that the elevated intrathoracic pressure is transmitted to the syrinx and makes it expand.
  ○ Spinal dural fistula may be associated with acute chest pain. At other times pain is not prominent and there is just progressive leg weakness and numbness on standing or walking. A dural fistula affected a baritone opera singer whose

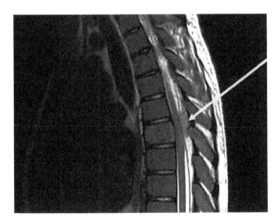

FIGURE 10.4: Cord compression in a 16-year-old man with thalassemia major causing extramedullary hematopoiesis. MRI sagittal T2-weighted image shows a posterior epidural bony mass (arrow) resulting in cord compression at T6. Reproduced with permission from Soman et al. (2009), Figure 3.

legs collapsed repeatedly whenever he stood up to sing (see later discussion).
- o Acute epidural hemorrhage (see Figure 10.8).
- ▶ *Neck pain, stiffness, and dysphagia suggest the DISH syndrome* (diffuse idiopathic skeletal hyperostosis).Figure 10.6, left)

This poorly understood condition is associated with massive overgrowth of osteophytes. If this happens anteriorly, there is pressure on the upper esophagus and dysphagia for solids. Posterior osteophyte extension may cause cord compression. The condition is diagnosed easily by lateral X-ray of the cervical spine.

Ossification of the posterior longitudinal ligament (OPLL) is related to the DISH syndrome. It is common among Japanese and Asian individuals, and, when severe, results in cord compression (see Figure 10.6 right). The symptoms are those of progressive cervical cord compression and pain. Some have obstructive sleep apnea.

- ▶ *Unilateral sore throat, dysphagia, and tinnitus with pain on one side of the face, neck, or ear suggests the Eagle syndrome* (Figure 10.7).

This is caused by an elongated styloid process that presses on CN V, VII, IX, or X. Pressure on the internal carotid artery may result in a contralateral hemiparesis or carotid dissection (see Figure 9.8).

- ▶ *Predominant upper limb weakness, spinothalamic sensory loss, and bladder*

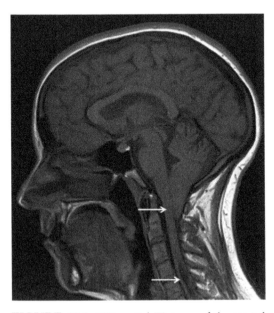

FIGURE 10.5: MRI sagittal T2 image of the cervical spine to show syringomyelia (lower arrow) with Chiari type 1 malformation (upper arrow). Courtesy Bart's Health Neuroimaging Department.

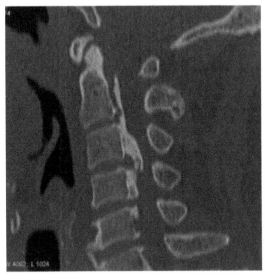

FIGURE 10.6: **Left**: Lateral X-ray of the cervical spine showing marked overgrowth of osteophytes in the mid-cervical spine. **Right**: Lateral CT of the cervical spine showing ossification of the posterior longitudinal ligament. This is particularly marked at C2–C3, where it was causing cord compression. Reproduced with permission from Radiopedia, Case 1, courtesy Dr. Frank Gaillard.

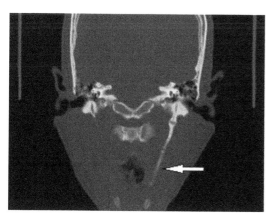

FIGURE 10.7: Eagle syndrome. Coronal CT scan of the head shows an elongated left styloid process (arrow). Reproduced with permission from Radiopedia, ID 13791, courtesy Dr. P Dharmesh.

impairment following neck hyperextension injury suggests the central cord syndrome.

One explanation is pinching of the cervical cord by a hypertrophied ligamentum flavum (posteriorly) or disk protrusion (anteriorly) and subsequent hemorrhage into the central cord.

▶ *Paraparesis in a patient with hemorrhagic diatheses, trauma, or anticoagulant therapy suggests spinal epidural hematoma.*

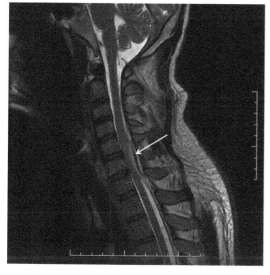

FIGURE 10.8: Sagittal spinal T2 MRI showing spontaneous epidural hematoma in a 26-year-old man. The posterior epidural lesion (arrow) was isointense on T1-weighted images but markedly hypointense on T2 images. Reproduced with permission from Radiopedia, ID 13061, courtesy Dr. Sachin Pathak.

Typically, there is acute spinal pain that radiates to the limbs, associated with paraparesis. Some patients have an underlying vascular anomaly (Figure 10.8). The history of trauma may be minor, and many cases occur spontaneously due to hemorrhage from epidural veins. Urgent surgical decompression is traditional management, although smaller collections may be managed conservatively.

▶ *Painless limb burns* suggest syringomyelia, self-inflicted lesions, leprosy, hereditary sensory neuropathy, or congenital indifference to pain (Figure 10.9).

▶ *Myelopathy in a cancer patient* suggests vertebral metastases with cord compression, radiation myelitis, or infectious and paraneoplastic causes.

▶ *Back pain that is worse in bed at night* suggests spinal malignancy.

This probably happens because of increased edema around the tumor in the recumbent position. The situation is the opposite of lumbar spondylosis, where pain tends to be worse with daytime activity and relieved by bed rest.

▶ *Marked spasticity with normal or near-normal power* is typical of pure (classic) hereditary spastic paraplegia (HSP; see Chapter 7), primary lateral sclerosis, hydrocephalus, and HTLV-1 myelopathy.

Although patients with HSP walk stiffly, in the typical variety they are rarely badly

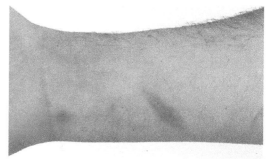

FIGURE 10.9: Painless burns. The forearm of an 18-year-old cook. Note several recent burns sustained in the kitchen, but they were never painful. The upper limb deep tendon reflexes were absent so syringomyelia is high on the diagnostic list. Sensory testing and demonstration of upper motor neuron signs in the lower limbs should clinch the diagnosis.

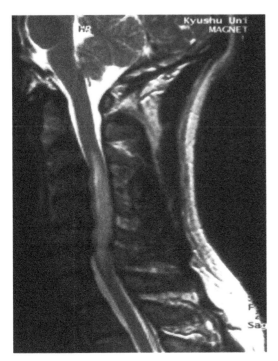

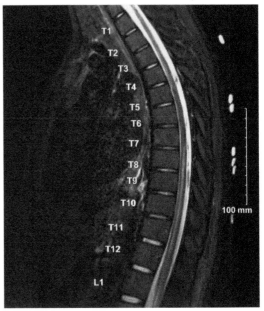

FIGURE 10.11: Surfer's myelopathy. MRI short T1 inversion recovery image of the thoracic spine shows a hyperintense cord lesion extending from the distal thoracic cord to the conus. Reproduced with permission from Chang et al. (2012).

FIGURE 10.10: Atopic myelitis. Sagittal MRI T2-weighted image of the cervical spinal cord. Apart from loss of cervical lordosis there is a longitudinally extensive lesion in the cervical cord. The IgE level was extremely high. Courtesy Jun-ichi Kira, Kyoto.

disabled and power is usually quite good. They often have an easily obtainable Babinski sign with sparing of the bladder, arms, and face, even when the legs are affected severely.

▶ *Cervical inflammatory lesion with very high blood IgE suggests atopic (eosinophilic) myelitis* (Figure 10.10).

The presentation is that of a clinically isolated syndrome thus simulating MS but does not recur. There is usually a history of allergic disorder such as eczema. It is more common among Japanese people and thought to result from allergy to an insect bite (mite).

▶ *Acute onset of weak legs in a surfer favors surfer's myelopathy.* (Figure 10.11)

The usual person is a beginner who presents with abrupt-onset low back pain followed by paraparesis evolving over 15–60 minutes. The likely mechanism is spinal cord ischemia.

▶ *Patients (without hip disease or hemorrhoids) who sit on one buttock likely have an S1 radiculopathy on the opposite side.*

They do this to avoid pressure on the affected sciatic nerve.

▶ *Longitudinally extensive (>3 vertebral segments) cervical or thoracic lesion on MRI* with coincident optic neuritis suggests Devic's disease (neuromyelitis optica; see also Chapter 4, Demyelination).

MS also needs to be considered, but the lesions are usually smaller, not as confluent, and extend over no more than two vertebral segments. As discussed in Chapter 4, at disease onset there may be yawning, nausea, vomiting, and intractable hiccups. Long spinal cord lesions without optic neuritis have many causes, also discussed in Chapter 4.

▶ *Abrupt reversible leg weakness on neck flexion* is usually caused by MS (McArdle's sign; O'Neill et al. 1987; see Chapter 4).

It probably happens in other cervical demyelinating conditions.

▶ *Seizures and myelopathy suggest multiple cavernomas* (spinal and cerebral), syringomyelia with hydrocephalus, or mitochondrial disorder.

▶ Note that cavernomas are often familial, and many patients are Hispanic Americans. Remember that hydrocephalus itself is associated with a tendency to seizures.

▶ *Myelopathy, ataxia, deafness, and anosmia favor superficial siderosis.*

There is usually a history of head trauma, evidence of blood seepage from a cerebral or spinal vascular anomaly or neurosurgical procedures in these areas. Cognitive changes are recognized. The abnormalities on CT or MRI scans are diagnostic (Figure 12.14). An alternative possibility is mitochondrial disorder, but anosmia would be unusual.

▶ *Myelopathy following long-term use of denture fixative cream or bariatric surgery* suggests copper deficiency myelopathy.

Until recently, some denture fixative creams contained zinc, which competes with copper for absorption and may result in copper deficit myelopathy, a disorder with similarity to vitamin B_{12} deficiency. Patients may have predominantly posterior column signs with pseudoathetosis. Copper shortage may follow gastric bypass surgery (Gletsu-Miller et al. 2012), probably related to malabsorption. Indeed, malabsorption elsewhere in the gastrointestinal tract may be responsible. Paradoxically, overzealous treatment of Wilson's disease with zinc sulfate may lead to copper deficiency.

○ Be aware that shortage of copper may coexist with vitamin B_{12} deficiency and that gastrointestinal surgery may have been undertaken several years before onset of symptoms.

○ The anemia of vitamin B_{12} deficiency (if present) is megaloblastic with slight increase in bilirubin, and some develop an encephalopathy.

○ The anemia in copper myelopathy is normocytic, macrocytic, or microcytic with sideroblasts, and there is no encephalopathy.

▶ *Paraparesis following nitrous oxide exposure* suggests subacute combined degeneration of the spinal cord.

This may happen after anesthesia for dental and obstetric procedures or recreational abuse of nitrous oxide from whipped cream canisters (whippets). Lhermitte's sign may be prominent. There is usually prior subclinical vitamin B_{12} deficiency before nitrous oxide administration. A characteristic finding on spinal MRI is the inverted-V sign that suggests a lesion in the posterior columns (Figure 10.12).

▶ *Spastic paraparesis following radiotherapy* months or years previously suggests delayed radiation myelopathy.

This is a gradually progressive condition that follows radiation to the neck, chest, or breast. If the pelvis has been irradiated, then the symptoms are lower motor neuron and result in a lumbosacral radiculopathy or plexopathy.

▶ *Exaggerated leg reflexes with normal plantar reflexes* is likely:
○ Severe anxiety
○ Thyrotoxicosis
○ Spinal muscular atrophy or ALS
○ Dopa-responsive dystonia

The abdominal and cremasteric reflexes may be preserved as well.

▶ *Bilateral extensor plantar responses with strictly unilateral symptoms* is usually caused by MS.

Thus the patient complains of a numb or heavy leg and insists that the other leg is normal, but both plantar responses are found to be extensor. The reason lies in the multiplicity of subclinical plaques in MS, only a few of which may rise to symptoms.

HANDLES FOR SPECIFIC DISORDERS

Spinal Dural Arteriovenous Fistula

All honest neurologists have missed one case in their careers. They may be overlooked even on spinal MRI unless specifically searched for (see Figure 10.13). The spinal dural fistula is the more common malformation and causes gradually progressive or stepwise

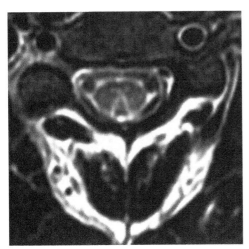

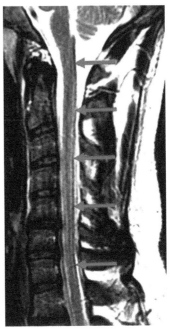

FIGURE 10.12: Nitrous oxide myelopathy. **Left**: Axial T2 MRI at the C3 level demonstrating bilateral symmetric T2 hyperintensities (inverted V or rabbit ear sign) in the lateral aspects of the dorsal columns, characteristic of nitrous oxide myelopathy. Similar changes occur in myelopathies associated with HIV or deficiencies of copper, vitamin B_{12}, and vitamin E. **Right**: Sagittal MRI of cervical cord, demonstrating a T2 hyperintensity (arrows) extending from the caudal medulla to C7. Reproduced with permission from Sotirchos et al. (2012), Figures 1 and 2.

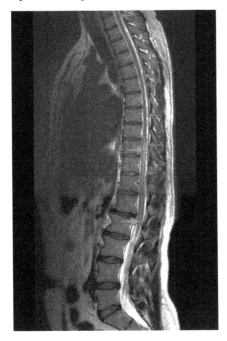

FIGURE 10.13: Spinal dural arteriovenous fistula. The conus and lower thoracic cord (from T9/10) demonstrate increased intrinsic T2 signal (blue arrows). Along the dorsal aspect of the cord numerous tortuous filling defects are demonstrated (red arrows). Reproduced with permission from Radiopedia, ID 19594, courtesy Dr. Frank Galliard.

paraparesis, usually with bladder involvement. The intramedullary arteriovenous malformation is a more acute process characterized by pain, often in a sciatic nerve distribution. Both may cause stepwise deterioration in neurological function, and patients sometimes describe progressive weakness and numbness on standing (neurogenic claudication), probably from intraspinal venous engorgement.

Following are some Handles for dural fistulas to help prevent you from having an embarrassing moment.

▶ *Myelopathy made worse by steroids* (Lee et al. 2009)
  Various mechanisms have been proposed for this clinical observation, including increased venous congestion around the fistula, but the actual cause of this valid clinical observation is unclear. A typical scenario is a patient with presumed myelitis, thought to be early MS, is given steroids, fails to respond, or actually deteriorates. It is so easy to ascribe this to "steroid resistance." This is where a Red Flag should really fly!

Also note:

▶ *Myelopathy helped by steroids* is not necessarily inflammatory in origin.
It could result from reduction of edema around a spinal tumor.
▶ *Burning leg pain and fasciculation*
The burning pain is due to spinothalamic involvement. Fasciculation presumably results from ischemia of the anterior horn cells. Thus, a patient with weak legs and fasciculation may be given a wrong diagnosis of early ALS, especially when the sensory symptoms are minimal. Be sure to test for pain and temperature loss in this setting.

Note:

◀ *Burning leg pain is not typical of degenerative spinal disease.*
▶ *Claudication when upright*
Here the patient is relatively symptom-free when seated but, after being vertical for several minutes, develops low back pain, perhaps with burning leg discomfort, progressive weakness, and sensory loss. It is easy to blame this on spinal stenosis (postural claudication) or a lumbar disc protrusion. The cause is probably progressive venous congestion that results in increased pressure on the spinal parenchyma and/or cauda equina.
▶ *Leg weakness when singing upright*
This concerns the baritone singer whose legs gave way whenever he stood up to sing (Khurana et al. 2002). The likely mechanism is increased spinal venous pressure during singing, transmitted to the dural fistula. In theory, any Valsalva-type maneuver could replicate this phenomenon.
▶ *Postprandial weakness*
The patient finds that after eating a heavy meal the legs become weak for a matter of hours. The likely mechanism is normal diversion of blood from the spinal cord into the gut, thus aggravating cord ischemia in the patient with a dural fistula. A comparable history may be obtained in those with anterior spinal artery stenosis and possibly brainstem ischemia.
▶ *Urinary incontinence on exercise or exertion*

▶ *Sciatic pain with normal lumbar spine MRI*
▶ *Worsening symptoms around menstruation*

Claudication

There are three types of claudication, described next.

Vascular Claudication

This is characterized by exercise-related calf pain, relieved by rest, and due to poor circulation in the femoral, iliac, or aortic arteries. The foot pulses are absent or weak.

Neurogenic Claudication

This is superficially similar, in that patients experience increasing calf pain on walking, relieved by rest. Comparable symptoms may develop on prolonged standing, termed *postural claudication*. In general, it is caused by diffuse or focal narrowing of the lumbar canal. Neurological examination is often normal in both types, but in the vascular type the foot pulses are weak or absent. Exercise may reduce the strength of the ankle jerks. Rarer varieties, provoked by walking, are associated with progressive tingling (paresthetic form), weakness (myasthenic type), or unsteadiness (ataxic variant) (Hawkes & Roberts 1980).

Spinal Cord Claudication

This is the rarest type, first described by Dejerine in 1906, and due to spinal cord ischemia. Patients describe progressive stiffness on walking. Sometimes there is weakness and numbness on standing, or transient ischemic attack (TIA)-like episodes when the arms or legs become transiently weak on exertion. Some affected individuals have an underlying vascular anomaly, and there are usually upper motor neuron signs in the lower limbs. Thus,

▶ *Calf pain provoked by standing suggests postural claudication.* It relates to lumbar canal stenosis or an arteriovenous malformation.
▶ *Calf pain relieved by standing is likely vascular claudication.* This happens because gravity improves distal blood flow.

On walking, both vascular and neurogenic varieties of claudication are accompanied by progressive calf pain. Most people have to stop after a few hundred yards, but if the pain is relieved by leaning forward, this strongly favors the neurogenic type. Leaning forward increases the sagittal diameter of the lumbar canal and lessens the degree of stenosis. This principle explains these further Handles:

▶ *The patient who can cycle for miles but walks just yards likely has neurogenic claudication.*

This occurs because people lean forward when cycling. A similar paradox is recognized in parkinsonism, but the mechanism is related to basal ganglia dysfunction, and there are obvious signs of extrapyramidal disorder (see Chapter 8, Movement Disorders).

▶ *The patient who visits a supermarket and prefers to lean forward on a shopping cart probably has neurogenic claudication.*

Neurogenic claudication is eased by walking up a hill but aggravated by walking down a (steep) hill because of the need to extend the lumbar spine.

▶ *Leg pain at night, relieved by hanging the legs out of bed or walking about suggests vascular claudication.*

These maneuvers improve distal blood flow. Those with neurogenic claudication do not give this history.

▶ *A short-stature patient with neurogenic claudication may be an achondroplastic dwarf* (Figure 10.14).

Such patients have congenital narrowing of the entire spinal canal, and, when age-related degenerative changes commence in the lumbar region, they develop neurogenic claudication. There may be signs of cervical canal compression as well.

▶ *Be aware of the patient with McArdle's syndrome.* Some develop calf or thigh pain on exercise that simulates any variety of claudication.

Infectious Myelopathies

Numerous infections produce intrinsic and extrinsic lesions of the spinal cord. Some of the easier ones to spot follow:

▶ *Infection (especially TB) damages the disks and joints, whereas neoplasia affects the vertebral bodies.*

This is a general rule for spinal disease.

▶ *Blood transfusion followed by myelopathy is usually retroviral infection, namely, HTLV-1 or AIDS.*

The interval between transfusion and myelopathy can be several years.

▶ *Myelopathy in* Schistosoma mansoni *infection may be due to egg deposition in the spinal cord.*

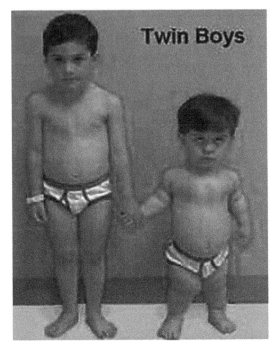

FIGURE 10.14: Twin boys. Achondroplasia affects the brother on the right. Note the normal-sized head but short limbs and digits. Reproduced with permission from Manbir Online: for Health & Fitness, http://manbir-online.com.

▶ Pulmonary TB followed by paraparesis suggests either

  ○ Pott's disease of the spine, where the intervertebral disks and then the vertebral body become infected, typically at the upper lumbar or lower thoracic level; this is followed by vertebral collapse and secondary spinal cord or cauda equina compression; or:

  ○ Tuberculomas in the spinal cord that cause compression or infarction of the anterior spinal artery from arteritis (Figure 10.15).

▶ The presence of choroid tubercles points to miliary TB (Figure 10.16).

About 25% of patients with miliary TB have tuberculous meningitis.

▶ *Back pain, myelopathy, and fever suggest epidural abscess* (Figure 10.17).

This triad is caused by systemic infection or introduction of organisms via contaminated medical equipment (e.g., epidural steroid injection). The abscess may be bacterial or fungal.

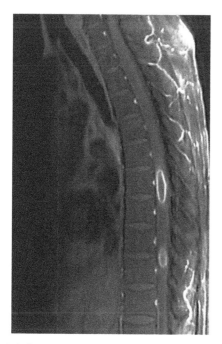

FIGURE 10.15: Spinal tuberculomas. Enhanced T1 sagittal MRI of the thoracic spinal cord shows two large enhancing tuberculous lesions. Reproduced with permission from Radiopedia, Image ID 13061, courtesy Dr. Sachin Pathak.

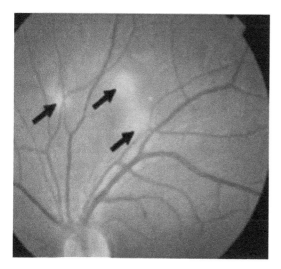

FIGURE 10.16: Choroid tubercles. This shows yellow fuzzy circular patches (arrows) about half the size of the optic disk and 2–3 disk diameters away from the optic disk. They are diagnostic of miliary TB. Reproduced from Ray et al. (2013).

- Presentation may mimic an acute abdomen and some patients even undergo unnecessary exploratory laparotomy.

Neurosyphilis

This may cause myelopathy in three ways:

- *Meningovascular type*, where there is ischemia secondary to arteritis of the spinal arteries. Inspection of the palms and soles may reveal a bronze-colored rash (Figure 10.18).
- *Spinal cord gumma.* This acts like a mass lesion.
- *Tabes dorsalis.* The reflexes, joint position sense, and deep pain are lost; Charcot joints develop, and there are Argyll-Robertson pupils.

Recurrent myelopathy is likely one of the following

- *Behçet's disease.* Look for orogenital ulceration, uveitis, and pathergy.
- *Multiple sclerosis.* Check for delayed visual evoked potentials, cerebrospinal fluid (CSF) oligoclonal bands, and characteristic white matter changes on brain MRI.
- *Devic's disease.* Measure aquaporin-4 antibodies.
- *Idiopathic recurrent myelopathy.* Oligoclonal bands are absent and there is male predominance.
- *Sjögren's syndrome.* Check for dry mouth, dry eyes, sensory neuropathy, and antibodies to Ro and La.

Recurrent Meningitis

Recurrent meningitis is associated with the following:

- *Mollaret's meningitis* (HSV-1 or HSV-2)
- *Relapsing polychondritis.* This can be diagnosed by the presence of floppy or puffy red swollen ears or nasal cartilage defects (see Figure 1.18).
- *Subacute pituitary apoplexy.* This is sometimes misdiagnosed as recurrent aseptic meningitis because of repeated small subarachnoid hemorrhages from an enlarged pituitary gland.
- *Nonsteroidal anti-inflammatory drugs and antineoplastic agents.* All of these may cause aseptic meningitis and CSF pleocytosis.
- *Recurrent CSF leakage*
- *Sarcoidosis, Behçet's disease, autoimmune disorders*

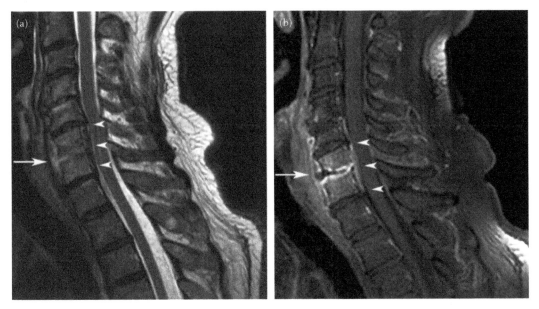

FIGURE 10.17: MRI of spondylodiscitis and epidural abscess. **Left**: T2-weighted image. **Right**: T1-weighted fat-saturated image after intravenous gadolinium. There is spondylodiscitis (large arrows) complicated by an epidural abscess at the C6–7 level (arrowheads). Reproduced from Sendi et al. (2008).

CEREBROSPINAL FLUID EXAMINATION

Here are some useful tips for a quicker understanding of spinal tap results.

- *High cell–protein ratio.* If there is a very high cell count with only modest increase in protein level, this favors meningitis, either bacterial or viral, but not TB.

- *Low cell–protein ratio.* This means that there is only mild elevation of cell count but a high protein level. This is typical of radiculopathy, such as the Guillain-Barré syndrome. It also happens with cerebral sinus thrombosis, cerebral abscess, spinal block, cauda equina tumor (e.g., ependymoma), meningeal infiltration, neurolymphomatosis, and viral encephalitis.

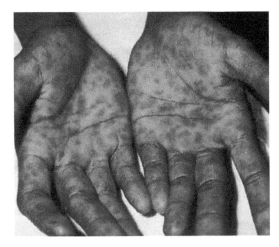

FIGURE 10.18: The bronze rash of secondary syphilis. Reproduced with permission from Manbir Online: for Health & Fitness, http://manbir-online.com.

- *Modest elevation of both cell and protein levels.* This is the hallmark of tuberculous meningitis. Usually the CSF glucose is moderately low. If a spinal block develops, from advanced TB or tumor, then the protein level becomes very high and the cell–protein ratio is low.
- *Chronic polymorphonuclear reaction* characterizes TB or *Nocardia* infection.
- *CSF eosinophilia.* The main causes are parasitic and fungal infection, CSF shunts, Hodgkin's disease, medication (ibuprofen and various antibiotics), and cholesterol emboli.
- *Low glucose.* This means a CSF glucose less than 50% of the blood level. There are three major causes:
  o Infection: bacterial, tuberculous, or fungal
  o Sarcoid
  o Carcinomatous meningitis

In general, the glucose is modestly lowered in TB but severely depressed in *untreated* bacterial infection. Rare causes of low CSF glucose are as follows:

- Viral infection
- GLUT-1 deficiency syndrome (De Vivo syndrome; see Chapter 6). This is mainly a disorder of infants and children, but it is recognized increasingly in adults.
- Histiocytosis. This causes diffuse meningeal thickening and presumably impairment of glucose transport.
- Ankylosing spondylitis and rheumatoid arthritis

Oligoclonal Bands

These are present in the following:

- All cases of clinically definite MS
- Infections: neurosyphilis, subacute sclerosing panencephalitis. AIDS, Lyme disease
- Autoimmune disease: for example, systemic lupus erythematosus, Sjögren's syndrome
- Sarcoidosis
- Primary CNS lymphoma
- Guillain-Barré syndrome
- Paraneoplastic disorders
- Carcinomatous meningitis
- ◀ Bands are rarely present in Behçet's disease.

Note that use of antibiotics for suspected bacterial meningitis prior to lumbar puncture may depress the cell count and lower the cell–protein ratio to a variable degree.

Dry Spinal Tap

The most common reason for a dry spinal tap is multiple failed attempts by inexperienced doctors or a technically difficult approach related to obesity, scoliosis, spondylosis, or previous surgery/metalwork. Sometimes the lumbar puncture is performed correctly but there is no fluid return—the true "dry tap." Assuming there has not been an attempted lumbar puncture within at least the previous 48 hours, the main causes are as follows:

- Epidural abscess or tumor (e.g., ependymoma)
- Spinal block, typically from tuberculous meningitis
- Intracranial hypotension
- Severe dehydration or systemic hypotension
- Arachnoid disorder (e.g., pachymeningitis [syphilis] or adhesive arachnoiditis)

SUMMARY

Handles for Localization

▶ Quadriparesis: lesion in the cervical cord
▶ Hemiparesis: lesion in the brain.
▶ Useless hand syndrome. Posterior column lesion usually resulting from MS
▶ Paraparesis with sacral sparing indicates an intrinsic spinal cord lesion.
▶ Paraparesis without sacral sparing suggests an extrinsic lesion. Use *ALS* mnemonic (arm, leg, sacrum)
▶ The spinal cord anatomical lesion is above the upper sensory limit due to oblique crossing of the spinothalamic fibers (classical teaching).
▶ A gradual transition at upper limit of sensory level is typical of an intrinsic lesion; an abrupt change characterizes an extrinsic disorder.
▶ A spinal sensory level apparently at the upper third of the sternum is not helpful since C4, T2, T3, and T4 levels overlap there.
▶ A patient who complains of a stiff or heavy leg on one side with a strong, burning/numb leg on the other side likely has a Brown-Sequard syndrome.
▶ An apparent sensory level on the anterior, but not posterior, chest wall may relate to a length-dependent neuropathy.

- ▶ Cape sensory loss ("suspended" sensory loss) suggests syringomyelia, paraneoplastic/traumatic lesions of the central cord, or porphyria.
- ▶ Brisk knee jerks, depressed ankle jerks, and extensor plantars:
  - ○ Subacute combined degeneration of the cord, ALS, widespread spinal spondylosis, syringomyelia, Friedreich's ataxia, taboparesis, copper deficiency, and neurofibromatosis
  - ○ HIV- or HTLV-1–related myeloneuropathy, spinal arteriovenous malformation, or dural fistula
  - ○ Adrenomyeloneuropathy, sarcoidosis
  - ○ With a completely normal sensory exam favors ALS.
  - ○ Reduced arm reflexes implicate cervical spondylosis and syringomyelia.
  - ○ Acute paraplegia, with cutaneous sensory level but preserved joint position sense, is most likely anterior spinal artery thrombosis.
  - ○ Lumbar Lhermitte sign
  - ○ Shoulder shrug sign
  - ○ Brisk limb reflexes with a normal jaw jerk favor a cervical cord lesion. If the jaw jerk is also brisk, the lesion must be above pontine level.
  - ○ Myelopathy hand sign
  - ○ Gradual-onset paraparesis with normal leg tone may be cortical.
  - ○ Hydrocephalus produces greater leg than arm weakness and hyperreflexia.
  - ○ Urinary urgency/incontinence about which the patient is unaware or unconcerned is characteristic of a frontal lobe lesion, whereas patients with spinal incontinence are embarrassed.
  - ○ The patient with back pain and depressed *knee* jerk may have a mid- or upper lumbar canal lesion (tumor or abscess). If the ankle jerk is preserved, think of plexopathy.

Handles That Might Lead to a Speedy Diagnosis

- ▶ Acute paraparesis with mainly motor symptoms and signs favors compression (prolapsed disk or tumor) rather than inflammation.
- ▶ Predominant sensory symptoms and signs with relatively little weakness favor an inflammatory cause.

- ▶ Acute spontaneous paraplegia in an Asian or Afro-Caribbean person suggests thalassemia major.
- ▶ Severe back pain and leg weakness after strenuous exercise favors: thoracic aortic dissection, ruptured inter-vertebral disk, rupture of the nucleus pulposus with fibrocartilaginous emboli, syringomyelia, spinal dural fistula, acute epidural hemorrhage.
- ▶ Neck pain, stiffness, and dysphagia suggest the DISH syndrome. Associated with obstructive sleep apnea
- ▶ Ossification of the posterior longitudinal ligament: progressive cervical cord compression and neck pain
- ▶ Unilateral sore throat, dysphagia, and tinnitus with pain on one side of the face, neck, or ear suggest the Eagle syndrome.
- ▶ Predominant upper limb weakness, spinothalamic sensory loss, and bladder impairment following neck hyperextension injury suggest the central cord syndrome.
- ▶ Paraparesis in a patient with hemorrhagic diatheses, trauma, or anticoagulant therapy suggests spinal epidural hematoma.
- ▶ Painless burns in the upper limb suggest syringomyelia, self-inflicted lesions, leprosy, hereditary sensory neuropathy, or congenital indifference to pain.
- ▶ Myelopathy in a cancer patient suggests vertebral metastases with cord compression, radiation myelitis, or infectious and paraneoplastic causes.
- ▶ Back pain that is worse in bed at night suggests spinal malignancy.
- ▶ Marked spasticity with normal or near-normal power is typical of HSP, primary lateral sclerosis, hydrocephalus, and HTLV-1 myelopathy.
- ▶ Cervical inflammatory lesion with very high blood IgE suggests atopic (eosinophilic) myelitis.
- ▶ Acute onset of weak legs in a surfer: surfer's myelopathy
- ▶ The patient (without hip disease or hemorrhoids) who sits on one buttock likely has S1 radiculopathy on the opposite side.
- ▶ Longitudinally extensive (>3 vertebral segments) cervical or thoracic lesion on MRI with coincident optic neuritis suggests Devic's disease.

- Abrupt reversible leg weakness on neck flexion is usually caused by MS (McArdle's sign).
- Seizures and myelopathy suggest multiple cavernomas (spinal and cerebral), syringomyelia with hydrocephalus or mitochondrial disorder.
- Myelopathy, ataxia, deafness, and anosmia favor superficial siderosis.
- Myelopathy following long-term use of denture fixative cream or bariatric surgery suggests copper deficiency myelopathy.
- Deficiency of copper may coexist with vitamin B_{12} deficiency.
- The anemia of vitamin B_{12} deficiency is megaloblastic with a slight increase in bilirubin, and some develop an encephalopathy. In copper myelopathy, the anemia is normocytic or microcytic with sideroblasts, and there is no encephalopathy.
- Paraparesis following nitrous oxide exposure suggests subacute combined degeneration of the spinal cord.
- Spastic paraparesis following radiotherapy months or years previously suggests delayed radiation myelopathy.
- Exaggerated leg reflexes with normal plantar responses are likely caused by anxiety, thyrotoxicosis, ALS/spinal muscular atrophy, or dopa-responsive dystonia.
- Bilateral extensor plantar responses with strictly unilateral symptoms usually indicate MS.

Handles for Specific Disorders
Spinal Dural Arteriovenous Fistula
- Myelopathy made worse by steroids
- Myelopathy that is helped by steroids is not necessarily inflammatory; it could be a spinal tumor.
- Burning leg pain and fasciculation
- Claudication when upright
- Leg weakness when singing upright
- Postprandial weakness
- Urinary incontinence on exertion or exercise
- Worsening symptoms around menstruation
- Sciatic pain with normal lumbar spine MRI

Note: Burning leg pain is not characteristic of degenerative spinal disease

Claudication
There are vascular, neurogenic, and spinal varieties:

- Calf pain provoked by standing (postural claudication) suggests neurogenic claudication due to lumbar canal stenosis or dural fistula.
- Calf pain relieved by standing is likely vascular claudication.
- The patient who can cycle miles but walk just yards likely has neurogenic claudication.
- The patient who visits a supermarket and prefers to lean forward on a shopping cart probably has neurogenic claudication.
- Neurogenic claudication is helped by walking uphill but aggravated by walking down a (steep) hill.
- Night leg pain relieved by hanging the legs out of bed or walking about suggests vascular claudication.
- Be aware of the short-stature patient who has neurogenic claudication; the patient is likely to be an achondroplastic dwarf.
- Be aware of the patient with McArdle's syndrome, who may have symptoms on walking that simulate claudication.

Infectious Myelopathies
- Infection (especially TB) damages the joints; neoplasia affects vertebral bodies.
- Blood transfusion followed by myelopathy: HTLV-1 or AIDS
- Myelopathy in *Schistosoma mansoni* infection may be due to egg deposition in the spinal cord.
- Pulmonary TB followed by paraparesis: Pott's disease of the spine or tuberculomas of the spinal cord
- The presence of choroid tubercles points to miliary TB.
- Back pain, myelopathy, and fever: epidural abscess

Neurosyphilis
- Meningovascular type: bronze rash on palms, soles, or trunk
- Spinal cord gumma acts like a mass lesion.
- Tabes dorsalis: high-stepping, noisy gait with Charcot joints and Argyll-Robertson pupils

Recurrent Myelopathy

▶ Behçet's disease, MS, Devic's disease
▶ Idiopathic recurrent myelopathy
▶ Sjögren's syndrome

Recurrent Aseptic Meningitis

▶ Mollaret's meningitis (HSV-1 or HSV-2)
▶ Relapsing polychondritis
▶ Subacute pituitary apoplexy
▶ Nonsteroidal anti-inflammatory drugs and antineoplastic agents
▶ Recurrent CSF leakage
▶ Sarcoidosis, Behçet's disease, autoimmune disorders

Cerebrospinal Fluid Examination

▶ High cell–protein ratio: infection
▶ Low cell–protein ratio: radiculopathy (Guillain-Barré syndrome), cerebral sinus thrombosis, cerebral abscess, spinal block, cauda equina tumor, meningeal infiltration, neurolymphomatosis, viral encephalitis
▶ Modest elevation of both cell and protein level: TB
▶ Chronic polymorphonuclear reaction: TB or *Nocardia* infection
▶ CSF eosinophilia: parasitic and fungal infection, CSF shunts, Hodgkin's disease, medication, cholesterol emboli
▶ Low glucose
  ○ Infection (bacterial, viral tuberculous and fungal)
  ○ Sarcoid
  ○ Carcinomatous meningitis
  ○ GLUT1 deficiency
  ○ Histiocytosis
  ○ Ankylosing spondylitis and rheumatoid arthritis

Positive Oligoclonal Bands

▶ All clinically definite MS
▶ Infections: neurosyphilis, subacute sclerosing panencephalitis. AIDS, Lyme disease
▶ Autoimmune disease: systemic lupus erythematosus, Sjögren's syndrome
▶ Sarcoidosis
▶ Primary CNS lymphoma
▶ Guillain-Barré syndrome

▶ Paraneoplastic disorders
▶ Carcinomatous meningitis

Note: Bands are usually absent in Behçet's disease

Dry Spinal Tap

▶ Repeated prior attempts at lumbar puncture
▶ Epidural abscess or tumor
▶ Spinal block
▶ Intracranial hypotension
▶ Severe dehydration or hypotension
▶ Arachnoid disorder: pachymeningitis, adhesive arachnoiditis

SUGGESTED READING

Chang CW, Donovan DJ, Liem LK, et al. Surfers' myelopathy: a case series of 19 novice surfers with nontraumatic myelopathy. *Neurology.* 2012;79:2171–2176.

Gletsu-Miller N, Broderius M, Frediani JK, et al. Incidence and prevalence of copper deficiency following roux-en-y gastric bypass surgery. *Int J Obes (Lond).* 2012;36:328–335.

Hawkes CH, Roberts GM. Lumbar canal stenosis. *Br J Hosp Med.* 1980;23:498–505.

Khurana VG, Perez-Terzic CM, Petersen RC, Krauss WE. Singing paraplegia: a distinctive manifestation of a spinal dural arteriovenous fistula. *Neurology.* 2002;58:1279–1281.

Lee CS, Pyun HW, Chae EY, Kim KK, Rhim SC, Suh DC. Reversible aggravation of neurological deficits after steroid medication in patients with venous congestive myelopathy caused by spinal arteriovenous malformation. *Interv Neuroradiol.* 2009;15:325–329.

Nathan PW, Smith M, Deacon P. The crossing of the spinothalamic tract. *Brain.* 2001;124:793–803.

O'Neill JH, Mills KR, Murray NM. McArdle's sign in multiple sclerosis. *J Neurol Neurosurg Psychiatry.* 1987;50:1691–1693.

Ray S, Talukdar A, Kundu S, Khanra D, Sonthalia N. Diagnosis and management of miliary tuberculosis: current state and future perspectives. *Ther Clin Risk Manag.* 2013;9:9–26.

Sendi P, Bregenzer T, Zimmerli W. Spinal epidural abscess in clinical practice. *QJM.* 2008;101:1–12.

Soman S, Rosenfeld DL, Roychowdhury S, Drachtman RA, Cohler A. Cord compression due to extramedullary hematopoiesis in an adolescent with known beta thalassemia major. *J Radiol Case Rep.* 2009;3:17–22.

Sotirchos ES, Saidha S, Becker D. Neurological picture. Nitrous oxide-induced myelopathy with inverted V-sign on spinal MRI. *J Neurol Neurosurg Psychiatry.* 2012;83:915–916.

Chapter 11: Peripheral Neuropathy

This chapter will adopt a basic anatomical classification of peripheral neuropathy: mononeuropathy (one or more peripheral nerves affected), radiculopathy (nerve root or plexus involved), and polyneuropathy (disorder of most peripheral nerves).

MONONEUROPATHY

Upper Limbs

Median Nerve Lesions

You must have a basic knowledge of the median nerve anatomy (Figure 11.1).

Carpal Tunnel Syndrome

▶ *All numbness, pain, weakness or tingling in the hand (usually dominant, often both) is carpal tunnel syndrome (CTS) until proven otherwise.*

This is not a bad rule, and, in many aspects, it reflects the poor history given by patients (or taken by doctors!). CTS is very common so it's a good opening bet anyway.

In its advanced stage, this is an easy diagnosis as there is weakness and wasting of the thenar muscles and median territory sensory loss that spares the palm since the palmar branch does not go through the carpal tunnel (Figure 11.2). This is not the case in the earlier sensory phase. Patients rarely observe that their sensory symptoms affect the outer three and a half fingers and usually state that it affects the whole hand.

▶ *The patient with a hand that tingles, especially at night and is relieved by a downward flick likely has CTS.*

The "hand-flick" sign as described by Pryse-Phillips is reported by patients who wake at night with numbness of the fingers and flick the relevant hand downward to help "restore the circulation"
Also ask:
Are there sensory symptoms on raising the affected arm, as in driving, using a phone,

reading newspaper, shaving, washing hair? You can verify this by asking patients to raise their arms while squeezing both forearms. The tingling usually appears in the affected fingers within 20 seconds (Figure 11.3; Hawkes sign).

On examination look for the following:

- Tinel's sign
  Tap the center of the anterior wrist *gently* with a tendon hammer, and, when positive, the patient reports tingling or electrical sensation at the wrist that often radiates into one or more fingers. It is important to avoid excessive force as this will provoke a false-positive response.
- Weakness of opposition
  This is really an early motor sign, but it is subtle and easily overlooked. As shown in Figure 11.4, the patient is trying to oppose the thumb to the little finger with the hand pronated on a flat surface. If there is weakness of opposition, the thumb is only flexed across the palm such that the thumbnail is seen in side view throughout the movement. When opposition is normal, the thumb is rotated 90 degrees so that the anterior aspect of the thumbnail becomes visible.
- Phalen's sign
  Here the wrist is flexed fully by the examiner. Patients with CTS report tingling in the tips of the digits (usually middle and ring fingers) in less than 30 seconds, whereas normal subjects report tingling (if at all) after 45 seconds. This maneuver induces kinking and flexion of the median nerve against the flexor retinaculum and replicates the patient's sensory symptoms. If the test is executed correctly, it is reliable and more sensitive than the Tinel maneuver, which may be negative, especially in early cases.

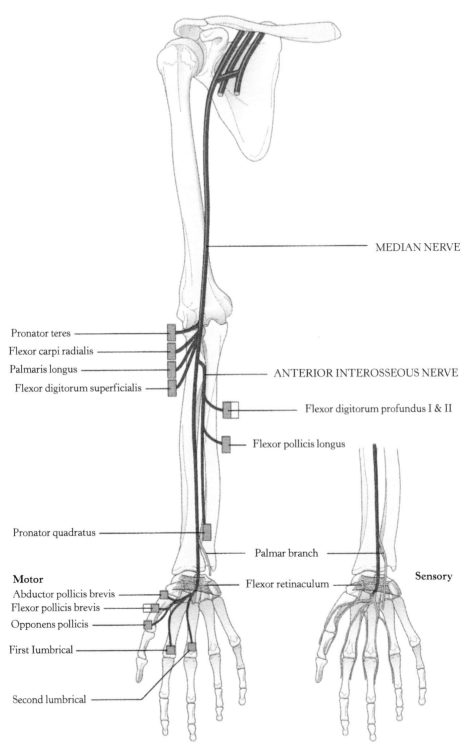

FIGURE 11.1: The main branches of the median nerve in the lower arm. Reproduced with permission from *Aids to The Examination of The Peripheral Nervous System*, 5th ed., Figure 35. Saunders Elsevier, 2010.

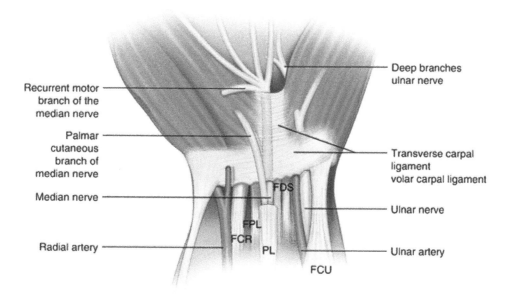

FIGURE 11.2: To show the relations of the left median nerve at the transverse carpal ligament. Note the palmar cutaneous branch which is purely sensory that does not pass through the carpal tunnel. Also note the recurrent motor branch as it hooks back to supply the muscles of the thenar eminence. FDS, flexor digitorum sublimis; FPL, flexor pollicis longus; FCR, flexor carpi radialis; PL, palmaris longus; FCU, flexor carpi ulnaris. Reproduced with permission from: Zezo Books

◀ *If the palm is numb, then isolated CTS is not the right answer.* This area is supplied by the palmar branch of the median nerve *before* it enters the carpal tunnel (Figure 11.2).

▶ *Isolated weakness and wasting of abductor pollicis brevis (APB) without sensory loss suggests a lesion of the recurrent motor branch of the median nerve* (Figure 11.2). This pure motor nerve escapes from the distal part of the transverse carpal ligament and hooks back to supply APB. Sustained pressure on the thenar eminence may damage this nerve (e.g., as in racing cyclists, although they usually press on the deep branch of the ulnar nerve).

▶ It should be distinguished from hypoplasia of the thenar eminence (Cavanagh's syndrome), a congenital disorder that is usually bilateral.

Anterior Interosseous Nerve Palsy

▶ *The patient who can squeeze a clothes pin (peg) but cannot pinch to pick up a needle or make the shape of a letter O has a palsy of the anterior interosseous nerve (AIN)* (Figure 11.5).

The AIN is a pure motor branch of the median nerve in the forearm (Figure 11.1) and supplies the following:

- Flexor pollicis longus: flexes the distal phalanx of the thumb

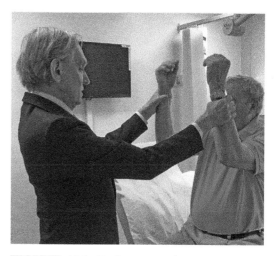

FIGURE 11.3: Hawkes test. Both arms are elevated slightly above shoulder height while the distal forearm is squeezed firmly just above the wrist. When positive the patient reports tingling of median-innervated fingers within 15 seconds.

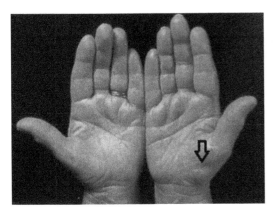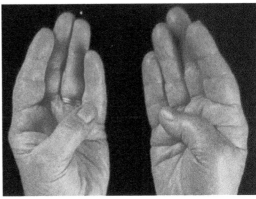

FIGURE 11.4: Carpal tunnel syndrome (CTS). **Left**: Note the wasting of abductor pollicis brevis in the right thenar eminence (arrow). **Right**: On attempted opposition, the right thumb flexes across the palm but it does not oppose, that is, rotate 90 degrees, like the normal left side. Reproduced with permission from *Atlas of Clinical Neurology*, 2nd ed., Figure 2.38a and b. GD Perkin, FH Hochberg, and DC Miller. Mosby Year Book Europe.

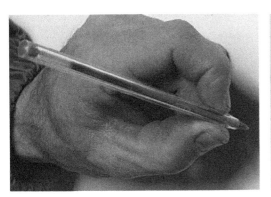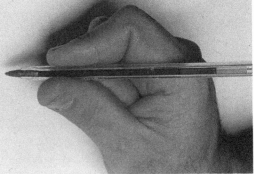

FIGURE 11.5: Anterior interosseous nerve palsy. This 30-year-old right-handed man complained of difficulty gripping a ballpoint pen. When the pen is gripped normally, a letter O shape is made with the left hand, but on the right side, the distal phalanges of digits I and II cannot be flexed, so that pinching is achieved only by flexor pollicis brevis, flexor digitorum sublimis and the first lumbrical This phenomenon is diagnostic of anterior interosseous nerve palsy. Remember that there is *no* sensory loss with this lesion.

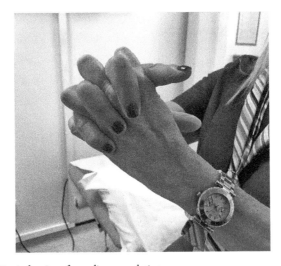

FIGURE 11.6: The pointing index sign of a median nerve lesion.

- Flexor digitorum profundus: flexes the distal phalanx of the index finger
- Pronator quadratus: pronates the forearm

Thus a lesion of the AIN takes away the ability to flex the distal phalanges of the thumb and index finger. There is no sensory loss.

▶ *If the fingers are interlocked and the index finger sticks out, this is a median nerve lesion*—the "pointing index" sign (Figure 11.6). It is due to weakness of flexor digitorum sublimis and seen in high median nerve lesions.

Ulnar Nerve Lesions

You must have working knowledge of the basic neuro-anatomy (Figure 11.7).

The usual presentations are (a) weakness and wasting of the first dorsal interosseous muscle in manual workers exposed to repeated elbow trauma or (b) fracture of the medial epicondyle. There may be clawing of the fourth and fifth fingers (Figure 11.8).

▶ *If the fingers are interlocked and the little finger sticks out, this is a high ulnar nerve lesion (elbow)* (Figure 11.9, *left*).
▶ *Patients who catch their little finger when putting a hand in their pocket likely have an ulnar nerve lesion* (Wartenberg's sign; Figure 11.9, *right*). The cause is weakness of the interossei resulting in passive abduction of the little finger, which catches on the pocket edge.
▶ Froment's sign (Figure 11.10)
  Ask the patient to pull a sheet of paper in opposite directions. On the normal side, adductor pollicis allows the paper to be gripped firmly. If there is an ulnar lesion, adduction is weak and the patient compensates by using the median-innervated flexor pollicis longus to squeeze the paper. Some learn to improve adduction by thumb rotation, thus allowing extensor pollicis longus to act as an adductor and improve grip.
▶ At the elbow, you should determine whether there is:
  ○ Full range of elbow movement. If not, there may be a problem with the elbow joint that could be compromising the ulnar nerve in its groove.
  ○ A superficially placed (possibly prolapsing) ulnar nerve. Check the carrying angle.

  ○ Nerve tenderness
  ○ Tinel's sign, by gentle percussion over the elbow groove just proximal to, at, or just distal to the medial epicondyle
▶ *If the sensory loss "splits" the ring finger, this suggests a lesion of the ulnar nerve and not C8.*
  To evaluate, test pin-prick or light touch on either side of the ring finger. A median nerve lesion also splits the ring finger but on its outer side, adjacent to the middle finger.
◀ *Ulnar sensory loss should not extend more than slightly above the wrist into the forearm.*
  The inner forearm skin is supplied by the medial cutaneous nerve of forearm, which is C8. The main catch is when there is a C8 *and* ulnar nerve lesion on the same side.

An ulnar nerve lesion at the elbow causes the following:

- Ulnar sensory impairment affecting the dorsum of the hand medially
  This happens because the posterior cutaneous branch of the ulnar nerve branches off in mid-forearm (Figure 11.7) so that the lesion must be above mid-forearm level. Most are 5 cm distal to the elbow in Osborne's canal. If there is no sensory loss over the dorsum of the hand, then the lesion is distal—most likely at wrist level
- Weakness and clawing of the distal phalanx of the fourth and fifth fingers
  This is caused by weakness of the fourth and fifth lumbricals and flexor digitorum profundus, which branches off in the upper arm.

Thus:

▶ If the distal phalanges of the fourth and fifth fingers are weak, then the ulnar lesion is at or above the elbow. If they are strong, the lesion is likely at the wrist.

Weak Wasted Hand with No Sensory Impairment

There are three main possible causes for this:

1. *Ulnar nerve lesion due to damage of the pure motor branch of the ulnar nerve in Guyon's canal near the pisiform bone. This is seen, for example, in the "handlebar palsy" of*

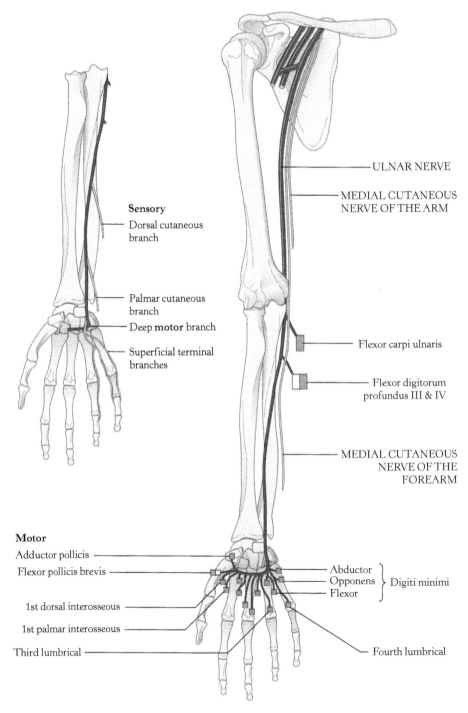

Sensory

Dorsal cutaneous branch

Palmar cutaneous branch

Deep **motor** branch

Superficial terminal branches

ULNAR NERVE

MEDIAL CUTANEOUS NERVE OF THE ARM

Flexor carpi ulnaris

Flexor digitorum profundus III & IV

MEDIAL CUTANEOUS NERVE OF THE FOREARM

Motor

Adductor pollicis

Flexor pollicis brevis

1st dorsal interosseous

1st palmar interosseous

Third lumbrical

Abductor
Opponens } Digiti minimi
Flexor

Fourth lumbrical

FIGURE 11.7: Anatomy of the ulnar nerve. Note that flexor digitorum profundus supplies the distal phalanges of the fourth and fifth fingers. Reproduced with permission from *Aids to The Examination of The Peripheral Nervous System*, 5th ed., Figure 45. Saunders Elsevier, 2010.

racing cyclists who put sustained pressure on the inner aspect of the palm. A heavy fall onto the palm of the hand is another cause. The thenar muscles remain strong except

for adduction and the tendon reflexes are normal.

2. *Amyotrophic lateral sclerosis (ALS)*. Apart from a history of fasciculation and cramp in the

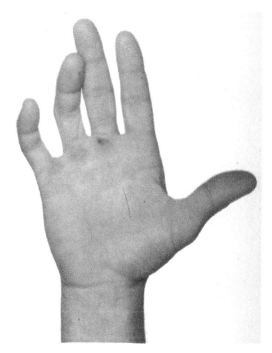

presence of brisk tendon jerks (upper motor neuron signs). See also the "split hand" sign in Chapter 7.

3. *Radiculopathy of C8 and T1.* Triceps and all intrinsic hand muscles are weak, and the triceps jerk is depressed.

A weak wasted hand without sensory loss due to syringomyelia is *almost* unheard of, hence the famous Red Flag:

▶ *No sensory loss, then no syrinx.*

Radial Nerve Lesions

Basic knowledge of the radial nerve anatomy is essential (Figure 11.11).

The most common presentation is wrist drop:

▶ *If there is mainly weakness of <u>finger</u> extension rather than <u>wrist</u> extension and no sensory loss and a normal triceps jerk, this is a lesion of the posterior interosseous nerve (PIN; Figure 11.12).*

▶ *If there is weakness of the wrist <u>and</u> finger extensors, the lesion is above the elbow.*

See Table 11.1 for other permutations of radial nerve lesions.

The PIN mainly supplies the finger extensors. It also contributes to extensor carpi ulnaris, so that, on wrist extension, you may observe radial deviation of the wrist, but the main deficit is finger extension.

FIGURE 11.8: Ulnar nerve palsy. Note the mild clawing of the fourth and fifth fingers and passive abduction of the little finger, which tends to catch when the hand is put in a pocket (Wartenberg's sign). There is usually sensory loss affecting the fourth and fifth fingers that splits the ring finger.

arms, there is usually exaggeration of tendon reflexes in the upper limbs, thus creating the classic paradox of weakness and wasting in the same limb (lower motor neuron signs) in the

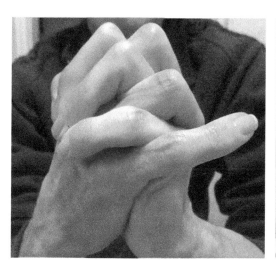

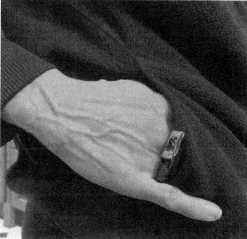

FIGURE 11.9: Left: Note that the right little finger is not fully flexed when the fingers are interlocked because of flexor digitorum profundus weakness. This is a sign of an ulnar lesion at elbow level. **Right:** The little finger sticks out when putting the affected hand in a pocket (Wartenberg's sign).

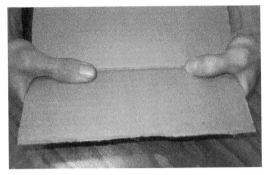

FIGURE 11.10: Froment's sign in ulnar palsy. This patient has a left ulnar palsy and has been asked to pull a piece of cardboard in opposite directions. Adductor pollicis is working normally on the right. Using the left hand, thumb adduction is weak and there is compensation with the median innervated flexor pollicis longus to pinch the card. Note the slight rotation of the thumb toward the palm, suggesting a trick movement that allows extensor pollicis longus to act as an adductor and improve grip.

▶ *Painless gradually progressive bilateral wrist drop could be lead poisoning.*
It is usually asymmetric and without sensory loss (Figure 11.13). Repetitive dorsiflexion movements by painters and their exposure to lead-based paint may render the radial nerve more susceptible. Lead exposure may also affect:
  o Bored children who chew lead-based paint on old window ledges ("pica")
  o Users of lead-containing Ayurvedic medicines prescribed as a health tonic or for psoriasis
  o Users of kohl eye shadow (predominantly Asians); this contains lead and occasionally cadmium.

Lead poisoning may be associated with the following:

- Foot drop
- Lead line, just outside the gingival margin (see Figure 1.40)
- Lead colic, simulating intestinal obstruction
- Encephalopathy
- Basophilic stippling on blood film (Figure 11.13)

Other causes of bilateral wrist drop:

- Multifocal motor neuropathy with block
- Atypical motor neuron disease

TABLE 11.1: SUMMARY OF MAIN FINDINGS IN WRIST DROP

Brachioradialis	Triceps jerk	Lesion
Strong	Normal	Posterior interosseous nerve
Weak	Normal	Lesion in spiral groove
Weak	Depressed	Above spiral groove: in brachial plexus or C7 and C8 roots

In wrist drop (Table 11.1), as a general rule:

- If brachioradialis is strong and triceps jerk is normal, the lesion is *below* the spiral groove and must involve PIN.
- If brachioradialis is weak and the triceps jerk is normal, the lesion is likely *in* the spiral groove.
- If brachioradialis is weak and the triceps jerk is impaired, the lesion is *above* the spiral groove and probably in nerve roots C7 and C8 or the brachial plexus.

▶ *An alcoholic with wrist drop likely has Saturday night palsy.*
The patient sleeps heavily on one side in a hard chair, compressing the radial nerve in the spiral groove. In *honeymooner's palsy* there is sustained pressure from the partner's head on the inside of the upper arm, resulting in proximal pressure on the radial nerve. The branch to triceps arises above the spiral groove thus the triceps jerk should be normal in Saturday night palsy but depressed in honeymooner's palsy.

Lower Limbs
Once more, knowledge of the basic anatomy of the peripheral nerves in the lower limbs is essential (Figure 11.14).
There are not many specific nerve or root Handles in the lower limbs, but here are the few we know about:

▶ *A patient who wakes from deep sleep unable to stand due to bilateral thigh weakness has the "dangling legs syndrome."*
This is seen typically in alcoholics who go into a prolonged deep sleep with both legs dangling over the side of the bed. This results in sustained stretching and pressure of both

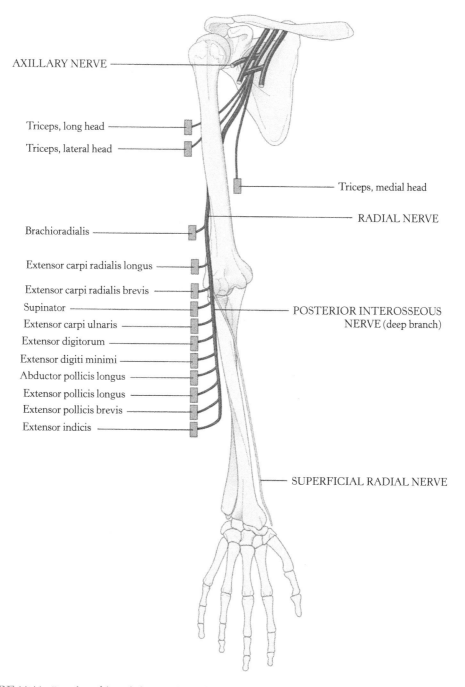

AXILLARY NERVE

Triceps, long head

Triceps, lateral head

Triceps, medial head

RADIAL NERVE

Brachioradialis

Extensor carpi radialis longus

Extensor carpi radialis brevis

Supinator

POSTERIOR INTEROSSEOUS
NERVE (deep branch)

Extensor carpi ulnaris

Extensor digitorum

Extensor digiti minimi

Abductor pollicis longus

Extensor pollicis longus

Extensor pollicis brevis

Extensor indicis

SUPERFICIAL RADIAL NERVE

FIGURE 11.11: Branches of the radial nerve. Reproduced with permission from *Aids to The Examination of The Peripheral Nervous System*, 5th ed., Figure 23. Saunders Elsevier, 2010.

femoral nerves where they cross the groin on their way to quadriceps. There will be minimal sensory loss (just in long saphenous nerve territory) and a depressed knee jerk (L3 and L4). Hip adduction is strong, in keeping with a femoral nerve lesion.

▶ *Foot drop after hip surgery is usually caused by trauma to the sciatic nerve.*
This nerve is a posterior relation of the hip joint and damaged occasionally during the operation. Pressure on the common

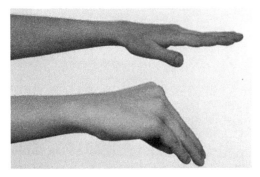 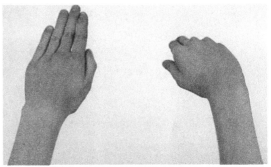

FIGURE 11.12: The **left** figure shows *finger* drop (but no *wrist* drop) of the subject's right hand, a sign that is pathognomic for a posterior interosseous palsy. Note the slight radial deviation of the hand in the **right** picture, due to weakness of extensor carpi ulnaris. Reproduced with permission from Atlas of Clinical Neurology, 2nd ed., Figure 2.16a and b. GD Perkin, FH Hochberg, and DC Miller. Mosby Year Book Europe Ltd.

peroneal nerve at the fibular head during surgery is a less frequent cause.

Unilateral Hip Flexor Weakness

This could be a lesion of (a) L2, L3, and L4 *nerve roots* (mainly L4) due to lumbar disk/tumor, or pelvic compression or (b) the *femoral nerve.*

The key tests are power of the hip adductors (L2 and L3) and ankle dorsiflexors (L4, L5). Thus:

▶ *If it is a root lesion, hip adduction and ankle dorsiflexion are weak.*

▶ *If it is a femoral nerve lesion, they are strong.*

▶ *Asymmetric pain, unilateral weakness, and wasting of the thigh muscles suggest proximal diabetic neuropathy* (diabetic amyotrophy).

It resembles a femoral neuropathy, but the damage is more widespread and hip adduction may also be weak. The typical misdiagnosis is prolapsed lumbar disk. Your suspicions should be aroused because anterior thigh pain is unusual in lumbar disk disease.

▶ *Wallet palsy*

Sciatic and posterior (femoral) cutaneous nerve lesions may be caused by a bulging wallet that imposes pressure on the buttock. It is found in taxi and bus drivers.

▶ *A misplaced injection into the buttock may cause sciatic palsy.*

▶ *Bilateral foot drop after childbirth in squatting position is likely a bilateral lesion of the common peroneal nerves.*

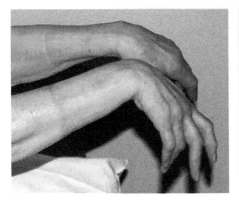 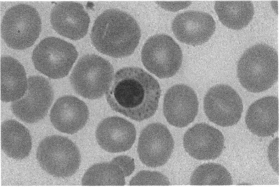

FIGURE 11.13: **Left:** Bilateral wrist drop due to lead poisoning. The lead source was from a contaminated water supply. **Right:** A nucleated red cell that shows basophilic stippling in the cytoplasm. Left image reproduced with permission from Pickrell et al. (2013).

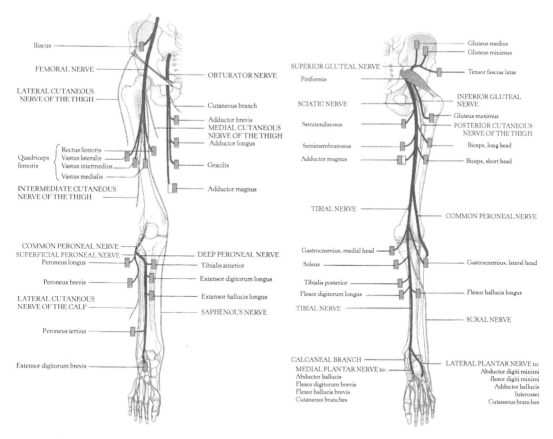

FIGURE 11.14: Left: Nerves of the front of the lower limb. **Right:** Nerves of the back of the lower limb. Reproduced with permission from *Aids to The Examination of The Peripheral Nervous System*, 5th ed., Figure 57. Saunders Elsevier, 2010.

This happens in women who squat for prolonged periods during labor. This crouched position causes pressure on the common peroneal nerve, as it lies between the biceps femoris and lateral head of gastrocnemius and the head of the fibula. A similar condition affects strawberry pickers— "strawberry picker's" foot drop. In "toilet sitter's" palsy there is compression of the sciatic nerve in the posterior thigh that may resemble a common peroneal palsy.

▶ *Flaccid foot drop and normal ankle jerk is likely a common peroneal nerve palsy.* Flaccid foot drop and depressed ankle jerk favors a proximal lesion.

To ensure an L5 lesion is not masquerading as a common peroneal nerve lesion, you should test hip abduction (gluteus medius, L5) and percuss the medial (short) head of hamstring for its reflex (L5). If the electromyogram (EMG) shows denervation of the medial head of biceps, gluteus medius, or tensor fascia lata (all fed by L5) this indicates a proximal lesion.

▶ *Unilateral painless foot drop could be a rare presentation of ALS.*

It may be hard to identify at first without an EMG. With time, upper motor neuron features and additional muscle wasting appear.

▶ *Acute groin pain in a patient receiving anticoagulants is likely a femoral neuropathy from bleeding into the iliacus muscle.*

To ease pain, the hip is passively flexed and laterally rotated, and there is tenderness to palpation over the inguinal canal and iliac fossa. Weakness of quadriceps develops after 1–2 days.

◀ Occasionally, there is no pain, and the leg weakness results in misdiagnosis of stroke.

▶ *Chronic inner groin pain in an athlete is likely obturator nerve entrapment.*

To confirm, test hip adduction, which should be weak.

MONONEURITIS MULTIPLEX

This term applies to conditions in which there is damage to several individual peripheral nerves. There are no really powerful Handles for these, just a list of etiologies:

- Diabetes
- Immune-based disorder: vasculitis (mainly rheumatoid arthritis and polyarteritis), lupus, Wegener's granulomatosis, Churg-Strauss syndrome
- Sarcoidosis
- Neoplastic and paraneoplastic disorder
- Leprosy, amyloid
- Neurofibromatosis

Note:

▶ *If there is a history of liver problems, then think of hepatitis C infection,* a disorder associated with cryoglobulinemic vasculitis.
▶ *Exposed nerves,* such as the ulnar at the elbow and common peroneal at the knee, are liable to pressure. If there are several or recurrent pressure palsies, this raises the possibility of *familial liability to pressure palsy* due to a mutation in *PMP22* (chromosome 17p).

Isolated Numb Patches

Many of these are associated with feelings of tinglings or burning. All are in essence a mononeuritis for which there are numerous causes. Only the main associations are mentioned.

▶ Outer thigh: meralgia paresthetica
This is caused by pressure on the lateral cutaneous nerve of thigh (lateral femoral cutaneous nerve) where it crosses under the inguinal ligament. Pregnancy, weight gain, iliac bone grafts, and pelvic surgery are related factors.
▶ Lateral thumb and first dorsal webspace: cheiralgia paresthetica (Figure 11.15)
This relates to pressure on distal branches of the radial nerve, which are purely sensory at this level. The most common cause is pressure from handcuffs!
▶ Interscapular: notalgia paresthetica
Figure 11.16)

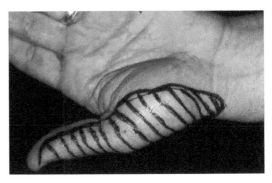

FIGURE 11.15: The sensory impairment of cheiralgia paresthetica. This was a 55-year-old man who was handcuffed by police the day before. The area of sensory loss shown here is more extensive than usually seen.

It is suspected that the thoracic dorsal cutaneous branches are compressed by the thick fascial planes in the back. If associated with severe persistent itching, it may indicate multiple endocrine neoplasia type 2A (Steinhoff et al. 2018).

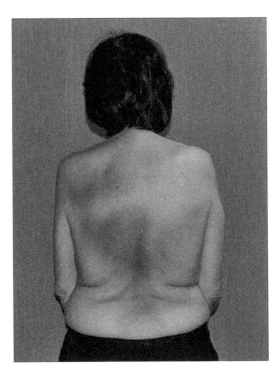

FIGURE 11.16: A 60-year-old woman with notalgia paresthetica that caused severe painless interscapular itching and sensory loss over T5 and T6 on left. Pigmented areas and scarring are secondary to scratching and use of capsaicin cream. Reproduced with permission from Lancet Neurology, Figure 2. Steinhoff M et al. (2018).

▶ Medial malleolus: saphenous neuropathy
In a surfer, this is due to a compression of the saphenous nerve where the ankle grips the back of the surfboard. In non-surfers, it could be an L4 root lesion or entrapment of the nerve in the femoral canal.

▶ Medial sole: tarsal tunnel syndrome.
Causes are fallen plantar arch, nerve tumor, athleticism

▶ Cheek: infraorbital nerve. Most are due to fracture of the orbital floor.

▶ Chin: mental nerve; "numb chin" (Roger syndrome) syndrome. Causes: local dental conditions including neoplasia, skull base neoplasm, mandibular metastases (usually from breast), systemic disease (sarcoid, diabetes, MS, sickle cell anemia)

▶ Unilateral occipital skin: occipital nerve.
Usually associated with pain (occipital neuralgia). Causes: local trauma; rarely, spinal fluid leak

▶ Palm or sole: leprosy

▶ Anterolateral leg: lateral sural cutaneous nerve. This is caused by entrapment (e.g., from prolonged kneeling)

▶ Multiple numb patches suggest Wartenberg's migratory sensory neuropathy. This is a pure sensory mononeuritis multiplex, with numbness in distribution of peripheral nerves, usually persisting several months.

▶ Patchy sensory loss affecting proximal and distal skin—scalp, thorax, abdomen, and buttocks—suggests a sensory ganglionopathy.
The chief causes are as follows:
  ○ Autoimmune disease: Sjögren syndrome, scleroderma, lupus
  ○ Paraproteinemia
  ○ Human T-lymphotropic virus (HTLV-1) infection
  ○ Fabry's disease
  ○ HIV
  ○ Pyridoxine excess
  ○ Neoplasia and paraneoplastic disorder

Tabes dorsalis is similar, with involvement of the anterior chest wall ("cuirass" distribution—a plate of armor), central face ("mask"), and shins ("greaves"—another piece of armor). However, the main pathology of tabes is thought to be in the dorsal

nerve roots and columns rather than the dorsal root ganglia.

RADICULOPATHY

Diagnosis of specific nerve root lesions can be straightforward, assuming one possesses a reasonable knowledge of neuroanatomy.

Compressive Lesions Affecting Upper Limbs

▶ *Depressed biceps jerk with sensory loss over the thumb suggests a C6 lesion.*
Biceps and radial wrist extension should be weak.

▶ *An inverted supinator or biceps jerk with hyperactive reflexes below this level is due to a spinal cord lesion at C6.*

▶ *Depressed triceps jerk and impaired feeling of the little finger and inner forearm suggests a C8 lesion.*
Triceps, forearm extensors, and the intrinsic hand muscles should be weak.

▶ *Most cervical root pain spreads into the shoulder or down the arms.* Characteristically:
  ○ C6 root pain spreads down the radial border of the arm into the thumb.
  ○ C7 root pain radiates to the second and third digits and medial to the scapula.
  ○ C8 root pain spreads down the inner aspect of the arm into the fourth and fifth fingers.

▶ *In cervical radiculopathy the affected nerve is painful and swollen.* This may extend out into the neck tissues. Palpation about halfway down and posterior to the sternomastoid muscle readily elicits pain.

▶ *An acutely painful shoulder with weakness and wasting typically of deltoid or serratus anterior 2–3 days later is acute brachial plexus neuropathy* (ABN, neuralgic amyotrophy).
  ○ A small patch of numbness over the outer aspect of deltoid is characteristic (Badge sign)

ABN often simulates a peripheral nerve lesion such as CTS, or ulnar or radial nerve lesion. The phrenic nerve may be involved, resulting in breathlessness when lying in bed or standing in deep water. Paralysis of the diaphragm may be confirmed on chest X-ray. The main triggers are the following:

- Vaccination
- Infections
- Surgery 1–2 weeks previously
- Mild trauma where the long thoracic nerve is stretched, resulting in scapular winging

Note: There is a rare, recurrent autosomal dominant form of ABN.

▶ *Bilateral, painful ABN and phrenic nerve involvement is often secondary to hepatitis E infection.*

Major causes of acquired noncompressive radiculopathies are the following:

- Infectious and postinfectious: Guillain-Barré syndrome (GBS), Lyme disease, neurobrucellosis, Elsberg syndrome (see later in this section)
- Immune-related: diabetic thoraco-abdominal radiculopathy and diabetic amyotrophy
- Infiltrative disease of meninges: neurolymphomatosis, metastatic lesions, syphilis
- Cervical or lumbosacral plexopathy

Handles for Noncompressive Radiculopathy

▶ *Muscle weakness is asymmetrical often more proximal than distal.*
▶ *Sensory loss is painful and patchy, affecting proximal and distal skin.*
▶ *Absent knee jerk with normal ankle jerk.*
▶ *Preserved sensory action potentials in territory of weak, denervated muscles.*

▶ *Loss of F and H reflexes*
▶ *EMG evidence of denervation in proximal muscles (e.g., paraspinal, glutei or rhomboids), which are affected last in axonal polyneuropathy*
▶ *Radiculopathy with target skin lesions is Lyme disease (Figure 11.17).*
▶ *Radiculopathy with perineal vesicles and urinary retention is Elsberg syndrome.*
▶ *Weak, pain-free swollen arm following radiotherapy for breast cancer given years previously is probably radiation-induced brachial plexopathy (RBP).*
Myokymia-like twitches in the affected limb are common. Distinction from metastatic plexus infiltration is difficult, but in general RBP is associated with the following:
   o High radiation doses
   o Little or no pain
   o Myokymia-like twitches
   o No Horner's syndrome
   o Preference for the upper trunk (C5, C6).
Conversely, if there are metastases, the radiation dose received is lower, pain is prominent, there is a Horner's syndrome, and preferential involvement of the lower trunk (C8, T1).
▶ *Sharp, burning pain in the shoulder radiating to the arm and hand following a blow to head, neck, or shoulder in a contact sport is a "stinger" or a "burner."*
Weakness involves biceps and shoulder girdle muscles. It resolves usually in a few minutes but exceptionally may persist. The site of damage is probably in the cervical cord or brachial plexus.

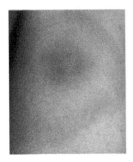 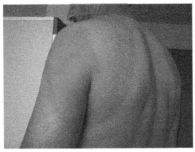 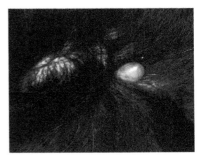

FIGURE 11.17: Erythema chronicum migrans. The characteristic spreading rash of Lyme disease. **Left**: The site of tick bite and developing rash. **Center**: The rash in a more advanced stage. Both figures show "target" lesions. **Right**: Engorged tick in the scalp with adjacent alopecia. Center image courtesy Jose Biller, Chicago. Right image reproduced from Figure 14.9 in the chapter Hair and Scalp Disorders, by S Lewis-Jones. Oxford University Press. DOI:10.1093/med/9780199208388.003.14.

▶ *Depressed shoulders in a woman with weakness, numbness, and pain in one or both upper limbs is the droopy shoulder syndrome* (Figure 11.18) (Swift and Nichols 1984).

Patients have low-hanging shoulders and a long neck, so that, on lateral cervical spine X-rays, the T4 vertebra (usually obscured by the shoulders), can be seen. Symptoms are worsened by downward traction on the arms and relieved by pushing the arms up. There is weakness and sensory impairment in the distribution of C8 and T1. There is no cervical rib or band; it arises from chronic stretching of the brachial plexus.

Lower Limbs

Handles to help localize a lesion

▶ *Depressed knee jerk with sensory loss over the inner leg and foot suggests a lesion of the femoral nerve or the L4 nerve root.*

Both lesions weaken quadriceps, but

• A femoral nerve lesion is associated with normal hip adduction and ankle dorsiflexion.

whereas

• An L4 root lesion is associated with
  ○ Weak ankle dorsiflexion and
  ○ Weak hip adduction and flexion from the semi-flexed position

▶ *Depressed ankle jerk with sensory loss over the little toe is a lesion of S1.*

▶ *Severe sciatic pain with a normal lumbar spine MRI scan is likely a lumbosacral plexopathy.*
Typically, this follows viral, autoimmune, or neoplastic involvement of the plexus. A similar syndrome occurs in:
  ○ Intravenous heroin addicts
  ○ Diabetes
  ○ Elsberg syndrome where there is acute urinary retention followed by myeloradiculopathy secondary to HSV-2 infection. Look for vesicles in the perineum and buttocks. Patients are usually women, and the cerebrospinal fluid (CSF) is cellular. The major leg nerves may be tender to touch, and the MRI scan may reveal swollen nerve roots
  ○ Possibly with a dural fistula

▶ Facet joint pain may simulate sciatica, but the pain does not usually radiate below the knee,

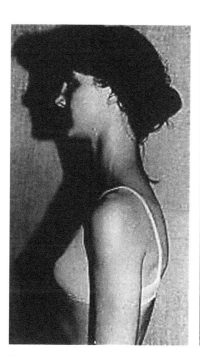
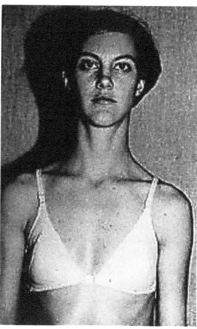

FIGURE 11.18: Droopy shoulder syndrome. Note long neck, low shoulders, and horizontal clavicles. This patient had severe upper extremity pain and numbness worse on the left where the shoulder is lower.

whereas sciatica typically spreads down to the ankle.

▶ Painful neurological relapse occurring months or years after pelvic radiation for malignancy is more likely tumor recurrence than radiation plexopathy.

▶ Acute-onset, generalized, severe weakness in a previously healthy child or adult with little or no sensory loss. Consider the following causes:
  ○ Neuropathies: GBS, porphyria
  ○ Psychiatric disease
  ○ Poliomyelitis
  ○ Neuromuscular transmission disorder; for example, myasthenia gravis, botulism
  ○ Acute myopathy with rhabdomyolysis
  ○ Demyelination: acute transverse my-elitis, Devic's syndrome, multiple sclerosis (MS)
  ○ Periodic paralysis
  ○ Tick paralysis
  ○ Organophosphate poisoning

POLYNEUROPATHY

In this condition, all major peripheral nerves are af-fected to varying degrees. Before going into detail, here are some Handles that can give you a head start on the diagnosis.   .

Pattern of Onset

▶ Rapidly evolving polyneuropathy is due to inflammatory, immune, toxic, or vas-cular causes. Conversely, a polyneuropathy evolving over several years suggests a heredi-tary or metabolic cause.

▶ Distal, symmetric polyneuropathy is usually metabolic, toxic, or inherited.
  These processes affect all nerves to an equal degree, and most are length-dependent—unlike the *immune- or infection-related neuropathies*, which tend to be *asymmetric*.
  Classic GBS is usually an easy diagnosis.
  • Onset about 2–3 weeks after viral or bacte-rial infection
  • Ascending symmetric weakness, sensory symptoms, spinal pain, and depressed reflexes.
  • Respiratory and autonomic involvement is common.

• CSF shows a raised protein and little or no elevation of cell count.

Red flags for apparent GBS:

◀ Normal CSF protein (unless very early in the disease course) or raised cell count. If CSF cell count is greater than 5/mm³, think of: HIV, Lyme disease, sarcoidosis, lymphoma

◀ Raised CK and proximal weakness in first few days suggests myositis. Later on muscle wasting raises the CK in GBS

◀ Abdominal pain during paralytic phase (rather than before). Suggests:
  • Lead/thallium/arsenic poisoning
  • Acute intermittent porphyria
  • Tyrosinemia (associated with ileus, extensor muscle rigidity, self-mutilation, keratitis)

◀ Preserved reflexes unless very early on in the disease course. Repeated exam may show that the reflexes become absent.

◀ Bladder or bowel involvement

◀ Distal neuropathic pain (rather than proximal or in back) suggests a vasculitic disorder

◀ Ataxia and ophthalmoplegia without pupil-lary changes suggest the Miller Fisher variant.

◀ Ophthalmoplegia, impaired pupillary reflexes, autonomic changes, and muscle weakness infers botulism. Check for skin lesions that characterize a drug addict.

◀ Hypokalaemia. This can mimic GBS.

▶ Polyneuropathy with arms affected before legs. Be careful to not overlook a pure motor disorder such as ALS and related syndromes, and always check for myotonia. If these are excluded this rare pattern suggests:
  ○ Lymphoma
  ○ GBS or multifocal demyelinating motor neuropathy
  ○ Diabetic radiculopathy or insulinoma
  ○ Hereditary causes: hereditary motor neu-ropathy type 5A and Charcot-Marie-Tooth disease type 2D.
  ○ In hereditary motor neuropathy type VII there is a hoarse voice due to involvement of the (longer) left recurrent laryngeal nerve
  ○ Copper deficiency (sensory ataxia usually with myelopathy) or lead (wrist drop)
  ○ Vasculitis, paraneoplastic sensory neuropathy
  ○ Amyloid, porphyria; both have autonomic dysfunction

Painful Polyneuropathy

There is a long checklist for this condition, but you can dissect out the answer with a bit more information. Most are due to a small fiber neuropathy. The main causes are the following:

- Thiamine (B$_1$) deficiency (usually alcoholic or nutritional)
- Diabetes
- HIV
- Sjögren's disease

Rare causes are as follows:

- Fabry's syndrome
- Sarcoidosis
- Vasculitis
- Amyloid
- Leprosy
- Paroxysmal extreme pain disorder (PEPD) and erythromelalgia
- Arsenic or thallium poisoning

The chief explanation for polyneuropathy secondary to thiamine deficiency is alcoholism, although there is probably a direct toxic effect from alcohol as well. Another thiamine deficiency syndrome that is overlooked easily occurs in early pregnancy from hyperemesis gravidarum. It usually baffles the obstetrician because the patient, if well enough to give a history, complains of tingling hands and feet. MS is a frequent misdiagnosis. People on hunger strike or malnourished individuals suffer the same condition.

Taken together, these three conditions constitute useful Handles:

- ▶ Painful tingling extremities associated with prolonged vomiting, alcoholism, or malnutrition are likely due to thiamine deficiency.

Note: In diabetes the pains are usually in the legs and feet and worse when warm in bed. Less often pain is felt in the trunk.

- ▶ Painful or burning distal predominantly sensory polyneuropathy is characteristic of HIV infection.
    There are many other varieties according to the phase of illness and whether antiretroviral drugs have been given.

Sjögren's syndrome is mainly a disorder of women that is associated with a sensory ganglionopathy and painful small fiber neuropathy. Less frequently, there is trigeminal neuropathy that is sometimes severe and mutilating. Thus:

- ▶ A woman with dry eyes, dry mouth, and burning feet, especially at night, likely has Sjögren's syndrome.

The clues for *Fabry's disease* (Figure 11.19, Figure 1.16, and Figure 9.26) are the bathing trunk rash due to angiokeratomas (sometimes confined to the perineum or absent), hypertension, and renal failure. A mnemonic is **F**ever, **A**rthralgia, **B**lood pressure, **R**enal failure, **Y**elling with pain, **S**kin changes. There is a useful Handle:

- ▶ If the pain is so pronounced that the patient will not permit an examination (i.e., severe allodynia), think of Fabry's disease. Severe allodynia is a feature of any small fiber neuropathy (e.g., HIV, diabetes, chronic regional pain syndrome, alcoholic), but Fabry's disease is probably the worst.

Check the skin for angiokeratomas and the eyes. There may be tortuous vessels in the conjunctiva and retina (Figure 1.16). With a slit lamp, you may see vortex keratopathy (Figure 11.19).

- ▶ Although Fabry's disease is X-linked and therefore primarily a disorder of men, it may present

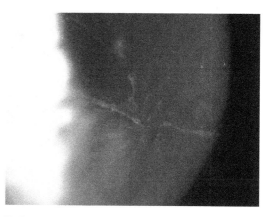

FIGURE 11.19: Vortex keratopathy as seen with a slit lamp in Fabry's disease. More common causes are drugs, such as amiodarone, chloroquine, and chlorpromazine. Reproduced with permission from *Training in Ophthalmology*, Venki Sundaram, Allon Barsam, Amar Alwitry, and Peng Khaw, eds. Figure 1.57 in the chapter External Eye Disease, by S Goyal, A Barsam, and S Tuft. Oxford University Press, 2009. DOI:10.1093/med/9780199237593.003.0001.

in middle-aged women as a relatively mild neuropathy with painful numb patches in the limbs.

▶ Frost-bitten appearance of the face (lupus pernio) is likely sarcoidosis (Figure 11.20, *left*). Skin biopsy, CT of the chest, or a PET scan may clinch the diagnosis. Also, granulomas developing in scars or tattoos are characteristic of sarcoidosis and may be a presenting feature (Figure 11.20, *right*).

▶ Restrictive cardiomyopathy and polyneuropathy suggest sarcoidosis, amyloidosis, Churg-Strauss syndrome, or Fabry's disease. The neuropathy (especially Fabry's disease) is often painful. Hemochromatosis also causes restrictive cardiomyopathy, but the neuropathy, if present, is secondary to diabetes.

▶ Polyneuropathy, asthma, and marked eosinophilia suggest the Churg-Strauss syndrome. This is now renamed *eosinophilic granulomatosis with polyangiitis* (EGPA). Painful mononeuritis multiplex is characteristic of the early stages. The diagnosis is confirmed by blood tests for antibodies against pANCA and myeloperoxidase with biopsy of the lung or a skin rash. Additional features are pulmonary/ cardiac infiltrates and nasal polyps. The neurological profile bears some similarity to that of Wegener's granulomatosis, but in the latter there is no asthma and hypereosinophilia is rare.

▶ Painful polyneuropathy with previous vitreous hemorrhage or lattice corneal dystrophy suggests amyloidosis (Figure 11.21).

▶ Lattice corneal dystrophy suggests the gelsolin mutation.

Often there are other clues:

  o Severe autonomic neuropathy with marked postural hypotension
  o Nerve enlargement
  o Loss of taste
  o Carpal tunnel syndrome
  o Family history of sudden death from restrictive cardiomyopathy

▶ Paroxysms of pain in the eye, jaw, or rectum with autonomic features (salivation, flushing) is *paroxysmal extreme pain disorder* (PEPD). This starts in children or young adults. Attacks are triggered by cold wind, eating, defecation, and emotion. It is a sodium channelopathy (NAV 1.7) that may overlap symptomatically with trigeminal neuralgia, although in PEPD there is often facial flushing (erythromelalgia) and hypersalivation.

▶ Bouts of red, painful, swollen hands, legs, ears, or face suggest erythromelalgia (Figure 11.22). The primary form is due to a mutation in NAV 1.7, as in PEPD. In the secondary variety, symptoms are comparable, but there is an underlying problem:

  o Small fiber polyneuropathy (especially diabetic)
  o Thrombocytosis
  o Reaction to medication (e.g., pergolide, verapamil, and nifedipine)

A useful Handle for all types of erythromelalgia is the following:

▶ Red, burning legs or palms, lessened by cooling or limb elevation, suggest erythromelalgia. You must check for underlying causes.

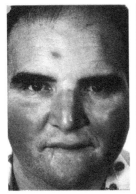 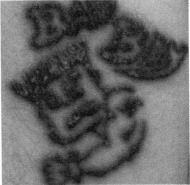

FIGURE 11.20: **Left**: This 55-year-old man was troubled by breathlessness and reddening of the face, including the nose, resembling frostbite. This is lupus pernio, and it is characteristic of sarcoidosis. A skin biopsy will usually reveal the diagnosis. **Right**: Scaly, inflamed skin over the tattoo of a 34-year-old man secondary to sarcoidosis. Left image courtesy John Pilling, Norwich, UK. Right image reproduced with permission from Post and Hull (2012).

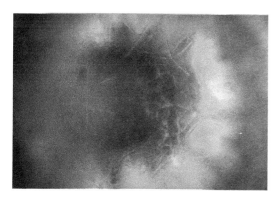

FIGURE 11.21: Lattice corneal dystrophy. This is a feature of familial amyloidosis due to the gelsolin mutation. Reproduced from Figure 1.65 in the chapter External Eye Disease, by S Goyal, A Barsam, and S Tuft. Oxford University Press. DOI:10.1093/med/9780199237593.003.0001.

Also note:

▶ Shooting leg pain at right angles to the skin along with a high-stepping, stamping gait suggests tabes dorsalis.
   The gait is high-stepping *and* stamping, and represents, in part, an attempt by the patient to provide more feeling to make up for the severely impaired joint position sense. Also, there are painless ulcers, Charcot joints, and positive treponemal serology.

Note:

▶ In bilateral foot drop with normal joint position sense, the foot is lifted high to clear the ground, but it is usually not stamped down.

Other tantalizing but rare causes of painful neuropathy are *arsenic* (Figure 11.23), *thallium*, and *mercury poisoning*. In mercury poisoning, remember the four P's mnemonic: **P**eripheral, **P**ainful, **P**aresthesias, and **P**erspiration. These disorders are worth considering if nothing else fits. In arsenic poisoning, always suspect the spouse!

▶ Be aware that some Ayurvedic medicines prescribed for treatment of diabetes or psoriasis may contain arsenic, lead, or mercury.

Neuropathic Itching

There is a long list of possibilities, but here are some of the leading contenders:

· Small fiber length-dependent polyneuropathy, particularly diabetic.
· Ehlers-Danlos syndrome
· Post-herpetic, particularly facial
· Multiple endocrine neoplasia type 2A.
· Ganglionopathy: Sjögren's syndrome, cancer (especially small-cell lung)
· MS, typically paroxysmal

Axonal or Demyelinating Polyneuropathy?

It is helpful to know whether you are dealing with a primary axonal or demyelinating polyneuropathy. Here are some Handles:

▶ Weakness with little wasting suggests a demyelinating neuropathy.

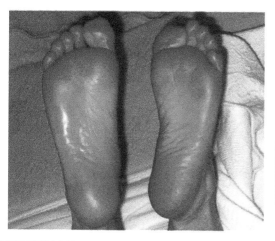

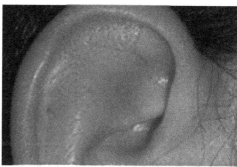

FIGURE 11.22: **Left**: Erythromelalgia involving the feet. The feet are typically painful, red, and swollen. Symptoms may be relieved by cooling or elevating the limb. **Right**: Reddening of the ear. The face and hands may be affected. Left image reproduced from Figure 16.4 in the chapter Neuropathic Pain Disorders with Autonomic Component, by ML Mauermann and W Singer. Oxford University Press. DOI:10.1093/med/9780199920198.003.0016.

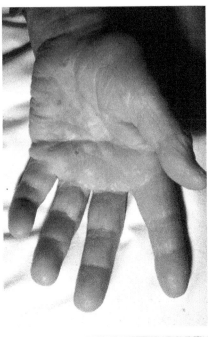
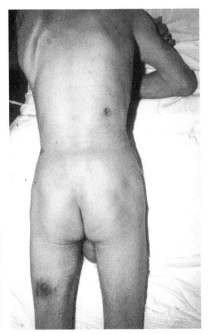

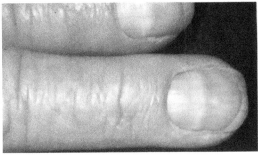

FIGURE 11.23: Arsenic poisoning. Note the thickened scaly, yellow patches on the hands. They were present on the soles of his feet as well. This was an elderly epileptic patient who received arsenicals in the 1930s when they were used to treat refractory seizures. He developed a painful peripheral neuropathy some 20 years after discontinuing arsenicals. The skin lesions are those of multiple squamous cell carcinomata—Bowen's disease—another complication of chronic arsenical exposure. A further clue is horizontal white lines in the nails as shown in the bottom picture. These are known as Mees lines. They are also seen in thallium poisoning.

Here, the motor neuron is in continuity with its anterior horn cell and it is able to function, at least partially. Nerve conduction studies show conduction block or slowing.

▶ Wasting associated with weakness in the early stages favors an axonal neuropathy.
  This happens because the axon is damaged and the connection between the cell bodies and their muscles is impaired, resulting in marked wasting.

Note:

▶ Early wasting of extensor digitorum brevis (EDB) favors axonal polyneuropathy.

▶ Axonal neuropathies are more common and likely painful, with greater weakness and wasting.
  They are harder to treat, and the overall prognosis is worse whereas:.

▶ Demyelinating neuropathies are rarer, unlikely to be painful, and display less weakness and wasting.
  The prospects of therapy and prognosis is better.

▶ Proximal leg weakness with absent reflexes is likely a demyelinating radiculo-neuropathy.
  For example, GBS or chronic inflammatory demyelinating polyneuropathy (CIDP).

In summary:

▶ Weakness with *mild* wasting suggests demyelinating neuropathy.
▶ Weakness with *marked* wasting favors axonal neuropathy.

Note:

▶ Bladder involvement is rare in demyelinating neuropathy and radiculopathy but more common in axonal neuropathy with autonomic dysfunction.

Main Causes of Chronic Demyelinating Polyneuropathy
1. Genetic

- Charcot-Marie-Tooth disease: types 1, 3 (Dejerine Sottas), 4, and CMTX
- Hereditary liability to pressure palsy
- ARSACS (autosomal recessive spastic ataxia of Charlevoix-Saguenay) and PHARC syndrome (polyneuropathy, hearing loss, ataxia, retinitis pigmentosa, and cataract) ((see Chapter 12)
- Refsum's disease
- Cerebrotendinous xanthomatosis (CTX)
- Leukodystrophies: metachromatic, adrenomyeloneuropathy, Cockayne's syndrome, Krabbe's disease, Pelizaeus-Merzbacher disease

2. Acquired

- CIDP
- Paraproteinemic
- Multifocal motor neuropathy with conduction block
- Medication: for example, amiodarone, perhexiline, bortezomib (although usually causes axonal neuropathy)
- Paranodopathies. These are similar to CIDP, but there are antibodies to contactin, neurofascin, or CASPR that are present in the paranodal area.
  Features: relapsing course; painful; severe weakness, sensory ataxia, and tremor; hypertrophied nerve roots. Resistance to immunoglobulin, but usually good response to rituximab.

Nerve Conduction Tests and Electromyography

Axonal neuropathies show the following:

- Less than 30% reduction of nerve conduction velocity; that is, not slower than 30 meters/second in the forearm or 20 meters/second in the leg.
- Marked reduction in amplitude of the compound muscle action potential (CMAP)

Demyelinating neuropathies show the following:

- Greater than 30% slowing of nerve conduction velocity; namely, slower than 30 meters/second in the forearm or 20 meters/second in the leg
- Conduction block. This means that the CMAP amplitude is relatively preserved when the nerve is stimulated distally but reduced by about 50% when stimulated proximally.

In the axonal variety, the EMG displays signs of denervation (fibrillations [acute phase], positive sharp waves, and a gapped interference pattern) but not in the demyelinating type, unless there is additional axonal degeneration.

Pure axonal or pure demyelinating varieties are rare; most neuropathies are mixed.

You can verify the diagnosis further by examination of the spinal fluid:

- In demyelinating neuropathies (and radiculopathies), the total protein is usually raised but not in most axonal varieties.
  As mentioned earlier for radiculopathy, the EMG will show:
▶ Preserved sensory action potentials in territory of weak, denervated muscles.
▶ Loss of F and H reflexes
▶ Evidence of denervation in proximal muscles (e.g., paraspinal, glutei, or rhomboids), which are affected last in axonal polyneuropathy

Length-Dependent (Long Fiber) or Non–Length-Dependent (Short Fiber) Neuropathy?

1. Length-dependent neuropathy (LDN). The longer peripheral nerves are affected first, thus
▶ First symptoms are in the toes, then the feet.

▶ When the leg is numb, the fingertips are
affected.
▶ On examination, there is symmetric sensory impairment up to the knee and wrist,
resulting in glove-and-stocking sensory loss.

As the disease progresses, the shorter nerves become progressively involved. This may cause

▶ Sensory loss on the anterior trunk, which may
be confused with a spinal cord sensory level,
but sensation over the back is preserved.

Many cases of LDN are due to *small (fine) fiber
neuropathy*, which has the following characteristics:

• Preserved reflexes
• Burning pain, worse at night
• Raised thermal threshold

The main causes of length-dependent symmetric
glove and stocking sensory motor polyneuropathies
are the following:

• Diabetes
• Alcohol-nutritional neuropathy
• Vitamin deficiencies: B_{12}, thiamine, B_6 (defi-
ciency or overuse) (Figure 11.24)
• Drug-induced, particularly antineoplastic
agents, Antabuse, thalidomide
• Metal poisoning: lead, arsenic, mercury, and
thallium
• Hereditary conditions such as Charcot-Marie-
Tooth disease, Refsum syndrome, Krabbe
disease, storage diseases
• POEMS syndrome (polyneuropathy,
organomegaly, endocrinopathy or edema, M
protein, and skin changes)
• Exposure to toxins such as ciguatera, ethylene
oxide, or snake bites
• IgM paraprotein

2. Non–length-dependent (short fiber)
neuropathy
In this variety, there is motor and sensory involvement, typically worse in the face and
areas covered by a short-sleeved shirt and
trunks. Ankle jerks may be preserved or
even hyperactive. Small or large fibers may
be involved. Routine nerve conduction
tests can be normal.

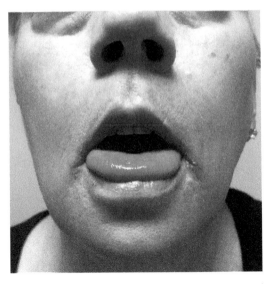

FIGURE 11.24: This woman presented on account of
memory difficulties. Note the angular stomatitis and smooth
tongue due to loss of fungiform papillae. She had deficiency of
vitamins B_1 and B_2 and a polyneuropathy.

The major causes of short fiber neuropathy are the
following:

• Diabetes (may affect either long or short
fibers)
• Immune-related disease: Sjögren's syndrome,
scleroderma, lupus
• HTLV-1, HIV, and hepatitis C infection
• Fabry's disease
• Neoplasia and paraneoplastic disorder
• Porphyria
• Acrylamide intoxication
• Tangier disease

Most of these conditions are described elsewhere in
this chapter.

▶ Relapsing polyneuropathy with orange-yellow
tonsils is Tangier disease (Figure 11.25). Other
features of Tangier disease are as follows:
  ○ Autosomal recessive inheritance
  ○ Relapsing mixed axonal and demyelinating
  peripheral neuropathy
  ○ Sensory loss in a cape distribution,
  simulating syringomyelia
  ○ Premature myocardial infarction and
  strokes
  ○ Low total and HDL cholesterol
▶ Polyneuropathy with preserved ankle reflexes
suggests:

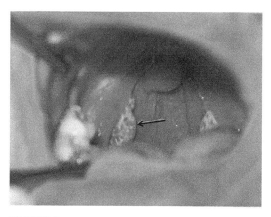

FIGURE 11.25: Tangier disease (familial alpha-lipoprotein deficiency, hypo-alpha-lipoproteinemia). Note the enlarged orange/yellow tonsils (arrow). Courtesy Dr. Federico Bigazzi, Dyslipidemias & Atherosclerosis Lab, Pisa, Italy.

- o Small fiber axonal neuropathy (e.g., porphyria or thalidomide)
- o Mild large fiber neuropathy
- o Additional CNS involvement

Pure Motor Polyneuropathy

There are few causes as follows:

- Diabetes
- Occasionally in GBS and CIDP
- Multifocal motor neuropathy
- Genetic: hereditary motor neuropathy, type 5A; if hoarse voice, type 7 Charcot-Marie-Tooth disease (type 2D)
- Diphtheria, porphyria
- ◀ Myotonic dystrophy (type 1) can simulate a pure motor polyneuropathy, so do not forget to check for myotonia. Also think of milder forms of ALS

Pure Sensory Polyneuropathy

These are the main causes:

- Diabetes (diabetic pseudo-tabes)
- CIDP
- Sjögren's disease (strictly a ganglionopathy)
- Drugs: pyridoxine intoxication (weight-lifters), cis-platinum
- Paraneoplastic (with anti-Hu antibodies)
- Hereditary sensory and autonomic neuropathy (HSAN)
- Cerebellar ataxia, neuronopathy, vestibular areflexia syndrome (CANVAS)

Inherited or Acquired?

If you are trying to determine whether the neuropathy is likely inherited or acquired, try the following guidelines.

- ▶ In general, peripheral neuropathy with sensory signs:
  - o Associated with positive phenomena such as tingling or pain is likely acquired
  - o Without positive phenomena is likely inherited

Thus, patients with Charcot-Marie-Tooth disease rarely complain of tingling because their sensory nerves have been abnormal since birth. If such a patient does report paresthesia, the diagnosis may be incorrect or there is an additional acquired neuropathy. This association is recognized, for example: Charcot-Marie-Tooth disease with subsequent CIDP (Marques et al. 2010).

- ▶ Pes cavus favors inherited neuropathy (Figure 11.26).
  Many people with pes cavus have an inherited neurological disorder. There is no generally agreed upon definition for pes cavus. It may be present from birth or result from acquired weakness of the intrinsic foot muscles.
- ▶ A useful additional clue for pes cavus is the presence of hammer-toe deformity (Figure 11.26).
- ▶ A man with apparent Charcot-Marie-Tooth disease type 1 that is transmitted only through his daughters likely has the Connexin

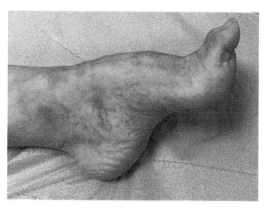

FIGURE 11.26: Pes cavus. There is hammer-toe deformity as well, a useful clue to the presence of pes cavus. Also note the convex upper border of the foot.

32 (*GJB1*) mutation. This is an X-linked dominant condition abbreviated to CMTX.

Thickened Peripheral Nerves

Thickened nerves may be detected clinically in the neck (great auricular nerve, over the upper part of sternomastoid), elbow (ulnar nerve), wrist (median nerve), or knee (common peroneal nerve, common fibular nerve), and over the dorsum of the hands and feet. MRI of the brachial/lumbar plexus or spinal canal may show thickened nerve roots (Figure 11.27). There are numerous causes of this:

- Neurofibromatosis type 1 (NF1)
- Acromegaly
- CIDP and paranodopathies
- Amyloid neuropathy
- Charcot-Marie-Tooth disease, demyelinating variety (hereditary motor and sensory neuropathy type 1)
- Leprosy (Figures 11.28 and 11.34); peripheral nerves may be calcified.
- Dejerine-Sottas disease
- Sarcoidosis
- Refsum's syndrome

Inspection of the skin will clinch several of these possibilities, as described later in this chapter.

Neurofibromatosis type 1 is usually easy to diagnose through the skin lesions and axillary freckling.

Acromegaly has characteristic coarsening of the facial appearance, bitemporal hemianopia, macroglossia, large hands, and often CTS. CIDP has been detailed already.

Following are more Handles for some of the other conditions:

▶ In amyloid neuropathy there is:
  o Severe autonomic neuropathy and ageusia
  o Neuropathic pain, thickened peripheral nerves
  o Vitreous hemorrhage, lattice corneal dystrophy (Figure 11.21); this type of corneal dystrophy is particularly common in the Finnish variety with the gelsolin mutation.
  o CTS (due to local amyloid deposits)
  o Family history of sudden cardiac death from restrictive cardiomyopathy
▶ In *Charcot-Marie-Tooth disease* (HMSN-1 and 2), the typical features are:
  o Claw hands, claw feet (Figure 11.37)
  o Absent reflexes
  o Family history of the disease in someone who, in general, is able to continue working until normal retirement age.
  o Markedly slowed nerve conduction velocity in type 1 (demyelinating variety); normal or slightly slowed conduction velocities in type 2 (axonal variety)

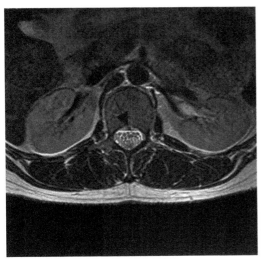 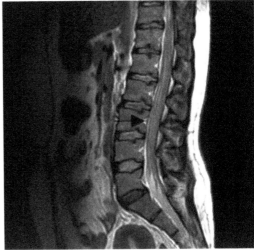

FIGURE 11.27: A 41-year-old woman with low back pain related to hypertrophic polyneuropathy. **Left**: Axial T2 weighted MRI at the level of L1. **Right**: Sagittal T2-weighted MRI (without contrast) of the cauda equina demonstrates marked nerve enlargement completely filling the spinal canal. Similar nerve root enlargement was seen throughout the cervical and thoracic spine. Reproduced with permission from Rowin (2010), Figure A.

▶ *Lepromatous neuropathy* (mainly axonal) needs consideration for someone who has lived in or visited endemic regions, such as South America or Asia. Typical features are as follows:
  ○ Painless foot ulcers (Figure 11.28)
  ○ Numb patches over cool areas of skin, for example pinnae of the ears, nose, cheeks, and upper lip, and extensor surfaces of arms and legs but sparing warmer regions of the body, including palms and soles. In theory plantar stimulation should be tickly, assuming it was tickly before disease onset!
  ○ Thickened peripheral nerves, particularly the great auricular nerve (see Figure 11.34)
▶ Patients with *Refsum's syndrome* have the following features:
  ○ Short stature
  ○ Anosmia
  ○ Retinitis pigmentosa causing poor night vision (Figure 2.2)
  ○ Ichthyosis, deafness, ataxia (Figure 11.29)
  ○ Short fourth metatarsal bones (Figure 3.11)
▶ In *sarcoid neuropathy* the patterns are diverse:
  ○ Asymmetric, non–length-dependent painful sensorimotor neuropathy
  ○ Slowly progressive distal to proximal weakness
  ○ Mononeuritis multiplex resulting in facial palsy, CTS, or sensorineural deafness
  ○ Acute generalized demyelinating motor neuropathy like GBS. It may be painful.
  ○ Look for inflamed scars or tattoos, alopecia, erythema nodosum, unidigital clubbing, lupus permio and conjunctival nodules.

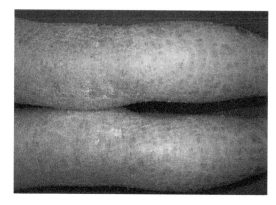

FIGURE 11.29: Refsum's disease. Marked ichthyosis is present on both lower limbs.

Nerve root hypertrophy may be detected on MRI of the spine or brachial plexus (Figure 11.27). This occurs most often in

- CIDP and paranodopathies
- Dejerine–Sottas syndrome (HMSN type III)
- Neurofibromatosis

Polyneuropathy with Tremor
You should first assess joint position sense. If this is normal, then the tremor is likely cerebellar or the essential variety. These conditions are considered in Chapter 12.

▶ Most polyneuropathies with tremor are demyelinating.

If joint position sense is impaired and there is little or no weakness, you are dealing with a sensory ataxia causing tremor, for which the main causes are:

- Anti-MAG (myelin–associated glycoprotein) polyneuropathy. Note: this disorder has the some of the slowest motor conduction velocities recordable.
- CIDP (Video 11.1, CIDP Tremor)
- Dejerine-Sottas syndrome (CMT3, HMSN III)
- Roussy-Levy syndrome. This is a variant of CMT type 1.

Tremor is found also in Kennedy syndrome (X-linked bulbospinal neuronopathy), but this is a neuronopathy.

Polyneuropathy with Skin, Hair, or Nail Lesions
Features of various diagnoses are listed next. More details follow subsequently or are provided elsewhere in this chapter.

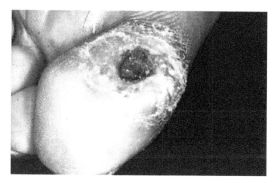

FIGURE 11.28: A perforating ulcer in leprosy (mal perforans). Similar ulcers occur in diabetic and other neuropathies in which there is severe reduction of pain sensation. Photo courtesy US Public Health Service Hospital, Carville, Louisiana.

- *Café-au-lait spots* (Figure 1.4), *cutaneous neurofibromas, axillary/inguinal freckles*: neurofibromatosis, type 1
- *Radiculopathy with target lesions*: Lyme disease (Figure 11.17)
- *Lupus pernio* (Figure 11.20), *erythema nodosum* (Figure 3.22), *unidigital clubbing* (Figure 1.1), *alopecia, granulomas in old scars and tattoos*: sarcoidosis (Figure 11.20)
- *Painless ulcers*: diabetes, leprosy (Figure 11.28), congenital indifference to pain, syringomyelia, HSAN
- *Heliotrope rash* (Figure 11.30): dermatomyositis, systemic lupus
- *Alopecia*: hypothyroidism, systemic lupus, amyloidosis, sarcoidosis, arsenic and thallium poisoning (Figure 11.33)
- *Angiokeratomas, anhidrosis*: Fabry's disease (Figure 9.26)
- *Thickened palms and soles, squamous cell carcinoma, Mees lines*: arsenic poisoning (Figure 11.23)
- *Ichthyosis*: Refsum's disease (Figure 11.29)
- *Hypomelanotic papules, painless ulcers, nodules, thickened dermis*: leprosy (see Figures 1.25, 11.28, and 11.34)
- *Hyperpigmentation, hirsutism, glomeruloid hemangiomas*: POEMS (Figure 11.31)
- *Pigmented rash, painless ulcers, loss of fungiform papillae on tongue*: HSAN (Figure 11.32)
- *Child with kinky hair*: Menkes's syndrome (Figure 11.35)

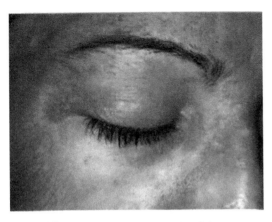

FIGURE 11.30: The heliotrope rash of dermatomyositis. Reproduced with permission from Plate 8 in the chapter Autoimmune Connective Tissue Diseases. Oxford University Press. DOI:10.1093/med/9780199229994.003.0008.

Here are some further possibilities that might permit a snap diagnosis:

- Polyneuropathy with swollen ankles and hirsutism is likely POEMS syndrome. Other striking skin changes are:
  - Generalized hyperpigmentation
  - Hirsutism particularly in the lower limbs
  - Glomeruloid hemangioma. These are pathognomonic lesions present on the trunk. They are small, dark red papules with a lighter red halo (Figure 11.31).

The polyneuropathy is length-dependent, and therefore distal and symmetric with a mixture of axonal and myelin damage.
Other features of POEMS are as follows:

- Paraprotein (IgG or IgA lambda)
- Sclerotic bone lesions (Figure 11.31)
- Raised blood vascular endothelial growth factor 1 (VEGF-1)
- Papilledema
- Autonomic features

Note that in vasculitic polyneuropathy (e.g., lupus) there is often hair *loss*, particularly from the scalp, a point that may help distinguish the two.

- Painful polyneuropathy with pigmented rash, painless ulcers, dysautonomia, skeletal abnormalities, and loss of fungiform papillae is HASN type IID (Figure 11.32)
- Polyneuropathy with alopecia (Figure 11.33)
  - Chemotherapy, for example, vincristine, carboplatin, taxanes
  - Lyme disease with tick in hair (Figure 11.17)
  - Arsenic, mercury, and thallium poisoning
  - Autoimmune disorders: hypothyroidism, systemic or discoid lupus erythematosus
  - Amyloidosis
  - Sarcoidosis
  - Leprosy
- Polyneuropathy with painless skin ulcers can occur in any severe small-fiber neuropathy, but the main ones are as follows:
  - Diabetes
  - Leprosy (Figure 11.28)
  - Congenital indifference to pain syndrome
  - Hereditary sensory neuropathy

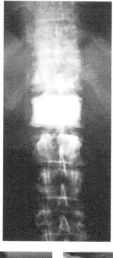
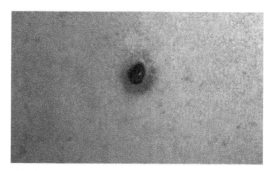
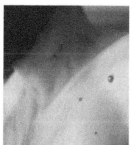
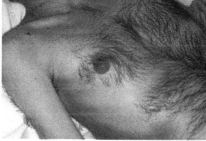
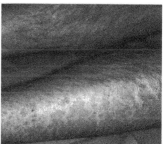

FIGURE 11.31: POEMS syndrome. **Top left:** Osteosclerotic myeloma affecting a lumbar vertebral body. **Top right:** Close-up of a glomeruloid hemangioma. Note the central dark area with a pink halo. **Lower left:** Glomeruloid hemangioma on chest and shoulder skin. **Lower center and lower right:** Hirsutism and scaling in the legs. Reproduced courtesy of the collection of the Department of Internal Medicine, Lille Nord-de-France University, France.

▶ Features of leprosy (Figure 11.34 and 11.28):
  ○ Iris pearls
  ○ Hypopigmented macules (Figure 1.25)
  ○ Thickened or calcified peripheral nerves
  ○ Alopecia
▶ A child with kinky hair and polyneuropathy has Menkes's syndrome (Figure 11.35). This is a recessive, infantile copper transport disorder. Giant axonal neuropathy is the main alternative diagnosis.

Polyneuropathy with Deafness

Deafness may occur acutely in the GBS and Fabry's disease, but, apart from these two, most polyneuropathies with deafness are chronic and inherited. There are multiple, mostly extremely rare associations, as follows:

- Refsum's disease. This is the most widely recognized cause.
- Charcot-Marie-Tooth disease, type 2
- Hereditary motor and sensory neuropathy Lom type (HMSNL or CMT4D). This affects Gypsies, with severe demyelinating polyneuropathy and deafness. Onset is in childhood, and most cases are reported from Bulgaria.
- Hereditary sensory neuropathy, type I (HSN-1)
- POLG mutations
- PHARC (demyelinating polyneuropathy, hearing loss, ataxia, retinitis pigmentosa and cataract)
- Hereditary autonomic neuropathy with sensory neuropathy, dementia, and deafness due to *DNMT1* mutations
- CMTX5 (Rosenberg-Chutorian syndrome). This is a variant of the X-linked form of

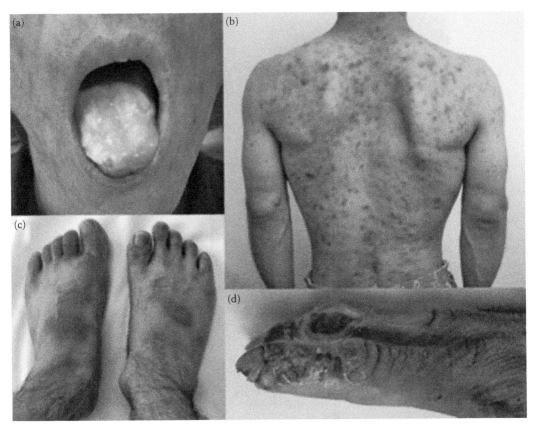

FIGURE 11.32: Hereditary sensory and autonomic neuropathy type IID caused by *SCN9A* mutation. (**A**) Reduced number of fungiform papilla on the tongue. (**B**) Patient's back showing a scattered rash, pigmentation, and short humerus. (**C**) Short right hallux. (**D**) Multiple painless ulcers and deformed joints in the fingers. Reproduced with permission from Yuan et al. (2013), Figure 1.

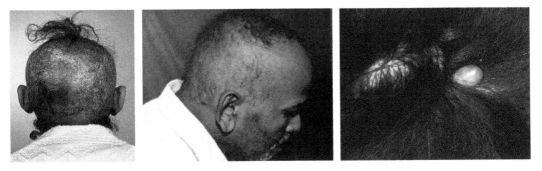

FIGURE 11.33: Alopecia. **Left**: Severe scarring alopecia secondary to systemic lupus erythematosus. **Center**: Secondary to thallium poisoning. **Right**: Mild alopecia secondary to tick infestation. Note the engorged tick on the scalp. Do not forget Lyme disease! Left image reproduced from Figure 19.11.2.4 in the chapter Systemic Lupus Erythematosus and Related Disorders, by A Rahman and DA Isenberg. Oxford University Press. DOI:10.1093/med/9780199204854.003.191102_update_003. Center image reproduced from Misra et al. (2003), Figure 3. Right image reproduced from Figure 14.9 in the chapter Hair and Scalp Disorders. Oxford University Press. DOI: 10.1093/med/9780199208388.003.14.

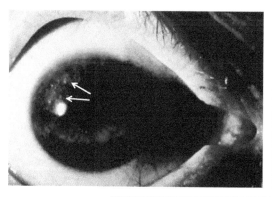

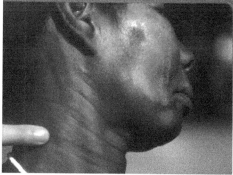

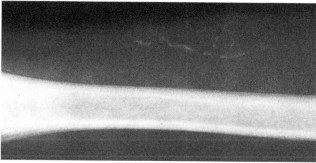

FIGURE 11.34: **Top left**: Iris pearls of leprosy. Note the small white dots (white arrows) between 9 and 12 o'clock over the iris. These are pathognomonic of lepromatous leprosy. **Top right**: Thickened greater auricular nerve (fingertip). **Bottom**: X-ray of the thigh shows calcification of a peripheral nerve, which is also characteristic of leprosy. Top left and bottom images Courtesy US Public Health Service Hospital, Carville, Louisiana. Top right image Courtesy Jose Biller, Chicago.

Charcot-Marie-Tooth disease. It is associated with optic atrophy.
- DOOR syndrome: deafness, onychodystrophy (absent nails), osteodystrophy, and mental retardation
- HHH syndrome (hyperornithinemia, hyperammonemia, and homocitrullinuria)
- SCA4 (spinocerebellar atrophy type 4). Sensory axonal neuropathy
- Sarcoidosis has a predilection for the auditory nerve and occasionally causes a polyneuropathy.

Polyneuropathy with Ophthalmoplegia
▶ Miller Fisher syndrome: acute bilateral ophthalmoplegia and ataxia; see Video 11.2, MFS (courtesy, Bryan Ho)
The Miller Fisher syndrome (one person), is a variant of the GBS that presents with ophthalmoplegia, ataxia, and areflexia, without limb muscle weakness. The ataxia is typically sensory rather than cerebellar. A key finding is preservation (usually) of pupillary reflexes, which

helps differentiation from botulism, in which the pupils are paralyzed. The confirmatory blood test is the ganglioside antibody, GQ1b.
▶ SANDO (sensory ataxic neuropathy, dysarthria, and ophthalmoplegia)

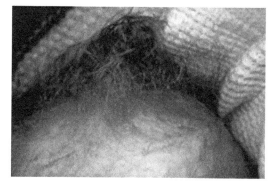

FIGURE 11.35: Menkes's syndrome in a baby. Note the sparse, wiry, refractile hairs, some with silvery sheen. Reproduced from Figure 3.24 in the chapter Disorders of Epidermal Appendages, by V Sybert. Oxford University Press. DOI:10.1093/med/9780195397666.003.0003.

This is an autosomal recessive condition caused by mutations in the mitochondrial gene, *POLG*. Onset is gradual and presentation may be in middle age or older.

▶ CANOMAD (chronic ataxic neuropathy, ophthalmoplegia, IgM paraprotein, cold agglutinins, and disialosyl antibodies). This is a rare, chronic immune-mediated demyelinating polyneuropathy.

Polyneuropathy and Anosmia

The main causes are:

* Refsum's disease
* Leprosy
* Wegener's granulomatosis

There are usually several other clues for *Refsum's disease*, such as short stature, retinitis pigmentosa, ichthyosis, deafness, and ataxia, so in theory the diagnosis should never be overlooked, but in practice it is. If you have a patient with retinitis pigmentosa (Figure 11.36), make sure you test the sense of smell. If this is impaired, then the diagnosis is Refsum's disease (Gibberd et al. 2004).

In *leprosy*, the distribution of sensory loss is unique, involving cooler areas like the upper face, dorsum of the hands and feet, posterior elbow. The nasal passages are also cooler than body temperature, thus encouraging bacterial growth, anosmia, and collapse of the nasal septum (Figure 1.25). The palms and soles are spared, and painless ulcers are characteristic. Once more it should be an easy diagnosis, but in practice it can be missed.

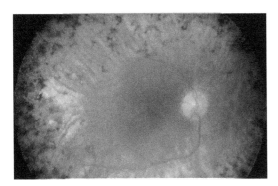

FIGURE 11.36: Retinitis pigmentosa in Refsum's disease. Reproduced with permission from *Training in Ophthalmology*, Venki Sundaram, Allon Barsam, Amar Alwitry, and Peng Khaw, eds. Figure 4.44 in the chapter by B Palil and P Pun. Oxford University Press. DOI:10.1093/med/9780199237593.003.0004.

Occasionally, in *Wegener's granulomatosis*, there is a sensory polyneuropathy, associated with crusting and blockage of the nasal passages leading to anosmia. There may be a saddle nose deformity and perforation of the nasal septum (Figure 1.6). Apart from the standard blood tests (cANCA, etc.), nasal mucosa biopsy may be diagnostic.

There are probably several other causes of polyneuropathy with anosmia, but until smell testing is adopted more widely, we shall never know.

Chronic Polyneuropathy and Ageusia

This combination suggests:

* Amyloid
* Diabetes
* Lepromatous neuropathy

In primary amyloid, ageusia may be a presenting symptom. If the polyneuropathy is acute and there is dysgeusia, your first diagnosis is GBS. The facial nerve will be affected at the same time.

Polyneuropathy with Cataract

* Diabetes
* PHARC syndrome
* CTX
* Refsum's disease
* Hypertrophic neuropathy (Dejerine-Sottas disease, HMSN type III)

Miscellaneous Handles

▶ Claw hands, claw feet (pes cavus) with depressed leg reflexes is usually Charcot-Marie-Tooth disease (CMT type 1 or 2); with brisk leg reflexes it is syringomyelia (Figure 11.37). Thus, in CMT, the pathology is predominantly in the peripheral nerves; hence, all reflexes will be depressed. In syringomyelia, the pathology is in the central gray matter of the spinal cord. It damages the anterior horn cells in the cervical cord, producing lower motor neuron signs predominantly in the arms. The syrinx in the lateral columns affects the corticospinal tracts, with upper motor neuron signs in the lower limbs (Figure 10.2). To repeat a related Handle:

▶ If you are considering syringomyelia and the arm reflexes are not depressed, then the diagnosis is probably wrong!

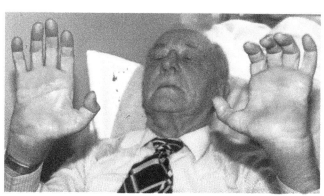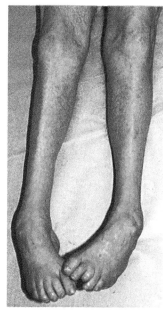

FIGURE 11.37: Charcot-Marie-Tooth disease (hereditary motor and sensory neuropathy, HMSN type 2). Note the claw hands and claw feet (pes cavus) although not clear in photo. There is severe wasting in the hands and legs. This picture could be seen in many inherited peripheral neuropathies, but HMSN types 1 or 2 are the most common. Similar changes are seen in syringomyelia, but here the lower limb reflexes are brisk and there is little wasting, whereas in HMSN and most peripheral neuropathies the reflexes would be reduced and there should be wasting. Therefore, testing the lower limb reflexes is a fast way of telling apart these two conditions.

▶ Obscure sensory demyelinating neuropathy in a middle-aged man is likely due to an isolated plasmocytoma.

This is a situation where you have done everything and found nothing other than a demyelinating neuropathy. Sometimes a bone scan or PET scan will give you the answer (Read & Warlow 1978).

▶ Sensory polyneuropathy in a weightlifter (Figure 11.38)

This suggests a pyridoxine-induced neuropathy from excess use of megadose vitamins.

▶ Polyneuropathy with mouth ulcers suggests Behçet's or HIV (Figure 11.39).

▶ Polyneuropathy with abdominal pains: lead, thallium, arsenic poisoning; porphyria; diabetes with gastroparesis; tyrosinemia

▶ Polyneuropathy with parotid enlargement:
   ○ Sarcoidosis
   ○ Sjögren's syndrome
   ○ Alcoholism
   ○ Diabetes

▶ Polyneuropathy with prominent autonomic features:

   ○ *Acute*: autoimmune ganglionopathy, paraneoplastic syndromes, GBS, botulism, toxic neuropathy, and porphyria
   ○ *Chronic*: diabetes, amyloid, inherited (e.g., HSAN); Fabry's disease; Sjögren's syndrome; toxic and infectious neuropathies

Note: unexplained chronic cough sometimes indicates autonomic dysfunction.

▶ Polyneuropathy in a veterinarian, slaughterhouse worker, or farmer after delivering a calf suggests brucellosis.

Other features:
   ○ Prominent lower motor neuron signs such as quadriceps fasciculation
   ○ Sacroiliitis
   ○ Deafness
   ○ Lymphocytic meningitis

▶ The patient who bobs up and down when standing but walks normally has plantar flexion weakness (Reilly's sign; Figure 11.40).

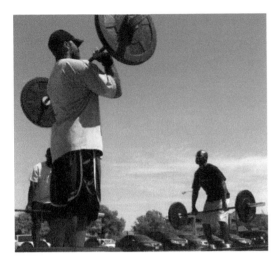

FIGURE 11.38: Weightlifters and other health fitness addicts who consume high doses of pyridoxine may suffer a predominantly sensory polyneuropathy. Reproduced from Wikipedia, under Creative Commons license.

In most polyneuropathies, standing is normal but walking is difficult because weak ankle dorsiflexion makes it necessary to raise the feet to clear the ground. In advanced Charcot-Marie-Tooth disease, for example, the plantar flexors eventually weaken and patients bob up and down at the knee when trying to stand because of intermittent fatiguing of the calf muscles (Rossor et al. 2012). In *early* polyneuropathies, if there is knee bobbing, you should think of *distal hereditary motor neuropathy type V* (really an anterior horn cell disorder) or *dysferlin myopathy*. This phenomenon has to be distinguished from asterixis

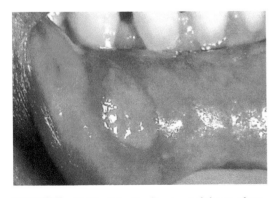

FIGURE 11.39: Behçet's disease. Aphthous ulceration of the oral mucosa in Behçet's disease. Reproduced from Figure 5.31 in the chapter Medical Ophthalmology, by E Hughes and M Stanford. Oxford University Press. DOI:10.1093/med/9780199237593.003.0005.

(negative myoclonus) that involves the knee flexors, as in posthypoxic myoclonus. The knee movement of orthostatic tremor is somewhat similar, but there is a rapid quadriceps tremor (typically around 16 Hz).

▶ Heroin addict who presents with a stiff jaw and neck

This is likely to be tetanus resulting from use of contaminated needles or "skin popping" because the person has run out of veins. There may be difficulty opening the mouth because of trismus.

Perform the *spatula test*, which may be diagnostic: you do a gag reflex in the usual way and instead of the expected gagging response, in those with tetanus the spatula is bitten because of trismus.

▶ History of night sweats usually indicates infection, especially TB or vasculitic disorder.

▶ Bouts of pyrexia without sweating

This suggests an autonomic neuropathy in which the innervation to sweat glands is at fault. Almost any autonomic neuropathy may be associated with this history. In young adults, consider congenital indifference to pain with anhidrosis: the CIPA syndrome.

▶ Polyneuropathy with raised eosinophil count

There are three main causes:

o Churg-Strauss syndrome

o Lymphoma

o Hypereosinophilic syndrome

▶ Polyneuropathy in someone with worn metallic hip replacement

This could be toxicity from cobalt-chromium alloy poisoning where the prosthesis has degenerated. The neuropathy is painful and mainly axonal.

▶ Acquired polyneuropathy with extremely slow but recordable distal motor latencies strongly suggests anti-MAG polyneuropathy. Tremor is usually present.

▶ Patient with intermittent distal tingling

This usually results from hyperventilation. The clues are that symptoms fluctuate and the tingling affects the central face. In an acute episode, say, a panic attack, *the hands are tightly clenched*, a feature not typical of metabolic alkalosis. There may be a positive Chvostek sign (as in hypocalcemia) and relief by breathing into a paper bag. Be alert to the

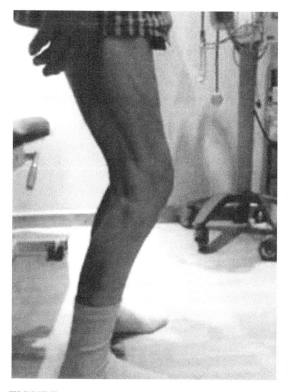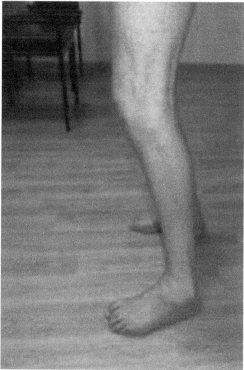

FIGURE 11.40: Shown here is the flexed knee posture characteristic of the knee bob sign (Reilly's sign) as seen in Charcot-Marie-Tooth patients with ankle plantar flexion weakness. Reproduced with permission from Rossor, Murphy, and Reilly (2012), Figure 1.

patient with dual pathology—someone who has physical disease (e.g., MS) *and* anxiety.

▶ Central facial numbness

If this is intermittent, the cause is likely anxiety/hyperventilation. The tingling sensation mainly involves the lips, sometimes the tongue and nose. Strangely, it can be asymmetric, and the extremities are not affected, at least according to patient reports. Rare physically based causes of intermittent central facial numbness include:

    ○ Basilar ischemia

    ○ Metabolic disorder such as hypoglycemia and hypocalcemia

    ○ Lambert-Eaton myasthenic syndrome

If the numb facial feelings are *continuous*, then think of the following:

    ○ Trigeminal neuropathy, such as Sjögren's syndrome or sarcoidosis

    ○ Tabes dorsalis

    ○ MS

    ○ Short fiber neuropathies

    ○ FOSMN (focal-onset sensorimotor neuronopathy); see Chapter 2

    ○ Ciguatera poisoning

    ○ Lambert-Eaton myasthenic syndrome

Remember that in syringobulbia the face is numb, but it is the peripheral not the central zones that are affected.

SUMMARY

Mononeuropathy

Median Nerve

The patient with a hand that tingles, especially at night and relieved by a downward flick likely has CTS. Sensory symptoms on raising the affected arm. Tinel, Hawkes, Phalen, and hand flick signs. Subtle weakness of opposition. Pointing index finger sign.

If the palm is numb, then isolated CTS is not the right answer. If there is isolated weakness and wasting of APB *without* sensory loss, then the diagnosis is a lesion of the recurrent motor branch of the median nerve. Distinguish from hypoplasia of the thenar eminence. The patient who can squeeze a clothes pin (peg) but cannot pick up a needle or is unable to make the shape of a letter O has anterior interosseous palsy.

Ulnar Nerve

Look for clawing of fourth and fifth fingers, Wartenberg's sign, and Froment's sign. Check mobility of elbow joint and carrying angle. In elbow groove: check ulnar nerve for tenderness, Tinel's sign, and prolapse of nerve.

Sensory loss should split the ring finger. Ulnar sensory loss in the hand should not extend into the forearm. Elbow lesion: sensory impairment affects the dorsum of the hand medially. Weakness of the distal phalanx of the fourth and fifth finger. Clawing of fourth and fifth fingers: proximal lesion. Weak wasted hand with no sensory impairment: (a) motor branch lesion of ulnar nerve in Guyon's canal or palm; (b) amyotrophic lateral sclerosis; (c) radiculopathy at C8 and T1. If there is no sensory loss, then no syrinx.

Radial Nerve

Mainly weakness of finger extension rather than wrist extension and no sensory loss and a normal triceps jerk is a posterior interosseous nerve lesion. Weakness of the wrist *and* finger extensors: lesion above the elbow. Unilateral painless wrist drop with normal triceps jerk: radial nerve lesion in or below the spiral groove. Painless, gradually progressive bilateral asymmetric wrist drop without sensory loss could be lead poisoning. Check for lead colic, foot drop, lead line, and basophilic stippling. Groups at risk: painters, bored children (pica), users of Ayurvedic medicine or lead-based eye shadow. Other causes of bilateral wrist drop: Multifocal motor neuropathy with block. Atypical motor neuron disease.

Localization: In wrist drop, as a general rule: If brachioradialis is strong and triceps jerk is normal, the lesion is *below* the spiral groove and must involve PIN. If brachioradialis is weak and the triceps jerk is normal, the lesion is likely *in* the spiral groove. If brachioradialis is weak and the triceps jerk is impaired, the lesion is *above* the spiral groove and probably in nerve roots C7 and C8 or the brachial plexus. An alcoholic with wrist drop likely has Saturday night palsy. Newly married couple: Honeymooner's palsy

Lower Limbs

Patient who wakes from deep sleep unable to stand due to bilateral thigh weakness: dangling legs syndrome due to bilateral femoral neuropathy. Foot drop after hip surgery: sciatic nerve trauma. Unilateral hip flexor weakness.

Hip adduction and ankle dorsiflexion weak: L2, 3, 4 root lesion. Hip adduction and ankle dorsiflexion strong: femoral nerve lesion.

Asymmetric pain, unilateral weakness and wasting of the thigh muscles suggest proximal diabetic neuropathy (diabetic amyotrophy). Wallet palsy: sciatic and posterior (femoral) cutaneous nerve lesion. A misplaced injection into the buttock may cause a sciatic palsy.

Bilateral foot drop after childbirth in squatting position is likely a bilateral lesion of the common peroneal nerve. Flaccid foot drop and normal ankle jerk: common peroneal nerve palsy. Flaccid foot drop and depressed ankle jerk: proximal lesion. Unilateral painless foot drop could be a rare presentation of ALS.

Acute groin pain in a patient receiving anticoagulants is likely a femoral neuropathy from bleeding into the iliacus muscle. Occasionally, there is no pain, and the leg weakness results in misdiagnosis of stroke. Chronic inner groin pain in an athlete is likely obturator nerve entrapment. Hip adduction should be weak.

Mononeuritis Multiplex

Causes: diabetes; immune based: rheumatoid arthritis; polyarteritis, lupus; Wegener's granulomatosis; Churg Strauss syndrome. Sarcoidosis; neoplastic and paraneoplastic disorder; leprosy; amyloid; neurofibromatosis. If there is a history of liver problems, think of hepatitis C infection. Recurrent pressure palsies suggest familial liability to pressure palsy.

Isolated numb patches. Outer thigh: meralgia paresthetica. Outer thumb: cheiralgia paresthetica. Interscapular: notalgia paresthetica. Medial malleolus: saphenous neuropathy. Medial sole: tarsal tunnel syndrome. Cheek: infraorbital nerve. Chin: mental nerve. Unilateral occipital skin: occipital nerve. Palm or sole: leprosy. Outer leg: lateral sural cutaneous nerve

Multiple numb patches: Wartenberg's migratory sensory neuropathy.

Patchy sensory signs affecting proximal and distal skin—scalp, thorax, abdomen and buttocks—is a sensory ganglionopathy. Causes: autoimmune disease: Sjögren's syndrome; scleroderma; lupus. Paraproteinemia; HTLV-1 infection, Fabry's disease. HIV; pyridoxine excess, neoplasia, and paraneoplastic disorder; tabes dorsalis.

Radiculopathy
Upper Limbs

Depressed biceps jerk with sensory loss over the thumb suggests a C6 lesion. Biceps and radial wrist extension should be weak. An inverted supinator jerk with hyperactive reflexes below this level is due to a spinal cord lesion at C6. Depressed triceps jerk and impaired feeling of the little finger and inner forearm suggests a C8 lesion. Triceps, forearm extensors, and the intrinsic hand muscles should be weak.

Most cervical root pain radiates: C6 root pain spreads down the radial border of the arm into the thumb; C7 root pain radiates to the second and third digits and medial to the scapula; C8 root pain spreads down the inner aspect of the arm into the fourth and fifth fingers. In cervical radiculopathy the affected nerve is painful and swollen.

An acutely painful shoulder with weakness and wasting, typically deltoid or serratus anterior 2–3 days later, is ABN. Patch of numbness over the outer aspect of deltoid is characteristic. Breathlessness suggests phrenic nerve involvement. Autosomal dominant form of recurrent ABN. Bilateral, painful ABN and phrenic nerve involvement may be secondary to hepatitis E infection

Major causes of acquired noncompressive radiculopathies: Infectious and post-infectious: GBS; Lyme disease; neurobrucellosis; Elsberg syndrome. Immune-related: diabetic thoraco-abdominal radiculopathy and diabetic amyotrophy. Infiltrative disease of meninges such as neurolymphomatosis; metastatic lesions; syphilis. Cervical or lumbosacral plexopathy

Handles for Noncompressive Radiculopathy
Muscle weakness is asymmetrical often more proximal than distal. Sensory loss is painful and patchy affecting proximal and distal skin. Absent knee jerk with normal ankle jerk

Preserved sensory action potentials in territory of weak, denervated muscles. Loss of F and H reflexes EMG evidence of denervation in proximal muscles e.g. paraspinal, glutei or rhomboids, affected last in axonal polyneuropathy. Radiculopathy with target skin lesions is Lyme disease. Radiculopathy with perineal vesicles and urinary retention is Elsberg syndrome

Weak, pain-free swollen arm following radiotherapy for breast cancer given years previously is likely RBP. Linked to high radiation doses, causes little or no pain, has myokymia-like twitches in upper limb and no Horner's syndrome, and preferentially involves the upper trunk (C5, C6). Prominent pain, Horner's syndrome, and preferential involvement of the lower trunk (C8, T1) favor metastases.

Sharp, burning pain in the shoulder radiating to the arm and hand following a blow to the head, neck,

or shoulder in a soccer, rugby, or football player is a "stinger" or "burner." Depressed shoulders in a woman with weakness, numbness, and pain in one or both upper limbs indicate the droopy shoulder syndrome.

Lower Limbs
Handles to Help Localize a Lesion
Depressed knee jerk with sensory loss over the inner leg and foot suggests a lesion of the femoral nerve or the L4 nerve root. Hip adduction and ankle dorsiflexion are normal in a femoral nerve lesion. Depressed ankle jerk with sensory loss over the little toe is a lesion of S1. Severe sciatic pain with a normal MRI scan lumbar spine is likely a lumbosacral plexopathy. Causes: viral/autoimmune plexopathy, intravenous heroin addiction, diabetes, Elsberg syndrome, possibly dural fistula. Facet joint pain may simulate sciatica

Painful neurological relapse occurring months or years after pelvic radiation for malignancy is more likely tumor recurrence than radiation plexopathy.

Acute-onset generalized, severe weakness in a previously healthy child or adult with little or no sensory loss. Causes: neuropathies; psychiatric disease; poliomyelitis; neuromuscular transmission disorder; acute myopathy; demyelination: periodic paralysis; tick paralysis; organophosphate poisoning.

Polyneuropathy
Pattern of Onset
Rapidly evolving polyneuropathy is inflammatory, immune, toxic, or vascular. Distal and symmetric polyneuropathy is usually metabolic, toxic, or inherited. Immune- or infection-related neuropathies tend to be asymmetric.

Patient with rapid-onset proximal weakness and raised CK is sometimes mistaken for polymyositis or hypokalemic periodic paralysis. The correct answer is usually GBS. Bladder involvement virtually excludes GBS

Polyneuropathy with arms affected before legs. Lymphoma; GBS or multifocal demyelinating motor neuropathy; diabetic radiculopathy or insulinoma; hereditary; copper deficiency; lead poisoning; vasculitis; paraneoplastic sensory neuropathy; amyloid; porphyria

Painful Polyneuropathy
Thiamine deficiency; diabetes; HIV; Sjögren's disease. Rare causes: Fabry's syndrome; sarcoidosis;

vasculitis; amyloid; leprosy; PEPD; arsenic or thallium poisoning.

Further clues: Painful tingling extremities associated with prolonged vomiting (especially hyperemesis gravidarum), alcoholism, or malnutrition is likely thiamine deficiency. Painful or burning distal predominantly sensory polyneuropathy is characteristic of HIV infection.

A woman with dry eyes, dry mouth, and burning feet, especially at night, likely has Sjögren's syndrome. If the pain is so severe that the patient will not permit an examination (allodynia), think of Fabry's disease. This may present in middle-aged women, with a relatively mild neuropathy with painful numb patches.

Frost-bitten face (lupus pernio) or granulomas developing in scars or tattoos: sarcoidosis. Restrictive cardiomyopathy and polyneuropathy: sarcoidosis; amyloidosis; Churg-Strauss syndrome; Fabry's disease; hemochromatosis if there is diabetes. Polyneuropathy, asthma, and marked eosinophilia: Churg-Strauss syndrome

Painful polyneuropathy with previous vitreous hemorrhage or lattice corneal dystrophy suggests amyloidosis. Other clues: Severe autonomic neuropathy with marked postural hypotension. Nerve enlargement. Loss of taste. CTS. Family history of sudden death.

Paroxysms of pain in the eye, jaw, or rectum with autonomic features is PEPD. Bouts of red, burning legs or palms lessened by cooling or elevation is erythromelalgia. Shooting leg pain at right angles to the skin along with a high-stepping, stamping gait suggests tabes dorsalis. In simple bilateral foot drop the foot is lifted high to clear the ground, but it is usually not stamped down if joint sense is preserved.

Ayurvedic medicines prescribed for diabetes or psoriasis may contain arsenic.

Neuropathic itching. Causes: small fiber length-dependent polyneuropathy, particularly diabetic. Ehlers-Danlos syndrome. Postherpetic, particularly facial. Multiple endocrine neoplasia type 2A. Ganglionopathy: Sjögren's syndrome, cancer (especially small cell lung), MS.

Axonal or Demyelinating Polyneuropathy?

Weakness with little wasting suggests a demyelinating neuropathy. Wasting associated with weakness in the early stages (especially extensor digitorum brevis) favors axonal neuropathy.

Axonal neuropathies are more common and more likely to be painful, with greater weakness and wasting. Demyelinating neuropathies are rarer and less likely to be painful and display less weakness and wasting. Proximal leg weakness with absent reflexes is likely a demyelinating radiculo-neuropathy. Bladder involvement is rare in demyelinating neuropathy and radiculopathy but common in axonal neuropathy

Main Causes of Chronic Demyelinating Polyneuropathy

Genetic: Charcot-Marie-Tooth disease: types 1, 3 (Dejerine Sottas), 4; and CMTX. Hereditary liability to pressure palsy; ARSACS and PHARC. Refsum's disease; CTX. Leukodystrophies: metachromatic, adrenomyeloneuropathy, Cockayne syndrome; Krabbe's disease, Pelizaeus-Merzbacher disease

Acquired: CIDP; paraproteinemic; multifocal motor neuropathy with conduction block; drugs, for example, amiodarone, perhexiline, bortezomib. Infection: for example, diphtheria

Nerve Conduction Tests and EMG

Axonal neuropathies: Less than 30% slowing of conduction velocity, marked reduction of CMAP amplitude. *Demyelinating neuropathies*: conduction velocity slowed >30% but CMAP amplitude is relatively preserved. Conduction block.

In axonal variety, the EMG shows denervation. In demyelinating neuropathies (and radiculopathies), the spinal fluid protein is usually raised, whereas in the axonal varieties it is not. In radiculopathy, the EMG will show: Preserved sensory action potentials in territory of weak, denervated muscles. Loss of F and H reflexes. Evidence of denervation in proximal muscles e.g. paraspinal, glutei or rhomboids, which are affected last in axonal polyneuropathy

Length-Dependent (Long Fiber) or Non–Length-Dependent (Short Fiber) Neuropathy?
Length-Dependent Neuropathy

First symptoms are in the toes, then feet. When the leg is numb the finger tips are affected next. Symmetric sensory impairment to the knee and wrist resulting in glove and stocking sensory loss. Sensory loss on the anterior trunk, may be confused with a spinal cord sensory level but sensation over the back is preserved. Many cases of length-dependent neuropathy are due to small (fine) fiber neuropathy characterized by preserved reflexes; burning pain, worse at night; and raised thermal threshold.

Main Causes of Long-Fiber Symmetric Glove and Stocking Sensory-Motor Polyneuropathies. Diabetes. Alcohol-nutritional neuropathy. Vitamin deficiencies: B_{12}, thiamine, B_6 (deficiency or overuse). Drug-induced. Hereditary. POEMS syndrome. Exposure to toxins such as ciguatera, ethylene oxide, or venom

Non–Length-Dependent (Short-Fiber) Neuropathy

Main causes: diabetes. immune-related. HTLV-1, HIV, and hepatitis C infection; Fabry's disease; neoplasia and paraneoplastic disorder; porphyria; acrylamide intoxication; Tangier disease. Tangier disease: relapsing polyneuropathy with orange-yellow tonsils

Polyneuropathy with preserved ankle reflexes suggests small fiber axonal neuropathy (e.g., porphyria, or thalidomide); mild large fiber neuropathy; additional CNS involvement.

Pure motor polyneuropathy. Causes: Diabetes. GBS and CIDP. Multifocal motor neuropathy. Genetic. Myotonic dystrophy (type 1) can simulate a pure motor polyneuropathy, so check for myotonia. Think of milder forms of ALS

Pure sensory polyneuropathy. Causes: Diabetes. CIDP. Sjögren's disease. Medication. Paraneoplastic. HSAN. CANVAS

Inherited or Acquired?

Peripheral neuropathy and sensory impairment: (a) with positive phenomena such as tingling or pain is acquired, (b) without positive phenomena is likely inherited. Pes Cavus favors inherited neuropathy. There is usually hammer-toe deformity. A man with Charcot-Marie-Tooth disease look-alike but only passed on to his daughters has the Connexin 32 mutation (CMTX).

Thickened Peripheral Nerves

Causes: neurofibromatosis type 1 (NF1); acromegaly, CIDP; amyloid neuropathy; Charcot-Marie-Tooth disease—demyelinating variety, especially Dejerine-Sottas disease; leprosy sarcoidosis and Refsum's syndrome. MRI of spine may be diagnostic. *Amyloid neuropathy*: severe autonomic neuropathy and ageusia; neuropathic pain, thickened peripheral nerves; vitreous hemorrhage, lattice corneal dystrophy; CTS; family history of sudden cardiac death from restrictive cardiomyopathy.

Charcot-Marie-Tooth disease (HMSN-1 and -2): claw hands, claw feet; absent reflexes; family history of the disease in someone who is able to continue working until normal retirement age. Markedly slowed nerve conduction velocity in type 1 (demyelinating variety). Normal or slightly slowed conduction velocities in type 2 (axonal variety). *Lepromatous neuropathy*: painless foot ulcers; numb patches over cool areas of skin-sparing warmer regions, especially palms and soles; thickened peripheral nerves. *Refsum's syndrome*: short stature; anosmia; retinitis pigmentosa; ichthyosis; deafness, ataxia; short fourth metatarsal bones. *Sarcoid neuropathy*: asymmetric; non-length-dependent painful sensorimotor neuropathy; slowly progressive distal to proximal weakness; mononeuritis multiplex resulting in facial palsy, CTS, or sensorineural deafness; acute generalized demyelinating motor neuropathy

Nerve root hypertrophy may be detected on MRI. Causes include CIDP, Dejerine-Sottas syndrome, and neurofibromatosis.

Polyneuropathy with Tremor

Usually demyelinating. Anti-MAG polyneuropathy. CIDP. Paranodopathy. Dejerine-Sottas syndrome (CMT3; HMSN III). Roussy-Levy syndrome. This is a variant of CMT type 1.

Polyneuropathy with Skin, Hair, or Nail Lesions

Café-au-lait spots, cutaneous neurofibromas, axillary freckles: neurofibromatosis, type 1. Radiculopathy with target lesions: Lyme disease.

Lupus pernio, erythema nodosum, unidigital clubbing, alopecia, granulomas in old scars and tattoos: sarcoidosis.

Painless ulcers: diabetes, leprosy, congenital indifference to pain, syringomyelia, HSAN

Heliotrope rash: systemic lupus, dermatomyositis.

Alopecia: hypothyroidism, systemic lupus, amyloidosis, chemotherapy, arsenic and thallium poisoning.

Angiokeratomas, anhidrosis: Fabry's disease.

Thickened palms and soles with squamous cell carcinomata and Mees lines: arsenic poisoning. Ichthyosis: Refsum's disease.

Hypomelanotic papules, painless ulcers, nodules, thickened dermis: leprosy. Hyperpigmentation, hirsutism, glomeruloid hemangiomas: POEMS.

Pigmented rash, painless ulcers, loss of fungiform papillae on tongue: HSAN.

Polyneuropathy with swollen ankles and hirsutism is likely POEMS syndrome.

Painful polyneuropathy with pigmented rash, painless ulcers, dysautonomia, skeletal abnormalities and loss of fungiform papillae is HSAN IID.

Polyneuropathy with painless skin ulcers: any severe small fiber neuropathy.

Features of leprosy: Iris pearls; hypopigmented macules; thickened or calcified peripheral nerves; alopecia.

Child with kinky hair: Menkes's syndrome

Polyneuropathy with Deafness

Occurs acutely in the GBS.

Refsum's disease. Charcot-Marie-Tooth disease, type 2. Hereditary motor and sensory neuropathy Lom type (Gypsy with severe demyelinating polyneuropathy and deafness). HSN-1, *POLG* mutations. Charcot-Marie-Tooth disease (type 2 and X-linked varieties). PHARC. Hereditary autonomic neuropathy with sensory neuropathy, dementia, and deafness due to *DNMT1* mutations. CMTX5 (Rosenberg-Chutorian syndrome). DOOR syndrome. HHH syndrome (hyperornithinemia, hyperammonemia, and homocitrullinuria). SCA4. Sarcoidosis

Polyneuropathy with Ophthalmoplegia

Acute bilateral ophthalmoplegia and ataxia. Miller-Fisher syndrome. Preserved pupillary reflexes.

Rapid-onset bilateral ophthalmoplegia with fixed dilated pupils. Botulism

SANDO

CANOMAD

Polyneuropathy and Anosmia

Refsum's disease; leprosy; Wegener's granulomatosis

Polyneuropathy and Ageusia

Chronic: amyloid; diabetes; lepromatous neuropathy. *Acute:* GBS

Polyneuropathy with Cataract

Diabetes; PHARC syndrome; CTX; Refsum's disease; hypertrophic neuropathy

Miscellaneous Handles

Claw hands, claw feet with depressed leg reflexes suggests Charcot-Marie-Tooth disease; with brisk leg reflexes is syringomyelia.

Obscure sensory demyelinating neuropathy in middle-aged man: isolated plasmocytoma. Sensory

polyneuropathy in a weightlifter: pyridoxine-induced neuropathy.

Polyneuropathy with mouth ulcers: Behçet's disease or HIV.

Polyneuropathy with abdominal pains. Lead, thallium and arsenic poisoning. Porphyria. diabetes with gastroparesis. Tyrosinemia.

Polyneuropathy with parotid enlargement: sarcoid, Sjögren's syndrome, alcoholism, diabetes.

Polyneuropathy with autonomic features: *Acute:* autoimmune ganglionopathy, paraneoplastic syndromes, GBS, botulism, toxic neuropathy and porphyria. *Chronic:* diabetes, amyloid, inherited (e.g., HSAN); Fabry's disease; Sjögren's syndrome; toxic and infectious neuropathy.

Polyneuropathy in a veterinarian, slaughterhouse worker, or farmer after delivering a calf suggests brucellosis. Also: prominent lower motor neuron signs such as quadriceps fasciculation. Sacroiliitis. Deafness. Lymphocytic meningitis

The patient who bobs up and down when standing but walks normally has plantar flexion weakness. Distal hereditary motor neuropathy type V or dysferlin myopathy.

Heroin addict with a stiff jaw and neck: tetanus. Confirm with spatula test.

History of night sweats usually indicates infection or vasculitic disorder.

Bouts of pyrexia without sweating: autonomic neuropathy.

Polyneuropathy with raised eosinophil count: Churg-Strauss syndrome; lymphoma and hypereosinophilic syndrome.

Polyneuropathy with worn metallic hip replacement: toxic neuropathy from degenerated cobalt-chromium alloy prosthesis poisoning.

Acquired polyneuropathy with extremely slow but recordable distal motor latencies: anti-MAG polyneuropathy. Tremor is usually present.

Central facial numbness with distal tingling. *Intermittent:* anxiety, basilar ischemia and metabolic disorder (hypoglycemia and hypocalcemia). *Continual:* trigeminal neuropathy; tabes dorsalis, MS; short-fiber neuropathies; FOSMN, ciguatera poisoning, Lambert-Eaton myasthenic syndrome

SUGGESTED READING

Gibberd FB, Feher MD, Sidey MC, Wierzbicki AS. Smell testing: an additional tool for identification of adult Refsum's disease. *J Neurol Neurosurg Psychiatry.* 2004;75:1334–1336.

Marques W Jr, Funayama CA, Secchin JB, et al. Coexistence of two chronic neuropathies in a young child: Charcot-Marie-Tooth disease type 1A and chronic inflammatory demyelinating polyneuropathy. *Muscle Nerve.* 2010;42:598–600.

Misra UK, Kalita J, Yadav RK, Ranjan P. Thallium poisoning: emphasis on early diagnosis and response to haemodialysis. *Postgrad Med J.* 2003;79:103–105.

Pickrell WO, Hirst C, Brunt H, Pearson OR. Peripheral neuropathy—lead astray? *Lancet.* 2013;381:1156.

Post J, Hull P. Tattoo reactions as a sign of sarcoidosis. *CMAJ.* 2012;184:432.

Read D, Warlow C. Peripheral neuropathy and solitary plasmacytoma. *J Neurol Neurosurg Psychiatry.* 1978;41:177–184.

Rossor AM, Murphy S, Reilly MM. Knee bobbing in Charcot-Marie-Tooth disease. *Pract Neurol.* 2012;12:182–183.

Rowin J. MR imaging of demyelinating hypertrophic polyneuropathy. *Neurology.* 2010;74:1155.

Steinhoff M, Schmelz M, Szabó IL, Oaklander AL. Clinical presentation, management, and pathophysiology of neuropathic itch. *Lancet Neurol.* 2018;17(8):709–720.

Swift TR, Nichols FT. The droopy shoulder syndrome. *Neurology.* 1984;34:212–215.

Yuan J, Matsuura E, Higuchi Y, et al. Hereditary sensory and autonomic neuropathy type IID caused by an *SCN9A* mutation. *Neurology.* 2013;80:1641–1649.

Chapter 12: Cerebellar Ataxia

A taxia means incoordination of voluntary movement. It has two main varieties: cerebellar and sensory. An unsteady gait may be seen when there is weakness, but the characteristics are quite different and these varieties are dealt with in other chapters. Falls may be a feature of parkinsonism or Huntington's disease, but there are other features such as bradykinesia, rigidity, or chorea that will normally allow distinction from primary cerebellar disorders.

The cerebellar variety results from any lesion in the cerebellum or its connections, which extend widely throughout the brainstem and spinal cord. Whether spinal cord lesions may cause a cerebellar ataxia ("spinal ataxia") is debatable. Remember that the cerebellum becomes active only when there is voluntary movement in progress. If the subject is completely at rest there should be no abnormalities.

The other major variety of ataxia, sensory ataxia, is due to impaired incoming signals from joint position receptors to the brain (thalamus and parietal cortex). To make a smooth voluntary movement there must be sensory feedback so that the brain knows exactly where in space are the body's limbs, eyes, tongue, and so on. In sensory ataxia, compensation by vision helps to lessen the incoordination, but when the eyes are closed, movements become clumsy. Thus, in a sensory ataxia affecting the upper limbs, the finger–nose test may be performed quite well with the eyes open, but once the eyes are closed, movements become irregular and the target (nose) is missed.

Note:

▶ *Romberg's sign is a test of joint position sense— not cerebellar function as popularly thought.*

When a patient with a cerebellar problem stands with the feet together, there is often some instability of stance. If the eyes are closed this changes little— *unless the patient is very nervous about falling.* In sensory ataxia, the stance is reasonable with the eyes open but deteriorates markedly when the eyes are shut because visual compensation has been removed. This is a positive Romberg's sign and classically it

indicates loss of joint position sense or in some cases a vestibular disorder.

Thus, in any patient with poor balance, it is essential to determine whether the ataxia is sensory or cerebellar using the approach just outlined.

◀ Be aware that some patients may have both sensory and cerebellar ataxia.

Handles related to sensory ataxia are dealt with in other chapters (see Chapter 11, Peripheral Neuropathy). The current chapter is devoted primarily to cerebellar ataxia. Note the following:

▶ If the patient has slurred speech, then you are likely dealing with a cerebellar rather than sensory ataxia. Spastic dysarthria also needs consideration.
▶ Cerebellar incoordination without nystagmus suggests a lesion of the cerebellar hemispheres.

In general, the brainstem vestibular nuclei or deep cerebellar nuclei must be involved to produce jerk nystagmus, so, in a sense, the term *cerebellar nystagmus* is a misnomer. A tumor in the cerebellar hemisphere is often associated with nystagmus, but usually that happens because of pressure effects on the deep cerebellar nuclei (flocculus, nodulus) or brainstem.

PATTERN

To analyze an ataxic patient rapidly, first determine whether the defect is unilateral or bilateral.

▶ Unilateral cerebellar ataxia is likely to be a structural lesion such as a tumor, infarct, or inflammatory or infectious process.
▶ Symmetric bilateral ataxia favors a metabolic, inherited, immunological, paraneoplastic, or infectious process. One example is leptomeningeal carcinomatosis (Figure 12.1) that is here associated with the sugar-coating sign. It is also found in meningeal infection.

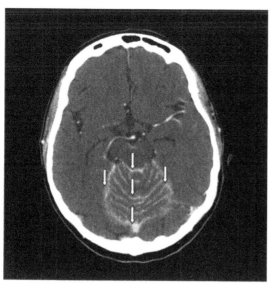 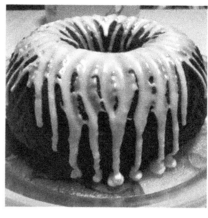

FIGURE 12.1: **Left**: Sugar-coating sign in a case of leptomeningeal carcinomatosis in a 54-year-old woman. The axial image of the gadolinium-enhanced MRI shows enhancement throughout the leptomeningeal spaces of the posterior fossa, highlighting the sugarcoating sign around the cerebellum and brain stem (white arrows). **Right**: a sugar-coated doughnut. Left image reproduced from Figure 1 with permission from: Metcalf C and Villa D (2013).

Also, it helps to know whether the time course of ataxia is (1) acute or subacute, (2) chronic or (3) episodic, or (4) rapidly progressive.

Acute or Subacute Ataxias

In general, acute-onset ataxia suggests intoxication or a vascular, an infective, or a structural cause. Following are some more specific associations with acute or subacute ataxia.

- ▶ Areflexia and ophthalmoplegia suggests Miller Fisher syndrome. See Video 11.2, Miller Fisher (courtesy Bryan Ho).
- ▶ Alcoholism or malnourishment favors thiamine deficiency.
- ▶ Glucose infusion is contraindicated as it increases the metabolic demand for thiamine.
- ◀ In a patient treated for epilepsy, ataxia is likely anticonvulsant toxicity (Figure 12.2).
- ▶ Intoxication or medication:
  - ○ Alcohol
  - ○ Lithium
  - ○ Amiodarone
  - ○ Chemotherapy (cyclosporin, tacrolimus, methotrexate)
  - ○ Metronidazole
  - ○ Recreational drugs, for example, organic solvents; see Figure 12.3 and Video 12.1, Toluene Toxicity (courtesy Shantanu Shubham)
  - ○ Serotonin syndrome
- ▶ Rigidity and myoclonic jerks suggests PERM (progressive encephalomyelitis with rigidity and myoclonus).
- ▶ Ataxia in a woman with type 1 diabetes is likely an autoimmune cerebellar ataxia.

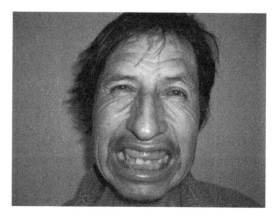

FIGURE 12.2: Massive gingival hypertrophy due to phenytoin use. Photo courtesy Ildefonso Rodriguez, MD.

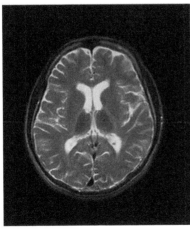 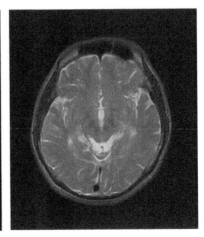

FIGURE 12.3: MRI T2 sagittal brain scan of a patient with toluene toxicity. **Left**: hypointensity in the thalamic nuclei and mild cerebral atrophy. **Right**: Hypo-intensity of the red nuclei and substantia nigra. In more advanced cases there are white matter lesions in the centrum semiovale and hypo-intensities in the putamen and caudate. Scans provided courtesy of Dr Chee Kok Yoon, Radiopaedia.org, rID: 17082.

▶ Childhood- or young adult–onset limb ataxia, worsening over 1–2 days, with fine horizontal head tremor, suggests viral cerebellitis often due to Coxsackie, varicella, Mycoplasma, or Epstein Barr infection.
▶ Malaria may present with cerebellar ataxia or Guillain-Barré syndrome.
▶ Hypoxic brain damage and hyperthermia

Rare causes: autoimmune, prion disorders, paraneoplastic processes, and inherited metabolic disorders may be subacute in onset.

Chronic Ataxia

Chronic ataxia is more in keeping with inherited or neurodegenerative conditions, and it is usually bilateral. The main exception for ataxia whether acute, subacute, or chronic is demyelinating disease such as multiple sclerosis.

One important cause of sporadic ataxia is multiple system atrophy (MSA)-C. There may not be any associated parkinsonism. Always check standing blood pressure and enquire about bladder dysfunction in patients with chronic sporadic ataxia.

Episodic Ataxia

This form is often inherited (see later in this chapter) but recurrent ataxia may be associated with drug intoxication and some metabolic disorders.

Rapidly Progressive Cerebellar Ataxia

Rapidly progressive cerebellar ataxia in the elderly suggests:

• Neoplastic or paraneoplastic conditions
• Prion-related disorder
• Infection
• Vascular disorder
• Hypomagnesemia. This is associated with alcoholism, vomiting, gastric bypass surgery, and use of proton pump inhibitors. It is easily misdiagnosed for Wernicke's encephalopathy

Neoplastic lesions that affect the cerebellum or brainstem are usually metastatic. For paraneoplastic syndromes, the main causes are cancers of the lung (especially small-cell carcinoma), breast, ovary, and lymphoma. The neurological condition usually precedes the diagnosis of the cancer by months or years.

INHERITED ATAXIAS

This section comprises (a) autosomal dominant inherited ataxias, (b) autosomal recessive inherited ataxias, (c) X-linked inherited ataxias, (d) inherited episodic ataxias, and (e) acquired episodic ataxias.

In general:

• If the age of onset is *greater than* 20 years, dominant inheritance is more likely.
• If the age of first symptoms is *less than* 20 years, then recessive inheritance is likely.

Autosomal Dominant Inherited Ataxias
Spinocerebellar Ataxias

All spinocerebellar ataxias (SCA) are autosomal dominant. There is an ever-expanding list of SCAs (more than 42 at present), and phenotypic classification can be difficult. Please refer to

TABLE 12.1: MAIN FEATURES OF AUTOSOMAL DOMINANT
SPINOCEREBELLAR ATAXIAS

Disease number	Gene	Age of onset (years)	Key features
1	ATXN1	20–40	Bulbar, pyramidal signs and peripheral neuropathy
2	ATXN2	20–40	Slow saccades, chorea, and neuropathy. Cognitive impairment. Some cases associated with ALS and parkinsonism. Occasionally levodopa responsive. *Alcohol sensitivity*
3	ATXN3	30–40	Synonym: Machado-Joseph disease. *Dystonia*, parkinsonism, pyramidal signs, and *bulging eyes*. Facial fasciculation. Dysautonomia. *Portuguese ancestry*
4	16p22.1	20–70	Sensory axonal neuropathy and deafness
5	SPTBN2	20–40	Early onset, slow progression. Some patients are *descendants of Abraham Lincoln*
6	CACNA1A	40–60	This is allelic with episodic ataxia type 2 and familial hemiplegic migraine. *Down-beating nystagmus*. Other features include parkinsonism and dystonia (Video 12.3, SCA6)
7	ATXN7	20–40	Visual loss due to *maculopathy*. Slow saccades. *Alcohol sensitivity*
8	ATXN81/80S	30–40	Pure ataxia of long duration
9	Not assigned		
10	ATXN10	30–40	Native American/Mexican origin. *Seizures*
11	TTBK2	20–30	Mild
12	PPP2R2B	30–40	Slow progression. Mild parkinsonism. Cognitive impairment. Predominant tremor, common in people from India
13	KCNC3	1–30	Mild cognitive impairment. Short stature
14	PRKCG	20–40	Early *axial myoclonus*. Very slow progression
15	ITPR1	30–40	Pure ataxia. Slow progression
16	SCA16	1–40	Head tremor. Allelic with SCA 15 and 29
17	TBP	30–40	Chorea and dementia *similar to Huntington disease*. (HDL type 4). Spasticity, dystonia.
18	7q22-q32	10–20	Sensorimotor neuropathy, pyramidal signs, fasciculations
19/22	KCND3	30–40	Slow progression. Myoclonus. Pyramidal signs
20	11p13-q11	40–50	Dysphonia, *palatal myoclonus*, and *dentate calcification. Coughing spasms* (may represent dysautonomia). Similar to progressive cerebellar ataxia with palatal tremor (PAPT). Hypertrophy of inferior olive.
26	EEF2	10–20	Ptosis and ophthalmoplegia
28	AFG3L2	Young adult	Slowly progressive ataxia, ptosis, nystagmus, ophthalmoplegia.
29	ITPR1	Infants	Hypotonia, motor delay, nonprogressive ataxia, cognitive impairment.
35	TGM6	40–50	Pyramidal signs. Cervical dystonia
36	NOP56	30–50	Fasciculation, *tongue atrophy*, increased reflexes

ALS, amyotrophic lateral sclerosis.

Handles are in italics.

Table 12.1 for the major associations with the cerebellar defect and average age of onset. Not every SCA is included in the table because either they are based on few families or there is insufficient information.
Note:

▶ Marked worsening of balance after small amounts of alcohol is a feature of SCA2 and SCA7. However:

◀ Alcohol sensitivity is seen also in lymphoma, porphyria, traumatic brain injury, and other causes of cerebral atrophy
▶ SCA mimics
   ○ SCA6 or SCA17 may present with specific focal dystonia.
   ○ SCA2 and SCA3 can manifest as young onset dopa-responsive PD.
   ○ SCA17 (homozygote) can look like Huntington's disease.

Other Autosomal Dominant Varieties Without SCA Number
Dentato-Rubral-Pallido-Luysian Atrophy (DRPLA)

This is characterized by ataxia, chorea, seizures, optic atrophy, dementia, and myoclonus and may simulate Huntington's disease. Most affected individuals are of Japanese descent.

Autosomal Dominant Cerebellar Ataxia with Deafness and Narcolepsy (ADCADN)

This is characterized by adult-onset progressive cerebellar ataxia, narcolepsy/cataplexy, sensorineural deafness, and dementia. The level of hypocretin in the cerebrospinal fluid (CSF) is low.

Ataxia with Coughing Spasms

This is an unusual middle-age–onset dominant cerebellar ataxia preceded by years of spasmodic coughing, described in Portuguese inhabitants. It may be related to SCA20. Recurrent cough is a feature of dysautonomia, which is possibly the explanation here.

Ataxia Followed by Dementia in Young Adult May Be Due to Presenilin Mutation

This is also autosomal dominant.

Autosomal Recessive Inherited Ataxias

Table 12.2 gives the main features with associated Handles. Just a few varieties are highlighted.

Some of the main features of the autosomal recessive ataxias are illustrated in videos given in the table and in Figures 12.4–12.14.

Ataxia telangiectasia is partly described in Chapter 1. Photographs of the conjunctival changes are shown in Figure 12.4.

Niemann-Pick type C is discussed in Chapter 8 (Movement Disorders).

Polyneuropathy, hearing loss, ataxia, retinitis pigmentosa, and cataract (PHARC) syndrome begins in teenagers and may resemble Refsum's disease. The polyneuropathy is unusual because it is demyelinating, like the autosomal recessive spastic ataxia of Charlevoix-Saguenay (ARSACS), whereas most other polyneuropathies with ataxia are axonal.

Two further Handles are the following:

▶ Friedreich's ataxia mimics: Bassen-Kornzweig syndrome, ataxia with vitamin E deficiency

(AVED, see Video 12.2); ARSACS syndrome, late-onset Tay-Sachs disease.
▶ Ataxia with demyelinating neuropathy: ARSACS and PHARC syndromes

X-Linked Ataxias

There are two varieties of these ataxias:

1. *X-linked sideroblastic anemia and ataxia (XLSA-A).* This is characterized by the following:
   ○ Nonprogressive early-onset cerebellar ataxia in males
   ○ Pyramidal signs
   ○ Hypochromic microcytic anemia
   ○ Ring sideroblasts in the bone marrow
2. *Fragile X–associated tremor-ataxia syndrome (FXTAS).* This is a premutation that presents in middle-aged or older men, but minor manifestations are seen in women who also suffer premature ovarian failure (see Video 8.38, FXTAS).

Diagnostic clues are as follows:

▶ Intellectual disability in a grandson (through the patient's daughter)
▶ Jerky tremor and cerebellar ataxia often mislabeled *essential tremor*
▶ Dysautonomia (bladder or bowel) causing confusion with MSA
▶ Dysexecutive syndrome

MRI may show increased signal in the middle cerebellar peduncles (Figure 12.5) although this is a nonspecific sign. See Chapter 8.

Inherited Episodic Ataxias with Variable Inheritance

Intermittent inherited cerebellar ataxia in an adult raises several possibilities, discussed next.

Autosomal Dominant Episodic Ataxia

There are currently seven varieties of episodic ataxia (EA) (see Table 12.3), but the more common are types EA1–3. These are characterized by attacks of imbalance of variable duration. If the ataxia lasts

▶ Seconds to minutes with myokymia this suggests EA1. This is a potassium channelopathy with a mutation in

TABLE 12.2: SUMMARY OF MAIN AUTOSOMAL RECESSIVE ATAXIAS

Disease name	Gene/Protein	Year of onset (Years)	Features
Friedreich's ataxia (FRDA)	FRDA	1–20	Progressive cerebellar and pyramidal signs. Cerebellar atrophy late feature. Skeletal deformities (scoliosis, pes cavus), prominent square-wave jerks, *cardiac arrhythmias or cardiomyopathy.* Inverted T waves. *Sensory axonal neuropathy essential for diagnosis;* 20% diabetic. Chorea is a Red Flag.
Ataxia telangiectasia (AT)	ATM	1–10	Choreoathetosis, telangiectases on conjunctiva or pinna (Figure 12.4). *Susceptibility to infection* (mainly sinopulmonary) and malignancy (leukemia and lymphoma). Head thrusts, premature graying of hair or skin. Raised α-fetoprotein, low IgA. *Death of sibling from malignancy at an early age*
AOA1 (ataxia with oculomotor apraxia type 1)	Aprataxin	1–20	Like AT with choreoathetosis, severe axonal motor neuropathy progressing to quadriplegia. Gaze-evoked nystagmus. Excess blinking. Apraxia leads to external ophthalmoplegia. *High total cholesterol,* low albumin. *α-fetoprotein normal. No telangiectases.* See Video 12.4, AOA1 (courtesy David Zee)
AOA2 (ataxia with oculomotor apraxia type 2)	SETX	10–30	Sensory-motor axonal neuropathy, *associated with juvenile ALS, raised α-fetoprotein. No telangiectases. Dystonic tongue movements*
Cerebrotendinous xanthomatosis (CTX)	CYP27A1	1–30	*Cataracts,* diarrhea, *tendon xanthomas.* Raised cholestanol. MRI: abnormal signal in the dentate nuclei See Figure 12.7. Treatable with chenodeoxycholic acid. Hypertrophy of inferior olive.
Abetalipoproteinemia (Bassen-Kornzweig syndrome)	MTTP	1–10	*Mimics FRDA.* Skeletal deformities, axonal polyneuropathy, retinitis pigmentosa, acanthocytes, *Low levels of cholesterol,* beta-lipoproteins, and vitamin E
AVED (Ataxia with vitamin E deficiency)	TTPA	1–20	*Mimics FRDA.* Mediterranean natives and Japanese. *Titubation, dystonia, paranoia, retinitis pigmentosa,* and poor vision. *Low vitamin E level.* Cardiomyopathy rare. See Video 12.2, AVED (courtesy Zain Guduru.)
ARSACS syndrome (autosomal recessive spastic ataxia of Charlevoix-Saguenay)	SACS	1–10	*Mimics FRDA or primary progressive MS.* French Canadian descent. Spastic ataxia due to pyramidal and cerebellar disorder; *demyelinating neuropathy. Thickened retinal nerve fiber layer* (Figure 12.6). MRI: atrophy of superior vermis and pontine hypointense horizontal stripes.
Niemann-Pick type C	NPC1	1–20	Dystonia, bulbar palsy, cognitive decline, *supranuclear vertical downgaze palsy. Cataplexy. Neonatal jaundice.* Deafness. Splenomegaly. Lysosomal storage disorder, treatable with cyclodextrin. See Video 8.35, Niemann Pick C (courtesy David Zee).
Late-onset Tay-Sachs disease	HEXA	10–40	Hexosaminidase A deficiency. *Mimics FRDA or juvenile ALS.* Bulbar palsy, axonal motor neuropathy. No cherry-red spot. Ashkenazi Jews susceptible. *Delayed visual-evoked potentials.* See Video 7.11, HexA.
Joubert syndrome	Multiple	1–10	*Irregular, sighing breathing.* Retinitis pigmentosa, skeletal malformations, seizures. *Molar tooth sign* on MRI (Figure 12.8). See Video 12.5, Joubert (courtesy Ildefonso Rodriguez).
Alpha-mannosidosis	MAN2B1	1–30	Intellectual disability, *patella dislocation,* skeletal changes (Charcot joints), hearing loss, and recurrent infections

(*continued*)

TABLE 12.2:   CONTINUED

Disease name	Gene/Protein	Year of onset (Years)	Features
PHARC	ABHD12	10–20	*Demyelinating polyneuropathy*, hearing loss, ataxia, retinitis pigmentosa, and *cataract. Resembles Refsum disease.*
MIRAS (mitochondrial recessive ataxia syndrome)	POLG	5–40	Axonal sensory neuropathy, ophthalmoplegia, Refractory seizures and migraine-like headache. *Valproate therapy leads to acute liver failure.* Common in Finland and Norway.
Marinesco-Sjögren syndrome	SIL1	5–25	Congenital *cataracts, facial and skeletal deformity*, hypotonia, muscle weakness, brittle nails. Severe cerebellar atrophy.
Gillespie syndrome	PAX6	Infancy and childhood	*Aniridia*, mental retardation, cerebellar atrophy. Some are autosomal dominant.
Oliver McFarlane syndrome	PNPLA6	Infancy and childhood	Progressive ataxia, reduced visual acuity, *retinitis pigmentosa*, bald, *thick curly hair, long eyelashes.*
CANVAS	Not known Probably recessive.	Late adult	Cerebellar ataxia, neuropathy and vestibular areflexia syndrome. Also, dorsal root ganglionopathy, orthostatic hypotension, coughing spasms, and neuropathic pain. Coughing may represent autonomic disorder. See Figure 12.9 and Video 12.6, CANVAS. (courtesy JA Petersen et al. 2013).

KCNA1. There is triggering by startle or noise.

▶ Hours or days with interictal downbeat nystagmus and migraine this favors EA2. This is a calcium channelopathy, with a mutation in the gene *CACNA1A*, the same gene responsible for SCA6 and familial hemiplegic migraine. Brain MRI shows vermis atrophy (Figure 12.10).

▶ About 10–30 minutes with episodes of tinnitus and vertigo is likely EA3.

This is a rarer variety, associated with headache, tinnitus, vertigo, and myokymia.

The gene is not yet identified but has been linked to 1q42.

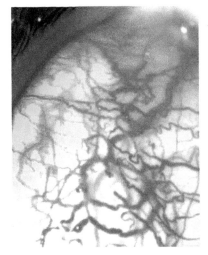
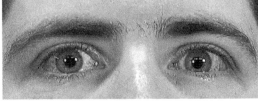

FIGURE 12.4: Ataxia-telangiectasia: **Left:** Dilated, tortuous vessels in bulbar conjunctiva in a 17-year-old boy. Reproduced from Figure 13-46 in the chapter Capillary Malformations, Hyperkeratotic Stains, Telangiectasias, and Miscellaneous Vascular Blots, by JB Mulliken. Oxford University Press. DOI:10.1093/med/9780195145052.003.0013. **Right:** Less florid telangiectases in an adult man. Courtesy Tania Jawad and Tim Lynch.

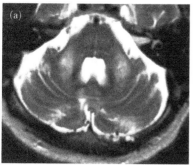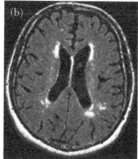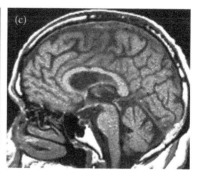

FIGURE 12.5: Fragile X tremor-ataxia syndrome (FXTAS) caused by a CGG premutation in a patient of 72 years. (**A**) Axial T2-weighted image demonstrating symmetric, increased signal within the middle cerebellar peduncles. (**B**) Axial FLAIR image reveals increased signal within the periventricular cerebral white matter. (**C**) Sagittal T1 image demonstrates mild atrophy of the caudal pons, mild cerebral volume loss, and thinning of the corpus callosum. Note: high signal in the middle cerebellar peduncle is not a specific sign for FXTAS and may be found in other ataxias such as sporadic olivopontocerebellar atrophy and spinocerebellar ataxia, metabolic diseases, adrenoleukodystrophy, Wilson's disease, and posterior reversible encephalopathy syndrome. Reproduced with permission from Hagerman and Hagerman (2007).

Types 2 and 3 respond to acetazolamide. Frequently, the diagnosis is delayed by several years, and, if there is headache, a wrong diagnosis of isolated migraine may be made.

Glucose Transporter Type 1 Deficiency Syndrome (De Vivo Disease)

See Video 12.7, GLUT-1 deficiency (courtesy Hanene Benrhouma) and Video 8.82, GLUT 1 deficiency). This is an autosomal dominant condition caused by

TABLE 12.3: FEATURES OF INHERITED EPISODIC ATAXIAS

Disease name	Gene	Age of onset (years)	Features
EA1	KCNA1	1–20	Myokymia; attacks lasting *seconds to minutes;* startle or exercise induced; no vertigo. *No response to acetazolamide.* AD
EA2	CACNA1A; CACNB4	1–30	Downbeat nystagmus; attacks *lasting minutes to hours;* vertigo; Permanent ataxia later. *Responds to acetazolamide.* Associated with FHM and allelic with SAC6. AD
EA3	1q42	20–20	Tinnitus, vertigo, myokymia. *Ataxia 10–30 minutes.* Headache. *Responds to acetazolamide.* AD
Maple syrup urine disease	Several	1–20	*Sweet smell to urine.* Encephalopathy, vomiting and seizures. Triggered by infection or high-protein meal. AR
Hartnup disease	SLC6A19	1–10	Failure to thrive. Nystagmus. *Light sensitive rash like pellagra* (Figure 12.11). AR
Ornithine transcarbamylase deficiency	OTC	1–20	Encephalopathic attacks, triggered by fever. *Headache after a high-protein meal.* Blood ammonia raised. XLR
Glucose transporter type 1 (GLUT1) deficiency. De Vivo disease	SLC2A1	1–10	Episodic ataxia or exercise-induced dyskinesia, anticonvulsant-refractory seizures. *Provocation by fasting and relief with sugary drink. Usually very low CSF glucose.* AD. See Video 12.7, GLUT-1 deficiency

AD, autosomal dominant; AR, autosomal recessive; FHM, familial hemiplegic migraine; XLR, X-linked recessive.

Important Handles are in italics.

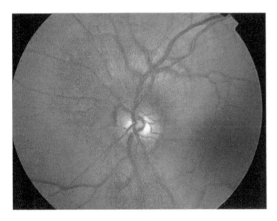

FIGURE 12.6: ARSACS (autosomal recessive spastic ataxia of Charlevoix Saguenay) syndrome. This fundus photograph shows blurring of the normally sharp-edged retinal vessels, with tortuosity near the optic disc. There are faint yellow streaks radiating from disk. Courtesy Fion Bremner, Moorfields Eye Hospital, London.

diminished activity of the glucose transporter protein (GLUT1). The classic presentation is acquired microcephaly, intellectual disability, and anticonvulsant-refractory seizures in infancy. Prolonged starvation may trigger status epilepticus, and some experience relief with a sugary drink. Classically, the CSF glucose level is low because of defective transport across the blood–brain barrier.

Note:

- Milder forms are not always associated with a low CSF glucose and sometimes misdiagnosed as refractory absence seizures resulting in preventable cognitive decline.

Atypical presentations include the following:

- Later onset
- Progressive ataxia

- Chorea, dystonia, or spasticity
- Exercise-induced dyskinesia

Acquired Intermittent Ataxias

More mundane *nongenetic* causes for adult-onset intermittent ataxia are the following:

- Multiple sclerosis
- Migraine
- Transient ischemic attacks
- Foramen magnum compression (e.g., Chiari malformation)
- Hydrocephalus from colloid cyst of third ventricle (Figure 12.12, *left*); aqueduct stenosis (Figure 12.12, *right*); tapeworm infestation (see Figure 6.11)
- Intoxicants: mercury, solvents, glue, repeated phenytoin toxicity

MISCELLANEOUS CEREBELLAR ATAXIAS

Mitochondrial Spinocerebellar Ataxia and Epilepsy

Mitochondrial spinocerebellar ataxia and epilepsy (MSCAE) is a mitochondrial disorder associated with mutations in *POLG-1*. Apart from cerebellar features, patients have seizures and there may be a family history of liver failure secondary to valproate exposure.

Coenzyme Q deficiency

This is an autosomal recessive disorder characterized by slowly progressive ataxia of childhood onset. Associated features are seizures, dystonia, and marked cerebellar atrophy on MRI. CoQ10 administration may help.

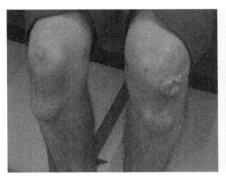 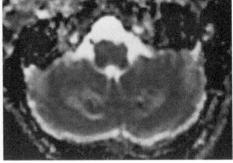

FIGURE 12.7: Cerebrotendinous xanthomatosis (CTX). **Left**: Tendon xanthomas over patellar tendons. **Right**: Abnormal MRI signal in the dentate in CTX. Left image courtesy GS Wali. Right image courtesy M Cesarini.

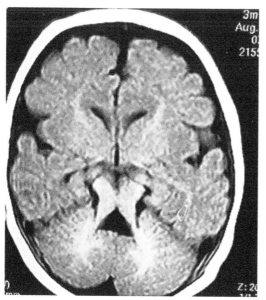
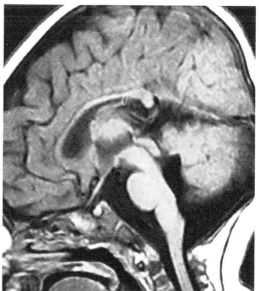

FIGURE 12.8: Joubert's syndrome. MRI T1 axial (**left**) and sagittal (**right**) images. On the axial image, note the small vermis, broad horizontal superior cerebellar peduncles, and narrow isthmus producing "molar tooth" sign. Irregular, sighing breathing is characteristic of Joubert syndrome (see also Video 12.5, Joubert Syndrome). Somewhat similar episodes (breath-holding) occur in Rett syndrome but the patient is not ataxic. Video and MRI courtesy Ildefonso Rodriguez.

Progressive Cerebellar Ataxia with Palatal Tremor

Progressive cerebellar ataxia with palatal tremor (PAPT) refers to the unusual combination of progressive ataxia and palatal tremor (Video 12.8, PAPT). It is often familial. Many cases represent Alexander disease due to *GFAP* gene mutations. Lower medullary and upper spinal cord atrophy

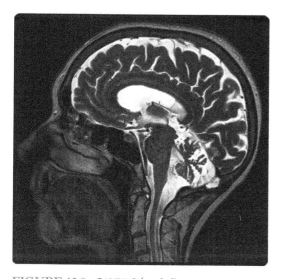

FIGURE 12.9: CANVAS (cerebellar ataxia, neuropathy, vestibular areflexia). The T2-weighted sagittal MRI shows marked cerebellar atrophy affecting the vermal lobules. There is also atrophy of the cervical spinal cord. Reproduced with permission from Petersen et al. (2013).

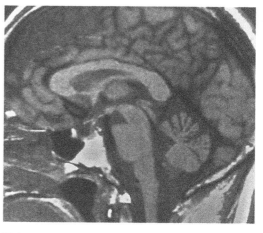

FIGURE 12.10: T1-weighted sagittal brain MRI in a patient with episodic ataxia type 2 showing atrophy of the cerebellar vermis. Reproduced from Figure 18–3 in the chapter Developmental and Genetic Disorders, by RW Baloh, V Honrubia, and KA Kerber. Oxford University Press. DOI:10.1093/med/9780195387834.003.0018.

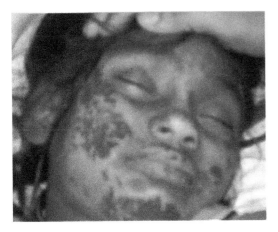

FIGURE 12.11: Hartnup disease. This shows the pellagra-type rash affecting the face. Reproduced from Patel and Prabhu (2008).

is characteristic, giving the "tadpole sign" (Figure 12.13).

In addition:

▶ Inferior olivary hypertrophy similar to that seen in symptomatic palatal tremor (SPT) is observed.

▶ Inferior olivary hypertrophy is also seen, rarely, in SCA20 and cerebrotendinous xanthomatosis (CTX).

Note: hypertrophy of the inferior olive is seen in several nondegenerative and non-genetic disorders of the brainstem that interfere with the Guillain-Mollaret triangle (e.g., hemorrhage, tumors, etc.).

▶ In SPT, ear clicks are not present because only the central palate is affected but:

▶ Ear clicks are heard in isolated (essential) palatal tremor due to contraction of the laterally placed tensor veli palatini muscle (CN V) that contracts the soft palate and opens the Eustachian tube.

▶ Isolated (essential) palatal tremor is usually psychogenic.

Sporadic causes of palatal tremor and progressive ataxia include brainstem disorder due to:

• Demyelination
• Neoplasia
• Vascular lesions, trauma, infection.

Progressive Cerebellar Gait Ataxia, Myoclonic Epilepsy, and Intention Tremor

The main causes of this combination are the "famous five":

• Neuronal ceroid lipofuscinoses (Batten's disease)
• Lafora disease
• Unverricht-Lundberg syndrome

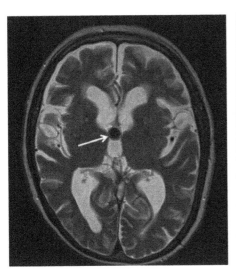
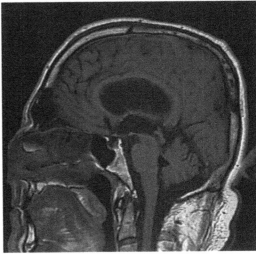

FIGURE 12.12: **Left**: T2 axial unenhanced MRI brain scan shows a colloid cyst (white arrow) at the level of the foramen of Monro. Note it is hypointense on T2 and hyperintense on T1 sequences. **Right**: Aqueduct stenosis. T1-weighted sagittal MRI brain scan. The lateral and third ventricles are dilated. The aqueduct is distended but stenosed caudally where it joins the fourth ventricle. Corpus callosum is stretched and thinned. Left image reproduced from Radiopedia, courtesy F Gaillard. Right image reproduced from Radiopedia, ID 9009, courtesy F Gaillard.

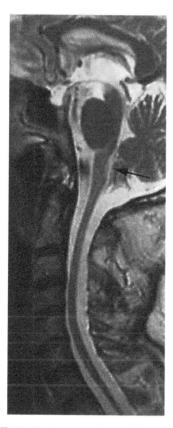

FIGURE 12.13: Alexander disease. This shows atrophy and signal abnormalities in the medulla oblongata (arrow); the hyperintensity fades away in the upper cervical spinal cord. The entire spinal cord is also atrophic. Sometimes this is called the "tadpole sign." Reproduced with permission from Pareyson et al. (2008), Figure 1a.

- Sialidosis type 1
- MERRF (myoclonus epilepsy and ragged red fibers)

A newly described addition (number 6!) is:

- *North Sea progressive myoclonus epilepsy,* so named because all patients described thus far live in countries bordering on the North Sea. It is due to homozygous mutation in the Golgi SNAP receptor complex 2 gene (*GOSR2*) on 17q. A combination of cortical myoclonus, ataxia, and areflexia is characteristic (Boisse et al. 2013). Other clues are pes cavus and kyphoscoliosis.

MISCELLANEOUS DISORDERS ASSOCIATED WITH ATAXIA

- *Myelopathy, deafness, and anosmia.* This suggests either superficial siderosis of the nervous system (Figure 12.14) or a mitochondrial disorder. See also Chapter 2.
- *Parkinsonism.* The main associations are SCA2, -3, -12, and -17; MSA-C; and the fragile-X syndrome.
- *Amyotrophy.* SCA 1, -2, -3, and -36. AOA2; GM2 gangliosidosis (see Video 7.11, HexA); and ARSACS
- *Deafness*
  - SCA4
  - ADCADN. Associated with narcolepsy and dementia

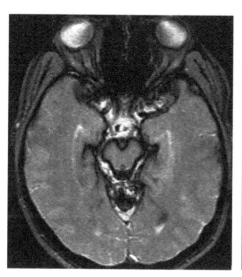
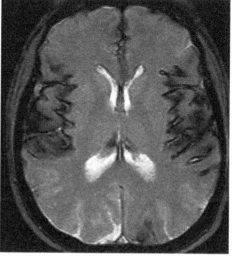

FIGURE 12.14: MRI brain images showing features characteristic of superficial siderosis. **Left**: T2-weighted inversion recovery image of the patient's brainstem outlined by a rim of hypointensity where hemosiderin has been deposited. **Right**: T2 hypointensity in the Sylvian and other sulci. MRI courtesy Ildefonso Rodriguez.

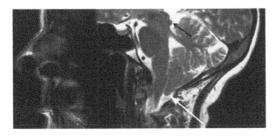

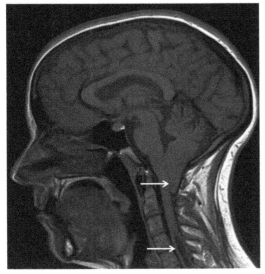

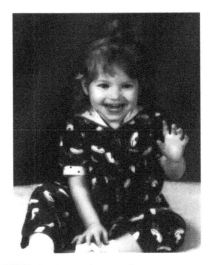

FIGURE 12.16: Angelman syndrome.

FIGURE 12.15: **Top**: T2-weighted sagittal brain MRI of Chiari type I malformation. White arrow points to the tip of the cerebellar tonsils. Also note peaking of the inferior colliculi (black arrow). **Bottom**: A more severe Chiari type 1 malformation (upper white arrow) associated with a syrinx in the mid-cervical region (lower white arrow). Top image reproduced from *Developmental and Genetic Disorders*, RW Baloh, V Honrubia, and KA Kerber, Figure 18–2. Oxford University Press.DOI:10.1093/med/9780195387834.003.0018. Bottom image courtesy Bart's Health Neuroimaging Department.

- o PHARC. Resembles Refsum's disease
- o Alpha mannosidosis
- o Superficial siderosis
- o Mitochondrial disorder (e.g., Kearns-Sayre syndrome), NARP
- o Cerebellar ataxia, areflexia, pes cavus, optic atrophy, sensorineural hearing loss (CAPOS) syndrome. This is due to mutation in *ATP1A3*, the same gene that causes rapid-onset dystonia-parkinsonism and alternating hemiplegia of childhood.
- *Hypoglossal palsy suggests a Chiari type 1 malformation.* The reason is that the hypoglossal nerve is vulnerable to pressure as it exits

from its foramen, that is close to the foramen magnum. Frequently there is peaking of the inferior colliculus, as seen in Figure 12.15. Vertebral or carotid artery dissection is an alternative diagnosis. In many cases the Chiari malformation is asymptomatic.

- *Sensory ataxia and dry mouth.* Sjögren's syndrome. If the unsteadiness is due to weakness or fatigue, then Lambert-Eaton myasthenic syndrome (LEMS) may be the answer.
- *Wide-based ataxic gait and normal arm coordination favors alcoholic or ischemic cerebellar atrophy.* This combination suggests a disorder of the anterior cerebellar lobe and vermis. Only the lower limbs and trunk are represented here, thus:
  - o The arms and extraocular movements are spared but there may be severe titubation.
  - o Patients with alcoholic cerebellar ataxia may also have a tendency to touch lightly a nearby wall to help walking balance.

The mechanism of this tendency is not understood.

- *Medication.* The same medication that produces acute ataxia may cause a chronic form. Thus, chronic intoxication with phenytoin, carbamazepine, metronidazole, and chemotherapy (cyclosporin, tacrolimus) are well-recognized associations.
- *High-stepping and stamping gait.* This is the classic sign of tabes dorsalis, where the patient is unaware of the position of the lower limbs unless they are observed directly. This is a sensory, not cerebellar ataxia. Note:

▶ Shoe wear in tabes is even.

This happens because the tabetic patient places down the foot squarely and does not drag it along. In the more common varieties of foot drop with preserved joint position sense the front of the sole is worn.

More common causes are vitamin B_{12} and copper deficiency (see Chapter 11).

Also note:

▶ High-stepping gait without stamping suggests *bilateral* foot drop, usually from a peripheral nerve lesion.

▶ *Seizures, frequent laughing, hand flapping, likely indicates Angelman's syndrome* (Figure 12.16). Sometimes the gait has a "prancing" character. Also, the child may have:
  ○ Red or blonde hair (usually)
  ○ Microcephaly
  ○ Speech impairment
  ○ Tongue thrusting
  ○ Fascination with water
- *Blood abnormalities*:
  ○ Acanthocytes and low cholesterol: Bassen-Kornzweig syndrome
  ○ High cholesterol: ataxia with oculomotor apraxia type 1 (AOA1) and AOA2
  ○ Raised cholestanol: CTX
  ○ Raised ammonia: ornithine transcarbamylase deficiency
  ○ GQ1b antibody: Miller Fisher syndrome
  ○ Low thiamine: malnutrition, chronic alcoholism
  ○ GAD antibodies in diabetic: autoimmune cerebellar ataxia or stiff person syndrome
  ○ Raised alpha-fetoprotein, low IgA: ataxia telangiectasia, AOA2
  ○ Sideroblastic anemia: X-linked sideroblastic anemia and ataxia syndrome
  ○ Hexosaminidase A deficiency: Tay-Sachs and related disorders
  ○ Low blood vitamin E: AVED and Bassen-Kornzweig syndrome

SUMMARY
- Romberg's sign is a test of joint position sense, not cerebellar function.
- If the patient has slurred speech, then you are likely dealing with a cerebellar rather than sensory ataxia.

- Cerebellar incoordination without nystagmus suggests a lesion of the cerebellar hemispheres.

Pattern
- Unilateral cerebellar ataxia is likely to be a structural lesion, such as a tumor, infarct, or inflammatory or infectious process.
- Symmetric bilateral ataxia favors a metabolic, inherited, immunological, or paraneoplastic process; Sugar-coating sign.

Acute or Subacute Ataxias
In general, acute-onset ataxia suggests intoxication or a vascular, an infective, or a structural cause.

Specific disorders associated with ataxia:

- Areflexia and ophthalmoplegia: Miller Fisher syndrome
- Alcoholism or malnourishment: thiamine deficiency
- Epilepsy: anticonvulsant toxicity
- Intoxication or medication: alcohol, lithium, amiodarone, chemotherapy (cyclosporin, tacrolimus), metronidazole, recreational drugs (e.g., organic solvents)
- Rigidity and myoclonic jerks: PERM
- In a woman with type 1 diabetes: autoimmune cerebellar ataxia with GAD antibodies
- Childhood- or young adult–onset limb ataxia, with fine horizontal head tremor suggests viral cerebellitis (chicken pox). Also occurs in some autoimmune or paraneoplastic processes, and inherited metabolic disorders
- Malaria may present with cerebellar ataxia or Guillain-Barré syndrome.

Chronic Ataxia
This form suggests inherited or neurodegenerative conditions, and it is likely bilateral. MSA-C is an exception.

Episodic Ataxia
This is often inherited but may be associated with drug intoxication and some metabolic disorders.

Rapidly Progressive Cerebellar Ataxia
Rapidly progressive cerebellar ataxia in the elderly suggests neoplastic or paraneoplastic conditions, a prion-related disorder, infection, hypomagnesemia, or vascular disorder.

Inherited Ataxias

In general: age of onset less than 20 years: recessive inheritance; age of onset greater than 20 years: dominant inheritance

Autosomal Dominant Inherited Ataxias

Learn Table 12.1. Other autosomal dominant varieties without a SCA number: DRPLA, ADCADN, ataxia with coughing spasms

Note: Alcohol sensitivity is a feature of SCA 2, SCA 7, porphyria, and lymphoma and many causes of cerebral atrophy.

SCA Mimics

- SCA6 or SCA17 may present with specific focal dystonia.
- SCA2 and SCA3 can manifest as young onset dopa-responsive PD.
- SCA17 (homozygote) can look like Huntington's disease

Recessively Inherited Ataxias

Learn Table 12.2.

- Friedreich's ataxia mimics: Bassen-Kornzweig syndrome, AVED, ARSACS syndrome, late-onset Tay-Sachs disease
- Ataxia with demyelinating neuropathy: ARSACS syndrome and PHARC

X-linked Ataxias

- With sideroblastic anemia: XLSA-A
- Fragile X tremor ataxia syndrome (FXTAS)

Intermittent Episodic Ataxias with Variable Inheritance

Learn Table 12.3.
Ataxia lasting:

- Seconds to minutes with myokymia suggests EA1.
- Hours or days with interictal downbeat nystagmus and migraine favors EA2.
- About 10–30 minutes with episodes of tinnitus and vertigo is likely EA3.

Acquired Intermittent Ataxias

- Multiple sclerosis, migraine, transient ischemic attacks, foramen magnum compression, hydrocephalus (colloid cyst, aqueduct stenosis, tapeworm infestation), intoxicants

Miscellaneous Cerebellar Ataxias

- *MSCAE. POLG1* mutation. Seizures and family history of liver failure secondary to valproate exposure
- *Coenzyme Q deficiency.* Slowly progressive ataxia of childhood onset, seizures, dystonia
- *Progressive cerebellar ataxia with palatal tremor.* Familial; PAPT including Alexander's disease (tadpole sign on MRI), SCA 20. Sporadic: demyelination, neoplasia, vascular brainstem lesions. Isolated (essential) palatal tremor is usually psychogenic.
- *Progressive cerebellar ataxia, myoclonic epilepsy, and intention tremor.* Batten's disease, Lafora disease, Unverricht-Lundberg syndrome, sialidosis type 1, MERRF, North Sea progressive myoclonus epilepsy
- CANVAS, Dysautonomia

Miscellaneous Disorders Associated with Ataxia

- *Myelopathy, deafness, and anosmia.* Superficial siderosis or mitochondrial disorder
- *Parkinsonism.* SCA2, -3, -12, and -17; MSA-C and the fragile-X syndrome
- *Amyotrophy.* SCA1, -2, -3, and -36. AOA2; GM2 gangliosidosis and ARSACS
- *Deafness.* SCA4, ADCADN, PHARC, alpha-mannosidosis, superficial siderosis, mitochondrial disorder (Kearns-Sayre syndrome, NARP), CAPOS syndrome, Refsum's disease (sensory ataxia)
- *Hypoglossal palsy.* Chiari type 1 malformation or vertebral/carotid artery dissection
- *Sensory ataxia with dry mouth.* Sjögren's syndrome. If the unsteadiness is due to weakness or fatigue, then LEMS may be the answer.
- *Normal arm coordination.* Alcoholic or ischemic cerebellar atrophy
- *Medication.* Chronic intoxication with phenytoin, carbamazepine, metronidazole, chemotherapy
- *High-stepping and stamping gait.* Tabes dorsalis. *High-stepping gait without stamping:* bilateral foot drop. Note: shoe wear in tabes is even.
- *Seizures, frequent laughing, hand flapping are likely Angelman's syndrome.* Other features

include red or blonde hair, microcephaly, speech impairment, tongue thrusts, and fascination with water.

- *Dysautonomia.* Fragile-X tremor ataxia syndrome, MSA, SCA 3, CANVAS
- *Coughing spasms.* CANVAS, SCA 20.
- Blood abnormalities:
  - Acanthocytes and low cholesterol: Bassen-Kornzweig syndrome
  - High cholesterol: AOA1
  - Raised cholestanol: CTX
  - Raised ammonia: ornithine transcarbamylase deficiency
  - GQ1b antibody: Miller Fisher syndrome
  - Low thiamine: malnutrition, chronic alcoholism
  - GAD antibodies in diabetic: autoimmune cerebellar ataxia or stiff person syndrome
  - Raised alpha-fetoprotein, low IgA: ataxia telangiectasia, AOA2
  - Sideroblastic anemia: X-linked sideroblastic anemia and ataxia syndrome
  - Hexosaminidase A deficiency: Tay-Sachs and related disorders
  - Low blood vitamin E: AVED and Bassen-Kornzweig syndrome

SUGGESTED READING

Boisse LL, Bayly MA, Hjalgrim H, et al. "North Sea" progressive myoclonus epilepsy: phenotype of subjects with GOSR2 mutation. *Brain.* 2013;136:1146–1154.

Franz DN, Glauser TA, Tudor C, Williams S. Topiramate therapy of epilepsy associated with Angelman's syndrome. *Neurology.* 2000;54:1185–1188.

Hagerman PJ, Hagerman RJ. Fragile X–associated tremor/ataxia syndrome—an older face of the fragile X gene. *Nat Clin Pract Neurol.* 2007;3:107–112.

Metcalf C, Villa D. Sugar coating of the cerebellum. *J Cancer Biol Res.* 2013;1(2):1010.

Pareyson D, Fancellu R, Mariotti C, et al. Adult-onset Alexander disease: a series of eleven unrelated cases with review of the literature. *Brain.* 2008;131:2321–2331.

Petersen JA, et al (2013). Wichmann WW, Weber KP. The pivotal sign of CANVAS. *Neurology.* 2013;81(18):1642–1643.

Patel AB, Prabhu AS. Hartnup disease. *Indian J Dermatol.* 2008;53:31–32.

Chapter 13: Dementia and Cognition

Dementia is one of the most complex areas in neurology, with a dire need for Handles and Red Flags. Major progress is being made in genetic aspects of dementia such that, in a few years, the diagnosis will be made (hopefully) by DNA analysis and sophisticated imaging rather than classic clinically based techniques. Until then, we list a few tips that might enhance your clinical prowess. For more a more detailed discussion, we suggest you refer to three reviews (Larner 2014; Rossor et al. 2010; Warren et al. 2013).

PRELIMINARY OBSERVATIONS

Following are some Handles to help you identify dementia and distinguish it from anxiety/depression.

▶ The patient who attends alone with suspected dementia is more likely to have anxiety/depression.

The patient who attends alone will have had to remember the appointment and its instructions, arrive by car or public transportation, navigated to your clinic without getting lost. If the patient is accompanied, then you may conclude less, but you should ask the accompanying person whether they thought the patient could have made their way to your clinic by themselves. The sensitivity of this sign is high at 0.93, with a negative predictive value of 0.93 for the presence of dementia (Larner 2009).

◀ Be aware that dementia and depression may coexist.

When the patient *is* accompanied, it is essential to take a detailed history from a relative or caregiver.

During your initial assessment, based on the referral letter and preliminary questions, you should try to determine whether the major issue relates to the following:

- Change in personality or behavior: frontal lobe problem
- Impairment of memory: temporal lobe disorder
- Disorder of vision (e.g., diminished visuospatial awareness, field loss): parietal lobe dysfunction
- In general, change in speech or language suggesting progressive aphasia (as in semantic dementia, where there is loss of word meaning): implicates the dominant temporal lobe and/or connections.
- In progressive nonfluent aphasia (PNFA), the dominant frontal lobe is affected; in logopenic progressive aphasia (LPA), it is the inferior parietal lobe.

One or more varieties may be present simultaneously, but it is nonetheless a useful preliminary approach.

It is often possible to spot dementia by asking just a few general questions about life history and current affairs.

▶ The patient with difficulty recalling the names and doses of their medication may have cognitive impairment.

If the patient is taking medication, the patient with memory failure may not be able to remember the names and doses of their tablets. This approach is a discrete way of checking episodic (short-term) memory, assuming they would normally have been able to recall such information. The depressed patient, perhaps with persuasion, will usually give an accurate list.

▶ Detailed recollection of lapses in memory and their circumstance suggests poor concentration and favors anxiety.
▶ Poor recall of objects, but accurate identification of cues and foils in psychometric tests, supports anxiety.

When the patient *is* accompanied:

▶ If the patient is more concerned than the informant, then anxiety/depression is more likely.
▶ Conversely, if the informant is more concerned than the patient, then dementia is more likely.

HANDLES AND RED FLAGS FOR ALZHEIMER'S DISEASE

Following are some Handles for Alzheimer disease's (AD)

▶ The patient with obvious memory difficulties yet well-dressed who retains their social graces, and conversation at a superficial level. An attentive caregiver may mask this sign.
▶ An individual who becomes lost near their home or on familiar routes.
▶ The head-turning sign

The patient who keeps turning the head to the accompanying person for an answer to questions is probably demented, most likely from AD. The reliability of this feature is less than the "attended alone" sign, but it is reasonably predictive of cognitive impairment, probably indicating an amnesic deficit.

▶ Delusion of theft may be an early feature.
▶ Loss of pleasure for reading. It probably results from a combination of memory impairment and visuospatial processing of text.
▶ Disruptive vocalizations (Video 13.1). These consist of screaming, abusive language, moaning, perseveration, and repetitive and inappropriate requests. It is a feature of the mid to late stages of AD and not specific.

Impaired visuospatial awareness is typical of AD and may be suggested by the following in someone with memory problems:

▶ Repeated minor traffic accidents or near misses. This suggests diminished visuospatial awareness from parietal lobe dysfunction due to AD or its posterior cortical atrophy variant.
▶ Problems in remembering personal names.

Note: prosopagnosia (face-blindness) is often thought to be a feature of AD but it is more typical of right temporal variant frontotemporal dementia (FTD).

▶ Difficulty in mastering a new TV remote controller or mobile phone.

Red Flags for AD

◀ Abrupt onset is rarely a dementia, more likely delirium or confusional state.
◀ The patient with a cold stare more likely has frontal dementia.
◀ Deterioration in social decorum (e.g., bad behavior in public, inappropriate vulgarity, emotional instability, loss of interpersonal warmth). Again, a frontal lobe characteristic.
◀ Preservation of a good sense of humor is unusual.
◀ Abnormal digit span in early stages. This is a late feature of AD unless it is the posterior cortical variant (see next section).
◀ Positive applause sign is atypical and favors progressive supranuclear palsy (PSP) and other types of parkinsonism, particularly corticobasal syndrome (see Chapter 8)
◀ Normal sense of smell identification. Nearly all patients with AD have impaired olfaction *on testing*. In the mid to late stages of disease, such testing is difficult because of impaired naming as well as identification.
◀ Confabulation. This is rare in AD, but common in the Korsakoff syndrome.
◀ The patient who keeps leaning forward as if deaf may have receptive aphasia or semantic dementia (Video 13.2, Wernicke). Conversely, an elderly person with progressive deafness may be thought erroneously to have dementia.

The Posterior Cortical Variant of Alzheimer's Disease

This entity affects younger patients than those with classic AD. It is characterized by progressive decline in visuospatial, visuoperceptual, literacy, and praxic skills. There are three useful Handles:

▶ Multiple visits to the optician
Despite several changes of prescription their visual problem cannot be corrected.
▶ "Failed" cataract operation
The patient complains of poor vision in one or both eyes, and, indeed, there are cataracts of varying severity. Surgery is undertaken,

which helps little. The underlying reason is a visuospatial problem or, rarely, an actual field defect that may have been overlooked or not evaluated properly before surgery.

▶ Difficulty in judging distances even though visual fields are normal.
This suggests optic ataxia, which is one component of Balint's syndrome, where the patient sees an object but cannot reach out and touch it accurately. As mentioned earlier, this may result in numerous minor traffic accidents. Visuospatial problems are more characteristic of the later stages of classic AD.

▶ Visual crowding and difficulty with visual search. Patients complain: "I cannot find objects that are right in front of me." This is strongly suggestive of the posterior cortical variant of AD.

Handles for Frontotemporal Dementia Variants

FTD affects patients who are younger than those with AD. In its early stages, it is characterized by varying degrees of frontal lobe dysfunction such as:

- Personality change
- Apathy
- Perseveration of motor tasks

The main variants of this disorder may be identified by the Handles presented next.

Semantic Dementia

In this variant there is

- Difficulty understanding the significance of familiar words and asking their meaning. For example, "What is asparagus?" is said to be pathognomonic of semantic dementia.
- Fluent but empty circumlocutory speech
- Obsession with timekeeping, numbers, or Sudoku!
- MRI scan shows atrophy in the anteroinferior and medial temporal lobe, usually more on the left.

Behavioral Variant FTD

Following are the main features of this variant:

- Rude conversation or behavior—in essence disinhibition.

- Cold stare. Loss of warmth and empathy toward others.
- Apathy and stereotyped/ritualistic behavior
- Changed food preferences, especially sweet food with gluttony. Also hyperorality (i.e., oral exploration of objects)
- Increased liking for sweet food sometimes with weight gain, whereas weight loss commoner in AD.
- Increased concern over timekeeping
- Obsession with new hobbies and easily distractible
- Relative preservation of posterior cortical function
- In later stages: primitive reflexes (e.g., forced grasping or rooting)
- MRI often shows asymmetric atrophy, particularly affecting the frontal and anterior temporal lobes.
- More likely to have a positive family history than AD or frontotemporal variants

Progressive Nonfluent Aphasia

- Stumbling over long words or stuttering
- Grammatical errors
- Effortful, speech
- Orofacial apraxia; for example, difficulty miming a yawn or cough
- If there is supranuclear gaze palsy, pure akinesia, and gait freezing, this suggests progressive supranuclear palsy variant
- MRI often shows atrophy in the perisylvian dominant hemisphere.

Logopenic Aphasia

- Hesitant, grammatically correct speech
- Word-finding pauses
- Difficulty in repetition of phrases more than single words
- MRI often shows left temporoparietal atrophy

Other Dementias
Vascular Dementias

Some clinicians doubt the existence of this variety and suggest that in many instances the correct diagnosis is AD with infarcts and chronic ischemic change. It is probably overdiagnosed. Following are the classic features:

- Elderly hypertensive arteriopath
- Gradual cognitive decline due to accumulation of lacunar infarcts in silent areas

- Less often, a step-wise decline in motor function due to repeated small strokes
- Pseudobulbar palsy
- Relatively late-onset memory impairment and cognitive slowing

Cerebral Amyloid Angiopathy

Cerebral amyloid angiopathy (CAA) is described in more detail in Chapter 9.

Note:

▶ If there is a history of apparent TIAs with *positive* rather than the usual negative symptoms, the patient may be describing *amyloid spells*, a precursor of CAA.

▶ The patient may give a history of lobar intracerebral hemorrhage rather than the usual deep location associated with hypertensive intracerebral hemorrhage.

▶ MRI often shows lobar micro-hemorrhages, cortical siderosis, prominent perivascular spaces, and predominantly posterior periventricular white matter signal change.

Extrapyramidal Diseases

- *Lewy Body disease.* Look for prominent fluctuations, rapid eye movement (REM) sleep behavioral disorder, intolerance of neuroleptics, and visual hallucinations.
- *Huntington disease.* Imbalance may be more obvious than chorea in the early phase.
- *Classic Parkinson disease (PD) and parkinsonism.* Dementia is common only in the mid to later stages of PD and PSP. Conversely, parkinsonian features are seen in the late stages of AD. The presence of parkinsonism raises the possibility of FTDP-17 dementia caused by a mutation in the MAPT gene (chromosome 17). This provides instructions for making tau protein.
- *Wilson disease.* Almost any movement disorder may be seen, but the typical varieties are dystonia, chorea, and parkinsonism.
- *Late-presenting Gaucher disease.* The main clues are Ashkenazi Jewish ancestry, parkinsonism, supranuclear horizontal gaze palsy, and conjunctival pingueculae (see Chapter 8, Movement Disorders).
- *Hereditary diffuse leukoencephalopathy with spheroids (HDLS).* This causes a corticobasal syndrome and results from mutations in the CSF1R gene.

▶ **Muscle wasting or fasciculation**

This points to:

- *FTD* with amyotrophic lateral sclerosis associated with the *C9ORF72* mutation.
- Hyperthyroidism
- Spino-cerebellar ataxia type 2 (SCA 2)

POINTS IN THE HISTORY

Communicating Hydrocephalus

This is suggested by a history of:

- Severe head injury with skull fracture or prolonged loss of consciousness
- Brain hemorrhage from aneurysm or stroke
- Bacterial meningitis

All these instances may allow blood to accumulate at the skull base and produce communicating hydrocephalus by obstructing the flow of cerebrospinal fluid (CSF) along the skull floor. The hydrocephalus may take months *or years* to develop and consequently may present late with:

- Memory failure
- Urinary problems
- Poor balance.

Large Arteriovenous Malformation

Rarely, dementia results from an arteriovenous malformation (AVM) that "steals" blood from other brain areas or causes mass effect. Very rarely, there is a parkinsonian syndrome that reverses after treatment of the AVM (See Chapter 8). It may also produce superficial siderosis (SS), as explained next.

Superficial Siderosis

This disorder is caused by accumulation of iron in the meninges secondary to chronic blood loss in the subarachnoid space causing local superficial neuronal damage.

The chief causes of SS include

- Repeated head injury
- Hemorrhage from an AVM, previous brain or spinal surgery

- Leakage of blood from a subdural hematoma, cavernoma, or dural tear

▶ The combination of myelopathy, ataxia, and deafness suggests superficial siderosis or mitochondrial disorder.

▶ SS may present years after injury. About a quarter of patients have cognitive impairment and most are anosmic.

Repeated Concussion (Chronic Traumatic Encephalopathy)

Boxers and other athletes who participate in contact sports may suffer repeated head trauma. They develop multiple parenchymal petechial brain hemorrhages and white matter lesions that, over the years, result in a delayed-onset ataxic-parkinsonian syndrome with dementia: the "punch drunk" syndrome or *dementia pugilistica* in the case of boxers.

This topic and the previously discussed points give a few useful Handles:

▶ Previous severe head injury, meningitis, or subarachnoid hemorrhage and recent dementia may be due to communicating hydrocephalus, chronic subdural hematoma, or superficial siderosis.

▶ Dementia associated with myelopathy, ataxia, deafness, cognitive decline, and anosmia is probably SS or less likely a mitochondrial disorder.

▶ Repeated concussion from boxing, American football, ice hockey, rugby, or wrestling may cause an ataxic-parkinsonian syndrome with progressive dementia.

Temporal Characteristics

You should try to determine from the history whether the dementia is continuous or intermittent and the rate of progression.

Episodic Confusion

Some patients with apparent dementia experience episodic confusion or memory impairment with normal behavior in between. The correct diagnosis may be one of the following:

- Delirium, for example, hepatic encephalopathy
- Transient ischemic attacks (TIAs)
- Transient global amnesia (recurrence is rare)
- Transient epileptic amnesia (TEA)

- Temporal lobe status
- Lewy body dementia
- Sleep apnea
- Channelopathies

Patients with a channelopathy (e.g., LGI1, glutamate, glycine, gamma-aminobutyric acid [GABA], N-methyl-D-aspartate [NMDA], α-amino-3-hydroxy-5-methyl-4-isoxazolepropionic acid [AMPA]) may experience intermittent confusion. Diagnostic clues are refractory seizures, low sodium levels, and movement disorders such as orofacial dyskinesias, stereotypies, chorea, myoclonus, dystonia, and rigidity. Thus:

▶ Recurrent episodes of amnesia with refractory seizures or movement disorders may be a channelopathy.

▶ Faciobrachial dystonic seizures characterize the voltage-gated potassium channel antibody syndrome (now termed LGI-1). See Chapter 6 (Epilepsy) and Video 6.10, Facio-Brachial-Dystonic Seizures).

▶ A low sodium level is a useful confirmatory Handle.

Patients with TEA classically have the following:

- Confusion after sleep. One explanation is that there is failure of hippocampal readout of memories into long-term storage, a process that is normally consolidated during sleep.
- Complete loss of memories for salient events such as holidays (vacational amnesia), family weddings, and funerals
- Olfactory hallucinations and microsmia

These aspects may allow differentiation from most degenerative forms of amnesia such as Alzheimer's disease, where at least some sketchy recall may be elicited with cueing. Diagnosis is important given that TEA is treatable with anticonvulsants. Thus:

▶ Confusion after sleep, severe loss of memory for salient events, and olfactory hallucinations support a diagnosis of TEA.

Dementia That Progresses over a Period of Months

The main possibilities in this category are the following:

- Creutzfeldt-Jakob disease (CJD)

- Fatal familial insomnia (prion disorder). This is associated with difficulty sleeping and prominent autonomic features.
- Korsakoff psychosis
- CNS infection (neurosyphilis, nocardia, and HIV)
- Medication (hypnotics, antipsychotic drugs, antianxiety agents, narcotics, and barbiturates)
- Deficiency states (thiamine, vitamin D, vitamin B_{12}, hypothyroidism)
- Paraneoplastic/autoimmune encephalopathy
- Cerebral vasculitis
- Chronic subdurals
- Normal pressure hydrocephalus (may take years to develop)

Creutzfeldt-Jakob disease
Handles for the classical form:

▶ Exposure to cadaveric human pituitary tissue corneal or dural grafts
▶ Rapidly progressing dementia.
▶ Myoclonus, cerebellar, extrapyramidal and pyramidal signs
▶ Periodic sharp waves ('clocking') on EEG. See Figure 6.16.
▶ CSF: Nonspecific tests: 14-3-3; S100b; neurone-specific enolase. Specific: Real-time quaking-induced conversion (RT-QUIC).

Red Flags:
◀ Unexplained fever suggests infection or lymphoma.
◀ Seizures. Favors autoimmune channelopathy.
◀ Low blood sodium. Usually implies LGI-1; occasionally, NMDA encephalitis.
◀ Facial movement disorder. Suggests NMDA encephalitis or Whipple's disease.
◀ Raised CSF cell count. More likely infection, neurosarcoidosis, vasculitis, lymphoma, and other malignancy
◀ On MRI: contrast-enhancing lesions outside striatum, thalamus, and cortex; suggests vascular disease, lymphoma, leukoencephalopathy

Variant CJD (vCJD)
◀ Consumption of infected beef or blood transfusion
◀ Psychiatric problems

◀ Sensory symptoms: nonspecific distal pain, tingling, and oversensitivity to touch, especially in legs
◀ Hockey-stick or pulvinar sign on MRI (Figure 13.1D)

Cancer Patient with Dementia
Assuming the MRI scan shows no sign of metastases, you should think of:

- Paraneoplastic limbic encephalitis
- Carcinomatous meningitis, and, if relevant:
- Radiation encephalopathy.

RARE COGNITIVE SYMPTOMS
It is important to be aware of these conditions given that they may be mistaken for a primary psychiatric disorder.

- *Simultanagnosia.* Inability to recognize multiple objects or events at the same time. Visual fields may be full. This may be detected by asking a patient to comment on a picture with several events (Figure 13.2). It has been described in lesions of the inferior left occipital lobe or both visual cortices. It may be part of Balint syndrome (nondominant parietal) which is found in AD and posterior cortical atrophy.
- *Akinetopsia* "motion blindness." Inability to see moving objects although items that are stationary are perceiving without difficulty. This has been described in traumatic brain injury and carbon monoxide poisoning.
- *Achromatopsia.* Inability to perceive colors (color blindness). In the acquired form, there are usually upper visual field defects associated with prosopagnosia. The lesions may be in the lower part of both occipital and temporal lobes, typically after traumatic brain injury but it has been described in AD.
- *Palinopsia* (Figure 13.3). This refers to one or more after-images (visual perseveration). It usually localizes to the right parieto-occipital cortex. It may be an illusion, as in migraine, or a hallucination due to a seizure. It is also described with hallucinogenic drugs such as lysergic acid (LSD), ecstasy, psychoses, and nonketotic hyperglycemia. It occurs in dementia with Lewy bodies, posterior cortical atrophy variant of AD, and CJD.

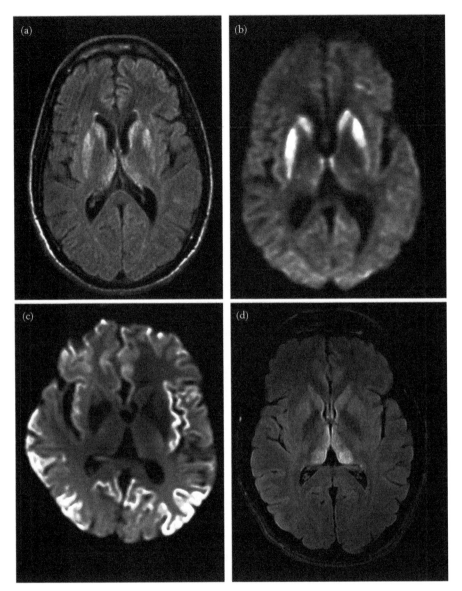

FIGURE 13.1: Characteristic MRI features of Creutzfeldt-Jakob disease (CJD). (A and B) Sporadic CJD showing typical basal ganglia signal return on FLAIR sequence (A), which is more obvious on diffusion-weighted sequences (B). (C) Diffusion-weighted imaging displaying striking cortical ribboning with normal basal ganglia in sporadic CJD. (D) Variant CJD showing pulvinar sign on the FLAIR sequence. Reproduced with permission from Mead and Rudge (2017).

- *Prosopagnosia.* Inability to recognize familiar faces (face-blindness). Some may be able to identify a person by voice or hairstyle. The lesion (atrophy) is usually in the fusiform gyrus on the undersurface of the temporal lobe. Prosopagnosia is not characteristic of AD (where the problem is more that of remembering personal names), but it is a feature of frontotemporal and semantic variants especially where there is right temporal lobe involvement.

- *Amusia.* Inability to perceive music or recognize familiar music. This suggests a lesion in the nondominant temporal lobe. The acquired form has been described in FTD.

PSEUDO-DEMENTIA

Pseudo-dementia refers to someone who appears to have memory loss but is really suffering from depression and/or anxiety. True dementia and

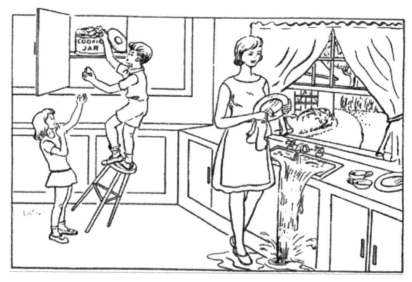

FIGURE 13.2: The Boston cookie-theft picture. A patient with simultanagnosia will only be able to describe one event at a time in the drawing

pseudo-dementia can be difficult to separate, but here are some clues to depression:

- Continual fatigue
- Frequent sighing or yawning suggest anxiety.
- Psychomotor underactivity; sometimes agitation with pacing or rocking movement at rest
- Poor sleep pattern: rapid sleep onset, early morning wakening, intrusive dreams, not refreshed in morning
- Unexplained physical symptoms
- With gentle probing, memory may be found reasonable but some have dementia *and* depression.
- Smell sense is usually normal in depression but impaired in AD. See later in this chapter.

DISSOCIATIVE FUGUE

This used to be called "fugue state" or "psychogenic fugue." It may be confused with a dementia especially the episodic variety.

Handles include:

- Loss of personal identity (rarely seen in dementia unless severe)
- One or more amnesic episodes during which the subject is alert and responsive, unlike complex partial seizures
- Sudden unplanned wandering or travel sometimes with creation of a new identity

- Impaired recall of past events, particularly stressful occurrences

EXAMINATION

It is important to perform a general neurological examination to determine whether there are any focal signs that might point to a space-occupying lesion, hemorrhage,

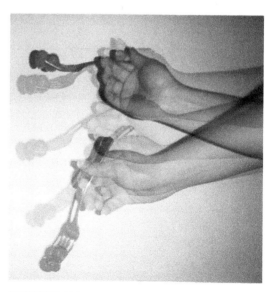

FIGURE 13.3: Palinopsia. A form of visual perseveration that suggests a lesion in the right parieto-occipital cortex. This is a feature of migraine, seizures and hallucinogenic drugs. It is found rarely in dementia with Lewy bodies and Creutzfeldt-Jacob disease.

demyelination, or the like. Much of the further examination process in dementia depends on qualitative bedside testing of cognition and psychometric tests.

Note:

◀ The Mini-Mental Status Examination (MMSE) and its shorter variants are relatively crude instruments and mostly unhelpful.

Diagnostic Clues

▶ Applause sign. This suggests frontal lobe dysfunction and typifies PSP; see Chapter 8 and Video 8.31, Applause.

The patient is asked to clap their hands 3–5 times. When positive, the hands are clapped more than the required number, suggesting motor perseveration. This phenomenon was described initially in PSP and parkinsonism. Apart from these disorders, it is found in subcortical dementia, such as Huntington disease, AIDS dementia, and some varieties of FTD.

▶ A positive applause sign excludes early AD.

▶ A positive snout or grasp reflex (if present) favors frontal lobe involvement and would be unusual in early AD

▶ Reflex asymmetry may alert you to a structural lesion.

▶ Testing the sense of smell may help distinguish dementia from depression.

Patients with AD, diffuse Lewy body disease, Parkinson's disease, or Huntington's disease all have significant olfactory loss. Thus, if the patient reports a normal sense of smell and you are able to confirm this with a standardized screening test (e.g., University of Pennsylvania Smell Identification Test or Sniffin' Sticks), then the dementias listed at the beginning of this paragraph are unlikely and the patient may have depression.

Red Flags

In any patient with cognitive impairment, you should be alert to the presence of the following:

◀ Extrapyramidal disease (rigidity, bradykinesia, and tremor)

◀ Muscle wasting or fasciculation

Either of these features would argue against AD, at least in the early stages, and suggest one of the following.

- *Lewy Body disease.* Look for prominent fluctuations, REM sleep disorder, and visual hallucinations.
- *Huntington's disease.* Imbalance may be more obvious than chorea in the early phase.
- *Classic Parkinson's disease (PD) and Parkinsonism.* Dementia is common in the late stages of PD and progressive supranuclear palsy. Conversely, parkinsonian features are seen in the late stages of AD.
- *Frontotemporal dementia* with
  - Amyotrophic lateral sclerosis suggests the *C9ORF72* mutation.
  - Parkinsonism suggests a tau mutation.
- *Wilson's Disease.* Almost any movement disorder may be seen, but the typical varieties are dystonia, chorea, and parkinsonism.
- *Late-presenting Gaucher's disease.* The main clues are Jewish ancestry, parkinsonism, supranuclear horizontal gaze palsy, and conjunctival pingueculae (see Chapter 8, Movement Disorders).
- *Hereditary diffuse leukoencephalopathy with spheroids (HDLS).* This causes a corticobasal syndrome.

Supranuclear Gaze Palsy

It is important to check the eye movements for a supranuclear defect. Dementia and supranuclear gaze palsy raise the possibility of the following:

- *Progressive supranuclear palsy.* There is a vertical supranuclear gaze palsy sometimes associated with utilization behavior (see later discussion).
- *Niemann-Pick disease type C* (Video 8.35, Niemann Pick C). Consider this in a young adult with dementia, *vertical* (predominantly downward) supranuclear gaze palsy, gait ataxia, and splenomegaly. There is sometimes a history of cataplexy and neonatal jaundice. This is an important condition not to miss, given the availability of treatment with, for example, cyclodextrin.
- *Adult onset Gaucher's disease.* Here there is cognitive impairment, extrapyramidal features, and *horizontal* supranuclear gaze palsy (Video 2.3, Gaucher disease). Another clue is the

presence of pingueculae in the conjunctiva (see Figure 8.10). Gaucher's disease may present to neurologists with a parkinsonian syndrome. It is a lysosomal storage disease for which treatment is available.

- *Spinocerebellar ataxia type 2.* Supranuclear vertical gaze palsy with slow saccades, chorea, neuropathy, and alcohol intolerance. Some cases are associated with amyotrophic lateral sclerosis (ALS) and parkinsonism.

Utilization Behavior

See Video 13.3, Utilization. Here, the patient may be unable to resist grasping or using an object placed in front of them, regardless of the context or environment. A characteristic feature in a patient who wears glasses is a tendency to put on another pair of spectacles, sometimes multiple pairs. If patients see a toothbrush, they may start brushing their teeth. This is usually a feature of frontal lobe disorder, particularly the behavioral variant of FTLD and the fronto-subcortical syndromes such as PSP.

Miscellaneous Dementias
Alcoholic Dementias

There are various patterns of dementia in alcoholism, and some instances relate to malnutrition rather than specific alcohol-induced dementia. The patient's history or relatives' report is a major clue, also the presence of a painful peripheral neuropathy. On occasion, the diagnosis is not straightforward when there is denial of alcohol excess by the patient or ignorance or concealment by the accompanying person.

- ▶ Confabulation. The patient boasts of unfounded achievements, possessions, and friendship with famous people.
- ▶ Confabulation is rare in AD but characteristic of Korsakoff syndrome.
- ▶ There is usually a wide-based gait ataxia with little or no incoordination on the heel-shin test and none in the arms.
  This happens because of selective alcohol-related damage to the anterior cerebellar lobule and vermis. These regions regulate coordination of leg and trunk but not arm movement.

Normal-Pressure Hydrocephalus

This somewhat ill-defined disorder is characterized by:

- Dementia, ataxia, and urinary problems. The hydrocephalus leads to cognitive impairment (Figure 13.4).
- Normal sulcal width (typically <3 mm) over the superior cerebral convexity in the presence of large ventricles
- Improvement in gait and cognition after lumbar puncture

Dementia with Cerebellar Features
- Prion disorder
- Early-onset AD due to presenilin-1 mutation. Spastic paraparesis is associated

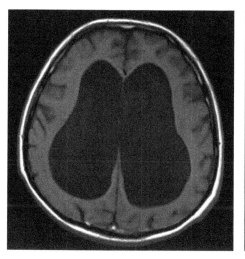
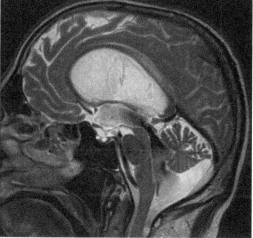

FIGURE 13.4: Normal-pressure hydrocephalus. **Left:** MRI T1 axial sequence. Note the massive symmetric enlargement of the lateral ventricles with relatively little peripheral cortical atrophy. **Right:** MRI T2 sagittal sequence. This shows upward bowing of the corpus callosum. Reproduced with permission from Radiopedia, courtesy Frank Gaillard.

- Spinocerebellar ataxias (SCA2, -12, and -17)
- Superficial siderosis
- Niemann-Pick disease type C
- Multiple system atrophy
- Alexander's disease
- Multiple sclerosis (MS)
- Fragile X tremor ataxia syndrome
- Paraneoplastic disorder
- Normal pressure hydrocephalus

Dementia with Pyramidal Signs

- MS
- FTD with motor neuron disease
- Alzheimer's disease with presenilin 1 mutation
- Spinocerebellar ataxias
- Hereditary spastic paraplegia (SPG4)
- Adrenoleukodystrophy
- Vanishing white matter disease
- Polyglucosan body disease
- Polycystic lipomembranous sclerosing leukoencephalopathy (PLOSL; Nasu-Hakola disease)

Dementia with Dystonia or Chorea

- Huntington's disease and Huntington's disease-like syndrome 1–3
- Wilson's disease
- Neuroacanthocytosis
- Neurodegeneration with brain iron accumulation (NBIA; see Chapter 8)
- Lesch-Nyhan syndrome
- Dentato-rubral-pallido-luysian atrophy (DRPLA)
- Corticobasal syndrome
- Neuroferritinopathy
- NMDA encephalitis
- Variant CJD

Dementia with Deafness

- Superficial siderosis
- Mitochondrial disorders
- Familial Danish dementia
- Alpha-mannosidosis; note the associated tendency to recurrent knee dislocation!
- Sialidosis

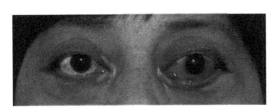
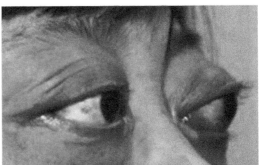
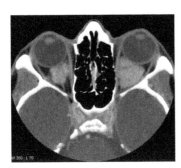
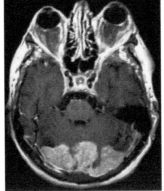
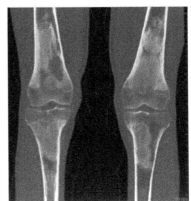

FIGURE 13.5: Erdheim-Chester disease (polyostotic sclerosing histiocytosis). This rare condition is a histiocytosis with widespread manifestations. Many have diabetes insipidus. **Top**: bilateral exophthalmos particularly in the left eye. **Bottom left**: Contrast-enhanced T2 MRI scan through the orbits that shows large granulomatous deposits. **Bottom center**: T1 axial MRI scan displays a mass involving the extra-axial compartment posterior to the cerebellum. These lesions may mimic meningiomas. **Bottom right**: Plain X-ray of the long bones shows symmetric metaphyseal sclerosis and cysts. Top images reproduced with permission from Yin et al. (2013). All lower images courtesy Frank Gaillard and Andrew Dixon, Radiopedia.

- Neurosarcoidosis
- Also Behçet's disease, neurosyphilis, Susac's syndrome, Niemann Pick disease

Dementia with Autonomic Features

- Lewy body disease
- Multiple system atrophy
- Fatal familial insomnia
- Porphyria
- Adrenoleukodystrophy
- NMDA receptor encephalitis
- Fragile-X tremor ataxia syndrome
- SCA3

Dementia with Bone Disorders

There are four causes of this unusual combination:

- PLOSL; Nasu-Hakola disease. This is caused by a mutation in the *TREM2* gene.
- Langerhans cell histiocytosis. There are aneurysmal bone cysts and CSF glucose is low. A fronto-temporal dementia is described. Some have cerebellar involvement.
- Erdheim-Chester disease, also known as polyostotic sclerosing histiocytosis. Major clues are the presence of diabetes insipidus, bone pain (due to cysts), exophthalmos, and retroperitoneal fibrosis (Figure 13.5). Cognitive impairment is an occasional feature (Estrada-Veras et al. 2017)
- Frontotemporal dementia with Paget's disease of bone and inclusion body myositis. This is a late adult-onset autosomal dominant condition associated with a distal myopathy due to a mutation in the valosin-containing protein gene, VCP (Kimonis et al. 2008).

Dementia with Buccolingual Mutilation

There are three possible causes for this:

- Neuroacanthocytosis
- Lesch-Nyhan syndrome. These conditions are described in Chapter 8.
- Secondary Tourette syndrome

SUMMARY

Preliminary Observations

- Attends-alone sign. Dementia and depression may coexist.

- Change in personality: frontal lobe; impaired memory: temporal lobe. Disorder of vision (e.g., diminished visuospatial awareness, field loss): parietal lobe. Change in speech or language: dominant temporal lobe or connections
- Difficulty recalling names of medication
- Detailed recall of lapses in memory and their circumstance suggests poor concentration and favors anxiety.
- Poor recall of objects but accurate identification of cues and foils in psychometric tests supports anxiety.
- If the patient is more concerned than the informant, then anxiety/depression is likely. If the informant is more concerned than the patient, then dementia is probable.

Handles for Alzheimer's Disease

▶ The patient with obvious memory difficulties, yet well-dressed, retains social graces, and can converse at a superficial level

▶ The patient who becomes lost near their home or familiar places

▶ The head-turning sign, delusion of theft, loss of pleasure for reading

▶ Disruptive vocalizations. Repeated minor traffic accidents/near misses.

▶ Problems in remembering personal names.

▶ Difficulty in mastering a new TV remote controller or mobile phone

Red Flags for Alzheimer's Disease

◀ Abrupt onset is rarely a dementia, more likely delirium or confusional state.

◀ The patient with a cold stare more likely has frontal dementia.

◀ Deterioration in social decorum (e.g., bad behavior in public, inappropriate vulgarity, emotional instability). Again, a frontal lobe characteristic.

◀ Preservation of a good sense of humor is unusual. Abnormal digit span in early stages.

◀ Positive applause sign is atypical and favors PSP or other types of parkinsonism.

◀ Normal sense of smell identification. Confabulation.

◀ The patient who keeps leaning forward as if deaf may have receptive aphasia, not dementia. Conversely, an elderly person with progressive deafness may be thought erroneously to have dementia.

Posterior Cortical Variant of Alzheimer's Disease

- Multiple visits to their optician
- "Failed" cataract operation
- Difficulty judging distances even though visual fields are normal (optic ataxia)
- Visual crowding and difficulty with visual search

Handles for Frontotemporal Dementia Variants
Semantic Dementia

▶ Difficulty understanding the sense of familiar words and asking their meaning

▶ Fluent but empty circumlocutory speech. Obsession with timekeeping, numbers, or Sudoku!

▶ MRI: atrophy in the anteroinferior temporal lobe, usually more on the left

Behavioral Variant FTD

▶ Rude conversation or behavior; loss of empathy. Cold stare. Apathy and stereotyped/ritualistic behavior

▶ Changed food preferences, especially sweet food with gluttony

▶ Weight gain. Weight loss common in AD

▶ Increased concern over timekeeping; obsession with new hobbies and easily distractible

▶ Relative preservation of posterior cortical function

▶ Later: primitive reflexes

▶ MRI: asymmetric atrophy (frontal and anterior temporal lobes)

▶ Positive family history

Progressive Nonfluent Aphasia

▶ Stumbling over long words or stuttering; grammatical errors

▶ Effortful speech; orofacial apraxia

▶ Supranuclear gaze palsy, pure akinesia, and gait freezing suggest PSP variant.

▶ MRI: atrophy in the perisylvian dominant hemisphere

Logopenic Aphasia

▶ Hesitant, grammatically correct speech

▶ Word-finding pauses; difficulty in repetition of phrases

▶ MRI: left-sided temporoparietal atrophy

Other dementias

- **Vascular dementias:** doubtful entity. Characteristics include elderly hypertensive arteriopath; in some, gradual cognitive decline; in others, step-wise decline in motor function; pseudobulbar palsy; relatively late onset of memory impairment. Cognitive slowing.

- **Cerebral amyloid angiopathy** (CAA): amyloid spells: TIA-like attacks with positive symptoms, are precursors of CAA. History of lobar intracerebral hemorrhage rather than the usual deep location associated with hypertensive intracerebral hemorrhage. MRI: lobar micro-hemorrhages, cortical siderosis, prominent perivascular spaces, and predominantly posterior periventricular white matter signal change

- **Extrapyramidal disease**: consider Lewy body disease, Huntington's disease, late stage parkinsonism or AD, FTDP-17, PSP, Wilson's disease, late-presenting Gaucher's disease, hereditary diffuse leukoencephalopathy with spheroids (HDLS).

- **Muscle wasting/fasciculation:** consider: FTD (C9ORF72 mutation)

Points in the History

Communicating hydrocephalus: suggested by severe head injury, hemorrhage from aneurysm or stroke, bacterial meningitis. Large arteriovenous malformation. Superficial siderosis. Chronic traumatic encephalopathy.

Temporal Characteristics

Episodic confusion: delirium, for example, hepatic encephalopathy. Transient ischemic attacks, transient global amnesia, transient epileptic amnesia. Temporal lobe status. Lewy body dementia. Sleep apnea. Channelopathies: faciobrachial dystonic seizures (voltage-gated potassium channel antibody syndrome; LGI-1). Low blood sodium confirmatory

Dementia That Progresses over a Period of Months

Prion disease: CJD, fatal familial insomnia. Korsakoff psychosis. CNS infection, deficiency states. Medication. Paraneoplastic/autoimmune encephalopathy. Cerebral vasculitis. Chronic subdural hematoma. Normal pressure hydrocephalus

Creutzfeldt-Jakob Disease

Handles for the classical form: Exposure to cadaveric human pituitary tissue or dural grafts. Rapidly progressing dementia. Myoclonus, cerebellar, extrapyramidal and pyramidal signs. Periodic sharp waves (clocking) on EEG. CSF: Nonspecific tests: 14-3-3; S100b; neurone-specific enolase. Specific: RT-QUIC

Red Flags:

◄ Unexplained fever. Seizures. Low blood sodium. Facial movement disorder. Raised CSF cell count. On MRI: contrast-enhancing lesions outside striatum, thalamus, and cortex.

Variant CJD (vCJD)

Consumption of infected beef or blood transfusion. Psychiatric problems. Sensory symptoms: nonspecific distal pain or tingling. Hockey-stick or pulvinar sign on MRI.

Cancer Patient with Dementia

With normal MRI brain scan: Paraneoplastic limbic encephalitis. Carcinomatous meningitis. Radiation encephalopathy.

Rare Cognitive Symptoms

Simultagnosia. Akinetopsia. Achromatopsia. Palinopsia. Prosopagnosia. Amusia.

Pseudo-dementia

Continual fatigue, frequent sighing or yawning. Psychomotor under- or overactivity. Poor sleep pattern: rapid sleep onset. Early morning wakening. Intrusive dreams. Not refreshed in morning. Unexplained physical symptoms. Memory may be reasonable.

Dissociative Fugue

May be confused with a dementia especially the episodic variety.

Features: loss of personal identity. Amnesic episodes during which the subject is alert and responsive, unlike complex partial seizures. Sudden unplanned wandering or travel sometimes with creation of a new identity. Impaired recall of past events, particularly stressful occurrences.

Examination

Applause sign, snout or grasp reflexes: frontal lobe involvement and unusual for AD. Reflex asymmetry:

possible structural lesion. Demented patent with normal sense of smell probably does not have AD and may be depressed.

◄ Extrapyramidal disease. Muscle wasting or fasciculation.

Be alert to LBD; Huntington disease; Parkinsonism; FTD with ALS or parkinsonism; Wilson disease; late-presenting Gaucher disease; HDLS'

Supranuclear Gaze Palsy and Dementia
- *Vertical:* Progressive supranuclear palsy; Niemann-Pick disease type C; SCA2
- *Horizontal:* Gaucher's disease

Utilization Behavior

Suggest frontal lobe disorder, particularly behavioral variant of FTLD and fronto-subcortical syndromes such as PSP.

Miscellaneous Dementias
- *Alcoholic dementia.* Wide-based gait ataxia with little or no incoordination on the heel-shin test and none in the arms. Confabulation is rare in AD but characteristic of Korsakoff syndrome.
- *Normal-pressure hydrocephalus.* Dementia, ataxia, and urinary problems. Hydrocephalus leads to cognitive impairment. Improvement after lumbar puncture.
- *Dementia with cerebellar features.* Prion disorder; early-onset AD due to presenilin-1 mutation; SCA2, -12, and -17; superficial siderosis; Niemann-Pick disease type C; MSA; Alexander's disease; MS; Fragile-X tremor ataxia syndrome; paraneoplastic disorder; normal-pressure hydrocephalus
- *Dementia with pyramidal signs.* MS; FTD with ALS; AD with presenilin mutation; spinocerebellar ataxias; hereditary spastic paraplegia (SPG4); adrenoleukodystrophy; vanishing white matter disease; polyglucosan body disease; polycystic lipomembranous sclerosing leukoencephalopathy
- *Dementia with dystonia or chorea.* Huntington's disease and HDL 1–3; Wilson's disease; neuroacanthocytosis; NBIA; Lesch-Nyhan syndrome; DRPLA; corticobasal syndrome; neuroferritinopathy; NMDA encephalitis; variant CJD

- *Dementia with deafness.* Superficial siderosis; mitochondrial disorders; familial Danish dementia; alpha-mannosidosis (note: recurrent knee dislocation); sialidosis; neurosarcoidosis; Behçet's disease; neurosyphilis; Susac's syndrome; Niemann Pick disease type C.
- *Dementia with autonomic features.* Lewy body disease; MSA; fatal familial insomnia; porphyria; adrenoleukodystrophy; NMDA receptor encephalitis. Fragile-X tremor ataxia syndrome. SCA3
- *Dementia with bone disorders.* PLOSL; Nasu-Hakola disease; Langerhans histiocytosis; Erdheim-Chester disease. FTD with Paget's disease of bone and inclusion body myositis
9. *Dementia with buccolingual mutilation.* Neuroacanthocytosis; Lesch-Nyhan syndrome

SUGGESTED READING

Estrada-Veras JI, O'Brien KJ, Boyd LC, Dave RH, Durham BH, Xi L, Malayeri AA, Chen MY, Gardner PJ, Enriquez JR, Shah N. The clinical spectrum of Erdheim-Chester disease: an observational cohort study. *Blood Adv.* 2017 Feb 14;1(6):357–366.

Kimonis VE, Mehta SG, Fulchiero EC, et al. Clinical studies in familial VCP myopathy associated with Paget disease of bone and frontotemporal dementia. *Am J Med Genet A.* 2008;146A:745–757.

Larner AJ. 'Attended alone' sign: validity and reliability for the exclusion of dementia. *Age Ageing.* 2009;38:476–478.

Larner AJ. Neurological signs of possible diagnostic value in the cognitive disorders clinic. *Pract Neurol.* 2014;14:332–335.

Mead S, Rudge P. CJD mimics and chameleons. *Pract Neurol.* 2017;17(2):113–121.

Rossor MN, Fox NC, Mummery CJ, Schott JM, Warren JD. The diagnosis of young-onset dementia. *Lancet Neurol.* 2010;9:793–806.

Warren JD, Rohrer JD, Rossor MN. Clinical review. Frontotemporal dementia. *BMJ.* 2013;347:f4827.

Yin J, Zhang F, Zhang H, et al. Hand-Schuller-Christian disease and Erdheim-Chester disease: coexistence and discrepancy. *Oncologist.* 2013;18:19–24.

Chapter 14: The Fast Neurological Examination

W e have left this chapter to the end because by now you should have digested the preceding chapters and have a pretty good idea of several diagnostic shortcuts. Neurological examination is a dying art and that is inevitable, sad as that may appear to the older generations. It was essential in the early part of the twentieth century because then the only investigations were X-rays and a few blood tests. We only know of a handful of neurologists who still use a two-point discriminator or Von Frey hairs, and they are all more than 80 years old! Even funduscopy is gradually moving over into the territory of ophthalmologists, although if a decent smartphone fundus camera becomes available that might change. Magnetic resonance imaging (MRI) trumps almost every bedside test!

What follows is a coalescence of material already detailed in earlier chapters but in a form that will save time in the clinic. Please note that our proposed approach is for the patient you wish to screen after having predicted from the history that there will be few physical signs. This would apply to most patients with nonspecific headache and dizziness for example. If the history suggests a peripheral neuropathy, then you will have your work cut out!

Also note that you will find considerable variation in technique from one neurologist to another, and favorite regimes and personal techniques are common among many experienced neurologists.

FIRST ENCOUNTERS

Re-read Chapter 1 so you can make a spot diagnosis based on the patient's physical appearance. Remember that the examination starts the moment you set eyes on your patient. It is a good plan to fetch the patient yourself and not buzz for a nurse. You can then observe the gait, involuntary movement, handshake, speech, and more. An experienced neurologist often diagnoses Parkinson's disease before the patient has entered the consulting room. If you are still at your desk, you should *not have your head buried in the case notes* when the patient comes in.

More than two accompanying persons can be a hallmark of functional disease, especially if the patient wears sunglasses indoors for no clear reason (migraine, recent eye surgery). Watch how the patient walks in, turns; listen to their speech and analyze their handshake. Look at the face critically for eye contact, excess frowning, weight loss, facial expression, blink rate, birthmarks, type of spectacles.

When taking the history, make a preliminary analysis of speech (i.e., fluency, clarity, hesitancy, vocabulary). Inspect the clothes informally during history taking for heavily creased garments and food stains, as in frontal dementia. Migraineurs are often meticulously dressed. Have a preliminary look at the fingernails for tell-tale signs of disease (Figure 1.1). Type of jewelry worn will give you an approximate measure of the patient's wealth (might be useful if you are due to submit an invoice!). A loose or tight-fitting ring might point to recent weight loss or gain, respectively. Finally, smelling the breath can alert you to consumption of alcohol, cigarettes, poor mouth hygiene, or illicit drug exposure.

CRANIAL NERVES

Detailed examination of all 12 cranial nerves is tedious. The problem is knowing what to leave out, so here is our schedule, once more, for the patient in whom you do not expect to find abnormalities.

- *Olfactory nerve.* Omit. It is worth doing if there is a history of head trauma, especially in a medicolegal context. If the patient has parkinsonism or dementia, then check olfaction, as it should be abnormal in classical Parkinson's disease and Alzheimer's disease. If it is normal *on testing* then review your diagnosis
- *Optic nerve.* We suggest examination of everything. Ideally get someone else to measure

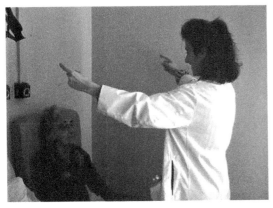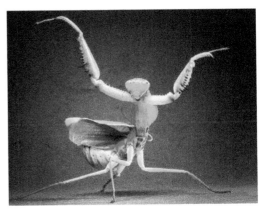

FIGURE 14.1: **Left**: Rapid screening of visual fields by the "praying mantis" technique. Ask the patient to look at your nose while you move your fingers simultaneously in the upper temporal then lower temporal fields. This will detect an absolute temporal field defect or visual inattention. If there is a suspected abnormality, then testing by the classic monocular method is required. This technique does not evaluate the nasal fields, but they are affected very rarely in isolation. **Right**: The praying mantis insect.

visual acuity—like the clinic nurse or a medical student! Check the visual fields by the "praying mantis" technique as shown in Figure 14.1. This will pick up significant temporal field loss and visual inattention. It does not detect nasal loss, but isolated nasal defects are very rare. Pupillary light reflexes are mandatory!

- *Oculomotor, trochlear, and abducens nerves.* Look for ptosis and asymmetry of the resting eye position by inspecting light reflection off cornea (Hirschberg test; see Figure 2.53). Assess eye movement to pursuit using the classical H-shaped trajectory. Then repeat using saccadic gaze, horizontal and vertical.
- *Trigeminal nerve.* Omit, unless there are facial sensory symptoms. Most patients dislike pinprick tests on the face. Do not perform the test for corneal reflex given the risk of corneal abrasion and its low diagnostic yield. A gentle stroke over the upper and lower face will suffice. Power testing and the jaw jerk: omit.
- *Facial nerve.* Look for facial asymmetry, especially the Cupid's bow sign (Figure 2.65) and asymmetry of the palpebral fissures. Ask the patient to show the teeth and simultaneously assess dental hygiene. You could omit raising the eyebrows as this movement is rarely affected in isolation; the main exception is leprosy.

- *Cochleovestibular nerve.* Ask the patient to repeat a whispered number about 5 cm from either ear. Whispering involves high frequencies, and most deafness affects this frequency band. The main exception is Ménière disease which affects low frequencies. If there are any abnormalities then Rinne's and Weber's tuning fork tests are required.
- *Glossopharyngeal and vagus nerves.* Inspect the soft palate and ask the subject to say "ah." Avoid the gag reflex for routine screening.
- *Accessory nerve.* Omit. Neck weakness is rarely present in isolation. If you need to do it, simply ask the patient to push on your hand, placed on the central forehead (Figure 2.76).
- *Hypoglossal nerve.* Ask the subject to protrude the tongue for inspection (wasting, fasciculation, ulcers, etc.), then move laterally for detection of abnormal movement.

UPPER LIMBS

Inspect the Limb

Remove any jackets and sweaters/jumpers! Look for wasting, fasciculation, involuntary movement at rest, birthmarks, contractures, scars, etc.

Check Tone

This should be done by alternate passive elbow supination/pronation and alternate wrist flexion and extension. Look out for a supinator catch, as in pyramidal tract disorder or cogwheeling as in extrapyramidal disease. Reinforcement by a hand-pumping move-ment of the non-test side may increase borderline cogwheeling.

- *Power 1. Hold arms out in front, palms down.* Inspect once more for birthmarks, nail changes, wasting, fasciculation, contractures, and involuntary movement. Wait a good 15 seconds in case of re-emergent tremor. Look for passive abduction of the little finger, as in lesions of the ulnar nerve or py-ramidal tract (Figure 3.3, myelopathy hand sign). Ask patient to spread out fingers. Look for *asymmetric* hyperextension at the metacarpophalangeal joint (Figure 3.6). When present, it suggests hypotonia as in cerebellar disorder and chorea. Symmetric hyperextension is normal in some races (e.g., Asians/Chinese), although it may be a feature of hypermobility as in Marfan's and Ehlers Danlos syndromes. If there is simulated weak-ness, the arm drops down vertically without rotation of the forearm.
- *Power 2. Ask patient to turn outstretched arms palms up.* Look for the pronator sign and minor elbow flexion that is typical of pyram-idal tract lesions (Figure 3.4). In genuine weakness, the arm may drift downward but pronation worsens. If simulated, the degree of pronation does not change. Note that formal power testing is not done. This saves a lot of time.
- *Check coordination with the finger–nose test.* This will detect most forms of involuntary movement. If normal, it is rarely necessary to check finger tapping, alternate pronation/supination, etc.
- *Check deep tendon reflexes.* Biceps, supinator, and triceps only.

- *Sensory testing.* If all the preceding is normal, then omit. If not, use a pin, light finger touch, or cotton wool to map out a sensory deficit, focusing on distal skin because that is where most pathology begins. If touch, pin-prick or vibration are intact over the fingertips, there is unlikely to be a more proximal deficit. For suspected root lesions, use the "hot spots" shown in Figure 3.29.

LOWER LIMBS

- *Inspect.* Ideally, the lower limbs should be exposed to the hip but for various reasons this is done rarely in practice. Once more, look for wasting, fasciculation, involuntary movement at rest, birthmarks, contractures, scars, etc. Do not forget to look at the *posterior* aspect of the limb.
- *Tone.* On the couch, rock the relaxed lower limb at the knee to observe passive ankle in-version/eversion (Figure 3.26). Then flick up the knee at the popliteal fossa to determine if the leg "hangs" before returning to the couch.
- *Power.* If there is no relevant history and the deep tendon reflexes are normal, then omit.
- *Coordination.* Perform the heel-shin test.
- *Deep tendon reflexes.* Check the knee and ankle jerks, then plantar response.
- *Sensory testing.* Omit, unless the history suggests a sensory problem. Screen for a sen-sory deficit with a pin or light touch/cotton wool over distal skin first. For suspected radiculopathy, check the hot spots as in Figure 3.29.

That's all there is to do.
If you still own a two-point discriminator, von Frey hairs, or temperature test tubes donate them to a museum!

APPENDIX: VIDEOS

INDEX

Page references followed by a *t* indicate table; *f* indicate figure.